SECOND EDITION

NURSING LEADERSHIP AND MANAGEMENT

for Patient Safety and Quality Care

Elizabeth Murray, PhD, RN, CNE

Program Director, MSN Nurse Educator

Associate Professor

Florida Gulf Coast University

School of Nursing

Fort Myers, Florida

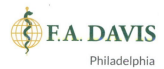

F.A. DAVIS

Philadelphia

F. A. Davis Company
1915 Arch Street
Philadelphia, PA 19103
www.fadavis.com

Printed in the United States of America

Last digit indicates print number: 10 9 8 7 6 5 4 3 2

Acquisitions Editor: Jacalyn Sharp
Senior Content Project Manager: Adrienne D. Simon
Design and Illustration Manager: Carolyn O'Brien

As new scientific information becomes available through basic and clinical research, recommended treatments and drug therapies undergo changes. The author(s) and publisher have done everything possible to make this book accurate, up to date, and in accord with accepted standards at the time of publication. The author(s), editors, and publisher are not responsible for errors or omissions or for consequences from application of the book, and make no warranty, expressed or implied, in regard to the contents of the book. Any practice described in this book should be applied by the reader in accordance with professional standards of care used in regard to the unique circumstances that may apply in each situation. The reader is advised always to check product information (package inserts) for changes and new information regarding dose and contraindications before administering any drug. Caution is especially urged when using new or infrequently ordered drugs.

Library of Congress Cataloging-in-Publication Data

Library of Congress Cataloging-in-Publication Data

Names: Murray, Elizabeth J., author.
Title: Nursing leadership and management for patient safety and quality
  care / Elizabeth Murray.
Description: Second edition. | Philadelphia, PA : F.A. Davis Company,
  [2022] | Includes bibliographical references and index.
Identifiers: LCCN 2021021676 (print) | LCCN 2021021677 (ebook) | ISBN
  9781719641791 (paperback) | ISBN 9781719646512 (ebook)
Subjects: MESH: Nursing Care—standards | Nursing Care—organization &
  administration | Patient Safety—standards | Quality Assurance, Health
  Care—methods | Leadership | Nurse's Role
Classification: LCC RT41 (print) | LCC RT41 (ebook) | NLM WY 100.1 | DDC
  610.73—dc23
LC record available at https://lccn.loc.gov/2021021676
LC ebook record available at https://lccn.loc.gov/2021021677

Dedication

This book is dedicated to my husband, Don, whose support and encouragement is unending and to my daughter, Angel, whose joyful spirit always brightens my day.

Additionally, I dedicate this book to my mother who taught me tenacity and persistence, two attributes that have served me well in life. I miss her every day, but I know we will be together some day in the future.

This book is also dedicated to Marydelle Polk, my mentor and friend, who shared so much with me and who had a great influence on my development as a faculty member and whom I miss dearly.

Finally, this book is dedicated to the hundreds of nurses and nursing students I have taught over the years for inspiring me to actualize my passion for nursing, quality, and patient safety through writing this book.

Epigraph

"It may seem a strange principle to enunciate as the very first requirement in a Hospital that it should do the sick no harm. It is quite necessary nevertheless to lay down such a principle."

Florence Nightingale, 1863
Notes on Hospitals

"The world, more specifically the Hospital world, is in such a hurry, is moving so fast, that it is too easy to slide into bad habits before we are aware."

Florence Nightingale, 1914
Florence Nightingale to Her Nurses

Preface

In 2000, the Institute of Medicine shocked the health-care community when it reported, in its landmark report, *To Err is Human*, that approximately 98,000 Americans die each year as a result of preventable adverse events. In response, many patient safety and quality initiatives were launched to make health care safer in the United States and globally. In 2013, James identified evidence suggesting that a more accurate estimate of deaths from preventable errors is 200,000 to 400,000 per year. More recently, Makary and Daniel (2016) suggest that these previous estimates were low and the incidence of deaths due to preventable adverse events between 1999 and 2013 is closer to 251,000 each year. There is no question that the health-care delivery system is undergoing major changes related to safety and quality. Nurses at all levels and in all settings have been identified as key to transforming health care to a safer, higher-quality, and more effective system. Front-line nurses are being charged with taking leadership and management roles in transforming care at the bedside. Nurse educators must prepare a new generation of nurses to step into these roles as well as manage safe and effective patient care. To that end, this book was written to provide a comprehensive approach to preparing nurses in the critical knowledge, skills, and attitudes in leadership and management needed for the current and future health-care environment.

This book is built on the premise that all nurses are leaders and managers regardless of their position or setting in which they work. First-level or front-line nursing leaders and managers are those leading and managing care of a patient or groups of patients at the bedside and clients or groups in the community. This level may also include charge nurses, patient care managers, and supervisors. Second-level nursing leaders and managers are those holding a formal position in the system such as unit manager. Their responsibilities include leading and managing material, economic, and human resources necessary for the care of a group of patients, as well as clients or groups in the community. The third-level nursing leaders and managers are those holding a formal position in the organization such as a director over several units and whose responsibilities are similar to those of the second-level manager but encompass a broader scope. The fourth level or executive level includes nursing leaders and managers in positions such as chief nursing officer (CNO) or Vice President of Nursing Services. Their responsibilities include administering nursing units in accordance with the mission and goals of the organization. Finally, many nurse leaders and managers hold positions outside direct care delivery such as nurses in academic settings, labor unions, political action groups, health-care coalitions, and consumer advocacy groups. This book provides an evidence-based approach to attaining the necessary knowledge, skills, and attitudes for nursing practice in today's dynamic health-care environment. It will be beneficial to prelicensure nursing students, RNs returning to school, new nurse leaders and managers, and nurses in any type of leadership and management position that affects health care and health-care recipients.

The underpinnings of this book are evidence-based practice, safety, quality, and effective nursing care. The book will assist students to understand a current perspective of nursing leadership and management theories, concepts, and principles. Evidence-based content is presented on topics relevant in today's ever-changing health-care environment, such as contemporary leadership and management theories, managing ethical and legal issues, leading and managing effectively in a culture of safety, improving and managing quality care, building and managing a sustainable workforce, leading change and managing conflict, creating and sustaining a healthy work environment, and managing resources.

The safety and quality of care depend greatly on our future nurses. I believe this book will help future nurses to attain leadership and management knowledge, skills, and attitudes critically needed to lead, manage, and provide safe, high-quality, and effective nursing care.

ELIZABETH J. MURRAY
Fort Myers, Florida

Contributors

Brett L. Andreasen, MS, RN-BC
Clinical Applications Analyst
Informatics Nurse Specialist
University of Washington
Medicine IT
Seattle, Washington

Paula M. Davis-Huffman, DNP, ANP-BC, PPCNP-BC, Emeritus CCRN
Assistant Professor
Florida Gulf Coast University
School of Nursing
Fort Myers, Florida

Linda K. Hays-Gallego, MN, RN
Lead Clinical Informatics Analyst, ORCA
Clinical Informatics and Support
University of Washington
Medicine IT
Seattle, Washington

Lynne Portnoy, MSN, RN, CNE
Instructor I
Florida Gulf Coast University
School of Nursing
Fort Myers, Florida

Contributors to Previous Edition

Rebecca Coey, MSN, RN, FNP
Family Nurse Practitioner
Fort Myers, Florida

Sara Jo Foley, RN, MSN, FNP
Family Nurse Practitioner
Fort Myers, Florida

Judith Walters, DNP, RN, PMHCNS-BC
Assistant Professor
Florida Gulf Coast University
School of Nursing
Fort Myers, Florida

Reviewers

Civita Allard, MS, RN, CAPT (ret), USNR NC
Professor, Nursing
Utica College
Utica, New York

Laurie Bladen, RN, PhD, MBA, CNE, FAACM
Associate Professor
Clarion University of Pennsylvania
Clarion, Pennsylvania

Linda Cassar, DNP, RNC-OB, CNE
Clinical Assistant Professor
The George Washington University School of Nursing
Ashburn, Virginia

Laura Crouch, RN, EdD, CPAN, CNE
Clinical Professor
Northern Arizona University
Flagstaff, Arizona

Terri Gibson, DNP RN-BC
Associate Professor, Nursing
Southwestern Adventist University
Keene, Texas

Rebecca Hegel, DNP, FNP-C, MS, RN
Interim Program Director, Department Chair
SUNY Empire State College
Saratoga Springs, New York

Debra Pile, DNP, APRN, PCNS
Associate Professor
Wichita State University
Wichita, Kansas

Rosemarie DiMauro Satyshur, PhD, MSN, BSN, DIP, RN
Assistant Professor, Course Director Leadership and
    Management
University of Maryland School of Nursing,
    Department of Family and Community Health
Baltimore, Maryland

Shelly Wells, PhD, MBA, APRN-CNS, ANEF
Division Chair and Professor
Northwestern Oklahoma State University
Alva, Oklahoma

Acknowledgments

I would like to thank Adrienne Simon and Jacalyn Sharp for keeping me on track amid unforeseen life challenges, a global pandemic, and overwhelming remote work responsibilities. You two are amazing and I am happy to have you in my corner.

Contents in Brief

Contents

Part III   Leadership and Management Functions

Introduction

This book reflects the notion that all nurses at all levels and in all health-care settings are leaders and managers. The purpose of this book is to provide an evidence-based approach to nursing leadership and management as well as practical applications to real-life situations that reflect today's dynamic health-care environment. By integrating content from the National Council of Boards of Nursing Licensure Examination (NCLEX) blueprint, the American Association of Colleges of Nurses (AACN) Essentials: Core Competencies for Professional Nursing Practice, the American Nurses Association (ANA) foundational documents for nursing practice, Quality and Safety Education for Nurses (QSEN), the American Organization for Nursing Leadership (AONL) standards, and various quality and safety initiatives, students will be introduced to leadership and management theories, concepts, and principles.

This book offers a comprehensive approach to prepare nursing students in the knowledge, skills, and attitudes needed to provide safe, quality, and effective nursing care. It is divided into four parts that organize evidence-based information and relevant topics for effective nursing leadership and management at various levels and settings.

Part I: Foundations and Background provides foundational information about health-care safety and quality, ethics and legal aspects, and nursing leadership and management. Students are introduced to historical perspectives of the quality and safety movement and the core competencies for safe, quality, and effective nursing care. Next, health-care policy and the health-care environment are addressed, and theories of nursing leadership and management are presented. Finally, an overview of critical thinking and decision making is presented along with various tools that effective nurse leaders and managers can use for decision making at various levels in the health-care system.

Part II: Promotion of Patient Safety and Quality Care focuses on patient safety and quality. Effective communication is reviewed, and types of communication in a health-care environment are discussed. Organizational theories are presented as well as high-reliability organizations. Next, an overview of medical errors, adverse events, and creating a culture of safety is presented. Last, models and tools for quality improvement and how informatics contributes to patient safety is discussed.

Part III: Leadership and Management Functions presents specific roles and functions that effective nurse leaders and managers must understand and develop to be able to create, manage, and sustain a healthy work environment that fosters a workforce that delivers safe, quality, and effective nursing care.

Part IV: Managing Your Future in Nursing provides guidelines for new nurses transitioning to practice and guidelines for career planning and development. Additional content on professional growth and transitioning from a staff nurse to a leader/manager role is presented. Finally, an overview of balancing personal and professional life is discussed.

Each chapter in this book provides learning activities and evidence that reflect current nursing research. This book is an excellent resource for nursing students, new nurses, new nursing managers, and nurses in leadership and management at any stage of their career.

Part I

Foundations and Background

Chapter 1

Core Competencies for Safe and Quality Nursing Care

Elizabeth J. Murray, PhD, RN, CNE

KEY TERMS

Advocacy
Care coordination
Care process
Clinical practice guidelines
Communication
Cultural competence
Disparity
Diversity
Documentation
Empowerment
Evidence-based management
Evidence-based practice
Health literacy
High-reliability organizations
Human errors
Human factors engineering
Informatics
Information management
Interdisciplinary
Interprofessional
Multidisciplinary
Nursing research
Optimal healing environment
Outcomes of care
Patient-centered care
Quality
Quality improvement
Reliability science
Safety

LEARNING OUTCOMES

- Describe the impact of the Institute of Medicine (IOM) reports on the quality of health care in the United States.
- Define the IOM competencies, outline the IOM's six aims for health care, and analyze the IOM's 10 rules for health care in the 21st century.
- Compare and contrast the IOM competencies and the Quality and Safety Education for Nurses (QSEN) core competencies.
- Identify and describe fundamental elements for each core competency for nursing.
- Discuss the importance of effective nursing leadership and management in providing safe and quality patient-centered care.

Safety culture
Self-management
Standardized practice

Standardized protocols
Structure or care environment
Teamwork and collaboration

Nurses at all levels are leaders in the patient safety movement. Every nurse must be educated to deliver patient-centered care as a member of an inter-professional team, emphasizing evidence-based practice, quality improvement approaches, informatics, and safety (Cronenwett et al., 2007; Greiner & Knebel, 2003). The modern patient safety movement began in 2000 when the Institute of Medicine (IOM; now the National Academy of Medicine) published its land-mark report, *To Err Is Human: Building a Safer Health System* (Kohn et al., 2000). With that publication, a quest for quality and safety in health care was launched that continues today. In 2003, the IOM published *Health Professions Education: A Bridge to Quality* (Greiner & Knebel, 2003), which identified five core competen-cies for all health-care professions. In response to the IOM report, the Quality and Safety Education for Nurses (QSEN) initiative was launched in 2005 with the primary goal of establishing a set of core competencies specific to the nurs-ing profession.

This chapter provides a foundation for the entire book and discusses the core competencies for health-care professionals identified by the IOM and adapted by the QSEN faculty to be integrated into basic nursing education. Because the QSEN core competencies are now being translated into practice, the fundamental elements of each competency are discussed to help nurse leaders and managers operationalize them in their work settings.

▶ INSTITUTE OF MEDICINE REPORTS

Established in 1970 as the health arm of the National Academies, the IOM was an independent nonprofit organization that worked outside the federal government to provide unbiased and authoritative advice on health and health care to decision makers and the public. In July 2015, the National Academy of Sciences changed the name of the Institute of Medicine to the National Academy of Medicine (NAM) to more effectively integrate the work of the National Academies of Science, Engi-neering, and Medicine (NAS, 2015). The mission of the NAM is "To improve health for all by advancing science, accelerating health equity, and providing indepen-dent, authoritative, and trusted advice nationally and globally" (NAM, n.d.). Since 2000, the IOM has published a number of reports related to the state of quality in the U.S. health-care system. Box 1-1 provides a list of the reports most relevant to the content of this book; select elements of the various reports are discussed here as well as in other chapters.

The IOM's first report, *To Err Is Human,* was groundbreaking in that it identified medical errors as the leading cause of injury and unexpected death in health-care settings in the United States. The purpose of the report was to present a strategy to improve health-care quality over the following 10 years. Contending that pre-ventable adverse events result in up to 98,000 deaths annually, three domains of

BOX 1-1 Institute of Medicine Reports	
1990 *Medicare: A Strategy for Quality Assurance: Executive Summary, Volume 1*	**2003** *Health Professions Education: A Bridge to Quality* *Priority Areas for National Action: Transforming Health Care Quality*
2000 *To Err Is Human: Building a Safer Health System*	**2004** *Keeping Patients Safe: Transforming the Work Environment of Nurses*
2001 *Crossing the Quality Chasm: A New Health System for the 21st Century*	*Patient Safety: Achieving a New Standard for Care* *Health Literacy: A Prescription to End Confusion*
2002 *Unequal Treatment: Confronting Racial and Ethnic Disparities in Health Care*	**2011** *The Future of Nursing: Leading Change, Advancing Health*

quality were identified: patient safety, practice consistent with current medical knowledge, and meeting customer-specific values and expectations. Additionally, patient safety was identified as a critical component of quality. The IOM outlined the following four-tiered approach to quality improvement (Kohn et al., 2000):

1. "Establishing a national focus to create leadership, research, tools, and protocols to enhance the knowledge base about safety" (p. 3)
2. "Identifying and learning from errors by developing a nationwide public mandatory reporting system and by encouraging health care organizations and practitioners to develop and participate in voluntary reporting systems" (p. 3)
3. "Raising performance standards and expectations for improvements in safety through the actions of oversight organizations, professional groups, and group purchasers of health care" (p. 4)
4. "Implementing safety systems in health care organizations to ensure safe practices at the delivery level" (p. 4)

Before the publication of *To Err Is Human*, in 1997, President Bill Clinton appointed the Advisory Commission on Consumer Protection and Quality in the Health Care Industry to advise him on changes occurring in the health-care system and to make recommendations on how to promote and ensure health-care quality as well as protect consumers and professionals in the health-care system. In response, the Commission drafted a consumer bill of rights, adopting the following eight areas of consumer rights and responsibilities (Advisory Commission on Consumer Protection and Quality in the Health Care Industry, 1997):

1. Information disclosure
2. Choice of providers and plans
3. Choice of health-care providers that is sufficient to ensure access to appropriate high-quality care
4. Access to emergency services
5. Participation in treatment decisions
6. Respect and nondiscrimination; confidentiality of health information

7. Complaints and appeals
8. Consumer responsibilities

Endorsing the eight recommendations for consumer rights and responsibilities adopted by the Commission, the IOM Committee on Quality of Healthcare in America (IOM, 2001) challenged all health-care organizations and professionals to work continually to reduce the burden of illness, injury, and disability of the people of the United States. Although health-care professionals were—and continue to be—dedicated to providing quality care, a gap remained. Asserting that the U.S. health-care system was in need of major restructuring, the IOM Committee on Quality of Healthcare in America called for an overhaul by outlining six aims for health-care improvement in the 21st century in its 2001 report, *Crossing the Quality Chasm: A New Health System for the 21st Century:* that health care should be safe, effective, patient-centered, timely, efficient, and equitable. The IOM Committee on Quality of Healthcare in America believed that addressing these performance characteristics would lead to narrowing the quality gap. Table 1-1 lists the descriptions of these six aims.

In addition to the six aims, the IOM Committee on Quality of Healthcare in America (2001) identified 10 rules to redesign and improve health-care delivery in the 21st century. Emphasizing that part of the quality gap reflects a lack of support of well-designed systems and the absence of an environment that fosters innovation and excellence, the IOM Committee on Quality of Healthcare in America contended that these 10 specific rules are necessary to achieve significant improvement in quality (IOM, 2001). These rules were implemented to have an impact on the health-care workforce and, in turn, require change in accountabilities, standards of care, and relationships between patients and health-care professionals (IOM, 2001). Box 1-2 compares the historical approach with the 10 rules for health care in the 21st century.

Building on the six aims for health-care improvement and the rules for health care in the 21st century, the IOM recognized health professions education as

Table 1-1	Institute of Medicine's Six Aims for Health Care in the 21st Century	
Health Care Should Be:	**Description**
Safe	Avoiding injuries to patients from the care that is intended to help them
Effective	Providing services based on scientific knowledge to all who could benefit and refraining from providing services to those not likely to benefit; avoiding overuse, underuse, and misuse of care
Patient-centered	Providing care that is respectful of and responsive to individual patients' preferences, needs, and values, and ensuring that patients' values guide all decisions
Timely	Reducing waits and sometimes harmful delays for both those who receive and those who give care
Efficient	Avoiding waste, in particular of equipment, supplies, ideas, and energy
Equitable	Providing care that does not vary in quality because of personal characteristics such as gender, ethnicity, geographic location, and socioeconomic status

Adapted from IOM, 2001, pp. 39–40.

BOX 1-2   Ten Rules for Health-care Delivery in the 21st Century

1. Care is based on a continuous healing relationship, *rather than* periodic individual face-to-face visits.
2. Care is based on patients' values and needs, *rather than* variations of care provided by health-care professionals based on different local and individual styles of practice and/or training.
3. The patient is the source of control over care, *rather than* health-care professionals.
4. Knowledge is shared, and information flows freely, *rather than* requiring the patient to obtain permission. The patient has access to information without restriction, delay, or the need to request permission.
5. Decision making is evidence based, *rather than* based on the education and experience of the health-care professionals.
6. Safety is a system property, in that procedures, job designs, equipment, communication, and information technology should be configured to respect human factors, make errors less common, and make errors less harmful when they do occur, *rather than* safety being an individual person's responsibility.
7. There is a need for transparency, *rather than* a need for secrecy.
8. Health-care professionals predict and anticipate needs, *rather than* reacting to problems and underinvesting in prevention.
9. Waste is continuously decreased, *rather than* resorting to budget cuts and rationing services.
10. Collaboration and teamwork are the norm, *rather than* professional prerogatives and roles.

Adapted from IOM, 2001, pp. 66–83.

the primary tactic to narrow the quality gap. Thus, its report *Health Professions Education: A Bridge to Quality* (Greiner & Knebel, 2003) outlined five essential competencies necessary for all future graduates of health professions education programs, regardless of discipline (pp. 45–46):

1. Provide patient-centered care.
2. Work in interdisciplinary teams.
3. Employ evidence-based practice.
4. Apply quality improvement.
5. Use informatics.

The competencies are interrelated and applied together. However, the IOM stresses that skills related to the competencies are not discipline-specific and that each profession may put them into practice differently (Greiner & Knebel, 2003). In response, the QSEN faculty adapted the IOM competencies for the nursing profession and identified the knowledge, skills, and attitudes for each competency that should be developed in prelicensure nursing education (Cronenwett et al., 2007).

LEARNING ACTIVITY 1-1

Apply the 10 Rules for Health Care

Think about a health-care experience you or your family have encountered. Apply the 10 rules for health care in the 21st century listed in Box 1-2 to various aspects of your experience. Can you identify examples of care that reflect the historical approach? Can you identify examples of care that reflect the 21st-century approach?

▶ QUALITY AND SAFETY EDUCATION FOR NURSES CORE COMPETENCIES

Although all health-care professionals have an obligation to provide safe and quality care, nurses have been directly linked to ensuring patient safety and quality care outcomes (Page, 2004). The national QSEN initiative has been funded by the Robert Wood Johnson Foundation since 2005 and was organized with the purpose of adapting the IOM competencies for nursing specifically to serve as guides for curricular development in formal nursing education, transitions to practice, and continuing education programs (Cronenwett et al., 2007, p. 124). In addition, the competencies provide a framework for regulatory bodies that set standards for licensure, certification, and accreditation of nursing education programs (Cronenwett et al., 2007, p. 124). In collaboration with a national advisory board, QSEN faculty adapted the five competencies outlined in *Health Professions Education: A Bridge to Quality* (Greiner & Knebel, 2003)—provide patient-centered care, work in interdisciplinary teams, employ evidence-based practice, apply quality improvement, use informatics—and added a sixth competency, safety. The overall goal for the QSEN project is to prepare future nurses with the knowledge, skills, and attitudes necessary to continuously improve the quality and safety of the health-care systems within which they work (Cronenwett et al., 2007). Definitions of the core nursing competencies and comparisons with the IOM competencies follow.

Patient-Centered Care

Patient-centered care is more than a one-size-fits-all approach to care (Frampton & Guastello, 2010). Health-care professionals must shift from disease-focused paternalistic care to ensuring that the patient is the source of control and facilitating shared decision making (Greiner & Knebel, 2003). The IOM defines **patient-centered care** as follows: "identify, respect, and care about patients rather than differences, values, preferences, and expressed needs; relieve pain and suffering; coordinate continuous care; listen to, clearly inform, communicate with, and educate patients; share decision making and management; and continuously advocate disease prevention, wellness, and promotion of healthy lifestyles, including a focus on population health" (Greiner & Knebel, 2003, p. 45).

The skills related to this competency identified by the IOM include the following (Greiner & Knebel, 2003, pp. 52–53):

- Share power and responsibility with patients and caregivers.
- Communicate with patients in a shared and fully open manner.
- Take into account patients' individuality, emotional needs, values, and life issues.
- Implement strategies for reaching those who do not present for care on their own, including care strategies that support the broader community.
- Enhance prevention and health promotion.

The nurse–patient relationship has changed over the years. Nurses no longer make all the decisions or provide total care for patients. Instead, patients and their families enter into a full partnership with nurses and other health-care professionals. Today, active involvement of patients and their families in the plan of care and decision making is considered a precursor to safe, effective, and quality care.

Patient safety and quality care require recognizing the patient as the source of control. Care is customized based on patients' values, needs, and preferences. The nursing core competency of patient-centered care is defined as the recognition of "the patient or designee as the source of control and full partner in providing compassionate and coordinated care based on respect for patients' preferences, values, and needs" (Cronenwett et al., 2007, p. 123). Nurses develop healing relationships with patients and families in which they share information and communication flows freely. The fundamental elements of the patient-centered care core competency include advocacy, empowerment, self-management, cultural competence, health literacy, and an optimal healing environment.

Advocacy

Advocacy is one of the philosophical underpinnings of nursing and encompasses caring, respect for an individual person's autonomy, and empowerment. **Advocacy** in nursing is defined as "a process of analyzing, counseling, and responding to patients' care and self-determination preferences" (Vaartio-Rajalin & Leino-Kilpi, 2011, p. 526). Nurses have an ethical obligation to advocate for patients. Further, an advocate defends patients' rights and ensures the safety of those who cannot advocate for themselves, including those who are children, unconscious, mentally ill, uninformed, illiterate, or intimidated and fearful of health-care professionals (Gerber, 2018, p. 56). The American Nurses Association (ANA) *Code of Ethics for Nurses With Interpretive Statements* asserts, "the nurse promotes, advocates for, and strives to protect the health, safety, and rights of the patient" (2015a, p. 9). Nurses often find themselves representing and/or speaking for patients who cannot speak for themselves. The nurse's role as advocate is discussed further in Chapter 4.

Empowerment

As part of patient-centered care, nurses are called to empower patients and their families to engage in self-care, decision making, and developing a plan of care. **Empowerment** is defined as "patients' perceptions of access to information, support, resources, and opportunities to learn and grow that enable them to optimize their health and gain a sense of meaningfulness, self-determination, competency, and impact on their lives" (Spence Laschinger et al., 2010, p. 5). To truly empower patients, nurses must engage with the patient in a supportive social climate that is respectful and includes mutual decision making and power sharing. This climate leads to patient "independence, increased self-confidence, self-reliance, and self-management" (Akpotor & Johnson, 2018, p. 748). A sense of empowerment is vital from the nurse's perception as well as the patient's perception. To empower patients, nurses must believe that they have the power to accomplish work in a meaningful way. Spence Laschinger and colleagues (2010) contend that empowered nurses empower their patients, with the result being better health-care outcomes.

Self-Management

Self-management is a priority area identified as needed for quality health care and in achieving patient-centered care (Adams & Corrigan, 2003). The major aim of **self-management** is "to ensure that the sharing of knowledge between clinicians and patients and their families is maximized, that the patient is recognized as the source of control, and that the tools and system supports that make self-management tenable [are] available" (Adams & Corrigan, 2003, p. 52). Further, there is strong evidence that support for self-management is critical to the success of chronic illness programs. Self-management support requires nurses to engage in a collaborative relationship with their patients to identify health goals, select actions to meet the goals, acquire needed information, and monitor progress toward goals (Kanaan, 2008). Nurses assist patients with self-management by helping them increase skills and confidence in managing their health problems. Health literacy, discussed next, plays a key role in self-management.

Health Literacy

A major barrier to patient-centered care is "the ability to read, understand, and act on healthcare information," or *health literacy* (Adams & Corrigan, 2003, p. 52). According to the Centers for Disease Control and Prevention (CDC), 9 out of 10 adult Americans struggle with understanding health information (CDC, 2019a). Poor health literacy affects Americans of all social classes and ethnic groups (Adams & Corrigan, 2003). According to the CDC (2019b, para. 3), even the most educated can have health literacy issues when:

- They are not familiar with medical terms or how their bodies work.
- They have to interpret statistics and evaluate risks and benefits that affect their health and safety.
- They are diagnosed with a serious illness and are scared and confused.
- They have health conditions that require complicated self-care.
- They are voting on an issue affecting the community's health and relying on unfamiliar technical information.

The IOM defines **health literacy** as "the degree to which individuals have the capacity to obtain, process, and understand basic information and services needed to make appropriate decisions regarding their health (Nielsen-Bohlman et al., 2004, p. 2). Low literacy skills are most prevalent among the elderly and the low-income population. Unfortunately, those people most in need of health care are the least able to read and understand information for self-management (Adams & Corrigan, 2003). Health literacy can be improved with clear communication strategies and techniques (CDC, 2019a). Advocating for patients and their families experiencing health literacy problems can make a major difference in their healthcare encounters.

LEARNING ACTIVITY 1-2

Assessing Health Literacy

Health literacy should be part of the health assessment performed by nurses as they begin their shift. Is health literacy part of the health assessment document in use in your clinical facility?

Cultural Competence

Patient-centered care requires nurses to provide acceptable cultural care and to respect the differences in patients' values, preferences, and expressed needs (American Association of Colleges of Nursing [AACN], 2008). **Cultural competence** is defined as "the attitude, knowledge, and skills necessary for providing quality care to diverse populations" (AACN, 2008, p. 1). Nurses have a moral mandate to provide culturally competent care to all, regardless of gender, age, race, ethnicity, or economic status. Moreover, nurses must develop the ability to effectively work within the patient's cultural context and recognize the economic and political conditions that produce health inequalities (AACN, 2021, p. 61).

Part of cultural competence consists of understanding and respecting diversity. Not everyone is alike, and nurses must acknowledge and be sensitive to differences in patients and coworkers. **Diversity** is the "broad range of individual, population, and social characteristics, including but not limited to age; sex; race; ethnicity; sexual orientation; gender identity; family structures; geographic locations; national origin; immigrants and refugees; language; any impairment that substantially limits a major life activity; religious beliefs; and socioeconomic status" (AACN, 2021, p. 63).

Disparity is another issue related to cultural competence and encompasses unequal delivery of care, access to care, and/or outcomes of care based on ethnicity, geography, or gender. **Disparity** is defined as "racial or ethnic differences in the quality of healthcare that are not due to access-related factors or clinical needs, preferences, and appropriateness of intervention" (Smedley et al., 2002, pp. 3–4).

▶ OPTIMAL HEALING ENVIRONMENT

In her book, *Notes on Nursing: What It Is and What It Is Not,* Florence Nightingale (1860; republished 1969) emphasizes the importance of the environment in what she calls the "reparative process." She describes nursing as more than "the administration of medicines and the application of poultices" (p. 8) and suggests that nurses should also focus on "proper use of fresh air, light, warmth, cleanliness, quiet, and the proper selection and administration of diet" (p. 8). Nightingale also recognized that there are times when nurses cannot control the environment in which they deliver care. She notes that "bad sanitary, bad architectural, and bad administrative arrangements often make it impossible to nurse" (p. 8). In essence, what she was describing was how to create an optimal healing environment. Who knew that more than 150 years later, the basic principles identified by Nightingale would reemerge as critical in the healing process and to establishing an environment essential to patient-centered care? Florence Nightingale was clearly a nurse ahead of her time.

An **optimal healing environment** is "designed to stimulate and support inherent healing capacity of patients, families, and their care providers" (Sakallaris et al., 2015, p. 40). Patient-centered care must be delivered in an environment that fosters healing; is safe and clean; guards patients' privacy; engages all the human senses with color, texture, artwork, music, aromatherapy, views of nature, and comfortable lighting; and considers the experience of the body, mind, and spirit of all who use the facility (Frampton et al., 2008, p. 170). Space is provided for loved ones to congregate and for peaceful contemplation, meditation, or prayer. "At the heart of the environment of care, however, are the human interactions that occur within the physical structure to calm, comfort and support those who inhabit it. Together the design, aesthetics, and these interactions can transform an institutional, impersonal, and alien setting into one that is truly healing" (Frampton et al., 2008, p. 170).

Teamwork and Collaboration

Nurses and other health-care professionals cannot work in a silo. Working in interdisciplinary teams requires a shift in the health-care culture from one of individual experts to a cooperative and collaborative team environment. Team members integrate expertise and optimize care for patients. The IOM defines work in **interdisciplinary** teams as follows: "cooperate, collaborate, communicate, and integrate care in teams to ensure that care is continuous and reliable" (Greiner & Knebel, 2003, p. 45). Although often used interchangeably, the terms *interdisciplinary, multidisciplinary,* and *interprofessional* do not mean the same thing. **Multidisciplinary** describes a team in which members function independently and then share information with each other (McCallin, 2001). Nurses are very accustomed to working with and within multidisciplinary teams. However, the IOM is calling for individual team members to be more involved with collaboration, coordination, and contribution to the team goals—in other words, not just sharing with team members. Currently, the term *interprofessional* is gaining popularity because it is more inclusive of all members of the health-care team. **Interprofessional** refers to members with specific disciplinary training and diverse perspectives working collaboratively in planning and implementing patient-centered care (Interprofessional Education Collaborative, 2016).

The skills related to this competency identified by the IOM include the following (Greiner & Knebel, 2003, p. 56):

- Learn about other team members' expertise, background, knowledge, and values.
- Learn individual roles and processes required to work collaboratively.
- Demonstrate basic group skills, including communication, negotiation, delegation, time management, and assessment of group dynamics.
- Ensure that accurate and timely information reaches those who need it at the appropriate time.
- Customize care and manage smooth transitions across settings and over time, even when the team members are in entirely different physical locations.
- Coordinate and integrate care processes to ensure excellence, continuity, and reliability of the care provided.
- Resolve conflicts with other members of the team.
- Communicate with other members of the team in a shared language, even when the members are in entirely different physical locations.

With the increasing complexity of care today necessary to keep pace with the dynamic needs of patients, interprofessional teams are critical. In the truest form, teamwork focuses on patient-centered care, transcends individual and discipline-specific needs, and generates a positive synergy that results in an advanced level of performance that would not have been possible if team members worked alone. Interdisciplinary or interprofessional teamwork results in enhanced quality of care, improved patient outcomes, and maximized resources (Galt & Paschal, 2011).

Although health-care professionals may approach collaboration from different world views, certain characteristics are shared, such as coordination, communication, and teamwork (Disch, 2017). Safe and quality care requires teamwork and collaboration among all team members as well as the patient and family. The definition of the nursing core competency of **teamwork and collaboration** is to "function effectively within nursing and interprofessional teams, fostering open communication, mutual respect, and shared decision-making to achieve quality patient care" (Cronenwett et al., 2007, p. 125). Teamwork and collaboration are discussed in more depth in Chapter 11; however, it is important to address them briefly here as they relate to the core competencies.

Interprofessional teamwork is defined as "the levels of cooperation, coordination, and collaboration characterizing the relationships between professions in delivering patient-centered care" (Interprofessional Education Collaborative, 2016, p. 8). Functioning as an effective team member requires nurses to collaborate with other team members, patients, and families, by using available evidence to inform shared decision making and problem-solving. Professional nursing's scope of practice is dynamic, often overlapping the practice of other health-care professionals, and requires cooperation and sharing of knowledge and ideas to deliver safe, quality care (ANA, 2010a). In addition, nurses collaborate with patients and families to assess, plan, implement, and evaluate safe and quality care (ANA, 2010a). Nurses are called to actively promote collaborative care planning to ensure availability and accessibility of quality health care to all persons who need it (ANA, 2015a). The fundamental elements of teamwork and collaboration include care coordination and communication.

Care Coordination

Nurse leaders and managers as well as all nurses coordinate care delivery as members of interprofessional and intraprofessional teams. Care coordination is a priority area needed for health-care quality improvement (Adams & Corrigan, 2003). Various organizations such as the National Quality Forum (NQF), the Agency for Healthcare Research and Quality (AHRQ), and the ANA are embracing its application to various patient care settings. The major goal of **care coordination** is "to establish and support a continuous healing relationship, enabled by an integrated clinical environment and characterized by the proactive delivery of evidence-based care and follow-up" (Adams & Corrigan, 2003, p. 49). The AHRQ describes it as "the deliberate organization of patient care activities between two or more participants (including the patient) involved in a patient's care to facilitate the appropriate delivery of health-care services. Organizing care involves the marshalling of personnel and other resources needed to carry out all required patient care activities, and is often managed by the exchange of information among participants responsible for different aspects of care" (McDonald et al., 2007, p. 41). The NQF (2006) defines care coordination as a "function that helps ensure that the patient's needs and preferences for health services and information sharing across people, functions, and sites are met over time" (p. 1). The ANA has endorsed NQF's definition because it addresses the priorities of "increasing patient-centered care and reimbursement structures based on patient outcomes" (McCammon & Francis, 2018).

The ANA identifies patient-centered care coordination as part of the independent scope of practice and a core professional standard and competency for all registered nurses (ANA, 2014). Care coordination includes organizing the components of the plan of care, coordinating the implementation of the plan of care, advocating for the delivery of dignified and holistic care, and documenting the coordination of care (ANA, 2015b). The ANA's (2015a) *Code of Ethics for Nurses With Interpretive Statements* establishes a primary commitment to the patient and the family and requires nurses to ensure the plan of care reflects the patient's wishes

EXPLORING THE EVIDENCE 1-1

Mellum, J. S., Martsolf, D., Glazer, G., Martsolf, G., & Tobias, B. (2018). A mixed methods study of the experience of older adults with multimorbidity in a care coordination program. *International Journal of Care Coordination, 21*(1–2), 36–46.

Aim

The aim of this mixed-methods study was to explore the experience of older adults with multimorbidity in care coordination programs.

Methods

A mixed-methods research design was used to understand the experience of care for older adults with multimorbidity. Quantitative data were collected using the Patient Assessment of Chronic Illness Care Plus (PACIC+). Qualitative data were collected using semistructured telephone interviews. Qualitative data were integrated with quantitative data from the PACIC+.

Key Findings

The investigators found two factors that influenced the experience of older adults were professional actions and professional attitudes. Patients' experiences were improved by professional actions of communication, coordination, and addressing fundamental problems. In addition, actions associated with self-management were also a positive influence on care experiences. The professional attitudes that improved care experiences were compassion, knowledge, mutual respect, and being positive and encouraging.

Implications for Nurse Leaders and Managers

Nurse leaders and managers involved in care coordination programs should ensure that all interventions foster communication, improve coordination among health-care providers, and provide adequate attention to older adults' problems. In addition, health-care providers should be compassionate, knowledgeable, respectful, positive, and encouraging in their care coordination for older adults.

and individuality. In addition, nurse leaders and managers should work to ensure that the relevant parties are involved and have a voice in decision making about patient care issues (ANA, 2015a).

Communication

Communication is a key aspect of teamwork and collaboration. It involves communicating with patients, families, and other health-care professionals by using effective techniques and tools. Effective communication is accurate and timely and enhances quality of care. Additionally, effective communication requires listening actively, encouraging input from others, and respecting opinions of all team members. Chapter 8 explores communication in greater depth.

There is a critical link between effective communication and patient safety. All aspects of patient care hinge on how health-care professionals, patients, and families interpret available information (Schuster & Nykolyn, 2010). Interprofessional and intraprofessional (made up of all nurses) team members make health-care decisions based on information communicated among all team members with input from patients and their families. Miscommunication and gaps in communication can jeopardize patient safety. The Joint Commission (TJC, 2015) cites communication errors as a leading cause of medical errors. Nurses need to create an atmosphere in which patients and their families feel valued, like an important part of the health-care team, and comfortable sharing personal information (Schuster & Nykolyn, 2010).

Evidence-Based Practice

Evidence-based practice promotes best practices, clinical expertise, patients' values, and patients' circumstances in health-care decisions and avoids underuse, misuse, and overuse of care (Greiner & Knebel, 2003). The IOM defines **evidence-based practice** as follows: "integrate best research with clinical expertise and patient values for optimum care, and participate in learning and research activities to the extent feasible" (pp. 45–46).

The skills related to this competency identified by the IOM include the following (Greiner & Knebel, 2003, pp. 57–58):

- Know where and how to find the best possible sources of evidence.
- Formulate clear clinical questions.
- Search for the relevant answers to those questions from the best possible sources of evidence, including those that evaluate or appraise the evidence for its validity and usefulness with respect to a particular patient or population.
- Determine when and how to integrate these new findings into practice.

Patient safety and quality care require the use of evidence-based practice to guide nursing practice and reduce variations in care. With that in mind, the nursing core competency of evidence-based practice is defined as "integrating best current evidence with clinical expertise and patient/family preferences and values for delivery of optimal healthcare" (Cronenwett et al., 2007, p. 126). Nurses should use evidence-based clinical decision making to individualize nursing care based on a patient's specific circumstances.

To integrate evidence into practice, nurses must best identify searchable clinical questions by using the seven-step approach outlined by Melnyk and Fineout-Overholt (2019). Step 0 involves cultivating a spirit of inquiry in the work environment. The organization must be supportive of evidence-based practice and provide needed resources for sustainability (Melnyk & Fineout-Overholt, 2019). Step 1 requires nurses to identify a clinical question. One technique is to use the PICOT method to ask a searchable question. (PICOT stands for Population/Patient Problem, Intervention, Comparison, Outcome, Time). In step 2, nurses must collect the best evidence relevant to the question using key words from the PICOT question to begin the search. During step 3, nurses should critically appraise the evidence before using it, by evaluating the studies for validity, reliability, and applicability. This step ensures the relevance and transferability of evidence to the specific population for whom nurses provide care (Melnyk & Fineout-Overholt, 2019). Step 4 requires integrating the evidence with the other aspects of evidence-based practice. During this step, nurses need to incorporate the evidence using their expertise and the patient's preferences to implement care. In step 5, nurses should evaluate their practice decision or change to determine whether it affected the patient's outcome. In step 6, the outcomes of the evidence-based decision or change should be disseminated.

It is important for nurses to remember that evidence can include a variety of research and nonresearch sources and that some sources of evidence are stronger than other sources. Sources of evidence are categorized into levels and are rated according to their strength (Melnyk & Fineout-Overholt, 2019; Polit & Beck, 2017). Figure 1-1 illustrates this pyramid of evidence.

There are numerous pre-appraised and non–pre-appraised resources available to nurses. Studies included in pre-appraised or filtered databases have been reviewed before inclusion, are updated regularly, and consist of the most methodologically sound and clinically important studies (Salmond, 2013). Popular filtered databases include the Cochrane Library (www.thecochranelibrary.com), Campbell Collaboration (www.campbellcollaboration.org), and Joanna Briggs Institute (www.joannabriggs.org). Non–pre-appraised or unfiltered databases consist of original studies of excellent to poor quality that require the nurse to critically appraise the research before using it in practice. Examples of unfiltered databases include the Cumulative Index of Nursing and Allied Health Literature (CINAHL) and the National Library of Medicine's MEDLINE.

Evidence should inform all nursing care. Safe and quality care requires basing nursing practice on the most current and best available knowledge. Evidence-based practice is critical in the quest for patient safety and quality care. The fundamental elements of evidence-based practice are nursing research, the relationship with quality improvement, clinical practice guidelines, and evidence-based management.

Relationship With Nursing Research

Evidence-based practice should not be confused with nursing research. **Nursing research** is a systematic inquiry that uses disciplined methods to answer questions, solve problems, and seek new nursing knowledge. The goals of nursing research

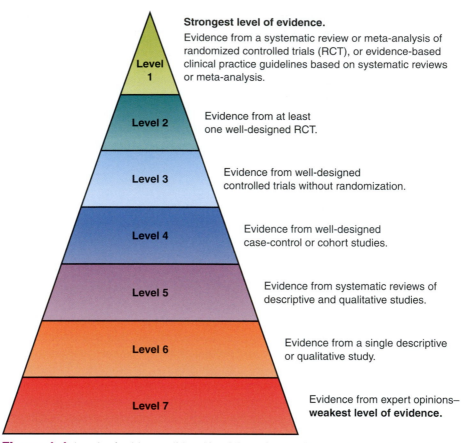

Strongest level of evidence.
Evidence from a systematic review or meta-analysis of randomized controlled trials (RCT), or evidence-based clinical practice guidelines based on systematic reviews or meta-analysis.

Level 1

Evidence from at least one well-designed RCT.

Level 2

Evidence from well-designed controlled trials without randomization.

Level 3

Evidence from well-designed case-control or cohort studies.

Level 4

Evidence from systematic reviews of descriptive and qualitative studies.

Level 5

Evidence from a single descriptive or qualitative study.

Level 6

Evidence from expert opinions—
weakest level of evidence.

Level 7

Figure 1-1 Levels of evidence. *(Adapted from DiCenso, Guyatt, & Ciliska, 2005; Melnyk & Fineout-Overholt, 2011; Polit & Beck, 2017.)*

include generating, testing, or evaluating knowledge and developing reliable evidence about issues important to the nursing profession (Polit & Beck, 2017). Nurses have a duty to advance the profession through knowledge development and dissemination as well as application to practice. "All nurses must participate in the advancement of the profession through knowledge development, evaluation, dissemination, and application to practice" (ANA, 2015a, p. 27). Rigorous nursing research provides one of the best sources for evidence-based practice.

Relationship With Quality Improvement

Quality improvement is also not the same as evidence-based practice. Although quality improvement is discussed later in this chapter and more thoroughly in Chapter 9, it is important to address its relationship with evidence-based practice here as well. **Quality improvement** is a cyclical process designed to monitor and evaluate workflow and work processes. It can include data collection and analysis but has no theoretical foundation. Quality improvement uses benchmarks to measure practice against established standards and provides methods to improve nursing practice continually. Hedges (2006) discusses the "three-legged stool" of nursing practice—evidence-based practice, quality improvement, and nursing research—and breaks down each element as inquiry processes that support nursing practice. She suggests that nurses can strengthen the foundation of nursing practice by using quality improvement to monitor nursing practice and patient outcomes, systematically reviewing the evidence using evidence-based practice, and conducting scientific studies through nursing research.

Clinical Practice Guidelines

Clinical practice guidelines are tools for clinicians to improve the quality and process of care delivery and patient outcomes and to reduce variations in care and health-care costs. These guidelines are "systematically developed statements to assist practitioner and patient decisions about appropriate healthcare for specific clinical circumstances" (IOM, 1990, p. 38). Clinical practice guidelines are systematically developed from the appraisal and summary evidence and attempt to address issues relevant to a clinical decision (Salmond, 2013). Nurses must be involved in developing practice standards "grounded in nursing's ethical commitments and developing body of knowledge... reflect nursing's responsibility to society" (ANA, 2015a, p. 28). The National Guideline Clearinghouse (www.guideline.gov), the CDC (www.cdc.gov), the Scottish Intercollegiate Guidelines Network (www.sign.ac.uk), and the Registered Nurses' Association of Ontario (rnao.ca/bpg) are major sources of clinical practice guidelines for nurses.

Evidence-Based Management

Using evidence-based clinical practice when caring for patients is critical in providing safe and quality care. Best practices and advances in organizational, leadership, and management research when carrying out leadership and management roles should also be considered. **Evidence-based management** is defined as "making decisions through the conscientious, explicit, and judicious use of four sources of information: practitioner expertise and judgment, evidence from the local context, a critical evaluation of the best available research evidence, and the perspectives of those people who might be affected by the decision" (Briner, Denyer, & Rousseau, 2009, p. 19).

The IOM asserts that evidence-based management is critical to achieving safety in health care (Page, 2004). Evidence-based management includes management strategies informed by rigorous research and requires managers "to search for, appraise, and apply empirical evidence from management research in their practice" (Page, 2004, p. 113). Evidence-based management is discussed throughout this text. Therefore, only a brief discussion as it relates to the core competency of evidence-based practice and nursing leadership and management is included here.

To foster an environment conducive to patient safety requires leadership capable of transforming both the physical environment and the beliefs and practices of health-care workers. The IOM identifies five management practices that consistently contribute to the success of patient safety initiatives in spite of a high risk for error (Page, 2004, p. 108):

1. Balancing the tension between production efficiency and reliability
2. Creating and sustaining trust throughout the organization
3. Actively managing the process of change
4. Involving workers in decision making pertaining to work design and flow
5. Using knowledge management practices to establish the organization as a learning organization

Despite the evidence that these essential practices minimize threats to patient safety, they are not applied consistently. Therefore, the IOM recommends promoting evidence-based management practices to identify and minimize management decisions on patient safety (Page, 2004). In addition, evidence-based management can improve patient outcomes, nurse satisfaction, organizational outcomes, and leadership success (Shingler-Nace & Gonzales, 2017).

Quality Improvement

Reports from the IOM since the 1990s document evidence of serious quality problems throughout the U.S. health-care system. In addition to substandard quality of care, the health-care industry is notorious for inefficiency and waste. Health-care professionals are called to provide quality care, but what exactly is quality? The IOM (1990) defines **quality** as "the degree to which health services for individuals and populations increases the likelihood of desired health outcomes and are consistent with current professional knowledge" (p. 4). The AHRQ (2005) suggests that providing quality health care involves striking the right balance of services by avoiding underuse and overuse and by eliminating misuse. Others posit that applying quality improvement methods used in the industrial sector can mitigate errors, waste, and inefficiency (Greiner & Knebel, 2003). Regardless, nurses must work to provide high-quality care to patients. Chapter 9 addresses quality improvement in detail; therefore, only a brief overview of quality improvement follows.

Quality improvement originated in the industrial sector as a method to reduce errors in production processes, but its adoption by health-care organizations has been slow. Constraints include lack of infrastructure and absence of leadership among health-care providers (Greiner & Knebel, 2003). The IOM has challenged the health-care system to build on the experiences of high-risk industries, such as aviation and nuclear power, that have demonstrated enhanced safety and quality by using quality improvement methods.

The IOM defines "apply quality improvement" as follows: "identify errors and hazards in care; understand and implement basic safety design principles, such as standardization and simplification; continually understand and measure quality of care in terms of structure, process, and outcomes in relation to patient and community needs; design and test interventions to change processes and systems of care, with the objective of improving quality" (Greiner & Knebel, 2003, p. 46).

The skills related to this competency identified by the IOM include the following (Greiner & Knebel, 2003, p. 59):

- Assess current practices and compare them with relevant better practices elsewhere as a means of identifying opportunities for improvement.
- Design and test interventions to change the process of care, with the objective of improving quality.
- Identify errors and hazards in care, and understand and implement basic safety design principles, such as standardization and simplification and human factors training.
- Both act as an effective member of an interdisciplinary team and improve the quality of one's own performance through self-assessment and personal change.

Patient safety and quality care require nurses to systematically identify potential and actual problems, explore potential and actual causes, and develop strategies for improvement. Quality improvement is the responsibility of all nurses regardless of position in the health-care system. The nursing core competency of quality improvement is to "use data to monitor the outcomes of care processes and use improvement methods to design and test changes to continuously improve the quality and safety of healthcare systems" (Cronenwett et al., 2007, p. 127). Quality improvement is a continuous process in which nurses collect quality data to establish standards for care delivery and monitor and evaluate those standards on an ongoing basis. The fundamental elements of quality improvement include structure or care environment, the care process, and outcomes of care.

Structure or Care Environment

The **structure or care environment** essentially means the setting *where* nursing care is provided. Examples include the physical environment (e.g., the unit, a patient room, a surgical suite, outpatient clinic, or a patient's home), equipment, staffing (including staff mix and staffing ratios), policies and procedures, the organizational culture, and management of the organization.

Care Process

The **care process** focuses on *how* nursing care is provided. Examples of care process include models of care delivery such as primary care, Transforming Care at the Bedside (TCAB), and case management. The care process also encompasses critical pathways, standardized clinical guidelines, actual physical care of patients, assessment, intervention, patient education, timeliness of care, counseling, and leadership and management activities.

Outcomes of Care

The **outcomes of care** include the *results* of all the nursing care provided and reflect the effectiveness of nursing activities. Examples of outcomes of care include length of stay, infection rates, patients' falls, postprocedure complications, and failure to rescue. Currently, approaches focus on nursing-sensitive outcomes, or outcomes linked directly to the quantity and quality of nursing care.

Informatics

Informatics is more than merely using information technology; rather, it includes the development and application of information technology systems to health-care problems, research, and education. Advances in technology have resulted in numerous innovations in health care, including electronic health records, telehealth, remote monitoring, and education through simulation (IOM, 2011). Successful use of informatics allows health-care professionals to manage knowledge and information, communicate more effectively, and reduce more errors than in the past. (Chapter 10 explores informatics in more depth.) The IOM defines **informatics** as follows: "communicate, manage knowledge, mitigate error, and support decision making using information technology" (Greiner & Knebel, 2003, p. 46).

The skills related to this competency identified by the IOM include the following (Greiner & Knebel, 2003, p. 63):

- Employ word processing, presentation, and data analysis software.
- Search, retrieve, manage, and make decisions using electronic data from internal information databases and external online databases and the Internet.
- Communicate using e-mail, instant messaging, LISTSERV, and file transfers.
- Understand security protections such as access control, data security, and data encryption, and directly address ethical and legal issues related to the use of information technology in practice.
- Enhance education and access to reliable health information for patients.

Informatics integrates data, information, and knowledge to support the interprofessional team and is linked consistently to patient safety and quality (Clancy & Warren, 2017; Greiner & Knebel, 2003). Safe and quality care requires information technology to facilitate effective communication and documentation. Nurses must develop and maintain their skills in informatics to use electronic health records, examine relevant evidence to support clinical decisions, solve patient and system problems, manage quality improvement data, and share information (Sherwood & Barnsteiner, 2017). In light of this, the nursing core competency of informatics is defined as the "use information and technology to communicate, manage knowledge, mitigate error, and support decision-making" (Cronenwett et al., 2007, p. 129). The incorporation of informatics in health care is inevitable, and nurses must develop the skills for entering patients' data and retrieving information for clinical decision making and quality improvement. Informatics is actually a thread through all of the QSEN competencies (Clancy & Warren, 2017). The fundamental elements of informatics are information management and documentation.

Information Management

Nurses depend on information to provide safe and quality care. How information is organized and presented influences how effectively and efficiently nurses deliver care (Sewell, 2016). The Technology Informatics Guiding Education Reform

(TIGER) was launched in 2006 to create a vision for the future of nursing in the digital age. Nine TIGER collaborative teams were formed to develop action plans related to key topic areas. The TIGER Informatics Computer Collaboration (TICC) team was charged with defining "the minimum set of informatics competencies that all nurses need to succeed in practice or education in today's digital era" (TIGER, 2009, p. 5). The TICC team developed a set of competencies related to information management and contended that all practicing nurses should "learn, demonstrate, and use information management competencies to carry out their fundamental clinical responsibilities in an increasingly safe, effective, and efficient manner" (TIGER, 2009, p. 11).

TIGER expanded globally in 2012 to help faculty, clinical educators, and students with coordination and synthesis of informatics competencies, pool educational resources, and foster international community development (O'Connor, Hubner, Shaw, Blake, & Ball, 2017, p. 79). The expansion of TIGER globally has resulted in a new interprofessional approach to health informatics. In 2016, TIGER joined the European Union (EU)–United States (US) Collaboration on eHealth to compile "a recommendation framework of health informatics competencies to measure, inform, education, and advance development of a skilled workforce throughout the EU, US, and around the world" (Healthcare Information and Management Systems Society, Inc. [HIMSS], 2020, para. 8).

Information management is an elemental process of collecting, analyzing, monitoring, manipulating, summarizing, storing, and communicating necessary information for health care (ANA, 2015c; Greiner & Knebel, 2003; TIGER, 2009). Access to online databases provides nurses and other health-care professionals with the literature and knowledge needed to implement evidence-based practice (Greiner & Knebel, 2003). Nurses manage information in a variety of ways, but "the preferred or required method is through information systems" (TIGER, 2009, p. 11). Nurses at all levels use information systems and patient care technologies in direct and indirect patient care. Nurses must "understand their role and value of their input in health information technology analysis, planning, implementation, and evaluation" (AACN, 2021, p. 48).

Documentation

Nurses have a professional responsibility to document care planning, actual care provided, and patient outcomes. **Documentation** is any written or electronically generated information about a patient that describes the care provided to that patient and offers an accurate account of what occurred and when it occurred. Nurses use documentation to communicate all interactions with patients including assessments, interventions, evaluations, and outcomes of care. Documentation is maintained in a health record, which may include paper or electronic documents such as electronic medical records, faxes, e-mails, audio or video records, and images.

Documentation is critical for effective intraprofessional and interprofessional communication. "Clear, accurate and accessible documentation is an essential element of safe, quality, evidence-based nursing practice" (ANA, 2010b, p. 3). Effective documentation provides a foundation for demonstrating nursing's valuable contributions to patient outcomes as well as to the organizations that provide and support quality patient care (ANA, 2010b). According to the ANA (2010b), documentation is critical to the nursing profession in the following areas:

- Communication within the health-care team and with other professionals
- Credentialing, legal, regulation, and legislation
- Reimbursement
- Research, quality process, and performance improvement

Nurses must consistently document all critical and necessary data and information regarding patient care. Nurse leaders and managers should ensure that staff are involved with decision making regarding documentation and provide clear guidelines, policies, and procedures for documentation (ANA, 2010b).

Safety

Although the IOM does not identify safety as a separate competency, it is included as one of the six aims critical to improving the overall quality of health care as well as safety for patients and health-care workers. The IOM's all-inclusive definition of **safety** is "freedom from accidental injury" (IOM, 2001, p. 45). As discussed earlier in this chapter, the IOM report, *To Err Is Human,* outlines recommendations for improving patient safety at the point of care delivery (Kohn, Corrigan, & Donaldson, 2000). The report also encourages health-care organizations to focus on creating environments that foster patient safety, or in other words, creating a safety culture. Key organizations committed to the patient safety movement include the AHRQ, NQF, TJC, and Institute for Healthcare Improvement (IHI).

Although the quest for safe and quality health care has been ongoing for more than two decades, health-care professionals continue to fall short. Chassin and Loeb (2011) suggested that the health-care system is at a critical intersection at which patients in the hospital are increasingly vulnerable to harm from medical errors, and, unfortunately, the complexity of health care today increases the likelihood of medical errors. Safety does not just happen; it must be carefully orchestrated and requires all staff to be adequately educated about patient safety and error prevention. Nurses, more than any other health-care professionals, have been identified as vital players in promoting patient safety.

Safety is another competency that is present in all other QSEN competencies and is a common theme throughout this book. The safety core nursing competency is defined as follows: "minimize risk of harm to patients and providers through both system effectiveness and individual performance" (Cronenwett et al., 2007, p. 128). The fundamental elements of safety include human errors and human factors, standardized protocols and practice, safety culture, and high-reliability organizations.

Human Errors and Factors

Given the high complexity of the health-care environment today, errors are inevitable. **Human errors** are acts of omission or commission leading to an undesirable outcome or the potential for an undesirable outcome (Wachter & Gupta, 2018). Acts of omission involve failing to do the right thing or omitting something that results in an error, such as a nurse forgetting to give a patient a prescribed medication. Acts of commission involve doing something wrong or committing an error, such as a nurse giving a patient the wrong medication. Human errors are discussed in more detail in Chapter 9.

Human factors engineering is an applied science that studies human capabilities and limitations and the interplay between humans, machines, and the work environment (Wachter & Gupta, 2018). It applies knowledge gleaned to the design of safe, effective processes and systems for humans with the goal of achieving effective, efficient, and safe care (Boston-Fleischhauer, 2008a). Human factors engineering assumes that well-designed processes and systems take into account human capabilities and limitations outside the control of those working with the processes and systems. Such limitations can be (1) physical, such as noise, climate, and lighting; (2) cognitive, involving short-term memory capacity and fatigue; and (3) organizational, such as job and task design (Boston-Fleischhauer, 2008a). Poorly designed processes and systems can result in increased potential for errors and decreased patient safety (Boston-Fleischhauer, 2008a). Nurses must monitor, evaluate, and improve processes and systems to ensure patient safety.

Reliability science is "the ability of an operation to be failure or defect free over time" (Boston-Fleischhauer, 2008b, p. 84). In other words, reliability science is employing deliberate strategies that make it difficult for nurses to do the wrong thing and easy to do the right thing. By designing simple processes and systems that are standardized and redundant, defy error, avoid reliance on memory, and employ continuous vigilance, the goal of safe, quality patient care can be realized. Simplicity and standardizing care can reduce the probability of errors by decreasing variability of care.

Standardized Protocols and Practice

Standardized protocols can decrease preventable adverse events and medical errors. Common standard protocols are used to prevent mislabeling of radiographs, to prevent wrong-site or wrong-patient procedures, and for labeling, packaging, and storing medications (AHRQ, 2005). The AHRQ (2005) identifies the use of evidence-based practice and standardized tools as critical aspects of patient safety improvement. **Standardized practice** reflects current research findings and best practices and outlines the minimally accepted actions expected from health-care professionals. Standardized practice is linked to several other competencies such as evidence-based practice and quality improvement.

Safety Culture

Patient safety and quality care require a culture of safety. The IOM describes a **safety culture** as one in which "an organization's care processes and workforce are focused on improving reliability and safety of care for patients" (Kohn, Corrigan, & Donaldson, 2000, p. 114). The goal in a safety culture is to balance accountability with the notion of "no blame" for errors (Wachter & Pronovost, 2009). Transparency is critical in a safety culture. Staff must feel comfortable to report errors, near misses, and potential for errors. Five principles are necessary for the design of a safe health-care environment (Kohn, Corrigan, & Donaldson, 2000):

- *Providing leadership:* Make patient safety a priority objective and everyone's responsibility. Make sure assignments are clear, with an expectation of safety oversight, and that there are effective mechanisms for identifying and dealing with unsafe practitioners. Provide human and financial resources for error analysis and system redesign.
- *Respecting human limits in the design process:* Design jobs for safety, and avoid reliance on memory and on vigilance. Simplify and standardize work processes.
- *Promoting effective team functioning:* Train health-care professionals expected to work in interprofessional teams with others who will be working with them.
- *Anticipating the unexpected:* Adopt a proactive approach. Identify threats to safety before an accident can occur, and redesign processes to prevent accidents.
- *Creating a learning environment:* Use simulation whenever feasible. Encourage transparency and reporting of errors without reprisals, and implement mechanisms for feedback and learning from errors. Develop a culture in which communication flows freely.

Creating a safety culture requires nurse leaders and managers to take ownership of patient and worker safety and to foster a work environment in which safety is a top priority. Nurse leaders and managers must understand the complexities of the health-care system and the limits of human factors (Barnsteiner, 2017).

High-Reliability Organizations

High reliability refers to consistent performance at high levels of safety over time (Chassin & Loeb, 2011). The first industries to embrace high-reliability concepts were aviation and nuclear power. **High-reliability organizations** create processes, systems, and a culture that radically reduce system failures and/or effectively respond when failures do occur (AHRQ, 2008). There are five characteristics fundamental to designing processes and systems for high-reliability organizations (AHRQ, 2008, p. 1):

1. *Sensitivity to operations:* Leaders and staff must be constantly aware of risks to patient safety and focus on preventing them.
2. *Reluctance to simplify:* Avoiding overly simple explanations of failures is essential to understand the true reasons that patient safety is in jeopardy.
3. *Preoccupation with failure:* Leaders and staff must view near misses as evidence that systems should be improved, rather than as proof that the system is working effectively.
4. *Deference to expertise:* Leaders and managers must listen and respond to the insights of frontline staff.
5. *Resilience:* Leaders and staff must be educated and prepared to respond when system failures do occur.

Overall, leaders, managers, and frontline staff must embrace a high-reliability mindset to become a high-reliability organization. High-reliability organizations foster a learning environment and promote a safety culture, evidence-based practice, and a positive work environment for nurses. In addition, they are committed to improving the safety and quality of care.

CURRENT STATE OF SAFETY AND QUALITY

There is strong evidence that links nursing practice to patient safety and quality of care (IOM, 2011). Since the publication of the IOM report *To Err Is Human,* there has been a diligent quest to improve the safety and quality of health care. However, some contend that progress has been frustratingly slow (James, 2013; Wachter & Gupta, 2018). There is some speculation that the IOM's estimate of 44,000 to 98,000 deaths from preventable adverse events was an underestimate and that far more lethal errors actually occur each year (Makary & Daniel, 2016; Wachter & Gupta, 2018). In his study, James (2013) contended that health care is experiencing a major epidemic of patient harm. He found that there are, at a minimum, 210,000 lethal preventable adverse events annually. However, Makary and Daniel (2016) suggest this is an underestimate of deaths due to preventable adverse events. They calculated the mean rate of deaths from medical errors using studies reported since the 1999 IOM document and contend that the incidence of deaths due to adverse events in studies between 1999 and 2013 is close to 251,000. Further, they suggest incidences are underestimated due to the fact that most studies rely on errors documented in health records and only include inpatient deaths (Makary & Daniel, 2016, p. 2). Makary and Daniel assert that medical errors are the third leading cause of death in the United States. Further, they suggest that when an adverse event results in death, the physiological cause of death as well as the adverse event should be identified in the medical record (p. 2).

Nurses play a critical role in preventing medication errors, decreasing infection rates, and safe transitions from hospital to home (IOM, 2011). The studies by James (2013) and Makary and Daniel (2016) further substantiate the continued need to prepare nurses with the necessary knowledge, skills, and attitudes to deliver patient-centered care as members of interprofessional teams, emphasizing evidence-based practice, quality improvement, and informatics (Cronenwett et al., 2007).

SUMMARY

Effective nursing leadership and management are critical to providing patients with safe, effective, reliable, and quality care. Care must be patient-centered, involving the patient and their family in all health-care decisions. In addition, the work environment must foster collaboration and teamwork and must include effective interprofessional and intraprofessional communication. Safe, reliable, and quality care requires nurses to base their practice on the most current available knowledge. Nurse leaders and managers must also employ management strategies that are informed by rigorous research to reduce threats to patient safety and to enhance the work environment for staff.

Quality of nursing care considers where the care is provided, how the care is provided, and the results or outcomes of the care provided. Nurses must learn to use technology to systematically identify potential and actual problems and their causes, and they need to develop strategies for prevention and improvement. The ultimate goal of quality improvement is patient and staff safety. Nurses are not expected to be perfect; they are human and will make errors. Nurse leaders and managers must strive for a culture of safety that recognizes the limitations of human factors and takes a proactive approach to prevention of errors.

NCLEX®-STYLE REVIEW QUESTIONS

Multiple Choice

1. The nurse is aware that the optimal healing environment, which is a component of the Patient-Centered Care Quality and Safety Education in Nursing (QSEN) competency, is designed to assist the patient in what way?
   1. Has enough room for family members
   2. Provides for privacy
   3. Helps the patient heal themselves
   4. Ensures a pleasant hospital experience

2. What is the first step that nurses should take in integrating evidence-based practice on a nursing unit?
   1. Research how other nursing units have implemented evidence-based nursing.
   2. Ensure that the evidence is relevant to the specific nursing unit.
   3. Evaluate the effectiveness of the evidence to patient care.
   4. Determine which clinical problem is to be researched.

3. Nurses are aware that the Quality and Safety Education in Nursing (QSEN) competency, Teamwork and Collaboration, requires what specific type of collaboration?
   1. Multidisciplinary
   2. Interdisciplinary
   3. Interprofessional
   4. Customized care

4. The nurse is aware that human factors engineering is utilized to accomplish what goal?
   1. Decrease errors in nursing care.
   2. Ensure that there is adequate staffing on a nursing unit.
   3. Determine whether the nursing unit is an optimal healing environment.
   4. Design more efficient ways for nurses to provide patient care.

5. The nurse understands that improvement of safety in nursing is dependent on evidence-based practice and which element of the safety competency?
   1. Resilience
   2. Human factors engineering
   3. High-reliability organizations
   4. Standardized protocols

6. The nurse manager has decided to use the strategies of the Institute of Medicine (IOM), *To Err Is Human,* to improve health care on the nursing unit. The nurse has identified that patient safety, practice consistent with current medical knowledge, and what other strategy must be implemented in this endeavor?
   1. Work in interdisciplinary teams.
   2. Work in intradisciplinary teams.
   3. Meet the expectations of the patient.
   4. Meet the expectations of the nurses.

7. The nurse leader as a part of the patient-centered care Quality Safety Education in Nursing (QSEN) competency has encouraged all nurses to be advocates for their patients. The nurse leader knows that this concept is understood by nurses when the patients state that:
   1. They believe they have access to information and resources and have the opportunity to learn and grow.
   2. They have all the supports necessary to manage their own disease.
   3. They have the ability to read, understand, and act on information about their diseases.
   4. The nursing staff knew about their desires and allowed them to make their own decisions.

8. The nurse manager, using the Institute of Medicine's 10 Rules for Healthcare Delivery in the 21st Century, knows that the policies and procedures should be based on what?
   1. Education of the staff nurses
   2. Research concerning best practices
   3. Education of the nurse manager
   4. Collective years of experience of the staff nurses

9. The nurse manager has encouraged the nurses to provide patients on the unit any toiletries that are needed but to determine whether the patient needs these supplies before providing them. Which one of the Institute of Medicine's Six Aims for Health Care in the 21st Century is the nurse manager using?
   1. Efficient
   2. Equitable
   3. Patient-centered
   4. Effective

10. The nurse manager recognizes that health-care organizations have been slow to accept the principles of quality improvement for what reason?
    1. Health-care organizations had programs comparable to quality improvement.
    2. Health-care organizations did not have sufficient infrastructure.
    3. Health-care organizations do not produce a product and therefore do not require quality improvement.
    4. Health-care organizations are considered low-risk organizations and have little need of quality improvement.

Multiple Response

12. The nurse manager is working to ensure that the Institute of Medicine's 10 Rules for Health-care Delivery in the 21st Century are in place on the medical-surgical unit by using which rules? *Select all that apply.*
    1. The patient may gain information after asking permission for records.
    2. Health-care professionals are to be transparent in all activities.
    3. Waste is controlled by budget cuts and rationing of services.
    4. The patient is the source of control over their own care.
    5. Health-care professionals anticipate needs of the patient.

13. The nurse manager is responsible for designing a new pediatric oncology unit and plans to ensure that it is designed with a culture of safety. The nurse manager is aware that this culture of safety requires what necessary principles to accomplish this task? *Select all that apply.*
    1. Patient safety must be the responsibility of the unit leadership team.
    2. Work processes are to be simplified.
    3. Train all members of the nursing unit to work as a team.
    4. Redesign work processes to prevent accidents.
    5. Discourage the use of simulation and focus on actual patient care.

14. The director of nursing has decided to begin a quality improvement program, and staff members with what skills should be included on the initial committee to ensure the success of this program? *Select all that apply.*
    1. Have experience in working with interdisciplinary teams
    2. Have experience in error justification
    3. Have experience in providing efficient care
    4. Have experience in performing self-assessment
    5. Have experience in designing and testing interventions to change a care process

REFERENCES

Adams, K., & Corrigan, J. (Eds.). (2003). *Priority areas for national action: Transforming health care quality.* National Academies Press.

Advisory Commission on Consumer Protection and Quality in the Health Care Industry. (1997). *Consumer bill of rights and responsibilities: Report to the President of the United States.* U.S. Government Printing Office.

Agency for Healthcare Research and Quality. (2005). *30 safe practices for better health care* [fact sheet]. www.archive.ahrq.gov/research/findings/factsheets/errors-safety/30safe/30-safe.practice.pdf

Agency for Healthcare Research and Quality. (2008). *Becoming a high reliability organization: Operational advice for hospital leaders.* AHRQ Publication No. 08-0022. Agency for Healthcare Research and Quality.

Akpotor, M. E., & Johnson, E. A. (2018). Client empowerment: A concept analysis. *International Journal of Caring Sciences, 11*(2), 743–750. www.internationaljournalofcaringsciences.org

American Association of Colleges of Nursing. (2008). *Cultural competency in baccalaureate nursing education.* Author. www.aacn.nche.edu/leading-initiatives/education-resources/competency.pdf

American Association of Colleges of Nursing (2021). *The essentials: Core competencies for professional nursing education.* https://www.aacnnursing.org/Education-Resources/AACN-Essentials

American Nurses Association. (2010a). *Nursing's social policy statement: The essence of the profession.* Author.

American Nurses Association. (2010b). *ANA's principles for nursing documentation: Guidance for registered nurses.* Author.

American Nurses Association. (2014). Care coordination and registered nurses' essential role. www.nursingworld.org/MainMenuCategories/Policy-Advocacy/Positions-and-Resolutions/ANAPositionStatements/Position-Statements-Alphabetically/Care-Coordination-and-Registered-Nurses-Essential-Role.html

American Nurses Association. (2015a). *Code of ethics for nurses with interpretive statements.* Author.

American Nurses Association. (2015b). *Nursing: Scope and standards of practice* (3rd ed.). Author.

American Nurses Association. (2015c). *Nursing informatics: Scope and standards of practice* (2nd ed.). Author.

Barnsteiner, J. (2017). Safety. In G. Sherwood & J. Barnsteiner (Eds.), *Quality and safety in nursing: A competency approach to improving outcomes* (2nd ed.). Wiley-Blackwell.

Boston-Fleischhauer, C. (2008a). Enhancing healthcare process design with human factors engineering and reliability science, part 1. *Journal of Nursing Administration, 38*(1), 27–32.

Boston-Fleischhauer, C. (2008b). Enhancing healthcare process design with human factors engineering and reliability science, part 2. *Journal of Nursing Administration, 38*(2), 84–89.

Briner, R. B., Denyer, D., & Rousseau, D. M. (2009, November). Evidence-based management: Concept cleanup time? *Academy of Management Perspectives.* https://journals.aom.org/doi/10.5465/amp.23.4.19

Centers for Disease Control and Prevention. (2019a). *Talking points about health literacy.* https://www.cdc.gov/healthliteracy/shareinteract/TellOthers.html

Centers for Disease Control and Prevention. (2019b). *Understanding health literacy.* https://www.cdc.gov/healthliteracy/learn/Understanding.html

Chassin, M. R., & Loeb, J. M. (2011). The ongoing quality improvement journey: Next stop, high reliability. *Health Affairs, 30*(4), 559–568.

Clancy, T. R., & Warren, J. J. (2017). Informatics. In G. Sherwood & J. Barnsteiner (Eds.), *Quality and safety in nursing: A competency approach to improving outcomes* (2nd ed.). Wiley-Blackwell.

Cronenwett, L., Sherwood, G., Barnsteiner, J., Disch, J., Johnson, J., Mitchell, P., Sullivan, D. T., & Warren, J. (2007). Quality and safety education for nurses. *Nursing Outlook, 55*(3), 122–131.

DiCenso, A., Guyatt, G., & Ciliska, D. (2005). *Evidence-based nursing: A guide to clinical practice.* Elsevier Mosby.

Disch, J. (2017). Teamwork and collaboration. In G. Sherwood & J. Barnsteiner (Eds.), *Quality and safety in nursing: A competency approach to improving outcomes* (2nd ed.). Wiley-Blackwell.

Frampton, S. B., & Guastello, S. (2010). Patient-centered care: More than the sum of its parts. *American Journal of Nursing, 110*(9), 49–53.

Frampton, S., Guastello, S., Brady, C., Hale, M., Horowitz, S., Smith, S. B., & Stone, S. (2008). *Patient-centered care improvement guide.* Planetree, Inc., and Picker Institute.

Galt, K. A., & Paschal, K. A. (2011). *Foundations in patient safety for health professionals.* Jones & Bartlett.

Gerber, L. (2018). Understanding the nurse's role as a patient advocate. *Nursing2018, 48*(4), 55–58.

Greiner, A. C., & Knebel, E. (Ed.) (2003). *Health professions education: A bridge to quality.* National Academies Press.

Healthcare Information and Management Systems Society, Inc. (2020). *Initiatives: TIGER initiative for technology and health informatics education.* https://www.himss.org/what-we-do-Initiatives/tiger

Hedges, C. (2006). Research, evidence-based practice, and quality improvement. *AACN Advanced Critical Care, 17*(4), 457–459.

Institute of Medicine. (1990). *Medicare: A strategy for quality assurance: Executive summary IOM committee to design a strategy for quality review and assurance in Medicare.* National Academies Press.

Institute of Medicine. (2001). *Crossing the quality chasm: A new health system for the 21st Century.* National Academies Press.

Institute of Medicine. (2011). *The future of nursing: Leading change, advancing health.* National Academies Press.

Interprofessional Education Collaborative. (2016). *Core competencies for interprofessional collaborative practice: 2016 update.* Interprofessional Education Collaborative. https://www.ipecollaborative.org/core-competencies

James, J. T. (2013). A new, evidence-based estimate of patient harms associated with hospital care. *Journal of Patient Safety, 9*(3), 122–127.

Kanaan, S. B. (2008). Promoting effective self-management approaches to improve chronic disease care: Lessons learned. Oakland, CA: California Health Care Foundation. www.chcf.org

Kohn, L. T., Corrigan, J. M., & Donaldson, M. S. (Eds.). (2000). *To err is human: Building a safer health system.* National Academies Press.

Makary, M., & Daniel, M. (2016). Medical error—the third leading cause of death in the US. *BMJ, 353,* 1–5. doi:10.1136/bmj.i2139

McCallin, A. (2001). Interdisciplinary practice—a matter of teamwork: An integrated literature review. *Journal of Clinical Nursing, 10*(4), 419–428.

McCammon, S., & Francis, R. (2018). Moving forward with nurse-led care coordination. *American Nurse Today, 13*(5), 23.

McDonald, K. M., Sundaram, V., Bravata, D. M., Lewis, R., Lin, N., Kraft, S., McKinnon, M., Paguntalan, H., & Owens, D. K. (2007). Volume 7: Care coordination. In K. G. Shojania, K. M. McDonald, R. M. Wachter, & D. K. Owens (Eds.), *Closing the quality gap: A critical analysis of quality improvement strategies: Technical Review 9* (Prepared by the Stanford University-UCSF Evidence-based Practice Center under contract 290-02-0017). AHRQ Publication No. 04(07)-0051-7. Agency for Healthcare Research and Quality.

Melnyk, B. M., & Fineout-Overholt, E. (2019). *Evidence-based practice in nursing and healthcare: A guide to best practice* (4th ed.). Lippincott Williams & Wilkins.

National Academy of Medicine. (n.d.). *About the National Academy of Medicine.* https://nam.edu/about-the-nam/

National Academy of Sciences. (2015). *Institute of Medicine to Become National Academy of Medicine.* https://www.nationalacademies.org/onpinews/newsitem.aspx?RecordID=04282015

National Quality Forum. (2006). *NQF-endorsed definition and framework for measuring and reporting care coordination.* National Quality Forum.

Nielsen-Bohlman, L., Panzer, A. M., & Kindig, D. A. (Eds.) (2004). *Health literacy: A prescription to end confusion.* National Academies Press.

Nightingale, F. (1969). *Notes on nursing: What it is and what it is not.* Dover Publications. (Original work published 1860.)

O'Connor, S., Hubner, U., Shaw, R., Blake, R., & Ball, M. (2017). Time for TIGER to ROAR! Technology informatics guiding education. *Nurse Education Today, 58*(2017), 78–81. doi:10.1016/j.nedt.2017.07.014

Page, A. (2004). *Keeping patients safe: Transforming the work environment of nurses.* National Academies Press.

Polit, D. F., & Beck, C. T. (2017). *Essentials of nursing research: Appraising evidence for nursing practice* (10th ed.). Wolters Kluwer Health; Lippincott Williams & Wilkins.

Sakallaris, B. R., MacAllister, L., Voss, M., Smith, K., & Jonas, W. B. (2015). Optimal healing environments. *Global Advances in Health and Medicine, 4*(3), 40–45. www.gahmj.com

Salmond, S. W. (2013). Finding the evidence to support evidence-based practice. *Orthopaedic Nursing, 32*(1), 16–22. doi:10.1097/NOR.0b013e31827d960b

Schuster, P. M., & Nykolyn, L. (2010). *Communication for nurses: How to prevent harmful events and promote patient safety.* F. A. Davis.

Sewell, J. (2016). *Informatics and nursing: Opportunities and challenges* (5th ed.). Wolters Kluwer.

Sherwood, G., & Barnsteiner, J. (Eds.) (2017). *Quality and safety in nursing: A competency approach to improving outcomes* (2nd ed.). Wiley Blackwell.

Shingler-Nace, A., & Gonzalez, J. Z. (2017). EBM: A pathway to evidence-based nursing management. *Nursing2017, 47*(2), 43–46. doi:10.1097/01.NURSE.0000510744.55090.9a

Smedley, B. D., Stith, A.Y., & Nelson, A. R. (Eds.). (2002). *Unequal treatment: Confronting racial and ethnic disparities in health care.* National Academies Press.

Spence Laschinger, H. K., Gilbert, S., Smith, L. M., & Leslie, K. (2010). Toward a comprehensive theory of nurse/patient empowerment: Applying Kanter's empowerment theory to patient care. *Journal of Nursing Management, 18*(1), 4–13.

Technology Informatics Guiding Education Reform. (2009). *The TIGER initiative: Collaborating to integrate evidence and informatics into nursing practice and education: An executive summary.* http://www.aacn.nche.edu/education-resources/TIGER.pdf

The Joint Commission. (2015). *Sentinel event data: Root causes by event type 2004-2Q 2015.* www.jointcommission.org/assets/1/18/Root_Causes_Event_Type_2004-2Q_2015.pdf

Vaartio-Rajalin, H., & Leino-Kilpi, H. (2011). Nurses as patient advocates in oncology care: Activities based on literature. *Clinical Journal of Oncology Nursing, 15*(5), 526–532.

Wachter, R. M., & Gupta, K. (2018). *Understanding patient safety* (3rd ed.). McGraw Hill Medical.

Wachter, R. M., & Pronovost, P. J. (2009). Balancing "no blame" with accountability in patient safety. *New England Journal of Medicine, 361*(14), 1401–1406.

To explore learning resources for this chapter, go to FADavis.com

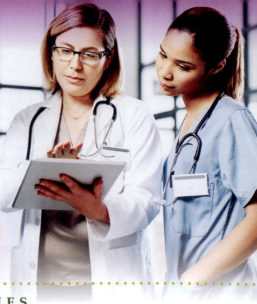

Chapter **2**

Health-Care Environment and Health Policy

Paula M. Davis-Huffman, DNP, ANP/PPCNP-BC

KEY TERMS

Affordable Care Act (ACA)
Emergency Medical Treatment and Active Labor Act (EMTALA)
Government health care
Health professional shortage area (HPSA)
Medicaid
Medicare
Medicare for All
National or universal health care
Nurses on Boards Coalition
Private health care
Public health care
Underinsured
Uninsured

LEARNING OUTCOMES

- Explore differences between private, public, and government-provided health care and insurance.
- Identify barriers experienced within the U.S. health-care system.
- Discuss the progression and future of the Patient Protection and Affordable Care Act (ACA).
- Describe the differences between Medicare and Medicaid.
- Discuss the concept of Medicare for All.
- Highlight the role of nurse leaders and managers, and nurses overall, in the area of health policy.
- Describe the importance of the Nurses on Boards Coalition.

The Knowledge, Skills, and Attitudes Related to the Following Are Addressed in This Chapter:

Core Competencies	• Patient-Centered Care • Teamwork and Collaboration • Evidence-Based Practice
The Essentials: Core Competencies for Professional Nursing Education (AACN, 2021)	**Domain 3: Population Health** • 3.4 Advance equitable population health policy (pp. 35–36). **Domain 7: Systems-Based Practice** • 7.2 Incorporate consideration of cost-effectiveness of care (pp. 46–47).
Code of Ethics with Interpretive Statements (ANA, 2015)	**Provision 7.3:** Contributions through nursing and health policy development (pp. 28–29) **Provision 8.2:** Collaboration for health, human rights, and health diplomacy (pp. 31–32) **Provision 9.4:** Social justice in nursing and health policy (pp. 36–37)
Nurse Manager (NMC) Competencies (AONL, 2015a) and Nurse Executive (NEC) Competencies (AONL, 2015b)	**NMC: Diversity (p. 6)** • Social justice • Maintain an environment of fairness and processes to support it **NEC: Communication and Relationship Building (p. 4)** • Relationship management • Build collaborative relationships • Create a trusting environment • Influencing behaviors • Facilitate consensus building • Promote decisions that are patient-centered • Community involvement **NEC: Knowledge of the Health Care Environment (p. 6)** • Health care economics and policy • Understand regulation and payment issues • Align delivery models with key economic drivers • Participate in legislative process on health care issues **NEC: Professionalism (p. 9)** • Advocacy • Represent perspective of patients and families • Advocate for optimal health care in the community
Nursing Administration Scope and Standards of Practice (ANA, 2016)	**Standard 1: Assessment** The nurse administrator collects pertinent data and information relative to the situation, issue, problem, or trend (pp. 35–36). **Standard 2: Identification of Problems, Issues, and Trends** The nurse administrator analyzes the assessment data to identify problems, issues, and trends (p. 37).

Continued

The Knowledge, Skills, and Attitudes Related to the Following Are Addressed in This Chapter:—cont'd

Standard 5B: Promotion of Health, Education, and a Safe Environment The nurse administrator establishes strategies to promote health, education, and a safe environment (p. 42).

Standard 7: Ethics The nurse administrator practices ethically (pp. 45–46).

Standard 8: Culturally Congruent Practice The nurse administrator practices in a safe manner that is congruent with cultural diversity and inclusion principles (pp. 47–48).

Standard 9: Communication The nurse administrator communicates effectively in all areas of practice (p. 49).

Standard 10: Collaboration The nurse administrator collaborates with healthcare consumers, colleagues, community leaders, and other stakeholders to advance nursing practice and healthcare transformation (p. 50).

Standard 11: Leadership The nurse administrator leads within professional practice setting, profession, healthcare industry, and society (pp. 51–52).

Standard 13: Evidence-Based Practice and Research The nurse administrator integrates evidence and research findings into practice (p. 54).

Sources: American Association of Colleges of Nursing. (2021). *The essentials: Core competencies for professional nursing education.* Author; American Nurses Association (ANA). (2015). *Code of ethics for nurses with interpretive statements.* Author; American Nurses Association (ANA). (2016). *Nursing administration: Scope and standards of practice* (2nd ed.); American Organization for Nursing Leadership (AONL). (2015a). *AONL nurse manager competencies.* Author; American Organization for Nursing Leadership (AONL). (2015b). *AONL nurse executive competencies.* Author; Cronenwett, L., Sherwood, G., Barnsteiner, J., Disch, J., Johnson, J., Mitchell, P., Sullivan, D. T., & Warren, J. (2007). Quality and safety education for nurses. *Nursing Outlook, 55*(3), 122–131; and Greiner, A. C., & Knebel, E. (Eds.) (2003). *Health professions education: A bridge to quality.* National Academies Press.

In the United States, the health-care environment is an extensive, rapidly changing, all-encompassing arena. This arena includes personal living spaces, providers' offices and clinics, hospitals, extended or skilled nursing care facilities, nursing homes and hospices, numerous service organizations related to health, private and public health systems, and a plethora of other locations and entities providing support and services. Service providers commonly include testing and ancillary services (laboratory, radiology, physical therapy, etc.), the pharmaceutical industry, medical equipment and device providers, and, more recently, expanding technology-linked health information and services, including electronic health records. According to Joy (2019), wearables, artificial intelligence, telehealth, virtual reality, and improved network performance are among new health-care trends.

Essentially, health care within the system can transpire at any time or in any location where health-care providers, or their surrogates, interact with persons needing or seeking health care or where their personal health information is gathered or accessed. As an example, wearables (activity trackers, Fitbit, Apple watch, etc.) are expanding exponentially and many devices generate an abundance of health data that could affect health care by promoting preventive health care and detailing health information; however, they could also overwhelm already stressed health-care providers (Joy, 2019).

The status of the health-care system in the United States was expected to change significantly with the passage of the Patient Protection and Affordable Care Act (2010), commonly referred to as the **Affordable Care Act (ACA)**. The number of uninsured persons was expected to decrease over time secondary to the ACA from a historic high of 44 million people being uninsured before the ACA.

The cost of health care and the quality of care provided continue to be of paramount importance to nurses, nurse leaders, and managers who are faced with the consequences of the rising costs of health care, decreasing reimbursement for health-care services, and limited resources. Equally important is that all nurses, students, bedside and community nurses, chief nursing officers, members of nursing organizations, and nursing researchers must develop leadership competencies, especially those related to health policy (Institute of Medicine [IOM], 2011). The **Nurses on Boards Coalition** (NOBC) (2018, 2020) has called for and has been working diligently toward a goal of 10,000 nurses on boards by 2020 to "increase nurses' presence and influence on corporate, health-related, and other boards, panels and commissions" (NOBC, 2018). Regardless of the fact that nurses are taught to treat all patients equally, despite their ability to pay, all nurses must understand what societal factors affect patients' health and that all nurses are called to be leaders "from the bedside to the boardroom" (IOM, 2011, p. 7).

Nurses at all levels play critical roles in advocating for health policy that impacts patients and the profession (American Association of Colleges of Nursing [AACN], (2021). Nurse leaders and managers determine policies, procedures, and resources for their staff members and facilities to provide safe quality care and ensure evidence-based interventions to assist in the control of costs and improve patient outcomes. Nurse leaders and managers must advocate for society by serving as experts in promoting and implementing health policies. Further, nurses are experts in health and should be at the table where and when policies are developed that affect the populations with which they interact.

This chapter discusses the current status of health care in the United States, the ACA, Medicare and Medicaid, health policy, and the role nurse leaders and managers play in these issues. The emerging topic of Medicare for All is also discussed.

▶ SYSTEMS WITHIN THE HEALTH-CARE ENVIRONMENT

Health care in most cases can be broken down into private and public health-care sectors. Private health-care sectors include companies, for profit and nonprofit, not associated directly with government agencies, whereas public health-care sectors are often funded by tax dollars.

Private health care is monetarily compensated health care that is provided to individuals seeking care within the health-care environment. The payment for private health care is usually predetermined and frequently negotiated with health-care providers. The cost of services can be paid directly to the provider by a monetary payment or rendered through government or commercial (private) health insurers, also known as third-party payers. Private health care is the predominant form of health care for persons residing in the United States. In 2018, employment-based health insurance covered 49% of the population, according to the Kaiser Family Foundation (KFF; 2018), a drop from 53.9% in 2013. The total percentage of people with health insurance was estimated at 86.6% in 2013 (Smith & Medalia, 2014). In 2018, the total percentage of health insurance coverage (including employer, nongroup, Medicaid, Medicare, and military coverage) had risen to 90% with 9% remaining uninsured (KFF, 2018).

The U.S. private health-care system is often referred to as "the greatest health-care system in the world" but was ranked 37th in the world, according to Murray and Frank in 2010. Life expectancy is often considered a measure of the adequacy of a health-care system's influence on its population. According to the World Health Organization (WHO, 2014), combined life expectancy in the United States was 79 years for both males and females (76 for males and 81 for females); however, it did not rank within the 10 top-ranked countries for life expectancy in either male or female categories in 2014. In 2017, life expectancy in the United States continued to rank lowest among comparable countries, with the average comparable country's life expectancy at 82.3 years whereas life expectancy in the United States was an average of 78.6 years (76.1 for men and 81.1 for women) (Organization for Economic Co-operation and Development [OECD], 2020).

Public health care, according to the Centers for Disease Control and Prevention (CDC) Foundation, "is the science of protecting and improving the health of families and communities through promotion of healthy lifestyles, research for disease and injury prevention and detection and control of infectious diseases" (CDC Foundation, 2016, para. 1). All states have public health departments that support this role and must report to U.S. government health agencies such as the CDC, which is a division of the U.S. Department of Health and Human Services (HHS). In certain states and communities, public health departments may provide primary care to indigent populations and underserved populations. Vaccination services and sexually transmitted disease clinics are frequently operated by state and county health departments. These services usually offer reduced payment options or free care for qualified individuals.

The Commissioned Corps of the U.S. Public Health Service, also a branch of the HHS, is a commissioned corps of health-care providers, including nurses, similar to the military with regard to rank and retirement. Members of this corps work in a number of public health-care arenas, including the CDC, National Institutes of Health, Indian Health Service, Food and Drug Administration, Agency for Healthcare Research and Quality (AHRQ), and many more.

Government health care in the United States is not provided directly by the government in most cases. The term actually refers to government-provided health insurance, such as Medicare and Medicaid (discussed later in this chapter), which is in most cases actually provided by the private health-care system.

The Veterans Health Administration, military hospitals, and clinics are directly funded by tax dollars and provide care directly to active duty military personnel and former service members of the armed services (Army, Navy, Marine Corps, Air Force, and Coast Guard). These are actual representations of government-provided health care within the Department of Veterans Affairs (VA) and Department of Defense (DOD) systems. Both agencies maintain numerous outpatient facilities and hospitals. The VA is primarily staffed by civilians, whereas the DOD has a considerable number of active duty military personnel staffing military clinics and hospitals in combination with civilians.

In the United States, charity care or reduced-cost care exists for persons who do not have adequate access to the private, public, or government health-care systems as a result of life circumstances (e.g., financial, geographic, lack of transportation). However, this care is very limited in scope and availability.

National or universal health care refers to health care or health insurance provided to citizens through their government, usually without the involvement of private health insurers. Currently, Australia, Canada, Taiwan, and the United Kingdom (England, Scotland, Wales, and Northern Ireland), as well as many European countries, provide this type of health care to their citizens. Although there are advocates for the implementation of a national or universal health-care insurance system in the United States, politically and culturally it is not likely to occur in the near future. In the 2020 election cycle, however, Medicare for All (discussed in more detail under Medicare) was the policy of some Democratic presidential candidates.

▶ CURRENT STATUS OF HEALTH CARE IN THE UNITED STATES

Although there have been changes to laws intended to improve the health-care system, specifically the ACA, the U.S. health-care system continues to be plagued by barriers stemming from an inability to access the system, the cost of care, and the quality of care provided (Davidson, 2013; Shi & Singh, 2019) (Fig. 2-1). In a poll conducted by Gallup, Newport (2019) reported for Gallup that "50% of Americans say they worry a great deal about the availability and affordability of health care" (Newport, 2019, para. 15).

Access to Health Care

Access to health care refers to the ability to obtain health-care services when needed (Shi & Singh, 2019). Accessibility to health care "is particularly hard to disentangle from considerations of health care quality in that it is a prerequisite to receipt of quality health care" (Docteur & Berenson, 2009, p 2). Health-care quality in the United States appears low in comparison with other countries with regard to prevention and care of chronic conditions. Access barriers experienced by the **uninsured** (those without

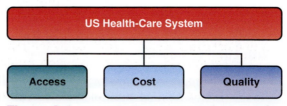

Figure 2-1 Barriers within the U.S. health-care system.

health-care insurance coverage) and the **underinsured** (those who have insurance coverage but lack adequate income to facilitate access to care because of high deductibles and co-payments) likely contribute to decreased health-care quality (Docteur & Berenson, 2009). Shi and Singh (2019) summarize this problem by stating that "access is linked to quality of care and the efficient use of needed services" (p. 509).

There are primarily two avenues through which health care can be accessed in the United States. The first is through a physician or care provider practice or clinic (usually referred to as primary care), and the other is through a hospital emergency department (ED). Provider practices and clinics are generally not required to accept patients with the inability to pay for services provided. EDs, conversely, are subject to the **Emergency Medical Treatment and Labor Act (EMTALA)**, which requires that "all Medicare participating hospitals with emergency departments provide stabilizing emergency care for all patients seeking help (including patients in labor), regardless of their insurance status or ability to pay" (La Couture, 2015, p. 1). Often this results in what is considered inappropriate use of the ED. In many cases, extended wait times and delays in transfer of patients to inpatient beds, leading to low patient satisfaction, result from this inappropriate use of the ED. Developing accurate models of ED service completion times is a critical first step in identifying barriers to patient flow and patient wait times (Ding et al., 2010).

Access to Care: Lack of Providers and Services

When viewing the U.S. health-care system from an individual perspective, three reasons can account for an inability to access the system: (1) living in an area with inadequate services, (2) lack of health insurance, and (3) cost prohibitions for those with health insurance as a result of out-of-pocket expenses (e.g., deductibles, co-payments) (Davidson, 2013) (Fig. 2-2).

Directly related to the issue of access to care is an inadequate supply of health-care providers and other health-care professionals, as well as hospitals and facilities, in certain areas. Most of these supply issues occur in rural areas (Davidson, 2013). The "availability of providers and services, coverage, benefits and affordability all come into play as potential explanations for different user experiences with the healthcare system and the outcomes attained" (Docteur & Berenson, 2009, p. 2).

Shortages of health professionals exist in all states, including urban areas. The Health Resources and Services Administration (HRSA) defines **health professional shortage areas (HPSAs)** as "areas or populations designated by HRSA as having too few primary care providers, high infant mortality, high poverty or a high elderly population" (HRSA, n.d.). Figure 2-3 shows HPSAs in primary care, which includes physicians, nurse practitioners, and physician assistants.

Access to Care: Lack of Health Insurance and Insurance With Limited Income

Before the implementation of the ACA, millions lacked health insurance even though many worked multiple jobs or full-time jobs (Jacobs & Skocpol, 2012). Millions of other individuals had health insurance but were considered underinsured. Out-of-pocket costs for the underinsured were estimated at 29.1% of total

E X P L O R I N G   T H E   E V I D E N C E   2 - 1

Morley, C., Unwin, M., Peterson, G. M., Stankovich, J., & Kinsman, L. (2018). Emergency department crowding: A systematic review of causes, consequences and solutions. *PLOS ONE, 13*(8), 1–42. https://doi.org/10.1371/journal.pone. 0203316

Aim

The aim of this systematic review was to critically analyze and summarize the findings of peer-reviewed research studies investigating the causes and consequences of, and solutions to, emergency department (ED) crowding.

Methods

A structured search of four databases (Medline, CINAHL, Embase and Web of Science) was undertaken to identify peer-reviewed research publications from 2000 to 2018 aimed at investigating the causes or consequences of, or solutions to, ED crowding. Two reviewers used validated critical appraisal tools to independently assess the quality of the studies.

Key Findings

1. Negative consequences of ED overcrowding are well established and include poorer patient outcomes and the inability to staff to adhere to guideline-recommended treatment.
2. There is a mismatch between causes and solutions.
3. The majority of the identified causes identified number and type of patients visiting the ED and timely discharge from the ED.
4. Solutions focused on efficient patient flow within the ED.
5. System-wide initiatives to meet timed patient disposition targets, as well as extended hours of primary care, demonstrated promising outcomes.
6. Increasing presentations by the elderly with complex and chronic conditions are an emerging and widespread driver of crowding.
7. More research is required to isolate precise local factors with system-wide solutions tailored to address identified causes.

Implications for Nurse Leaders and Managers

Nurse leaders and managers must also fully investigate barriers within the system that increase wait times and decrease patient flow in the ED and transfer to an inpatient bed. Considerations should include acceptable time frames for patients' discharge, staffing barriers preventing notification of housekeeping staff to prepare the room once the patient is discharged, admission timing from the ED to the inpatient bed, and adequate staffing of all personnel to facilitate these processes. Nurse leaders and managers must work to eliminate these barriers to ensure that care is safe, timely, efficient, equitable, evidence-based, and patient-centered.

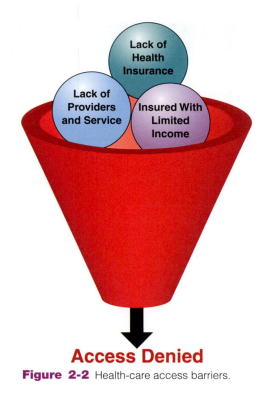

Access Denied

Figure 2-2 Health-care access barriers.

health-care costs in the United States in 2009 (Davidson, 2013). In the first half of 2014, the rate of the uninsured among adults 18 to 65 years of age decreased substantially. The ACA was credited with this decline (AHRQ, 2015). According to the KFF (2019), "the uninsured rate dropped to a historic low by 2016" and "coverage gains were particularly large among low-income adults in states that expanded Medicaid" (KFF, 2019). In 2017, the trend of decreasing numbers of uninsured had reversed and increased to 27.4 million people for the first time since the ACA was implemented (KFF, 2019). According to Witters (2019) reporting for Gallup from the *Gallup National Health and Well-Being Index* (2018), uninsured rates increased primarily for women, young adults, and lower income persons; however, all surveyed groups (age, gender, annual household incomes, and regions—except for the East) experienced a 1.3% to 4.8% increase in uninsured persons.

Individuals are often blamed for their own circumstances, including their inability to have an adequate income or to find better employment to obtain adequate health insurance. They are often stigmatized for health issues that could be managed by exercise and other lifestyle decisions (Davidson, 2013), yet the OECD found that the health-care system fell short with regard to incorporating these recommendations in primary care (OECD, 2015). Frequently, this is an example of the influence of social determinants of health that consist of patients' lifestyles and incorporate their social and physical environment. Lifestyle and environment are then modified by patients' access to public health services as well as medical and mental health care. Individual responses to these determinants interact with

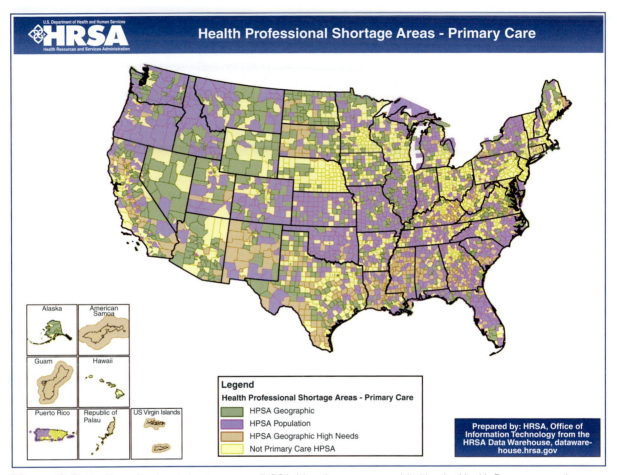

Figure 2-3 Health professional shortage areas (HPSAs) in primary care provided by the Health Resources and Services Administration data warehouse (additional interactive maps can be found at datawarehouse.hrsa.gov/topics/shortageAreas.aspx).

human biology to influence overall health status further (Arah et al., 2006). These individuals may be powerless to facilitate the changes necessary to overcome these obstacles and collectively have little support to facilitate change within the system.

Nurses at all levels must understand the implications of ineffective access to the health-care system. This may manifest as a patient who is seen in the ED, perhaps on numerous occasions, secondary to lack of insurance. This situation may translate into an inability to access more affordable care by a primary care provider. Traditionally, nurses have not concerned themselves with how a patient pays for services rendered because, in theory, care is provided to each patient in the same manner regardless of their ability to pay. Often, however, these patients are labeled as noncompliant, and caring for them in a busy ED can be stressful when more urgent needs are evident. This situation is grossly unfair to these patients and does affect how they are treated in the ED. Further, labeling and treating patients in this manner violate provision one of the American Nurses Association (ANA) *Code of Ethics for Nurses With Interpretive Statements* (2015): "The nurse practices with compassion and respect for the inherent dignity, worth, and unique attributes of every person" (p. 1). The same can be said for patients admitted to the hospital repeatedly for the same condition. Nurses should consider whether this occurs as a consequence of inadequate access or inability to afford medications or other needs for their condition.

Nurse leaders and managers set the vision for nursing practice in the delivery of safe and quality nursing care. To that end, nurse leaders and managers must have effective communication and relationship-building skills, according to the American Organization for Nursing Leadership (AONL, 2015a, 2015b). These skills would manifest in nurses' ability to influence behavior by asserting their views in a nonthreatening, nonjudgmental way and inspiring desired behaviors, while also managing undesired behaviors.

The Cost of Health Care

To understand health-care costs, it is helpful to define the included terms of cost, charge or price, and reimbursement. For instance, the term *cost* is defined by providers as "the expense incurred to deliver health-care services to patients"; to payers, the definition is "the amount they pay to providers for services rendered"; and to patients the term *cost* often means "the amount they pay out-of-pocket for health care services" (Arora et al., 2015, p. 1,046). The charge or price for health care is defined as the amount asked by a provider for health-care goods or services, which appears on a medical bill (Arora et al., 2015). Finally, reimbursement is the payment usually made by a third party to the provider of services and maybe delivered as a fee-for-service, for each day within a hospital or care facility, for each episode of hospitalization (e.g., diagnosis-related groups [DRGs]), or for each patient under the health-care provider's care (capitation) (Arora et al., 2015). Provider costs almost certainly incorporate additional expenses for personnel, equipment, and so on.

Overall cost per year for health care is another means for discussing the cost of health care, usually expressed as the amount a country spends each year on health care per person. In the year 2000, the United States was estimated to have spent $4,703 per person for health care; in 2010, that figure had increased to $8,233 per person (WHO, 2013); that figure further increased to $10,586 per person per year by 2017 (OECD, 2019). In 2018, U.S. health-care spending had increased to $11,172 per person and was reflected by the highest cost and fastest growth in the cost of health insurance ever (Centers for Medicare & Medicaid Services, 2018). According to OECD (2019), this amount of spending was higher than all other OECD countries by a considerable margin.

If one views the U.S. health-care system from the health-care provider's perspective (offices, clinics, hospitals) the revelation that "insurers do not cover provider costs" can be surmised (Davidson, 2013, p. 9). Any unpaid costs are commonly referred to as uncompensated care (Fig. 2-4). Davidson estimates that individuals without insurance pay or are billed amounts closest to actual charges, or approximately 90% of actual costs. The situation also occurs in situations where providers expect private payment or services not covered by insurance are delivered. This 90% assumes that whatever the person is billed is paid and therefore a cost far

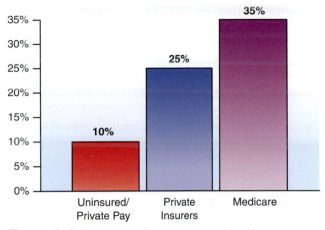

Figure 2-4 Percentage of uncompensated health-care costs. Uncompensated care is that portion of health-care expense that is not covered by insurance or other compensation. Note that the uninsured category is dependent on whether or not the private pay or uninsured person pays 90% of actual costs.

exceeding the 10% not covered may contribute to uncompensated care if the person does not have the resources to pay the provider. Those with private insurance pay approximately 65% to 75% of actual charges, depending on the insurer, and those with Medicare pay approximately 65% of actual provider costs. These expenses are covered by the persons themselves, the insurer, and the patient's out-of-pocket expenses (co-pays, deductibles, and costs not covered by the insurer). Medicaid has historically paid an even smaller percentage of actual provider costs; this applies to services at individual health-care practices as well as hospitals and other larger facilities (Davidson, 2013). Patients, regardless of which payment category they belong, are usually unaware of the actual cost of care (Shi & Singh, 2019).

Inconveniently, persons unable to access the health-care system through a provider's office or clinic often use the ED for care that could easily be provided in a primary care setting at a substantial cost reduction. This often results in excessive uncompensated costs for services that normally would cost much less if care had been provided by a primary care provider. Kaiser Health News (2019) estimates that more than $32 billion could be saved annually if patients whose medical problems were considered nonurgent were to take advantage of primary health care and not rely on EDs for their medical needs.

Inherent in the costs of these untenable situations is that inefficiency permeates the system, and individual service costs increase yearly, commonly in response to increased costs for supplies, medications, and professionals' compensation (Davidson, 2013).

The Cost of Care: Chronic Disease

Holman (2019) identified that 50% of the U.S. population has a chronic disease and that 86% of health-care expenditures can be attributed to these chronic diseases.

According to the OECD (2015), in comparing the United States with other member states, "the quality of acute care hospitals in the United States is excellent, but the U.S. health system is not performing very well in avoiding hospital admissions for people with chronic diseases" (OECD, 2015, p. 1). The OECD found that for conditions such as heart attack, stroke, and general lifesaving, the system performed well. For chronic conditions such as asthma, chronic obstructive lung disease, and diabetes, the United States fell short in areas involving patient self-care, providing effective counseling for diet, and the importance of regular exercise to moderate these chronic conditions.

In *Health at a Glance 2017: OECD Indicators* (OECD, 2017) the agency reported that obesity rates in the U.S. were the highest in the world and increasing. It reported that 38% of adults, compared with other OECD countries at 19.4%, were obese and that the United States had the second highest overall population of overweight or obese persons at 70%, exceeded only by Mexico at 72.9% of their total population. Obesity rates in the United States have increased by 65% since 2000, causing a high health and economic burden that disproportionally affects lower-educated populations.

Nurses play a central role in patient education, prevention of disease and readmission, and advancing patient self-care. In a study by Gilotra et al. (2016), the authors concluded that almost 50% of patients believed their hospitalization for heart failure was preventable and these patients were less likely to be readmitted within 30 days. Patients cited nonadherence and lack of knowledge as reasons their hospitalizations were preventable. This study demonstrates the necessity of patient education to prevent heart failure readmissions with concentration on self-care (adherence) and increased knowledge (patient education).

Cost Containment Efforts

There are numerous reasons for cost escalation within the U.S. health-care system, according to Shi and Singh (2019). Third-party payment, an imperfect market, the growth of technology, an increasing elderly population, the medical model of health-care delivery, the multipayer system, administrative costs, defensive medicine, waste and abuse, and practice variations are among many reasons for cost excesses. Increases in health-care expenditures result from unchecked price factors within these areas. The medical model of health care is based on interventions to cure sickness with less emphasis on prevention of illness (Shi & Singh, 2019). Nursing's model of health care is much different and includes a holistic vision of patients with a prevention focus concentrating on health and wellness of the overall person; however, nurses are generally not a party to cost containment efforts affecting the medical side of health care.

With the passage of the ACA, cost containment regulation intensified with regulation-based and competition-based cost containment strategies (Shi & Singh, 2019). Regulation-based strategies included supply-side controls (restrictions on expenditures—new construction, renovations and technology), price controls (reimbursement formulas, prospective payment systems, diagnosis-related groups, resource utilization groups) and utilization controls (peer-review organizations). Competition-based strategies included demand-side incentives (cost sharing—shared premium costs, deductibles, and co-payments), supply-side regulation (antitrust regulation), payer-driven competition among insurers and providers, and utilization controls, that is, managed care (Shi & Singh, 2019).

Not all cost containment regulations were successful. As an example, certificate of need (CON) statutes were state-enacted legislation requiring prior approval and demonstration of a community need before capital expenditures for additional services. In 2018, HHS encouraged state action to repeal CON laws stating that these laws restricted choice and significantly increased health-care costs (National Law Review, 2019). By May 2019, 12 states had repealed their CON requirements and 4 states had limited their CON programs.

In a more familiar example for nurses, a diagnosis-related group (DRG) is a patient classification system that standardizes prospective payments to hospitals for certain diagnoses. The use of the DRG payment system "encouraged the shift to outpatient care from traditional inpatient care, which is generally considered cost saving" (Mihailovic et al., 2016, p. 4).

Nurses at all levels must be aware of the limitations under which health-care systems operate. Labor is the largest component of total costs, with nursing being the largest of that component. In hospitals, labor correlates closely with total expenses. Hospital operating margins, the comparison of the operating budget compared with total income, vary per system, but usually operations leave less than 5% to 6% of total income available for profit (Health Leaders Media, 2015). Nurses must be cognizant of their contribution to increasing costs to the system and make a concerted effort to be good stewards of available resources in the delivery of safe and quality nursing care. Nurses should not maintain a dispassionate concern for the cost of health care, especially as the largest component of total costs within hospitals and other health-care systems.

Nurse leaders and managers are accountable for nursing expenditures, budgets, and outcomes. Skills required, according to the AONL (2015a), include financial management, human resources management, strategic planning, and information management and technology. Financial management includes management of annual operating budgets and long-term expenditures and education of patient care team members in relation to financial implications of patient care decisions. Human resources management includes the development of educational programs, workforce planning or employment decisions, corrective discipline, employee satisfaction, reward and recognition programs, promotion of healthy work environments, and compliance with legal and regulatory guidelines.

Strategic planning includes defending the business component of nursing, the analysis of market data in relation to supply and demand, and promotion of the image of nursing and the organization through effective media. Information management and technology consist of using technology to support clinical and financial improvements, collaborating to establish information technology resources, evaluation of technology in practice settings, the use of data management systems for decision making, demonstrating skills in assessing data integrity and quality, and leading the adoption and implementation of information systems (AONL, 2015a).

Quality of Care

The IOM defined *quality health care* as "the degree to which health services for individuals and populations increase the likelihood of desired health outcomes and are consistent with current professional knowledge" (Lohr, 1990, p. 128). The AHRQ states that "quality health care means doing the right thing at the right time in the right way for the right person and having the best results possible" (1998, p. 1). Quality of care typically reflects the positive effects of health care and performance of health-care systems (Docteur & Berenson, 2009).

High quality implies excellent health outcomes, and there is the assumption that "Americans with good insurance coverage uniquely benefit from prompt availability and accessibility of cutting-edge medical procedures, medicines, and devices, as well as highly educated and well-trained health-care professionals, who know and consistently do what is best for their patients" (Docteur & Berenson, 2009, p. 2).

The preparation of a National Quality Strategy (NQS) was mandated by the ACA in 2010. The NQS established three overarching aims initially that built on the Institute of Healthcare Improvement's Triple Aim® (improving the patient experience, improving the health of populations, and reducing the per capita cost of health care) with six priorities that addressed the most common health concerns in the United States. In addition, NQS designated nine propositions (measurement and feedback, public reporting, learning and technical assistance, certification, accreditation and regulation, consumer incentives and benefit designs, payment and health information technology, innovation and diffusion, and workforce development) to align business and organizational functions to drive improvement on the aims and priorities. The NQS, as a separate entity, was transitioned to the National Healthcare Quality and Disparities Report (NHQDR) in 2015 (AHRQ, 2019). The three aims of the original NQS have been incorporated into the NHQDR as "Better Care, Healthy People/Healthy Communities, and Affordable Care" (AHRQ, 2015, p. 1).

The six priorities of the NHQDR are as follows:

1. *Patient Safety:* Making care safer by reducing harm caused in the delivery of care.
2. *Person-Centered Care:* Ensuring that each person and family is engaged as partners in their care.
3. *Care Coordination:* Promoting effective communication and coordination of care.
4. *Effective Treatment:* Promoting the most effective prevention and treatment practices for the leading causes of mortality, starting with cardiovascular disease.
5. *Healthy Living:* Working with communities to promote wide use of best practices to enable healthy living.
6. *Care Affordability:* Making quality care more affordable for individuals, families, employers, and governments by developing and spreading new health-care delivery models (AHRQ, 2015, p. 2). (See Table 2-1 for status of NHQDR through 2017.)

Patient Safety

According to the WHO (2019), patient safety is a serious global public health risk with an estimated risk of patient death at 1 in 300. In comparison, the risk of dying while traveling by airplane is 1 in 3 million. James stated that "serious harm seems to be 10–20 fold more common than lethal harm" (James, 2013, p. 122). In

Table 2-1 NHQDR Priority Results Through 2017	
Priority	**Status Through 2017**
Patient Safety	13 measures improving; 7 measures without change; **1 measure worsening:** Adults who reported a home health provider asking to see all the prescription and over-the-counter medicines they are taking, when they first started getting home health care
Person-Centered Care	13 measures improving; 6 measures without change; 0 measures worsening
Care Coordination	3 measures improving; 4 measures without change; **2 measures worsening:** Home health-care patients who had an emergency department visit and then hospitalized; and home health-care patients who had an emergency department visit without hospitalization
Effective Treatment	16 measures improving; 15 measures without change; **3 measures worsening:** Emergency department visits involving opioid-related diagnoses per 100,000 population; hospital inpatient stays involving opioid-related diagnoses per 100,000 population; and suicide deaths among persons age 12 and over per 100,000 population
Healthy Living	35 measures improving; 22 measures without change; **2 measures worsening:** Women ages 21–65 who received a Pap smear in the last 3 years; and women ages 50–74 who received a mammogram in the last 2 years
Care Affordability	0 measures improving; 5 measures without change; 0 measures worsening

Note: Data from 2018 National Healthcare Quality and Disparities Report (AHRQ, 2019).

high-income countries, the WHO (2019) found that as many as 1 in 10 patients were harmed when hospitalized, with nearly 50% of these instances considered preventable, and 1 of the 10 leading causes of death and disability in the world. In addition, the WHO estimates that 4 out of every 10 patients are harmed in primary care clinics and outpatient health-care settings, where the majority of services are received.

Hospital-acquired infection (HAI) is another source of patient harm, affecting up to 10 out of every 100 hospitalized patients globally—7 per 100 in high-income countries and 10 in 100 in low- to middle-income countries (WHO, 2019). Patients with methicillin-resistant *Staphylococcus aureus* (MRSA), the most common HAI, accounts for a 64% greater likelihood of patient death compared with those patients without an HAI. Complications and death from surgery are another source of medical harm, with more than 1 million patients dying globally on an annual basis, and 7 million surgical patients suffer significant complications annually. Even though deaths related to surgical complications have decreased over the past 50 years they remain 2 to 3 times higher in low- to middle-income countries compared with high-income countries (WHO, 2019).

Unsafe medication practices, as well as medication errors (incorrect dosages or infusions, unclear instructions, use of abbreviations, and inappropriate prescriptions) harm millions and cost billions of dollars each year and are the leading cause of avoidable harm from health care (WHO, 2019). Inaccurate diagnosis is another common cause of patient harm, again affecting millions of patients. Inaccurate diagnoses occur in about 5% of adults in the United States in outpatient care settings, with 50% having the potential to cause severe harm. Diagnostic errors account for approximately 10% of patient deaths in the United States. Canada spends at least $1 out of every $7 (Canadian) treating the effects of patient harm from hospitalization (WHO, 2019), and in 2008, "medical errors cost the United States $19.5 billion" (Andel et al., 2012, p. 39).

Fatalities resulting from medical errors in the United States were estimated to be 98,000 per year by the IOM in 1999. A newer, evidenced-based estimate was provided by James (2013), with a lower estimate as high as 210,000 fatalities per year and an upper estimate of premature death from medical harm as high as 400,000 per year. In addition, James stated that "serious harm seems to be 10–20 fold more common than lethal harm" (James, 2013, p. 122). Makary and Daniel (2016) analyzed all available studies regarding fatalities from medical errors. They calculated a total of 251,454 deaths per year with the caveat that "we believe this understates the true incidence of death due to medical error because the studies cited rely on errors extractable in documented health records and include only inpatient deaths" (Makary & Daniel, 2016, p. 2). Their conclusion was that medical error is the third most common cause of death in the United States.

Investment in patient safety can lead to significant cost savings and improved patient outcomes because the cost of prevention is typically much lower than the costs associated with treatment after harm has occurred (WHO, 2019). Safety improvements in the United States have saved an estimated $28 billion for hospitals accepting Medicare between 2010 and 2015. Greater patient involvement, a key element of the NHQDR priorities (AHRQ, 2019) and the Quality and Safety Education in Nursing (QSEN) project, can be the key to safer care. The WHO states that "engaging patients is not expensive and represents a good value. If done well, it can reduce the burden of harm by up to 15%, saving billions of dollars each year—a very good return on investment" (WHO, 2019, p. 6).

Of the measures improving in the NHQDR priorities (AHRQ, 2019) patient-centered care is the only measure that showed significant improvements without worsening measures. Improvements were also seen in providers explanations to patients in offices and clinics, including using easy to understand explanations; providers spending enough time with patients; providers respecting what patients said; offices and clinics providing easy-to-understand instructions concerning patients' illnesses or health conditions; asking patients to describe how they will follow up; providers asking patients to assist with decision making when a choice exists for treatments; improvements in overall ratings of health care in offices and clinics; and decreases in the number of providers who sometimes or never listened carefully to patients. In the hospital setting, improvement were seen in communication regarding medications they received while in the hospital setting. An area without improvement in offices and clinics was health-care providers offering assistance filling out forms.

Improvements were also seen among home health-care providers in regard to explaining health care in easy-to-understand ways; informing patients what care and services they would receive when initiating home health; and the courtesy and respect that home health-care providers displayed when caring for patients in the home setting (AHRQ, 2019). Multiple areas regarding home health care had not changed since the prior year in regard to getting help or advice patients needed; consistently receiving gentle treatment in the home health setting; and listening and keeping patients informed in the home health setting. Worsening measures from NHQDR can be reviewed in Table 2-1.

Nurses at all levels need to be familiar with the safety and quality of care they provide patients and the issues associated with safe provision of quality nursing care. Knowledge deficits were noted by James (2013) to be a major contributor to individual and system deficiencies leading to medical errors and patient harm. These deficiencies can be rectified with comprehensive continuing education within all of the health professions (James, 2013).

Nurse leaders and managers may need to assist staff in acquiring adequate continuing education with a focus on evidence-based practice (EBP). EBP and the skills and methods by which it is implemented continue to face challenges for new nurses, as well as older staff members. Disler et al. (2019) identified abundant barriers in undergraduate students' nursing education, including perceptions of the lack of autonomy of nursing, perceived limited availability and utility of evidence, lack of knowledge regarding findings, and understanding the steps of EBP. One of the biggest obstacles found by the authors was the inability to critically appraise the evidence available. Nurse leaders and managers should be aware of their own knowledge of EBP as well as that of entry-level nurses and older staff members. Additional instruction in the importance of EBP and how to become involved in bringing forth policies and procedures that are evidence based should be commonplace in the work environment.

According to the AONL (2015b), clinical practice knowledge is a core competency. Leaders and managers are responsible for demonstrating "knowledge of current nursing practice and the roles of patient care team members" (AONL, 2015b, p. 6). The following are central to leadership roles: communication of patient care standards; compliance with state nurse practice acts, as well as accreditation, regulatory, and quality agency requirements; and adherence to professional standards of nursing practice. These requirements will need to be written into policies and procedures while integrating bioethical and legal requirements (AONL, 2015b).

Impact of the Coronavirus Pandemic (COVID-19)

It is premature to determine the permanent effects that COVID-19 will have on the health-care system and health policies. The total economic and human costs of the pandemic will be high. One way to reflect on the coronavirus pandemic (SARS-CoV-2) is to view it as a stress test with the understanding that the health-care system had evolved over decades with a concentration on economic efficiency (Spriggs, 2021). In addition to hospitals operating with economic efficiency, another resource that was critically underfunded at the time of the pandemic was the public health system including the CDC, local, and state health departments (Maani & Galea, 2020). According to Maani & Galea (2020), underinvestment in the public health infrastructure and underinvestment in the health of the U.S. population were critical factors. Prior to the pandemic, funding for the public health infrastructure had been cut by the federal government by as much as 40% from 1970 to 2015 with additional cuts coming from state and local governments (Maani & Galea, 2020). As the largest human resource, the nursing profession was prominently affected. In addition to the initial shortage of personal protective equipment, the human cost in terms of patient deaths was devastating to frontline staff as they cared for patients and provided emotional support when families were not permitted in hospitals or isolation areas. On top of an existing nursing shortage, the pandemic resulted in increases in daily critical staff shortages. Critical staff shortages increased stress in already stressful environments with immediate and future ramifications on the mental and physical health of nurses and other frontline workers (Maunder et al., 2006). The Guardian and Kaiser Health News (KHN) documented the ongoing number of deaths within frontline workers during the pandemic at *Lost on The Frontline*. Of the thousands of health-care workers who died from COVID-19, nurses experienced the largest at 32% (The Guardian/KHN, 2021).

▶ THE PATIENT PROTECTION AND AFFORDABLE CARE ACT

Many believed that the ACA would transform the health-care system in the United States and provide safer, higher-quality, more affordable, and more accessible care (IOM, 2011).

Enacted into law on March 23, 2010, after a lengthy political battle, the ultimate goal of the ACA was to reduce the number of uninsured persons in the United States by expanding Medicaid and implementing health-care exchanges. The health-care exchanges would allow the uninsured and other eligible persons to select health insurance coverage, which would include essential health benefits (Box 2-1) through state or federal exchanges. Many eligible persons would also receive government subsidies that would make health care affordable to those who qualified based on their income (Henry J. Kaiser Family Foundation, 2016).

Provisions included in the ACA guaranteed availability of insurance with the elimination of preexisting conditions as a means of denial for insurance. Other requirements of the ACA included the following: no annual limits on coverage; mandated coverage by employers with at least 50 full-time employees; extension of coverage to adult children to age 26 years with individual and group health policies; the inclusion of preventive services without cost sharing (if recommended by the U.S. Preventive Services Task Force); and limitation of annual cost sharing to the maximums allowed for health savings accounts ($5,950 for individual plans and $11,900 for families) (Henry J. Kaiser Family Foundation, 2016).

Lesser-known stipulations of the original ACA were annual taxes for individuals without health insurance coverage (repealed by the 2017 Tax Cuts and Jobs Act [TCJA], a 10% tax on indoor tanning services, an annual fee paid by the pharmaceutical industry ($2.8 billion in 2019 and thereafter), an excise tax of 2.3% on medical devices (repealed in 2019 by H.R. 1865), and a fee of no less than $2,000 (failure to offer coverage) to $3,750 (failure to offer coverage that is affordable) per employee for an employer not offering health insurance (Bechtold, 2018; Henry J. Kaiser Family Foundation, 2016).

BOX 2-1 Ten Essential Health Benefits Required by the Affordable Care Act	
1. Ambulatory patient services	6. Prescription drugs
2. Emergency services	7. Rehabilitative services and devices
3. Hospitalization	8. Laboratory services
4. Maternity and newborn care	9. Preventive and wellness services and chronic disease management
5. Mental health and substance use disorder services, including behavioral health treatment	10. Pediatric services, including oral and vision care

From Centers for Medicare & Medicaid Services (2011).

On June 28, 2012, the U.S. Supreme Court, in *National Federation of Independent Business v. Sebelius,* determined that the ACA was constitutional with the exception of the portion requiring states to participate in Medicaid expansion. This portion was deemed coercive because all Medicaid funds would be at risk, and states were not given adequate notice to consent voluntarily (Holahan et al., 2012). The requirement to expand Medicaid by the states was left to the discretion of each individual state after the court's ruling. In 2015, 21 states had continued to decline expansion of Medicaid secondary to the Supreme Court's ruling. In 2020, 14 states had not expanded Medicaid and 10 states were in the process of expanding Medicaid, but using an alternative to traditional expansion put in place by the Trump administration. Medicaid expansion by states can be tracked at www.nashp.org/states-stand-medicaid-expansion-decisions.

Efforts began to repeal the ACA within the Congress of the United States immediately after the 2010 midterm elections, although a Democratic-controlled Senate declined to take them up. In total, Republican-led efforts to repeal, modify, or otherwise curb the ACA since its inception had occurred 70 times through 2017 (Mattina, 2017). In December 2019 a Texas District Court judge declared the ACA unconstitutional in the *Texas v. U.S.* case. This decision was appealed and is working its way through the judicial system; however, the Supreme Court determined that it would not consider the case until after the 2020 election (Musumeci, 2020).

LEARNING ACTIVITY 2-1

How Health-Care Reform Affects Nurses

Review the ANA's information on health-care reform at www.nursingworld.org/MainMenuCategories/Policy-Advocacy/HealthSystemReform. Identify two to three ways the nursing profession is affected by health-care reform.

▶ MEDICARE AND MEDICAID

In the United States, **Medicare** and **Medicaid** are forms of government-provided health insurance, primarily for disabled persons, older persons, and economically disadvantaged persons, including children. Both programs are overseen by the Centers for Medicare and Medicaid Services (CMS), a division of HHS. To be eligible for Medicare without a disability, U.S. citizens must have worked a minimum of 10 years and paid into the Medicare Trust Fund. As of 2020, the eligibility age was 65 years, although there has been discussion about amending eligibility criteria for many years (Medicare.gov, 2020). Medicare provides health insurance for disabled persons and persons age 65 and older and consists of four components: Parts A, B, C, and D. Table 2-2 provides brief explanations of the components of Medicare, including individual costs and restrictions of coverage.

Medicaid provides health-care coverage to low-income people (primarily for children, nondisabled adults, and pregnant women) and is one of the largest payers for health care in the United States. The Children's Health Insurance Program, also known as CHIP, is the Medicaid program for children and provides federal matching funds to states who provide health-care coverage to children in families who cannot afford private insurance but have incomes too high to qualify for Medicaid. As of

Table 2-2 Costs of Medicare Components in 2020			
Component	**Basic Cost**	**Deductible**	**Coverage Type**
Part A Original Medicare	"Premium Free" for most; up to $458 per month for others (income based)	$1,408 per benefit period* • 0–60 days ($0 per benefit period) • 61–90 days ($352 per day per benefit period) • 91 or more days† ($704 per day)	Medicare Part A (hospital insurance) covers inpatient care at a hospital, skilled nursing facility (SNF), and hospice; Part A also covers services such as laboratory tests, surgery, doctor visits, and home health care
Part B	$144.60/month	$198 per year	Medicare Part B (medical insurance) covers doctor and other health-care providers' services, outpatient care, durable medical equipment, home health care, and some preventive services
Part C Medicare Advantage	Varies by plan	Varies by plan; may include monthly premium in addition to Medicare Part B premium; yearly deductible; co-pays per each visit or service	Each year, plans establish the amounts charged for premiums, deductibles, and services; the plan (rather than Medicare) decides how much is charged for covered services; the plan may change only once a year, on January 1
Part D Medications	Tiered drug plan with premiums based on income and IRS tax return	Formulary based; co-pays vary by plan/tiers and income/tax filing status	Services dependent on plan specifics; plan premium only if income less than $85,000 per year (single or married filing jointly)

*Benefit period: Day of admission to hospital or SNF until 60 days in a row when the recipient has not received inpatient hospital or SNF care; there is no limit to the number of benefit periods.
†Lifetime reserve days: Up to a maximum of 60 days per lifetime.
From Medicare.gov, 2020

May 2018, there were more than 9.46 million children enrolled in CHIP (Medicaid.gov, n.d.).

At the time the ACA became law, provisions were provided to allow greater access to Medicaid, although many states were allowed to opt out of expanding Medicaid, a key provision within the law, as a result of the Supreme Court ruling in June 2012. Although this situation denied a large percentage of the uninsured access to the system, pressure from health-care providers and pressure from health-care systems were thought likely to prevail in expanding Medicaid after initial implementation (Jacobs & Skocpol, 2012). The opposite, however, was actually the case.

In January 2020 the Trump administration unveiled a plan that would change Medicaid by allowing states to select a block grant to provide Medicaid services. In its current form states would have the option to accept a block grant, and those states that had expanded Medicaid under provisions of the ACA could opt out and continue expanded Medicaid services through the ACA. Although it is too soon to determine the actual effects of the state block grant plan, provisions could potentially include a Medicaid work requirement, increased cost-sharing provisions (co-pays and premiums), decreased access to medications, and elimination of some benefits, including covering children, covering the disabled, and eliminating long-term care for those over age 65 by allowing states, instead of CMS, to determine Medicaid benefits (Pradhan & Galewitz, 2020).

A key provision of the ACA's Medicaid expansion was the eligibility of adults without dependent children to qualify for Medicaid. Before the ACA, Medicaid eligibility was available only to low-income individuals such as children, older adults, or disabled persons. The income eligibility level for Medicaid, before the ACA, was significantly less than required by the ACA, which extended eligibility to 138% of poverty guidelines (Kaiser Commission on Medicaid and the Uninsured, 2014). The Kaiser Commission on Medicaid and the Uninsured (2014) identified another unfortunate consequence of states' not expanding Medicaid. The original law required Medicaid expansion by all states and did not anticipate the gap that would occur between those eligible for Medicaid at current state levels and those who would not be eligible for Medicaid if a state opted out of Medicaid expansion. The persons within this gap would subsequently not qualify for marketplace tax credits, even though they were not eligible for Medicaid. Those numbers equated to 5.2 million persons nationwide who would be denied access to health care through the ACA (Kaiser Commission on Medicaid and the Uninsured, 2014).

▶ MEDICARE FOR ALL

During the 2020 election cycle, several presidential candidates adopted platforms that would implement **Medicare for All** for all people living in the United States (including to immigrants and those not born in the United States), according to National Nurses United (NNU, 2019). NNU, founded in California in 2009, is the largest union and professional association of registered nurses (NNU, n.d.). The concept of Medicare for All includes five key principles: (1) universal coverage; (2) a single public program; (3) comprehensive benefits; (4) no costs at the point of service; and (5) a just transition program for workers. Item 5, a just transition program for workers, would result from the underlying need to eliminate private health insurers and their employees, making Medicare the only health insurer. Under these proposals, current Medicare would require significant changes in order to provide universal coverage. Medicare for All under Senator Bernie Sanders would be a single-payer model providing payment for all health-care services by expanding the Medicare program currently in place (with changes referenced previously).

The most significant point to the proponents of Medicare for All is likely to be the fact that a President of the United States alone cannot enact legislation to make any changes to Medicare in its current form; only the Congress of the United States can enact such legislation, consisting of the House of Representatives and the Senate. In November 2019, there were two Medicare for All legislative proposals (Senate Bill 1129 and House of Representatives Bill 1384). Unfortunately, these bills both faced strong opposition from the Trump administration and approximately 50% of Democrats had not cosigned the legislation, despite up to 67% of Americans polled supporting single-payer health care and 55% of physicians supporting single-payer health care (Cai et al., 2020).

Despite the rhetoric from proponents, opponents, and the presidential candidates themselves, it is not difficult to tabulate the cost of health care in the United States ($11,000+ per person/year) multiplied by the population, 327.2 million in

2018. It is difficult to envision that a better system could not be imagined with these amounts of money. According to Cai et al. (2020), the results of their systematic review of economic analyses found that when comparing 22 single-payer plans for the United States and individual states, 19% estimated that costs would fall in the first year and all predicted long-term cost savings. The largest savings would be seen from simplified billing and lower drug costs. The authors also noted that organizational studies across the political spectrum estimated savings for a single-payer system. The authors' conclusions found "near-consensus in these analyses that single-payer would reduce health expenditures while providing high-quality insurance to all U.S. residents" (Cai et al., 2020, p. 2).

▶ HEALTH POLICY

Health policy is developed at the local, state, national, and international levels. It can be developed by citizens' actions, local policies and proceedings (city and county), legislation at the state or federal level, or international arrangements and policies of international groups, such as the WHO. The incorporation of walking or biking paths in a locality is an example of implementation of local health policy. State health policies are developed by the local health department or through the legislative body of state government. The ACA is a legislative action or health policy conducted at the national level. Medicare for All could be adopted by state or national legislation. International health policies are often the result of foundations, such as the Bill and Melinda Gates Foundation (#1 in the nation), or individual philanthropy. Some organizations are primarily devoted to the business of health policy, such as the Robert Wood Johnson Foundation (#6 in the nation) or the Henry J. Kaiser Family Foundation (#80 in the nation). The WHO develops many policies associated with international public health.

A call has been made for nurses to be active in the formation of public health policy. As Byrd et al. found, "the importance of nurses' involvement in shaping public policy to promote population health is widely documented in nursing and public health" (2012, p. 433). In fact, the AACN established specific requirements addressing health policy through their *Essentials* documents that guide schools of nursing in developing curricula at all levels: *The Essentials of Baccalaureate Education for Professional Nursing Practice* (2008), *The Essentials of Master's Education in Nursing* (2011), and *The Essentials for Doctoral Education for Advanced Nursing Practice* (2006), as well as the recently endorsed document, *The Essentials: Core Competencies for Professional Nursing Education* (2021).

Nurses at all levels must be involved in health policy to advance health care in the United States. It is critical for all nurses to see health policy "as something they can shape rather than something that happens to them. Nurses should have a voice in health policy decision making and participate in implementation efforts" (IOM, 2011). Further, nurses, nurse leaders and managers have an ethical responsibility to be involved in health policy development and implementation by serving on committees within their practice settings and beyond. Nurse leaders and managers can contribute to health policy by serving as elected or appointed representatives in health-care activities at the local, state, national, and global levels (ANA, 2015).

E X P L O R I N G   T H E   E V I D E N C E   2 - 2

Thomas, T., Martsolf, G., & Puskar, K. (2020). How to engage nursing students in health policy: Results of a survey assessing students' competencies, experiences, interests, and values. *Policy, Politics, & Nursing Practice, 21*(1), 12–20. https://doi.org/10.1177/1527154419891129

Aim

The purpose of this study was to assess nursing students' perceptions of their competencies, previous experiences, levels of interest, and values concerning health policy (p. 12).

Methods

Between September and November 2018, the researchers conducted a cross-sectional descriptive online survey study among baccalaureate, masters, and Doctor of Nursing Practice students at a Midwestern U.S. nursing school (University of Pittsburgh School of Nursing). Participants completed a questionnaire corresponding to their nursing program based on the respective AACN Essentials (p. 13).

Key Findings

1. There was a 9% response rate with 89 students completing the survey (p. 16).
2. All students reported a moderate level of preparedness relevant to their respective AACN Essentials. Students perceived themselves as being most prepared to advocate for the nursing profession (p. 17).
3. Students were least prepared in the areas of health policy concerning reimbursement, health-care organization and finance, legislative and regulatory processes, the development and implementation of policy, and leadership in health policy that shapes health-care financing, regulation, and delivery (p. 17).
4. The most frequent responses for previous health policy experiences included voting in elections, belonging to student organizations, and regularly following nursing and health-care issues (p. 17).
5. Less than half of students indicated that they belonged to any health-related professional or advocacy organization, and less than a third of students belonged to national health-related organizations (33.7%) compared with local organizations (16.9%) or state organizations (27%). Only two students had held leadership positions within any organization (p. 18).

Implications for Nurse Leaders and Managers

Nursing students are prepared to become engaged in health policy throughout their careers. Nurse leaders and managers should foster interest among nurses to join and participate in professional organizations as well as in health policy at the local, state, and national levels.

► SUMMARY

Nurses at all levels are affected by the rapidly changing health-care environment, rising costs of care, safety and quality issues, and access to care. Nurses must be aware of the consequences of inadequate access to health care for patients. Nurse leaders and managers need to develop effective communication and relationship-building skills to be able to advocate for patients as they attempt to navigate health-care systems. All nurses must have a basic understanding of the broader context of health care and health-care policy. The ACA was intended to assist those who are uninsured or underinsured and help with controlling costs of health care, expanding access to care, addressing the Medicaid gap, and improving the safety and quality of care. Population heath is fueled by health policy. Effective nurse leaders and managers will develop competencies in financial management, human resource management, strategic management, and information management and technology. Further, nurse leaders and managers have an ethical responsibility to take an active role in developing and implementing health policy.

NCLEX®-STYLE REVIEW QUESTIONS

Multiple Choice

1. A nurse educator is discussing the implementation of the Patient Protection and Affordable Care Act and shares with the students which aspect of the law that has had a major impact on access to health insurance?
   1. Individuals may remain on a parent's health insurance until age 26
   2. Inclusion of preventive services such as mammograms
   3. Imposition of a tax on persons without health insurance
   4. Inability for health insurers to deny service due to preexisting conditions

2. The nurse is discussing health-care reimbursement with a group of student nurses. Which statement by a student nurse indicates an understanding of the reimbursement system?
   1. Individuals without insurance pay approximately 50% of the actual provider costs.
   2. Individuals with private insurance pay approximately 90% of the actual provider costs.
   3. Individuals with Medicare pay approximately 65% of actual provider costs.
   4. Individuals with Medicaid pay approximately 75% of actual provider costs.

3. The nurse is counseling a 20-year-old male who is unemployed and has no health insurance and is concerned that he may have contracted a sexually transmitted disease. What facility or agency would be the most appropriate place for the nurse to refer this patient?
   1. Emergency department of the local hospital
   2. County health department
   3. 24-hour urgent clinic
   4. Private physician's office

4. The nursing student correctly identifies which country that does not offer universal health care to its citizens?
   1. France
   2. United Kingdom
   3. United States
   4. Australia

5. The nurse manager is studying the 2018 National Healthcare Quality and Disparities report and notes that improvements have been made in all but which priority?
   1. Person-centered care
   2. Care coordination
   3. Healthy living
   4. Care affordability

6. The nurse is talking with a patient who was just admitted to an acute care health facility and just recently enrolled in Medicare Parts A, B. The patient is concerned that Medicare benefits will not cover hospitalization, and the nurse knows that which statement is true concerning this individual?
   1. The patient is not covered because Part C is necessary for hospital benefits.
   2. The patient is covered because Part A covers hospital benefits.
   3. The patient is covered because Part B covers hospital benefits.
   4. The patient is not covered because Part D is necessary for hospital benefits.

7. The nurse manager knows that more effort needs to be made to increase attention to what type of disorders to help avoid repeated hospital admissions?
   1. Childhood communicable disorders
   2. Traumatic injuries caused by sports
   3. Chronic disorders such as diabetes and chronic obstructive pulmonary disease (COPD)
   4. Dementia in the geriatric population

Multiple Response

8. A nondisabled client who will turn 65 years of age in 6 months asks the nurse about Medicare. Which statements by the nurse are true concerning Medicare eligibility? *Select all that apply.*
   1. "Individuals become eligible for Medicare at 65 years of age."
   2. "To be eligible for Medicare, an individual must have worked a minimum of 5 years."
   3. "The individual must have paid into the Medicare Trust Fund while employed."
   4. "Children who are disabled are eligible for Medicare."
   5. "Medicare is available for all persons who have low income."
9. The nurse is trying to explain the requirements of the Patient Protection and Affordable Care Act (ACA) and knows that which provisions are required of the act? *Select all that apply.*
   1. There is a $500,000 annual limit on coverage.
   2. Employers must provide health insurance if the company has more than 50 employees.
   3. Children may stay on their parent's health plans until age 26.
   4. Cost sharing is eliminated.
   5. Insurance coverage cannot be denied because of preexisting conditions.
10. A parish nurse is working with a local faith community to open a reduced-cost/free clinic for patients with limited or no insurance coverage. The nurse explains to the group that this type of health-care organization has which characteristics? *Select all that apply.*
    1. The clinic is staffed primarily by volunteers.
    2. The clinic will be able to offer many services.
    3. The clinic will need to rely on contributions or grants for funding.
    4. The clinic is subject to the EMTALA Act.
    5. The clinic can expect to be open 7 days/week.

REFERENCES

Agency for Healthcare Research and Quality. (1998). *Your guide to choosing quality health care.* www.archive.ahrq.gov/consumer/qnt

Agency for Healthcare Research and Quality. (2015). *National healthcare quality and disparities report.* AHRQ Pub. No. 15-0007. Author.

Agency for Healthcare Research and Quality. (2019). *2018 National healthcare quality and disparities report: Introduction and methods.* AHRQ Pub. No. 19-0070-EF. Author.

American Association of Colleges of Nursing (AACN). (2006). *The essentials for doctoral education for advanced nursing practice.* Author.

American Association of Colleges of Nursing (AACN). (2008). *The essentials of baccalaureate education for professional nursing practice.* Author.

American Association of Colleges of Nursing (AACN). (2011). *The essentials of master's education in nursing.* Author.

American Association of Colleges of Nursing. (2021). *The essentials: Core competencies for professional nursing education.* Author. https://www.aacnnursing.org/Portals/42/AcademicNursing/pdf/Essentials-2021.pdf

American Nurses Association. (2015). *Code of ethics for nurses with interpretive statements.* Author.

American Nurses Association (ANA). (2016). *Nursing administration: Scope and standards of practice* (2nd ed.). Author.

American Organization for Nursing Leadership (AONL). (2015a). *AONL nurse manager competencies.* Author.

American Organization for Nursing Leadership (AONL). (2015b). *AONL nurse executive competencies.* Author.

Andel, C., Davidow, S. L., Hollander, M., & Moreno, D. A. (2012). The economics of health care quality and medical errors. *Journal of Health Care Finance, 39*(1), 39–50.

Arah, O. A., Westert, G. P., Hurst, J., & Klazinga, N. S. (2006). A conceptual framework for the OECD Health Care Quality Indicators Project. *International Journal for Quality in Health Care, 18*(Suppl. 1), 5–13.

Arora, V., Moriates, C., & Shah, N. (2015). The challenge of understanding health care costs and charges. *American Medical Association Journal of Ethics, 17*(11), 1046–1052.

Bechtold, A. (2018). *ACA watch 2018 (employer limits and penalties).* https://www.onedigital.com/blog/aca-limits-fees-and-penalties-2019/

Byrd, M. E., Costello, J., Gremel, K., Schwager, J., Blanchette, L., & Malloy, T. E. (2012). Political astuteness of baccalaureate nursing students following an active learning experience in health policy. *Public Health Nursing, 29*(5), 433–443. http://doi.org/10.1111/j.1525-1446.2012.01032.x

Cai, C., Runte, J., Ostrer, I., Berry, K., Ponce, N., Rodriguez, M., Bertozzi, S., White, J. S., & Kahn, J. G. (2020). Projected costs of single-payer healthcare financing in the United States: A systematic review of economic analyses. *PLOS Medicine, 17*(1): e1003013. http://doi.org/10.1371/journal.pmed.1003013

CDC Foundation. (2016). *What is public health?* www.cdcfoundation.org/content/what-public-health

Centers for Medicare & Medicaid Services. (2011). *Essential health benefits bulletin: Center for consumer information and insurance oversight.* https://www.cms.gov/CCIIO/Resources/Files/Downloads/essential_health_benefits_bulletin.pdf

Centers for Medicare & Medicaid Services. (2018). *National health expenditures 2018 highlights.* https://www.cms.gov/files/document/highlights.pdf

Cronenwett, L., Sherwood, G., Barnsteiner, J., Disch, J., Johnson, J., Mitchell, P., Sullivan, D. T., & Warren, J. (2007). Quality and safety education for nurses. *Nursing Outlook, 55*(3), 122–131.

Davidson, S. M. (2013). *A new era in U.S. health care: Critical next steps under the Affordable Care Act.* Oxford University Press.

Ding, R., McCarthy, M., Desmond, J. S., Lee, J. S., Aronsky, D., & Zeger, S. L. (2010). Characterizing waiting room time, treatment time, and boarding time in the emergency department using quantile regression. *Academic Emergency Medicine, 17*(8), 813–823.

Disler, R. T., White, H., Franklin, N., Armari, E., & Jackson, D. (2019). Reframing evidence-based practice curricula to facilitate engagement in nursing students. *Nurse Education in Practice, 41*(8), 102650.

Docteur, E., & Berenson, R. A. (2009, August). *How does the quality of U.S. health care compare internationally? Timely analysis of immediate health policy issues.* Robert Wood Johnson Foundation Urban Institute. https://www.rwjf.org/en/library/research/2009/08/how-does-the-quality-of-u-s--health-care-compare-internationally.html

Gilotra, N., Shpigel, A., Okwuosa, I. S., Tamrat, R., Flowers, D., & Russell, S. D. (2016). Patients commonly believe their heart failure hospitalizations are preventable and identify worsening heart failure, nonadherence, and a knowledge gap as reasons for admission. *Journal of Cardiac Failure, 23*(3), 252–256. http://dx.doi.org/10.1016/j.cardfail.2016.09.024

Greiner, A. C., & Knebel, E. (Ed.) (2003). *Health professions education: A bridge to quality.* National Academies Press.

Health Leaders Media. (2015.). *Factfile: Drivers of operating margin.* http://www.healthleadersmedia.com/internal/drivers-operating-margin

Health Resources and Services Administration. (n.d.). *MUA find.* datawarehouse.hrsa.gov/tools/analyzers/muafind.aspx

Henry J. Kaiser Family Foundation. (2016). *Health reform implementation timeline.* www.kff.org/interactive/implementation-timeline

Holahan, J., Buettgens, M., Carroll, C., & Dorn, S. (2012). *The cost and coverage implications of the ACA Medicaid expansion: National and state-by-state analysis, executive summary.*

Holman, H. R. (2019). The relation of the chronic disease epidemic to the health care crisis (commentary). *ACR Open Rheumatology, 0*(0), 1–7. http://doi.org/10.1002/acr2./11114

Institute of Medicine. (2011). *The future of nursing: Leading change, advancing health.* National Academies Press.

Jacobs, L. R., & Skocpol, T. (2012). *Health care reform and American politics: What everyone needs to know.* Oxford University Press.

James, J. T. (2013). A new, evidence-based estimate of patient harms associated with hospital care. *Journal of Patient Safety, 9*(3),122–128. http://doi.org/10.1097/PTS.0b013e3182948a69

Joy, K. (2019). 5 healthcare tech trends to watch in 2020. https://healthtechmagazine.net/article/2019/12/5-healthcare-tech-trends-watch-2020

Kaiser Commission on Medicaid and the Uninsured. (2014). *The coverage gap: Uninsured poor adults in states that do not expand Medicaid.* Henry J. Kaiser Foundation.

Kaiser Family Foundation. (2018). *Health insurance coverage of the total population.* Henry J. Kaiser Foundation.

Kaiser Family Foundation. (2019). *The uninsured and the ACA: A primer - Key facts about health insurance and the uninsured amidst changes to the Affordable Care Act.* https://www.kff.org/report-section/the-uninsured-and-the-aca-a-primer-key-facts-about-health-insurance-and-the-uninsured-amidst-changes-to-the-affordable-care-act-how-many-people-are-uninsured

Kaiser Health News (2019). *The cost of unwarranted ER visits: $32 billion a year.* https://khn.org/morning-breakout/the-cost-of-unwarranted-er-visits-32-billion-a-year/

La Couture, B. (2015). *The Emergency Medical Treatment and Active Labor Act (EMTALA) and its effects.* American Action Forum.

Lohr, K. N. (ed.) (1990). *Medicare: A strategy for quality assurance, volume II: Sources and methods.* National Academies Press.

Maani, N., & Galea, S. (2020). COVID-19 and underinvestment in the public health infrastructure of the United States. *The Millbank Quarterly, 98.* https://www.milbank.org/quarterly/articles/covid-19-and-underinvestment-in-the-public-health-infrastructure-of-the-united-states/#_ednref11

Makary, M., & Daniel, M. (2016). Medical error—the third leading cause of death in the US. *BMJ, 353,* 1–5. doi:10.1136/bmj.i2139

Mattina, C. (2017). *Infographic: A brief history of ACA repeal and replace efforts.* https://www.ajmc.com/newsroom/infographic-a-brief-history-of-aca-repeal-and-replace-efforts

Maunder, R. G., et al. (2006). Long-term psychological and occupational effects of providing hospital healthcare during SARS outbreak. Emerging infectious diseases, 12(12), 1924 -1932. https://doi.org/10.3201/eid1212.060584

Medicaid.gov. (n.d.). *Children's health insurance program.* https://www.medicaid.gov/sites/default/files/2019-12/fy-2018-childrens-enrollment-report.pdf

Medicare.gov. (2020). *2020 Medicare costs.* https://www.medicare.gov/pubs/pdf/11579-medicare-costs.pdf

Mihailovic, N., Kocic, J., & Jakovljevic, M. .(2016). Review of diagnosis-related group-based financing of hospital care. *Health Services Research and Managerial Epidemiology, 16*(3), 1–8. https://doi.org/10.1177_2333392816647892

Murray, C. J., & Frank, J. (2010). Ranking 37th: Measuring the performance of the U.S. health care system. *New England Journal of Medicine, 362*(2), 98–99.

Musumeci, M. (2020). *Explaining* Texas v. U.S.: *A guide to the case challenging the ACA.* http://files.kff.org/attachment/Issue-Brief-Explaining-Texas-v-US-A-Guide-to-the-Case-Challenging-the-ACA

National Law Review. (2019, July 1). *Florida repeals significant portions of certificate of need law.* https://www.natlawreview.com/article/florida-repeals-significant-portions-certificate-of-need-law

National Nurses United. (n.d.). *About National Nurses United.* https://www.nationalnursesunited.org/about

National Nurses United. (2019). *Medicare for all.* https://www.nationalnursesunited.org/medicare-for-all

Newport, F. (2019). *Americans' mixed views of healthcare and healthcare reform.* Gallup: Polling Matters. https://news.gallup.com/opinion/polling-matters/257711/americans-mixed-views-healthcare-healthcare-reform.aspx

Nurses on Boards Coalition. (2018). *Infographic: To improve the health of communities and the nation through the service of nurses on boards and other bodies.* https://www.nursesonboardscoalition.org/wp-content/uploads/NOBC_Infographic_123118.pdf

Nurses on Boards Coalition. (2020). *Infographic: 2020 year in review.* https://documentcloud.adobe.com/link/track?uri=urn:aaid:scds:US:2bca840a-26d4-4e48-ad0d-ad7fe5f5745e#pageNum=1

Organization for Economic Co-operation and Development. (2015). *Health at a glance 2015: How does the United States compare?* Organization for Economic Co-operation and Development.

Organization for Economic Co-operation and Development. (2017). *Health at a glance 2017: OECD indicators. How does the U.S. compare?* Author. https://www.oecd.org/unitedstates/Health-at-a-Glance-2017-Key-Findings-UNITED-STATES.pdf

Organization for Economic Co-operation and Development. (2019). *Health at a glance 2019: OECD indicators.* OECD Publishing. https//doi.org/10.1787/4dd50c09-en

Organization for Economic Co-operation and Development. (2020). *Life expectancy at birth (indicator).* https://doi.org/10.1787/27e0fc9d-en

Pradhan, R., & Galewitz, P. (2020). *5 things to know about Trump's Medicaid block grant plan.* https://khn.org/news/5-things-to-know-about-trumps-medicaid-block-grant-plan/

Shi, L., & Singh, D. A. (2019). *Delivering health care in America: A systems approach* (7th ed.). Jones & Bartlett Learning.

Smith, J. C., & Medalia, C. (2014). *Health insurance coverage in the United States: 2013.* U.S. Department of Commerce, Economics, and Statistics Administration, U.S. Census Bureau. www.census.gov/content/dam/Census/library/publications/2014/demo/p60-250.pdf

Spriggs, W. E. (2021). Post-pandemic: Economics. *Issues in Science and Technology: Arizona State University, 1*(21), 38-41. https://issues.org/postpandemic-economics/

The Guardian & Kaiser Health News. (2021). Lost on the frontline: Thousands of U.S. healthcare workers have died fighting Covid-19. https://www.theguardian.com/us-news/ng-interactive/2020/aug/11/lost-on-the-frontline-covid-19-coronavirus-us-healthcare-workers-deaths-database

Witters, D. (2019). *U.S. uninsured rate rises to four-year high.* https://news.gallup.com/poll/246134/uninsured-rate-rises-four-year-high.aspx

World Health Organization. (2013). *World health statistics: 2013: Indicator compendium.* World Health Organization. www.who.int/gho/publications/world_health_statistics/WHS2013_IndicatorCompendium.pdf

World Health Organization. (2014). *World health statistics: 2014.* Author. apps.who.int/iris/bitstream/10665/112738/1/9789240692671_eng.pdf

World Health Organization. (2019). *Patient safety fact file.* Author. https://www.who.int/features/factfiles/patient_safety/patient-safety-fact-file.pdf?ua=1

 To explore learning resources for this chapter, go to FADavis.com

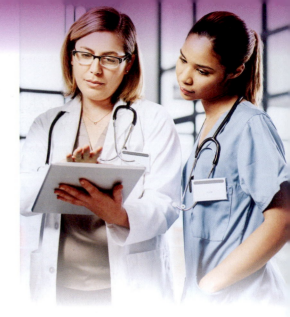

Chapter 3

Theories and Principles of Nursing Leadership and Management

Lynne Portnoy, MSN, RN, CNE

KEY TERMS

Authentic leadership
Behavioral theories
Complexity leadership
Connective leadership
Emotional intelligence
Followership
Mentorship
Quantum leadership
Self-awareness
Servant leadership
Transactional leadership
Transformational leadership

LEARNING OUTCOMES

- Examine the historical development of leadership and management theories.
- Describe contemporary leadership and management theories.
- Describe primary characteristics of leaders and managers.
- Examine the value of self-awareness and emotional intelligence in leadership.
- Determine how leaders can identify different types of followers.
- Explain how leaders and managers can be effective mentors.

The Knowledge, Skills, and Attitudes Related to the Following Are Addressed in This Chapter:	
Core Competencies	• Patient-Centered Care • Teamwork and Collaboration
The Essentials: Core Competencies for Professional Nursing Education (AACN, 2021)	**Domain 9: Professionalism** • 9.5 Demonstrate the professional identity of nursing (pp. 54–55). **Domain 10: Personal, Professional, and Leadership Development** • 10.3 Develop capacity for leadership (pp. 57–58).
Code of Ethics with Interpretive Statements (ANA, 2015a)	**Provision 1.5:** Relationships with colleagues and others (p. 4) **Provision 2.3:** Collaboration (p. 6)
Nurse Manager (NMC) Competencies (AONL, 2015a) and Nurse Executive (NEC) Competencies (AONL, 2015b)	**NMC: All Competencies (pp. 4–7)** **NEC: All Competencies (pp. 4–11)**
Nursing Administration Scope and Standards of Practice (ANA, 2016)	**All Standards of Practice (pp. 35–44)** **All Standards of Professional Performance (pp. 45–59)**

Sources: American Association of Colleges of Nursing. (2021). *The essentials: Core competencies for professional nursing education.* Author; American Nurses Association (ANA). (2015a). *Code of ethics for nurses with interpretive statements.* Author; American Nurses Association (ANA). (2016). *Nursing administration: Scope and standards of practice* (2nd ed.). Author; American Organization for Nursing Leadership (AONL). (2015a). *AONL nurse manager competencies.* Author; American Organization for Nursing Leadership (AONL). (2015b). *AONL nurse executive competencies.* Author; Cronenwett, L., Sherwood, G., Barnsteiner, J., Disch, J., Johnson, J., Mitchell, P., Sullivan, D. T., & Warren, J. (2007). Quality and safety education for nurses. *Nursing Outlook, 55*(3), 122–131; and Greiner, A. C., & Knebel, E. (Eds.) (2003). *Health professions education: A bridge to quality.* National Academies Press.

Because nurses embody the largest number of professionals in health care, they are most often the closest to the patient and therefore offer a unique perspective of the entire system of care surrounding the patient. This places nurses in a prime position to be leaders. The Institute of Medicine (IOM) report *The Future of Nursing: Leading Change, Advancing Health* (2011) contended that strong nursing leadership is critical to addressing the demands of the increasingly complex health-care system. Further, "the nursing profession must produce leaders throughout the health care system, from the bedside to the boardroom, who can serve as full partners with other health professionals and be accountable for their own contributions to delivering high-quality care while working collaboratively with leaders from other health professions" (IOM, 2011, p. 221).

To navigate the evolving health-care landscape, all nurses must recognize and embrace their leadership responsibilities and understand nursing leadership competencies. All nurses, regardless of their positions, must develop leadership skills with an emphasis on effective decision making, initiating and maintaining effective working relationships, using respectful communication, collaborating on interprofessional and intraprofessional teams, coordinating care effectively, and developing delegation skills and conflict resolution strategies (American Association of Colleges of Nursing [AACN], 2008).

Additionally, all nurses are managers in some way. They may be in a formal management position or managers at the bedside. Nurses in formal management positions are typically in a hierarchical position with subordinates. In this role, they focus on the following: order, consistency, and planning; organizing and budgeting; establishing and enforcing rules; and taking corrective action. The responsibilities of managers at the bedside include the following: managing care transitions; actively participating on interprofessional and intraprofessional teams; identifying system issues; and developing working skills in delegation, prioritization, and overseeing patient care (AACN, 2008, p. 35).

Leadership and management, in fact, are not interchangeable. In the best scenario, a manager is a true and effective leader; however, an excellent leader may not have any management responsibilities within an organization. Although there are many similarities between leadership and management—both involve the direction and influence of others, and both entail the accomplishing of tasks and goals of an organization—there are significant differences. Leadership is a process of influencing others through effective relationship skills, whereas management is a formal position with specific functions. Ideally, a nurse can be both a leader and a manager simultaneously.

This chapter is designed to assist in preparing nurses to perform as leaders by providing information on historical perspectives, current leadership theories, characteristics of leaders, and followership. In addition, leadership and management competencies, mentoring, and self-awareness will be discussed.

▶ HISTORICAL DEVELOPMENT OF LEADERSHIP AND MANAGEMENT

Management and leadership in nursing were first discussed by Florence Nightingale in her *First Formal Letter to the Nurses* (1872). In this letter she stated, "A person in charge must be felt more than she is heard—not heard more than she is felt" and "A person... in charge must have a quieter and more impartial mind than those under her, in order to influence them by the best part of them and not by the worst" (Nightingale, 1872, p. 13). More recently, many of these traits have been named self-awareness, moral leadership, and authenticity (Goleman, 1998; Grossman & Valiga, 2020). Since the mid-20th century and beyond, the profession of nursing has adapted the management and leadership styles popular in business, psychology, sociology, and anthropology (Clark & Clark, 1999). Management theories were developed as a means to enhance productivity in business with leadership theories growing from the science of management. One clear definition follows: "Leadership is an activity or set of activities, observable to others, that occurs in a group, organization or institution and which involves a leader and followers who willingly subscribe to common purposes and work together to achieve them" (Clark & Clark, 1999, p. 25). According to Bennis and Nanus (2004, as cited in Grossman & Valiga, 2020) more than 850 definitions are available. Historical perspectives on leadership and management are still relevant today because modern theories of leadership incorporate some of the ideas first introduced almost a century ago.

Trait Theories

One early leadership theory from the 19th century was "The Great Man Theory," focused on the traits of a leader and noting that certain men were born leaders (Raelin, 2015). The focus of leadership research during this time involved the study of popularly identified great leaders. The goal was to identify what traits these individuals possessed, with the aim of being able to identify new potential leaders more quickly.

Behavioral Theories

The next phase in the development of leadership theories (1940 to 1960) concentrated on the identification of styles of leadership. The emphasis of study was on what leaders *did*, rather than on innate traits, and these theories were also known as **behavioral theories** (Raelin, 2015). These theories centered on how leaders and managers conducted themselves. Primary leadership styles were identified as autocratic (authoritarian), democratic (participative), and laissez-faire (Lewin, 1951). Table 3-1 notes characteristics associated with these primary leadership and management styles.

Table 3-1	Primary Styles of Leadership and Management
Style	**Characteristics**
Autocratic	• Makes decisions without input from the team
	• Does not consider valuable suggestions from team members' input
	• Potentially demoralizes team members
Democratic	• Expects team members to contribute to the decision-making process
	• Encourages team input
	• Enables individual growth and development
	• Analyzes and makes final decisions
	• Increases participation in projects and creative solutions
	• Brings about higher production and satisfaction
Laissez-faire	• Provides advice, support, and timelines with low-level involvement
	• Lacks focus or time management, resulting in high job satisfaction with risk of low productivity
	• Risks the potential of team members not having the knowledge to execute the tasks
	• May find intrateam disagreements common, which may produce disharmony

Situational and Contingency Leadership Theories

From 1950 to 1970, building on behavioral theories, researchers began to identify new contributing factors to leadership theories. One idea that evolved at this time was that situational factors contributed to the leadership style one embraced. This approach considers that a leader may be effective in certain situations and less effective in others. Another model, contingency leadership, holds that the leader's style is flexible to the needs of an organization at a particular point in time and relates to their followers and the tasks to be completed (Fiedler, 1967).

▶ CONTEMPORARY THEORIES OF LEADERSHIP

There are numerous contemporary leadership theories that grew from examining the multiple factors that contribute to successful leadership. Many modern theories continue to include concepts developed in earlier research but have expanded to include a multidimensional approach. In the late 20th century, leadership theorists started to notice that for leaders to be effective, the values and beliefs of the environment needed to be considered. Change cannot occur simply by a talented leader's imposing it; rather, relationships within the organization need to be cultivated to promote a productive and healthy environment. This marked a significant shift in leadership theories from those based on industrial models to theories that are more relationship focused. This progression is noteworthy for nursing because it incorporates the multifaceted nature of health-care organizations. Nurses find themselves being called to leadership in ever-changing, complex environments where there are multiple stakeholders, increasing pressures of cost containment, and pay-for-performance initiatives. In the past, leadership theories were broken down into two types: relational and attribution. Currently, leadership theories have become multifactorial.

Relational Leadership Theories

Relational leadership theories focus primarily on the relationship that occurs between the leader and the team member. There is less emphasis on a leader's traits, the situation or context, or the end result and more emphasis on the leader's relations with others. Relational theories such as quantum, transactional, transformational, complexity, and connective share the objective of optimizing the rapport among team members and building effective resilient teams.

Quantum Leadership

Quantum leadership involves the premise of an increasingly complex, dynamically changing health-care environment. Quantum leadership draws some of its basic tenets from quantum theory in physics: The transition has begun in moving from views that are orderly and linear to those that are holistic and relational (Porter-O'Grady, 1999, p. 38). Traditionally, leaders have looked at work activities from the basic perspective of identifying tasks, jobs to be completed, and roles to be performed. The quantum leader looks at the system, the processes, and the relationships between workers and tasks to determine efficiency and job performance. The unpredictability of a world dominated by chaos mandates models of leadership that incorporate flexibility and adaptability. Nurses as leaders today are faced with ever-increasing complexity in both job duties and technological advances. Quantum leadership offers nursing a framework within which to develop leadership skills to assist in advancing the goals of their organizations.

Transactional Leadership

Transactional leadership is one of the most common styles of leadership in health-care organizations. The transactional leader focuses on the goals of the organization, with a directive style establishing expectations for team members and motivating with rewards. With this type of leadership, both the leader and the team member gain something from the interactions, although theirs is not necessarily a shared vision. The leader is focused on getting the job done, and the team member is motivated by the reward earned. This approach limits innovation and the ability for team members to truly engage in the outcomes of their work. Given the focus of task completion, the concrete rewards that followers receive are more generally limited to a sense of a job well done (Burke et al., 2006).

Transformational Leadership

As health care has evolved and increased in complexity, it has become necessary for leadership models to address identified aims of quality improvement, particularly in keeping with the recommended aims of the IOM: the provision of safe, effective, patient-centered, timely, efficient, and equitable care (IOM, 2001). One leadership theory that fits well with these aims is transformational leadership.

Transformational leadership involves an active involvement of both the leader and team members. It is a process in which leaders and team members "motivate each other to attain and achieve levels of success" (O'Neill, 2013, p. 179). There is a unified investment in achieving the goals of the organization with shared values. A transformational leader guides staff in creating an environment in which all members contribute to meeting the mission of the organization. The leader provides a vision that has included the input of all members, thus encouraging members to reach their highest potential and often exceed expectations. Transformational leaders transform organizations. In the process, all nurses at all levels of the organization are involved in decision making. Transformational leaders are able to help followers grow by responding to needs, empowering individuals, and aligning goals and objectives across all levels in an organization (ANA, 2013).

Transformational leaders are comfortable with challenging themselves, learn from their failures, and consistently demonstrate effectiveness in organizational change and innovation (O'Neill, 2013). Transformational leadership is viewed as an effective type of leadership for nurses to lead the change necessary to meet the demands of the current health-care system. This type of leadership has been identified as one of the five components of the Magnet Recognition Program, discussed in Chapter 7.

Connective Leadership

Although transformational leadership attends to the creation of relationships by consensus building, resolving conflict, and establishing common goals, another popular theory focuses on caring. **Connective leadership** incorporates the needs of diverse stakeholders within the health-care environment through acknowledgment and use of the strengths of members and by including them in the leadership process (Lipman-Blumen, 1992). Nurse leaders and managers must consider not only *whom* they are guiding but *where* they may be leading them. Today's healthcare environment demands a seamless continuity of care across multiple settings. Connective leaders identify and foster the strengths of team members by including them in the processes of change within the organization (Klakovich, 1996). A successful connective leader can develop future leaders who begin contributing early in their career, well before undertaking a formal nursing leadership position.

Complexity Leadership

Complexity leadership has been defined by Uhl-Bien, Marion, and McKelvey as "a leadership paradigm that focuses on enabling the learning, creative and adaptive capacity of complex adaptive systems within a context of knowledge-producing organizations" (Uhl-Bien et al., 2007, p. 298). Hospitals are indeed knowledge producing and can be complicated and complex organizations to navigate. Crowell (2020) describes a complex leader as one who is "in the midst of the action, cultivating relationships, accepting feedback, tolerating uncertain situations, seeking diverse opinions, listening to multiple views, and as much as possible remaining calm and centered" (p. 5). The framework for this theory is rooted in the premise that the technological era is vastly different from the industrial age. In order to be flexible and creative, three types of leadership occurs within the framework: adaptive leadership, enabling leadership, and administrative leadership (Uhl-Bien et al., 2007). This leadership theory may be most effective in the fast-paced world that hospitals have become, with patients more acutely ill and their care more technical than ever before. Complexity leadership has been described as a dynamic, emergent, and interactive process when applied to nurse management (Henriksen, 2016). Rather than depending on an authoritative approach, this type of leadership allows for adaptation and learning within social systems. Complexity leadership allows the nurse manager to focus on alignment of objectives, resources, strategies, and conflicts (Henriksen, 2016). In addition, nurse managers using this style create conditions that foster invention, encourage flexibility, and increase the sharing of expertise.

Nurse leaders must possess special characteristics to supervise others in complex environments. The following characteristics provide the foundation for complexity leadership: expert, visionary, mentor, achiever, communicator, and critical thinker.

Attribution Leadership Theories

Attribution leadership theories encompass many similarities with relational theories and share the historical perspective of trait theories, by considering the characteristics or attributes of the leader as the cornerstone within leadership relationships. In contrast to trait theories, attribution theories also take into consideration either the context or the interrelational aspects. Nurse leaders are neither born nor practicing within a vacuum. Attribution leadership theories used in nursing are authentic leadership and servant leadership.

Authentic Leadership

Leaders engaged in **authentic leadership** hold firmly to their values, beliefs, and principles and inspire their followers. The determination and courage of the authentic leader in difficult and challenging times create an environment that is predictable, efficient, and steadfast. In addition, the integrity of the leader is evidenced by a strong commitment to truth telling, thereby decreasing ambiguity in the system and increasing efficiency and productivity (Shirey, 2006). When a leader's integrity is at a high point, a healthier work environment is achievable. According to Gardner et al. (2005), "A key factor contributing to the development of authentic leadership is the self-awareness or personal insight of the leader… by reflecting through introspection, authentic leaders gain clarity and concordance with respect to their core values, identity, emotions, motives and goals" (p. 245).

The health-care environment can present challenges from multiple conflicting stakeholders with competing agendas, and these challenges require fortitude and steadfastness from leaders. For example, financial pressures may be placed on nurse leaders and managers to adjust nursing care to fit within specific parameters that are not in keeping with their own value system, and the recommendations of national organizations (e.g., being asked to change nurse/patient ratios to unacceptable levels). Authentic leaders will be challenged to hold steady to their beliefs and values, and do so with the knowledge that they are upholding the tenets of the nursing profession.

The authentic leader must embrace self-awareness and self-regulation to enhance moral leadership (Waite et al., 2014, p. 283). In moral leadership, the core ethical principles of nursing are held in highest regard. Authentic leaders, while holding these principles in mind, "develop heart and compassion by getting to know the life stories of those with whom they work and by engaging co-workers in shared meaning" (Shirey, 2006, p. 261). The five distinguishing characteristics of authentic leaders are purpose, heart, self-discipline, relationships, and values (p. 260).

Servant Leadership

Beginning in the 1970s, **servant leadership** emerged as a new concept. Robert Greenleaf (1977) introduced the "nature of legitimate power and greatness" as being the ability to lead, not from any innate ability, but by the desire to serve others. Greenleaf's work has been subsequently studied and refined to 10 key factors: (1) the empowerment and promotion of people, (2) authenticity, (3) humility, (4) accepting people for who they are, (5) providing direction, (6) healing, (7) listening, (8) awareness, (9) being a conscientious custodian of resources, and (10) building community (Grossman & Valiga, 2020). The servant leadership style fits well within the nursing profession as these factors are necessary to promote the personal responsibility that is integral to the profession. "The leader needs two intellectual abilities that are usually not formally assessed in an academic way; (s)he needs to have a sense for the unknowable and be able to foresee the unforeseeable" (Greenleaf, 1977, p. 21). This ability of foreseeing what may occur with patients is indeed a cornerstone of what nurses do on a daily basis, through assessment, nursing diagnosis, and creating care plans. Nursing is about service to others as a primary intent (ANA, 2015a). Nurse managers must be able to support these skills and empathize with both colleagues and patients in our care.

Serving as a way to lead others is a humanistic approach. Greenleaf (1977) argues that having an optimistic view of employees and believing that they will respond in a positive manner to servant leadership will create a best self in employees. Servant leadership motivates others to react positively to leaders who demonstrate servant leadership traits. According to Fields et al.(2015), servant leadership creates a reassuring and kind workplace. In addition, the ethical conduct displayed by servant leaders creates a climate of trust and acceptance even when errors are made. This conduct is congruent with the ANA *Code of Ethics for Nurses With Interpretive Statements* (ANA, 2015a). This contributes to a healthy work environment and inspires joy in work and fidelity to the workplace.

▶ EMERGING LEADERSHIP THEORIES

The newest and latest developments in nursing leadership and management involve aspects such as "strategic agility" (Shirey, 2015) and "system leadership" (Senge et al., 2015). Although the health-care industry is constantly undergoing change and being required to adapt, it is the nurse leader and manager's responsibility to ensure safety and quality. Nurse leaders and managers must "incorporate strategic agility to be bold and mindful" (Shirey, 2015, p. 305). In contrast to the singular focus on the leader's responsibility, there is the case for system leaders to "develop in order to foster collective leadership" (Senge et al., 2015), to provide a broader perspective to solve larger problems. The current development of leadership theories is moving toward a more comprehensive view, incorporating flexibility and adding broader perspectives. In fact, according to Porter-O'Grady and Malloch (2018), "the success of the leader is more closely linked to personal authenticity, self-awareness, and genuineness than to a particular leadership style… it is the leader's authenticity not the leadership style that really matters" (p. 322).

▶ PROFESSIONAL COMPETENCE IN NURSING LEADERSHIP

According to the ANA (2015a), the public has a right to expect all nurses to demonstrate competence throughout their careers. Nurses are individually accountable for attaining and maintaining professional competence. Nurses need to develop leadership competencies that "emphasize ethical and critical decision-making, initiating and maintaining effective working relationships, using mutually respectful communication and collaboration within interprofessional teams, care coordination, delegation, and developing conflict resolution strategies" (AACN, 2008, p. 13). The ANA (2015b) believes that competence in nursing practice can be defined, measured, and evaluated. Further, ANA (2013) believes competence in nursing leadership can also be defined and measured.

No one document or organization encompasses all required competencies for nursing leadership and management. However, many share the same themes (ANA, 2016). In *Nursing: Scope and Standards of Practice* (2015b), the ANA identifies leadership as a standard of professional performance for all nurses, stating that "the registered nurse leads within the professional practice setting and the profession" (p. 75). The registered nurse:

- Contributes to the establishment of an environment that supports and maintains respect, trust, and dignity.
- Encourages innovation in practice and role performance to attain personal and professional plans, goals, and vision.
- Communicates to manage change and address conflict.
- Mentors colleagues for the advancement of nursing practice and the profession to enhance safe, quality health care.
- Retains accountability for delegated nursing care.
- Contributes to the evolution of the profession through participation in professional organizations.
- Influences policy to promote health.

The ANA developed the Leadership Institute for all nurses with career goals of excelling in their role, refining leadership knowledge, skills, and attitudes, and enhancing leadership impact (ANA, 2013). The Leadership Institute identified specific leadership competencies that transcend those developed by other nursing organizations and identify leadership competencies across the course of professional development (ANA, 2013, p. 5). The competencies are organized by three domains: Leading Yourself, Leading Others, and Leading the Organization.

▶ LEADERSHIP CHARACTERISTICS

It is no longer a prevailing belief that leaders are born. Leaders must constantly learn new skills and competencies. Although certain innate qualities can make a person a better leader, leaders today cannot rely on natural instincts alone to lead successfully. Common characteristics exhibited by successful leaders are illustrated in Box 3-1.

BOX 3-1 Common Characteristics of Successful Leaders		
Action-oriented	Emotionally intelligent	Resilient
Ambitious	Fair-minded	Self-aware
Broadminded	Forward-looking	Self-confident
Caring	Goal-oriented	Self-controlled
Competent	Honest	Self-directed
Compassionate	Imaginative	Self-regulating
Cooperative	Independent	Sociable
Courageous	Inspiring	Straightforward
Creative	(Have) Integrity	Supportive
Decisive	Intelligent	Visionary
Dependable	Loyal	
Determined	Mature	

⚙ **American Organization for Nursing Leadership Nurse Leader Competencies**

The American Organization for Nursing Leadership (AONL) (previously known as the American Organization for Nurse Executives [AONE]), a subsidiary of the American Hospital Association, was established in 1967 to "promote nursing leadership excellence and shape public policy for health care nationwide" (AONL, 2019). The AONL mission—"to shape the future of health care through innovative and expert nursing leadership" (AONL, 2019)—applies to all nurses, whether the nurse functions in a frontline nurse position or as a nurse executive. The AONL has stood as a guiding light for nursing leadership in the health-care field and has functioned as an advocate through research, education, and professional development. The AONL is committed to developing and disseminating leadership competencies for nurses at all levels of responsibility and in a variety of settings.

Nurse Executive

The AONL (2015b) competencies for nurse executives outline the knowledge, skills, and attitudes current and aspiring nurse leaders and managers can use to guide practice, identify areas for growth, and plan for future careers. The nurse executive is "influential in improving the patient experience of care (including quality and satisfaction), improving the health of populations and reducing the per capita cost of health care" (p. 3). The core competencies for leadership are organized according to five distinct domains: (1) communication and relationship-building, (2) knowledge of the health-care environment, (3) leadership, (4) professionalism, and (5) business skills (AONL, 2015b). Each domain is broken down into specific knowledge and skills that nurse leaders and managers need to develop to achieve this competency.

Nurse Manager

The AONL (2015a) competencies for nurse managers outline the knowledge, skills, and attitudes nurse leaders and managers with responsibility for direct care units. Nurse leaders and managers at this level provide the vital link between the administration and the point of care. They need to create safe and healthy environments that support the work of the health care team and promote optimal patient outcomes. The core competencies are organized according to the Nurse Manager Learning Domain Framework: The Science: Managing the Business; The Leader Within: Creating the Leader in Yourself; and The Art: Leading the People.

Five core characteristics common to the basis of leadership are character, commitment, connectedness, compassion, and confidence (Kowalski & Yoder-Wise, 2004). A person's character is anchored in their values, based on standards established over time. A leader with character incorporates moral accountability while never losing sight of human dignity, humility, and caring. Character forms the backbone of a leader.

As an aspect of leadership, commitment encompasses a leader's ability to make a promise, keep it, and carry through with the promise. Commitment is measured by how well a leader can be trusted to keep their word. Both character and commitment can really be gauged only within the context of connected relationships, or connectedness. The strength of the connections a leader makes lies in respect and authenticity and will determine the effectiveness of their leadership.

Compassion is a hallmark of nursing and an essential aspect of leadership. Some nurse leaders and managers are able to recognize the individual strengths and weaknesses of team members and coordinate the most effect use of their skill set. Confidence, the sense of self-assurance without arrogance, provides nurse leaders and managers with an ability to lead through difficult times.

Self-awareness, the ability to self-reflect on one's beliefs and biases and adapt behavior accordingly, is another important characteristic of leaders. Nurse leaders and managers should perform a self-assessment of their leadership and management qualities and then have colleagues rate these same qualities. This information can provide valuable insight. According to Vitello-Cicciu (2019), the goal is "to ensure that the environment supports open discourse, has room for conflict and resolution, and is a safe environment for speaking up even when it differs from the leaders' position. It is about ensuring dialogue" (p. 202). Self-assessment is often measured through emotional intelligence testing.

Emotional intelligence itself is considered by many to be a significant characteristic of effective nurse leaders and managers. **Emotional intelligence** can be conceptualized generally as self-awareness and other awareness in terms of emotions, feelings, and points of view (Momeni, 2009). Nursing involves highly emotional interactions, whether in relation to providing care to patients or working with fellow nurses and other professionals in the health-care environment. As nurses develop leadership skills, conducting a critical consideration of emotional intelligence is useful. Self-awareness, empathy, and compassion are the cornerstones of nursing. Nurse managers and leaders capable of handling their own emotions in tense or volatile situations display emotionally intelligent leadership. Emotional intelligence includes five components: (1) self-awareness, (2) self-regulation, (3) motivation, (4) empathy, and (5) social skills (Goleman, 1998).

Emotional intelligence develops as a person ages and can be enhanced through educational activities. Individuals with high emotional intelligence are typically successful and emotionally healthy (O'Neill, 2013). Emotional intelligence is believed by many to be more important than intelligence quotient (IQ) and other personality or learned skills (Goleman, 1998; O'Neill, 2013). Many organizations perform an emotional intelligence survey of their employees who demonstrate leadership ability. One example is a 360-degree survey in which an individual is assessed based on ratings from direct reports and supervisors, as well as their own ratings (Goleman, 1998).

Nurse leaders and managers must realize that they are in charge and accountable and that their leadership style and behavior affect the overall performance of their team. A nurse leader and manager who perceives their leadership abilities in the highest regard predictably has the lowest perception of effectiveness by others. The most self-aware, successful leaders develop techniques not only to understand their own emotional intelligence but also to seek a way to solicit open and honest critique of their leadership performance. Nurse leaders and managers who have an accurate understanding of their own capabilities will have a team that can provide better results. Emotionally intelligent nurse leaders have an impact on staff, peers, patient satisfaction, and organizational success.

Further discoveries about self-awareness in leadership have been made specifically with regard to gender differences that occur in the personal rating of self-awareness and knowledge of self (Van Velson et al., 1993). Beliefs about gender differences in leadership were traditionally rooted in the stereotypical gender differences in values: women have generally been noted to value affiliation, acceptance, and dependence, whereas men have been seen as valuing competition, power, and independence. Historically, leadership theories were rooted in masculine value structures (Grossman & Valiga, 2020). Despite how much society has tried to move to gender neutrality in the workplace, it cannot be denied that there is a gender bias. As a predominantly female profession, nursing now includes more men. The numbers of men entering nursing leadership roles will continue to increase, and this change will affect how leaders are viewed. Fortunately, current leadership theories embrace both feminine and masculine values, which should lead to more successful models of leadership.

LEARNING ACTIVITY 3-1

Leadership Self-Assessment

Visit https://hbr.org/2015/06/quiz-yourself-do-you-lead-with-emotional-intelligence self-assessment.

1. Take the self-assessment for emotional intelligence.
2. Did your results surprise you?
3. Discuss with your group or your class.

▶ FOLLOWERSHIP

An integral part of leadership is the concept of **followership**. Where would a leader be without followers? An unsavvy leader may possibly view their followers as an identical, like-minded group of individuals who will blindly and without criticism execute the leader's objectives (Frisina, 2005); followers then become seen as a mindless herd. A Freudian approach to followership focused on the dysfunctional (disruptive) follower (e.g., impulsive, compulsive, masochistic, or withdrawn subordinate) (Zaleznik, 1965). In contrast, an exemplary follower has the right to decide whether they follow the leader (Kelley, 1992).

Several leadership theories previously discussed address the relationship between leaders and followers (team members), but with the conceptual lens that the leader bears the responsibility for the relationship. One study presented the concept that leadership is a co-construction of the leader and followers, and researchers found that "leaders are sometimes followers, and *vice versa*, suggesting that following and leading are interdependent activities to be found in both groups: leaders and followers" (Kean et al., 2011, p. 515). Following can fall into the categories of "doing following," "standing by," or "resisting following" (Kean et al., 2011, p. 515). In essence, those in the "doing following" group represent positive role models and potentially could be groomed for leadership. The "standing by" group member is someone who is participating in the group but responds best with detailed guidance. The "resisting following" group member would appear to bring negative energy to the group dynamic. It is this last team member who potentially distracts from the performance of the team. A leader with the ability to assess types of followers could either provide opportunities of improvement for their team members or provide consequences for their actions, when appropriate.

There has been much discussion of what it takes to be a good or even a great leader, but what makes a good follower? Just as the commonly held belief claims

Tyczkowski, B., Vandenhouten, C., Reilly, J., Bansal, G., Kubsch, S., & Jakkola, R. (2015). Emotional intelligence (EI) and nursing leadership styles among nurse managers. *Nursing Administration Quarterly, 59*(2), 172–180.

Aim

The aim of this study is to determine the level of relationship between emotional intelligence (EI) and leadership style among nurse managers.

Methods

A descriptive, exploratory study was conducted using a convenience sample of nurse managers from six Midwestern health systems. Standardized leadership and EI questionnaires were administered.

Key Findings

A significant relationship was found between EI and a transformational leadership style, as well as outcomes of leadership such as extra effort, effectiveness, and satisfaction. There was no significant relationship between the EI characteristics of decision making, interpersonal relations, or happiness and specific leadership styles.

Implications for Nurse Leaders and Managers

Health-care institutions strive for excellence in the provision of care, with leadership being a key component in reaching that goal. Acknowledging the relationship between EI and leadership style allows nursing executive management to facilitate the leadership potential of nurses earlier in their career by fostering the development of EI. An additional implication of this study is the important finding of a lack of relationship between the EI area of decision making and leadership style. Nurse leaders and managers are faced with critical decision-making tasks on a daily basis. More current leadership theories focused on the implications of relationships within health-care systems may shed light on this area of emotional intelligence.

that good leadership can improve quality and safety, it is becoming clear that good followership also affects quality and safety (Whitlock, 2013). Followers are not passive participants who go along for the ride. It is also imperative that a follower does not undermine the goals of a leader. This can create not only a hostile work environment but also an unsafe one. As with leaders, there is more known now about what constitutes a good follower. A good follower is a member of the team who contributes to the success of the organization. As with leadership skills, followership skills can be learned and developed. The good follower can interpret the overt and subtle objectives and adjust their work behavior to provide the best results for the organization's improvement of quality and safety.

Followers can also be broken down into four types: (1) effective or exemplary, (2) alienated, (3) conformist, and (4) passive (Kelley, 1992, p. 97). Along with these general characteristics, the behavioral attributes of passiveness versus activeness and independent critical thinking versus dependent uncritical thinking tie into types of followers. For example, the effective or exemplary follower is an active participant who functions independently while using critical thinking, and a passive follower shows passiveness and is a dependent, uncritical thinker.

No matter the type of follower, it is important to recognize the significant role that the follower plays within the organization or team. Nurses, as part of the health-care team, must take their position very seriously, whether it is as primary leader or primary follower within a given time and circumstance. A good leader recognizes opportunities to adjust roles from leader to follower fluidly and has an understanding that followership enhances team functioning. Box 3-2 provides a list of characteristics that make a good follower.

Leaders must always remember that followers wield tremendous influence in an organization. Effective followers engage in healthy dialogue with leaders, whereas ineffective followers dialogue in a manner that can result in unsafe or unhealthy situations, thus resulting in organizational chaos. A nurse leader and manager can use an effective follower to better the team. For example, a savvy leader or manager will pair a new hire with a preceptor who is a part of the "doing following" group. This ensures that the new team member will be exposed to proper policies and procedures and encourages a positive, rapid start.

▶ MENTORSHIP

Across all industries, mentoring and apprenticeships have always been primary tools of training. **Mentorship** in nursing developed over time from the traditional apprenticeship-style approach to a less formal process in which two people engage in a relationship designed to support the growth and development of the less experienced party. As nurse leaders and managers grow and mature, mentoring relationships will change. An understanding of the roles of mentor and mentee are important in leadership. A leader may at any time be both a mentor to less experienced nurses and a mentee in a relationship to foster his or her own growth and development.

Nurse leaders and managers are charged with mentoring "colleagues for the advancement of nursing practice, the profession, and quality health care" (ANA, 2016, p. 52). In the role of mentor, a nurse leader and manager focuses on the exchange of information to assist the mentee in advancing clinical competencies, research skills, or leadership abilities, depending on the predetermined needs

---

BOX 3-2   Characteristics of a Good Follower

- Able to receive and give feedback
- Courageous
- Creative
- Critical thinker/knowledgeable
- Dependable
- Ethical
- Flexible
- Humble
- Lifelong learner
- Responsible
- Risk-taker
- Thoughtful
- Understands they are an essential part of a team
- Visionary

E X P L O R I N G   T H E   E V I D E N C E   3 - 2

Kean, S., Haycock-Stuart, E., Baggaley, S., & Carson, M. (2011). Followers and the co-construction of leadership. *Journal of Nursing Management, 19,* 507–516.

Aim

The aim of this study was to discover the perceptions of leadership by community nurses, as well as gain an understanding of the impact of policy changes in leadership development.

Methods

This study used a qualitative research design consisting of individual interviews and focus groups. Interview questions focused on describing leadership for nurses, the impact and outcomes of leadership, and how community nurses are supported in developing effective leadership. In all, 39 subjects were recruited and reflected a broad demographic of urban, rural, and mixed communities.

Findings

A major theme found was that the act of following is involved in the process of leadership. A leader can move in and out of the follower role, depending on the situation. A leader's participation may vary over time and can include "standing by," "doing following," or "resisting following." Leadership and followership are two intertwined concepts that are key to successful management. Encouraging strong followership is an important component of leadership competencies.

Implications for Nurse Leaders and Managers

A major consideration for nurse leaders and nurse managers is the achievement of goals established within their work environment. Inspirational leaders have the ability to facilitate the creation of strong followers who will take the action steps that lead to success. Nurse leaders and managers who have the ability to recognize the process of developing followership skills can have a positive impact on leadership and its resulting success.

established within the mentoring relationship (McCloughen et al., 2009). A mentee seeking to advance in leadership must embrace open-minded dialogues with other nurse leaders and managers. It is within these relationships that a mentee can experience the inside view of an organization and develop a more in-depth understanding of system functioning.

Nursing as a profession benefits from mentoring relationships by ensuring continued growth of future nursing leaders as well as ensuring continuity of highly skilled workers. Because the nursing workforce is aging, it is imperative that more experienced leaders pass on their knowledge and skills. Nurse leaders and managers are often in positions to function as mentors and can teach mentees the finer arts of nursing, such as interprofessional collaboration and teamwork. Mentoring brings benefits of increased job satisfaction, higher nurse retention, and professional advancement (Barker et al., 2006). When nurse leaders are supported in mentoring new nurses to create healthy work environments, some of the burden of supervision of new nurses is lifted from the manager.

► SUMMARY

All nurses are leaders and managers regardless of practice setting. Leaders are neither strictly born nor created. Research into leadership and management theories, both historical and contemporary, offers many clues to the successful characteristics of effective nurse leaders and managers. Health care today is constantly evolving and requires nurses to embrace leadership roles to ensure high-quality care. Nurse leaders and managers will be challenged to stay abreast of the constantly evolving health-care system while simultaneously increasing patient and staff satisfaction and quality care. Knowledge of leadership theories offers a perspective and guide for leading and managing, and in particular, transformational leadership has been identified as an effective style to meet today's ever-changing health-care system. Although many leadership styles and theories have been discussed in this chapter, nurse leaders and managers must develop the key leadership characteristics of self-awareness and emotional intelligence to lead and manage today.

NCLEX®-STYLE REVIEW QUESTIONS

Multiple Choice

1. The nurse leader is working with a team to develop a more effective admission assessment process. Which team member is an example of one who participates in the team by "standing by"?
   1. A team member who often works with team members who are new to the team and helps to mentor them in their role
   2. A team member who appears to function against the goals set up by the team leader
   3. A team member who is flexible and ready to make any needed changes
   4. A team member who requires detailed instructions concerning the leader's expectations
2. The nurse leader believes that a mentorship program for new nursing graduates would benefit the organization in what way?
   1. New nurses will require no supervision after the mentorship program is completed.
   2. Mentorship leads to new nurses remaining with the organization longer than those nurses who did not engage in a mentorship program.
   3. The nurse who completes the mentorship program will understand better how to care for patients without assistance.
   4. Engaging in a mentorship program helps that individual to work longer hours without fatigue.

3. A nurse is aspiring to move from a staff nurse's position to a leadership and management role. What activity would be most helpful to this nurse in achievement of this goal?
   1. Complete a leadership survey.
   2. Enroll in a graduate leadership program.
   3. Read a leadership book.
   4. Request a change in position weekly from the charge nurse.

4. A new chief operating executive believes that patients will receive better care and be more satisfied in a unit that is specific to their disorder. A nurse manager heads a unit that has functioned for the last 10 years as a general medical-surgical unit but will now become a specialty unit for patients with chronic respiratory issues. What is the nurse manager's priority responsibility during this transition?
   1. Assist the staff to feel more comfortable in their new roles.
   2. Ensure that the patients receive safe care by qualified staff.
   3. Survey the patients daily to determine whether needs are being met.
   4. Hold briefings daily with the staff to determine common problem areas.

5. A staff nurse approached the director of nursing to discuss steps that would be helpful in moving to an administrative position. The director of nursing told the staff nurse not to consider leadership because this nurse was not a "born leader." What leadership theory is the director of nursing using to make this judgment?
   1. Behavioral theory
   2. Situational leadership theory
   3. Contingency leadership theory
   4. Great Man theory

6. A new nurse leader has adopted a laissez-faire style of leadership that may result in what characteristics of those who report to this leader?
   1. Team members may be very good at time management but poor on job satisfaction.
   2. The staff may be very knowledgeable but have a lack of focus on the job at hand.
   3. Team members experience disagreements among themselves.
   4. Productivity is high with low job satisfaction.

7. The nurse student is aware that what feature is now a part of the newest nursing leadership theories?
   1. Self-discipline
   2. Flexibility
   3. Motivation
   4. Visionary

8. The nurse manager is aware that what aspect of leadership relates to the ability to make a promise, keep it, and carry through on that promise?
   1. Compassion
   2. Confidence
   3. Connectedness
   4. Commitment

9. The nurse manager is evaluating several nurses who have expressed an interest in leadership activities and knows that the nurse who demonstrates which type of followership has the most potential for a leadership role?
   1. Standing by
   2. Doing following
   3. Resisting following
   4. Passive follower

10. A nurse seeking to advance to a leadership position within the health-care organization has become the mentee of a nurse manager. What is the primary responsibility of the mentee in this relationship?
    1. Follow the mentor in all activities.
    2. Work to dialogue with other nurse leaders and managers.
    3. Request a monthly meeting with the mentor to discuss leadership attainment.
    4. Ask the mentor to place the mentee in a minor leadership position.

11. A nursing student is required to take a nursing leadership course and questions why this type of course is necessary when the initial primary role of the graduate nurse is to perform bedside patient care. What is the nurse educator's best response to this student?
    1. "It is a part of the curriculum that is required by all state boards of nursing."
    2. "Though new graduates begin at the bedside, most take on leadership positions within the first 6 months of employment."
    3. "Leadership competencies are required even at the bedside to help in navigating the evolving health-care landscape."
    4. "All nurses report to someone, so you have to understand leadership so you know who you report to."

Multiple Response

12. A nurse who is endeavoring to increase emotional intelligence knows that what are the core components necessary to the development of this leadership characteristic? *Select all that apply.*
    1. Empathy
    2. Motivation
    3. Intellectual skills
    4. Leadership
    5. Self-awareness

13. A nurse manager has begun to use transformational leadership theory and knows that this theory uses what aims of the Institute of Medicine (IOM)? *Select all that apply.*
    1. Nurse-centered
    2. Efficient
    3. Timely
    4. Safe
    5. Inexpensive

REFERENCES

American Association of Colleges of Nursing (AACN). (2008). *The essentials of baccalaureate education for professional nursing practice.* Author.

American Association of Colleges of Nursing. (2021). *The essentials: Core competencies for professional nursing education.* Author. https://www.aacnnursing.org/Portals/42/AcademicNursing/pdf/Essentials-2021.pdf

American Nurses Association (ANA). (2013). *ANA Leadership Institute: Competency model.* https://learn.ana-nursingknowledge.org/template/ana/publications_pdf/leadershipInstitute_competency_model_brochure.pdf

American Nurses Association (ANA). (2015a). *Code of ethics for nurses with interpretive statements.* Author.

American Nurses Association (ANA). (2015b). *Nursing: Scope and standards of practice* (3rd ed.). Author.

American Nurses Association (ANA). (2016). *Nursing administration: Scope and standards of practice* (2nd ed.). Author.

American Organization for Nursing Leadership (AONL). (2015a). *AONL nurse manager competencies.* Author.

American Organization for Nursing Leadership (AONL). (2015b). *AONL nurse executive competencies.* Author.

American Organization for Nursing Leadership (AONL). (2019). *About American Organization for Nursing Leadership.* https://www.aonl.org/about/overview

Barker, A. M., Sullivan, D. T., & Emery, M. J. (2006). *Leadership competencies for clinical managers: The renaissance of transformational leadership.* Jones & Bartlett Learning.

Burke, C. S., Stagl, K. C., Klein, C., Goodwin, G. F., Salas, E., & Halpin, S. (2006). What type of leadership behaviors are functional in teams? A meta-analysis. *Leadership Quarterly, 17*(3), 288–307.

Clark, K. E., & Clark, M. B. (1999). *Choosing to lead* (2nd ed.). Center for Creative Leadership.

Cronenwett, L., Sherwood, G., Barnsteiner, J., Disch, J., Johnson, J., Mitchell, P., Sullivan, D. T., & Warren, J. (2007). Quality and safety education for nurses. *Nursing Outlook, 55*(3), 122–131.

Crowell, D. M. (2020). *Complexity leadership: Nursing's role in health-care delivery* (3rd ed.). F. A. Davis.

Fiedler, F. (1967). *A theory of leadership effectiveness.* McGraw-Hill.

Fields, J. W., Thompson, K. C., & Hawkins, J. R. (2015). Servant leadership: Teaching the helping professional. *Journal of Leadership Education* (Special Ed.), 92–103. doi:10.12806/V14/I4/R2

Frisina, M. E. (2005). Learn to lead by following. *Nursing Management, 36*(3), 12.

Gardner, W. L., Avolio, B. J., Luthans, F., May, D. R., & Walumbwa, F. (2005). "Can you see the real me?" A self-based model of authentic leader and follower development. *Leadership Quarterly, 16,* 343–372. doi:10.1016/j.leaqua.2005.03.003

Goleman, D. (1998). *Working with emotional intelligence.* Bantam Books.

Greenleaf, R. K. (1977). *Servant-leadership: A journey into the nature of legitimate power and greatness* (pp. 1–59). Paulist Press.

Greiner, A. C., & Knebel, E. (Ed.) (2003). *Health professions education: A bridge to quality.* National Academies Press.

Grossman, S. C., & Valiga, T. M. (2020). *The new leadership challenge: Creating the future of nursing* (6th ed.). F. A. Davis.

Henriksen, J. (2016). An alternative approach to nurse manager leadership. *Nursing Management, 47*(1), 53–55. doi.10.1097/01.NUMA0000475636,82881.75

Institute of Medicine. (2001). *Crossing the quality chasm: A new health system for the 21st century.* National Academies Press.

Institute of Medicine. (2011). *The future of nursing: Leading change, advancing health.* National Academies Press.

Kean, S., Haycock-Stuart, E., Baggaley, S., & Carson, M. (2011). Followers and the co-construction of leadership. *Journal of Nursing Management, 19*(4), 507–516.

Kelley, R. (1992). *The power of followership.* Bantam Doubleday.

Klakovich, M. D. (1996). Registered nurse empowerment: Model testing and implications for nurse administrators. *Journal of Nursing Administration, 26*(5), 29–35.

Kowalski, K., & Yoder-Wise, P. (2004). Five C's of leadership. *Nursing Leadership, 17*(1), 3645.

Lewin, K. (1951). *Field theory in social science: Selected theoretical papers.* Harper & Row.

Lipman-Blumen, J. (1992). Connective leadership: Female leadership styles in the 21st century work-place. *Sociology Perspectives, 25*(1), 183–203.

McCloughen, A., O'Brien, L., & Jackson, D. (2009). Esteemed connection: Creating a mentoring relationship for nurse leadership. *Nursing Inquiry, 16*(4), 326–336.

Momeni, N. (2009). The relation between managers' emotional intelligence and the organizational climate they create. *Public Personnel Management, 38*(2), 35–48.

Nightingale, F. (1872). *Florence Nightingale to her nurses* (p. 13). McMillan & Co. https://books.google.com/books?hl=en&lr=&id=pqw-AAAAYAAJ&oi=fnd&pg=PR5&dq=Florence+Nightingale+First+letter+to+the+nurses+1872&ots=8gVQrnMA9R&sig=Iv9mU_S36ipdnHmj56aul_iaa9U#v=onepage&q=Florence%20Nightingale%20First%20letter%20to%20the%20nurses%201872&f=false

O'Neill, J. A. (2013). Advancing the nursing profession begins with leadership. *Journal of Nursing Administration, 43*(4), 179–181.

Porter-O'Grady, T. (1999). Quantum leadership: New roles for a new age. *Journal of Nursing Administration, 29*(10), 37–42.

Porter-O'Grady, T., & Malloch, K. (2018). *Quantum leadership: Creating sustainable value in healthcare* (5th ed.). Jones & Bartlett.

Raelin, J. A. (2015). Rethinking leadership. *MIT Sloan Management Review, 56*(4), 96.

Senge, P., Hamilton, H., & Kania, J. (2015). The dawn of system leadership. *Stanford Social Innovation Review.* www.ssireview.org/articles/entry/the_dawn_of_system_leadership

Shirey, M. R. (2006). Authentic leaders creating healthy work environments for nursing practice. *American Journal of Critical Care, 15*(3), 256–267.

Shirey, M. R. (2015). Strategic agility for nursing leadership. *Journal of Nursing Administration, 45*(6), 305–308.

Tyczkowski, B., Vandenhouten, C., Reilly, J., Bansal, G., Kubsch, S. M., & Jakkola, R. (2015). Emotional intelligence (EI) and nursing leadership styles among nurse managers. *Nursing Administration Quarterly, 59*(2), 172–180.

Uhl-Bien, M., Marion, R., & McKelvey, B. (2007). Complexity leadership theory: Shifting leadership from the industrial age to the knowledge era. *Leadership Quarterly, 18*, 298–318.

Van Velson, E. V., Taylor, S., & Leslie, J. B. (1993). An examination of the relationship among self perception accuracy, self-awareness, gender, and leader effectiveness. *Human Resource Management, 32*(2–3), 249–263.

Vitello-Cicciu, J. M. (2019). Am I an authentic nursing leader for healthy workplace environments? *Journal of Management and Nursing Leadership, 17*(3), 201–203. http://dx.doi.org/10.1016/j.mnl.2019.03.011

Waite, R., McKinney, N., Smith-Glasgow, M. E., & Meloy, F. A. (2014). The embodiment of authentic leadership. *Journal of Professional Nursing, 30*(4), 282–291.

Whitlock, J. (2013). The value of active followership. *Nursing Management, 20*(2), 20–23.

Zaleznik, A. (1965). The dynamics of subordinacy. *Harvard Business Review, 118*, 119–131.

To explore learning resources for this chapter, go to FADavis.com

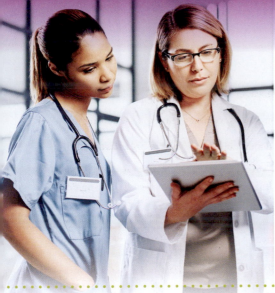

Chapter 4

Ethical Aspects of Nursing Practice

Elizabeth J. Murray, PhD, RN, CNE

LEARNING OUTCOMES

- Discuss the five core professional nursing values.
- Describe several ethical theories and principles crucial to nursing practice.
- Define moral distress and discuss its consequences.
- Identify strategies to build moral resilience.
- Explain the role of ethics committees.
- Analyze the types of ethical issues nurse leaders and managers may face.

KEY TERMS

Advocacy
Autonomy
Beneficence
Code of ethics
Deontology
Ethical dilemma
Ethical principles
Ethics
Fidelity
Justice
Moral courage
Moral distress
Moral integrity
Moral obligation
Moral resilience
Moral uncertainty
Morals
Nonmaleficence
Nursing autonomy
Paternalism
Principlism
Professionalism
Social justice
Utilitarianism
Values
Values clarification
Veracity

The Knowledge, Skills, and Attitudes Related to the Following Are Addressed in This Chapter:

Core Competencies	• Patient-Centered Care • Teamwork and Collaboration • Evidence-Based Practice • Safety
The Essentials: Core Competencies for Professional Nursing Education (AACN, 2021)	**Domain 1: Knowledge for Nursing Practice** 1.2 Apply theory and research-based knowledge from nursing, the arts, humanities, and other sciences (p. 27). **Domain 2: Person-Centered Care** 2.1 Engage with the individual in establishing a caring relationship (pp. 28–29). **Domain 9: Professionalism** 9.1 Demonstrate an ethical comportment in one's practice reflective of nursing's mission to society (p. 52). 9.5 Demonstrate the professional identity of nursing (pp. 54–55). 9.6 Integrate diversity, equity, and inclusion as core to one's professional identity (p. 55).
Code of Ethics with Interpretive Statements (ANA, 2015)	**All provisions of the Code of Ethics (pp. 1–37)**

Nurse Manager (NMC) Competencies (AONL, 2015a) and Nurse Executive (NEC) Competencies (AONL, 2015b)	**NMC: Personal and Professional Accountability (p. 7)**
	• Practice ethical behavior—including practice that supports nursing standards and scopes of practice
	NEC: Leadership (p. 8)
	• Foundational thinking skills
	  • Address ideas, beliefs or viewpoints that should be given serious consideration
	NEC: Professionalism (p. 9)
	• Ethics
	  • Uphold ethical principles and corporate compliance standards
	  • Hold self and staff accountable to comply with ethical standards of practice
	  • Discuss, resolve, and learn from ethical dilemmas
	• Advocacy
	  • Represent the perspective of patients and families
	  • Advocate for optimal health care in the community
	NEC: Business Skills (p. 10)
	• Human resource management
	  • Evaluate the results of employee satisfaction/quality of work environment surveys
	  • Promote healthful work environments
	  • Address sexual harassment, workplace violence, verbal and physical abuse

The Knowledge, Skills, and Attitudes Related to the Following Are Addressed in This Chapter:—cont'd

Nursing Administration Scope and Standards of Practice (ANA, 2016)	**Standard 1: Assessment** The nurse administrator collects pertinent data and information relative to the situation, issue, problem, or trend (pp. 35–36).
	Standard 5: Implementation The nurse administrator implements the identified plan (p. 40).
	Standard 7: Ethics The nurse administrator practices ethically (pp. 45-46).
	Standard 9: Communication The nurse administrator communicates effectively in all areas of practice (p. 49).
	Standard 13: Evidence-Based Practice and Research The nurse administrator integrates evidence and research findings into practice (p. 54).

Source: American Association of Colleges of Nursing. (2021). *The essentials: Core competencies for professional nursing education.* Author; American Nurses Association (ANA). (2015). *Code of ethics for nurses with interpretive statements.* Author; American Nurses Association (ANA). (2016). *Nursing administration: Scope and standards of practice* (2nd ed.). Author; American Organization for Nursing Leadership (AONL). (2015a). *AONL nurse manager competencies.* Author; American Organization for Nursing Leadership (AONL). (2015b). *AONL nurse executive competencies.* Author; Cronenwett, L., Sherwood, G., Barnsteiner, J., Disch, J., Johnson, J., Mitchell, P., Sullivan, D. T., & Warren, J. (2007). Quality and safety education for nurses. *Nursing Outlook, 55*(3), 122–131; and Greiner, A. C., & Knebel, E. (Eds.) (2003). *Health professions education: A bridge to quality.* National Academies Press.

Nursing care is undoubtedly an intimate activity. Interactions with patients are very personal and occur at a time when patients are in an extremely vulnerable state. In turn, the career of nursing comes with a myriad of ethical considerations. Establishing nurturing relationships with patients and their families while maintaining professional boundaries is an important goal of nursing, as is delivering care without prejudice and respecting human needs and values. All nurses must practice nursing in accordance with professional codes of ethics and recognized standards of professional practice. Nurse leaders and managers must ensure staff members maintain competence and provide safe, effective, and ethical care. In addition, nurse leaders and managers assist with ethical decision making related to patient care, managing and allocating resources, and administrative practices (American Nurses Association [ANA], 2016a).

In this chapter, nurse leaders and managers learn the ethical aspects of nursing practice, including their essential roles in developing, maintaining, and promoting "compassionate systems of care delivery that preserve and protect health care consumer, family, and employee dignity, rights, values, beliefs, and autonomy" (ANA, 2016a, p. 45). In addition, ethical principles and theories along with common ethical issues nurse leaders and managers may face are presented.

▶ NURSING ETHICS

Respect for the individual is the ethical underpinning of nursing practice, and most nurses use a combination of ethical morals, values, principles, theories, codes, and laws to guide practice (Murray, 2003). Ethical nursing practice requires nurses to be sensitive enough to recognize when they are faced with an ethical issue (Butts & Rich, 2020). **Ethics** in nursing is "the examination of all kinds of ethical and bioethical issues from the perspective of nursing theory and practice, which, in turn, rest on the agreed core concepts of nursing, namely: person, culture, care, health, healing, environment, and nursing itself" (Johnstone, 2016, p. 15). By applying ethics, nurses can determine the best course of action in specific situations. Ethics is core to professional nursing practice and guides a nurse's behavior (American Association of Colleges of Nursing [AACN], 2021). Nurse leaders and managers are obligated to model the values of the nursing profession and conduct themselves in a truthful and open manner (ANA, 2016a).

Morals

The terms *morals* and *ethics* are often, incorrectly, used interchangeably. **Morals** are defined as "conduct, character, and motives involved in moral acts and include the notion of approval or disapproval of a given conduct, character, or motive that we describe by such words as good, desirable, right, worthy, or conversely bad, undesirable, wrong, evil, unworthy" (Davis et al., 2010, p. 1). Morals are ingrained in one's consciousness, provide people with established rules of conduct based on societal customs and habits, and reflect what is right or wrong and good or bad. In comparison, ethics reflects what actions people should take in a specific situation based on their own morals. Both morals and ethics are influenced by personal life experiences and value systems. Nurses must maintain moral integrity and fulfill their moral obligation to patients, regardless of the setting.

Moral Integrity

Moral integrity refers to quality of character and involves acting consistently with personal and professional values (Butts & Rich, 2020). Nurses with moral integrity are honest and trustworthy, consistently do the right thing, and stand up for what is right despite the consequences (Laabs, 2011). In addition, nurses with moral integrity have a sense of self-worth because they have clearly defined values that are congruent with their actions (Epstein & Delgado, 2010). Moral integrity is a positive attribute for nurses in leadership and management positions and is critical to ethical decision making. Nurse leaders and managers with moral integrity own their beliefs and values, respect the beliefs and values of others, and, despite possible differences, avoid compromising their moral integrity. When a nurse behaves in a way that is not congruent with professional moral beliefs, moral integrity is in jeopardy.

Moral Obligation

An obligation is a duty to or responsibility for another human being. Nurses enter a relationship of trust with a patient that involves a **moral obligation** or duty to provide care in a nondiscriminatory manner. A nurse's primary commitment is to the recipient of care (ANA, 2015a). Once a nurse–patient relationship has been established, a nurse has a duty to the patient and cannot abandon a patient in need of care (ANA, 2015b). At times, nurses are challenged to balance professional obligations and personal risks. Although nurses have a moral obligation to care for patients at all times, situations may arise in which nurses could face potential personal harm. Therefore, nurses must be able to critically think and analyze certain situations in which the risk may outweigh the moral obligation to care for a patient. In such cases, it is a nurse's decision to accept personal risk that exceeds the limits of their moral obligation. The ANA asserts that nurses are morally obligated to care for patients when the following four criteria are present (ANA, 2015b, pp. 2–3):

1. The patient is at significant risk of harm, loss, or damage if the nurse does not assist.
2. The nurse's intervention or care is directly relevant to preventing harm.
3. The nurse's care will probably prevent harm, loss, or damage to the patient.
4. The benefit the patient will gain outweighs any harm the nurse may incur and does not present more than an acceptable risk to the nurse.

If one or more of these criteria are absent, the nurse must evaluate the situation and choose whether or not to care for the patient as their moral obligation (ANA, 2015b). However, once a nurse accepts an assignment, they must fulfill the assignment or risk being charged with abandonment (Guido, 2014).

Values

Values are personal beliefs that influence behavior and give meaning and direction to life. Values evolve over time and reflect ethnic background, family life, cultural beliefs, environment, and societal norms. As a person matures, their value systems may change and grow to encompass personal, professional, and societal values. Nurses' values or core beliefs of worth and dignity inform their attitudes and guide their actions. Although individuals are not always conscious of how much their value system influences decision making, they are constantly making decisions based on values. "Nurses have a right and duty to act according to their personal and professional values" (ANA, 2015a, p. 20). Being aware of personal values helps nurses to make clear, thoughtful, and consistent decisions. The process one goes through to understand personal values is called *values clarification.*

Values Clarification

Values clarification is the process of reflecting on and analyzing values to better understand what is important. Self-reflection on personal and professional values requires a readiness and willingness to take an honest look at personal behaviors, words, actions, motivations, and any congruencies or incongruencies among them (Burkhardt & Nathaniel, 2014). Values clarification is an ongoing process of becoming self-aware of the personal and professional values that are important.

Through self-reflection, nurses can develop an insight into their value systems, thus enhancing their self-awareness and their ability to make value decisions in nursing practice (Burkhardt & Nathaniel, 2014). Nurses must become self-aware to be able to provide nonjudgmental care to patients and to develop and maintain a nonjudgmental approach to leadership and management. The nursing code of ethics, discussed later in this chapter, obligates nurses to deliver care with respect for human needs and values without prejudice. It is difficult to carry out this obligation without self-awareness.

LEARNING ACTIVITY 4-1

Values Clarification

Complete a values clarification activity online. Here are two links:

https://www.thebalancecareers.com/values-clarification-exercise-2275847
https://positivepsychology.com/values-questionnaire/

1. Reflect on your values.
2. What surprised you?
3. Why is self-awareness of values important to you professionally?

Core Professional Values for Nurses

Professionalism in nursing is defined as "the consistent demonstration of core values evidenced by nurses working with other professionals to achieve optimal health and wellness outcomes in patients, families, and communities by wisely applying principles of altruism, excellence, caring, ethics, respect, communication, and accountability" (AACN, 2008, p. 26). Being a professional nurse involves accountability for oneself and one's nursing practice and a duty to provide safe and quality care. Professional values and associated behaviors are critical to professional nursing practice and professional identity (AACN, 2008; AACN, 2021; ANA, 2015a). There are five core professional values nurses must follow (AACN, 2008, pp. 27–28):

1. *Altruism:* A concern for the welfare and well-being of others. In professional practice, altruism is reflected by a nurse's concern and advocacy for the welfare of patients, other nurses, and other health-care providers.
2. *Autonomy:* The right to self-determination. Professional practice reflects autonomy when the nurse respects a patient's right to make health-care decisions.
3. *Human dignity:* Respect for the inherent worth and uniqueness of individuals and populations. In professional practice, concern for human dignity is reflected when the nurse values and respects all patients and colleagues.
4. *Integrity:* Acting in accordance with an appropriate code of ethics and accepted standards of practice. Integrity is reflected in professional practice when the

nurse is honest and provides care based on an ethical framework that is accepted within the profession.

5. *Social justice:* Acting in accordance with fair treatment regardless of economic status, race, ethnicity, age, citizenship, disability, or sexual orientation.

Nurses must become self-aware and understand their personal values to better recognize situations that may result in inner conflict between personal and professional values.

Ethical Theories

Ethical theories assist nurses in understanding the origin of ethical thinking and behavior in the context of culture and moral norms (Burkhardt & Nathaniel, 2014). Although various ethical theories are used in nursing, many experts consider utilitarianism, deontology, principlism, and virtue ethics as the most relevant to nursing practice (Bandman & Bandman, 2002; Burkhardt & Nathaniel, 2014; Butts & Rich, 2020; Davis et al., 2010; Joel, 2006; Volbrecht, 2002). These four ethical theories provide the foundation for ethical decision making by nurse leaders and managers.

Utilitarianism

Utilitarianism is a form of teleologic theory, from the Greek word *telos* meaning "the end." The basic premise of utilitarianism is the notion that acting morally should increase human happiness and make the world a better place. The principle of utility provides the foundation of utilitarianism, which assumes it is possible to balance good and bad. Utilitarianism is a theory of consequentialism in which the moral rightness of an action is determined by the consequences of that action (Burkhardt & Nathaniel, 2014; Volbrecht, 2002). The belief of utilitarians is that increasing happiness means maximizing pleasure and minimizing pain. In other words, the end justifies the means.

In nursing, the utilitarian approach is used in situations in which benefits should be maximized for the good of the greatest number of people, such as the funding of health care and the delivery of care (Black, 2014; Davis et al., 2010). A drawback to utilitarianism is that, although the goal is the greatest happiness for the greatest number of people, this approach can overlook the rights of an individual. Nurse leaders and managers may rely on a utilitarian approach when establishing staffing schedules, when honoring time-off requests, or in times of high census when determining whom to discharge to make room for patients requiring care that is more acute. Because the emphasis of utilitarianism is to produce the greatest good for the greatest number of people, it is one of the most common ethical approaches used in public health nursing (Butts & Rich, 2020).

Deontology

Deontology comes from the Greek word *deon,* meaning "that which is obligatory." The basic premise of deontology is that the rightness or wrongness of an action often depends on the nature of the act rather than the consequences of the act

(Burkhardt & Nathaniel, 2014; Davis et al., 2010). The principle of duty provides the foundation of deontology, which assumes a person is moral when they act from a sense of duty. Deontology recognizes the dignity and autonomy of individuals and negates paternalism. Deontology supports the notions that all individuals must respect their own humanity and that a person is never to be treated as a means to an end. Most codes of ethics are rooted in deontology. Deontology stresses equal treatment of all people, respect, freedom, and human dignity (Bandman & Bandman, 2002). A drawback to the deontologic approach is that it can be rigid and does not assist nurses in choosing alternatives to solve an ethical dilemma (Butts & Rich, 2020).

Nurse leaders and managers may rely on a deontologic approach when needing to maintain an objective approach to making hiring decisions, making daily staff assignments, and promoting the most qualified staff members.

Virtue Ethics

Virtues are learned attributes of moral character that influence nurses to meet their moral obligation of doing what is right (ANA, 2015a). The ANA (2015a) defines *virtue* as "a habit of character that predisposes one to do what is right; what we are to be as moral agents; habituated, learned" (p. 46). Specific virtues of moral character are expected of nurses such as patience, compassion, knowledge, skill, wisdom, honesty, altruism, and courage (ANA, 2015a). Virtue ethics is "concerned with being good and having moral character rather than doing good and following rules or focusing on duties" (Butts & Rich, 2020). Whereas deontology and utilitarianism provide a framework to use to seek the morally correct solution, virtue ethics suggests that a person's actions are based on the person's character and an action is right if it is what a virtuous person would do (Sakellariouv, 2015). The virtuous person does not act based on principles but rather based on innate morals (Burkhardt & Nathaniel, 2014).

Principlism

Although utilitarianism and deontology are the predominant theories used to guide nursing practice, neither approach is adequate in all ethical situations at all times. A principle-based approach uses rule-based criteria for conduct that stem from the identification of obligations and duties (Butts & Rich, 2020). Principles are sets of rules, ideals, standards, and values characteristic of a group (Jameton, 1984). **Principlism** is a theory in which one or more ethical principles are used to analyze and resolve an ethical issue or dilemma. For example, nurses use the principles of beneficence and nonmaleficence, balancing the benefit of nursing care and avoiding harm to patients, in everyday practice. Nurse leaders and managers apply principlism when they respect the rights, responsibilities, and professional autonomy of their nursing staff members.

Principles

Ethical principles are basic moral truths that guide a person's actions. Valuing human dignity, respecting individuals, and believing in an individual's right to be self-governing are the foundation of ethical principles. All nurses must have an understanding of ethical principles and be able to apply them in a meaningful manner in a variety of settings and situations (Burkhardt & Nathaniel, 2014). The principles of autonomy, beneficence, nonmaleficence, justice, fidelity, veracity, privacy, and confidentiality guide everyday nursing practice, regardless of roles or settings. Table 4-1 provides a brief definition for each ethical principle.

Autonomy

The principle of **autonomy** refers to self-governance/self-determination and is defined as "rational self-legislation and self-determination that is grounded in informedness, voluntariness, consent, and rationality" (ANA, 2015a, p. 41). An individual makes autonomous decisions based on their own values, adequate and appropriate information, and freedom from coercion. An autonomous person has the capacity to understand, reason, deliberate, manage, and independently choose a plan of care (Beauchamp & Childress, 2019).

Patients have a moral and legal right to self-determination, including "the right to accept, refuse, or terminate treatment" (ANA, 2015a, p. 2). In turn, nurses have an obligation to understand and support the moral and legal rights of patients.

Nurses respect autonomy by supporting a patient's health-care choices, obtaining informed consent, allowing a patient to refuse treatments, and maintaining privacy and confidentiality. Autonomy for nurses means "determining [their] own actions through independent choice, including demonstration of competence, within the full scope of nursing practice" (ANA, 2010, p. 39). Nurse leaders and managers are responsible for promoting and protecting patient autonomy as well as professional autonomy among staff. Nurses at all levels also have autonomy in their practice. **Nursing autonomy** is "the capacity of a nurse to determine her or his own actions through independent choice, including demonstration of competence, within the full scope of nursing practice" (ANA, 2016a, p. 61).

Beneficence

The principle of **beneficence** is a core principle of patient advocacy and refers to any action intended to benefit another—in other words, one's actions should

Table 4-1	Ethical Principles
Principle	**Description**
Autonomy	Respecting a person's right to self-determination
Beneficence	Adhering to the duty to do good
Nonmaleficence	Adhering to the duty to do no harm
Justice	Treating others with fairness
Fidelity	Keeping promises
Veracity	Telling the truth
Privacy	Respecting a person's right to keep information about themselves from being disclosed to others
Confidentiality	Preventing the disclosure of a person's private information

always promote good. Promoting good in nursing is exemplified several ways, such as encouraging a patient to undergo painful treatment if it will increase quality and quantity of life or honoring a patient's wish to die (Guido, 2014). Some forms of beneficence are obligatory and include moral rules such as the following (Beauchamp & Childress, 2019, p. 219):

1. Protect and defend the rights of others.
2. Prevent harm from occurring to others.
3. Remove conditions that will cause harm to others.
4. Help persons with disabilities.
5. Rescue persons in danger.

Nurse leaders and managers must frequently apply the principle of beneficence professionally when establishing staffing plans to ensure patient safety and avoid nurse fatigue, when conducting staff performance appraisals, and when assisting an employee in establishing a plan for professional growth.

Nonmaleficence

The principle of **nonmaleficence** refers to the moral obligation to do no harm or injury to another person. Nurses honor the principle of nonmaleficence by following standards of care and implementing best practices. Nonmaleficence also involves an obligation to avoid imposing risks of harm to another and includes moral rules such as the following (Beauchamp & Childress, 2019, p. 159):

1. Do not kill.
2. Do not cause pain or suffering.
3. Do not incapacitate.
4. Do not cause offense.
5. Do not deprive others of goods of life.

Nonmaleficence differs from beneficence in that nonmaleficence morally prohibits people from causing harm to anyone; beneficence is failing to help or benefit another, but it is not always considered immoral (Beauchamp & Childress, 2019). Some situations result in a conflict between beneficence and nonmaleficence and present challenges for nurses and other health-care professionals. A common example is the administration of chemotherapy. Chemotherapeutic agents destroy cancer cells but also healthy cells and have extremely uncomfortable side effects. When providing chemotherapy, nurses violate the principle of nonmaleficence in the short term to produce a good outcome or benefit the patient in the long term. Table 4-2 presents a comparison of the rules of beneficence and nonmaleficence.

Related to the principles of beneficence and nonmaleficence is **paternalism**, which is "the intentional overriding of one person's preferences or actions by another person" (Beauchamp & Childress, 2019, p. 231) or, in the health-care world, controlling a patient's choices. Many nurses often justify paternalism in the name of beneficence and nonmaleficence. Many times a nurse, because of their knowledge, education, and experience, may believe that they know what is best for the patient and act accordingly regardless of the patient's wishes. This

Table 4-2	Comparison of the Moral Rules of Beneficence and Nonmaleficence	
Moral Rules of Beneficence	**Moral Rules of Nonmaleficence**
1. Present positive requirements for action	1. Present negative requirements for action
2. Do not need to be followed impartially	2. Must be followed impartially
3. Generally do not provide reasons for legal punishment when rules are not followed	3. Provide moral reasons for legal prohibitions in certain forms of conduct

From Beauchamp & Childress, 2019.

interferes with the patient's autonomy and right to self-determination. Nurses must be able to differentiate between controlling patient choices, or paternalism, and assisting patients in making informed choices, or respecting autonomy. For example, when a nurse decides not to tell a patient that their temperature is elevated or their heart rate is irregular because the nurse believes that the news will upset the patient, that nurse is acting in a paternalistic manner. The nurse is deciding for the patient whether they should be told this information.

Justice

The principle of **justice** refers to the obligation of nurses to provide fair, equitable, and appropriate treatment to all patients based on their needs and without prejudice. Justice is about treating everyone equally and fairly and giving people what they deserve. Nurses apply the principle of justice when they deliver care to patients without bias. However, the principle of justice can be very complicated, especially when considering inequalities in access to health care and health insurance. **Social justice** is "the expectation that everyone deserves equal economic, political, and social rights and opportunities" and includes equity, access, participation, and human rights (AACN, 2021, p. 71). Nurse leaders and managers apply justice professionally when they promote giving staff members adequate compensation commensurate with education, experience, and responsibilities (ANA, 2016a).

Fidelity

The principle of **fidelity** refers to being faithful or loyal by keeping promises to others. Further, fidelity requires a commitment in relationships, it is fundamental for the nurse–patient relationship, and requires nurses to be loyal, truthful, fair, and advocates for patients. When nurses receive their nursing license, they accept the mandate to practice nursing within established scope and standards of practice, which includes keeping promises to patients (Burkhardt & Nathaniel, 2014).

Nurse leaders and managers apply fidelity professionally when they keep promises to staff by maintaining a culture of safety and a healthy work environment, one that is empowering and satisfying. A healthy work environment is discussed in detail in Chapter 12. Nurse leaders and managers must be mindful of the health and safety of both patients and their staff members.

Veracity

The principle of **veracity** is defined as telling the truth. Veracity is related to autonomy and fidelity and suggests that patients have a right to truthful information. Patients expect nurses to be truthful when under their care. Overall, society trusts health-care professionals; moreover, for the 18th consecutive year, Americans ranked nurses the most ethical and honest among a list of professions (Reinhart, 2020). Nurses must establish relationships of trust (ANA, 2015a).

Telling the truth encompasses respect, open communication, trust, and shared decision making, all elements of the nurse–patient relationship. When nurses enter the nurse–patient relationship, they must speak truthfully and not be deceptive. Nurse leaders and managers apply the principle of veracity professionally when they are truthful with employees and avoid intentionally deceiving or misleading staff.

Privacy and Confidentiality

Respecting a patient's privacy and confidentiality is essential to maintaining a trusting relationship between nurses and patients (ANA, 2015a). Privacy is the right to control access to personal information, including the choice to disclose or not disclose information. Confidentiality is the nondisclosure of personal information shared within the nurse–patient relationship (ANA, 2015a). Although privacy and confidentiality are ethical principles, they are also legal rights of patients protected by the Health Insurance Portability and Accountability Act (HIPAA), which is discussed in detail in Chapter 5.

Codes of Ethics

A **code of ethics** is an essential requirement for any profession. It reflects the values and beliefs shared by members, informs the public of the standards of ethical conduct for the profession, and provides rules and principles for self-regulation (Bandman & Bandman, 2002; Burkhardt & Nathaniel, 2014; Guido, 2014). Codes of ethics for nurses serve as ethical guides for all practicing nurses in all settings and they are nonnegotiable. Box 4-1 is a partial list of nurses' associations worldwide with specific codes of ethics. Many nurses' associations worldwide have specific codes of ethics for nurses; the International Council of Nurses *ICN Code of Ethics for Nurses,* the Canadian Nurses Association (CNA) *Code of Ethics for Registered Nurses,* and the ANA *Code of Ethics for Nurses With Interpretive Statements* will be further discussed here. In reviewing these codes of ethics, it is clear that globally, nursing focuses on respect for patients and their dignity and right to autonomy. Each code of ethics is similar in its focus on the nurse's obligation to uphold professional standards, maintain competence, promote patient safety, participate in ongoing lifelong learning, and collaborate with health-care team members. Nurse leaders and managers have an obligation to ensure that nursing care provided by those they supervise reflects the guidelines set forth in the various codes of ethics.

BOX 4-1 **Nurses Associations Worldwide With Nursing Professional Codes of Ethics: A Partial List**	
NURSES ASSOCIATIONS	**WEB SITES**
American Nurses Association	https://www.nursingworld.org/practice-policy/nursing-excellence/ethics/code-of-ethics-for-nurses/
Australia Nursing and Midwifery Federation	https://www.nursingmidwiferyboard.gov.au/Codes-Guidelines-Statements/Professional-standards.aspx
Canadian Nurses Association	https://www.cna-aiic.ca/en/nursing-practice/nursing-ethics
European Nurse Directors Association	https://enda-europe.com/wp-content/uploads/2019/04/enda-proto-code-of-ethics.pdf
International Council of Nurses	https://www.icn.ch/sites/default/files/inline-files/2012_ICN_Codeofethicsfornurses_%20eng.pdf
Nursing Council of Hong Kong	https://www.nchk.org.hk/en/code_of_conduct_and_practice/code_of_professional_conduct_and_code_of_ethics_for_nurses_in_hong_kong/index.html
Nursing Council of New Zealand	https://www.nursingcouncil.org.nz/Public/Nursing/Code_of_Conduct/NCNZ/nursing-section/Code_of_Conduct.aspx
Nursing and Midwifery Council (United Kingdom)	https://www.nmc.org.uk/standards/code/
Philippine Nurses Association, Inc.	http://www.pna-ph.org/component/jdownloads/summary/3-policies-laws/4-code-of-ethics-for-nurses
Singapore Nurses Board	https://www.healthprofessionals.gov.sg/docs/librariesprovider4/publications/code-for-nurses-and-midwives-april-2018.pdf
Taiwan Nurses Association	http://www.ngo.e-twna.org.tw/nursing_policy_1.php

International Council of Nurses Code of Ethics for Nurses

The *International Council of Nurses (ICN) Code of Ethics for Nurses* was first adopted in 1953 and has been revised numerous times since, most recently in 2012, and is currently under revision (Stievano & Tschudin, 2019). The purpose of the *ICN Code of Ethics for Nurses* is to provide "a guide for action based on social values and needs…. The Code must be understood, internalised, and used by nurses in all aspects of their work" (ICN, 2012, p. 5). The *ICN Code of Ethics for Nurses* recognizes that the need for nursing is universal and delineates four fundamental responsibilities of nurses: "to promote health; to prevent illness; to restore health; and to alleviate suffering" (p. 2). This code of ethics also provides four elements that outline the standards of ethical practice: nurses and people, nurses and practice, nurses and the profession, and nurses and coworkers. It is a global document and, as such, applies to nurses from countries where national nursing organizations are ICN members (Johnstone, 2016).

Canadian Nurses Association Code of Ethics for Registered Nurses

The *Canadian Nurses Association (CNA) Code of Ethics for Registered Nurses* serves as a foundation for nurses' ethical practice and provides a statement of ethical values for nurses and their commitment to those with health-care needs and those receiving nursing care. The CNA's *Code of Ethics* is divided into two sections. Part one addresses the core nursing values and responsibilities central to ethical nursing practice, including providing safe, compassionate, competent, and ethical care; promoting health and well-being; promoting and respecting informed decision making; honoring dignity; maintaining privacy and confidentiality; promoting justice; and being accountable. The core responsibilities "apply to nurses' interactions with all persons who have health care needs or are receiving care as well as with students, colleagues, and other health care providers" (CNA, 2017, p. 8). Part two describes the nurse's role in ethical endeavors related to broad societal issues (CNA, 2017). The CNA addresses the fact that ethical nursing practice is "focused on improving systems and society structures to create greater equity for all" (CNA, 2017, p. 8).

American Nurses Association Code of Ethics for Nurses With Interpretive Statements

The Nightingale Pledge, drafted in 1893 and modeled after the Hippocratic Oath, was the first code of ethics for nurses (ANA, 2015a). This pledge was revised and adopted as a "tentative code" and published in the *American Journal of Nursing* in 1940 but was never formally adopted until 1950 as the *Code for Professional Nurses*. It has been subsequently revised a number of times through the years: in 1956, 1960, 1968, 1976 (at which time it became *Code of Ethics for Nurses With Interpretive Statements*), 1985, 2001, and most recently in 2015 to reflect the influences of societal changes. The initial versions of this code of ethics reflected general attitudes toward nursing at the time and included values such as obedience, trustworthiness, loyalty, and adeptness in social etiquette, as well as obligations to carry out physicians' orders (Murray, 2003). Later versions emphasized nurses' responsibility to the patient, society, and the nursing profession. Although this code of ethics has evolved over the past century to mirror changes in society, health care, and the nursing profession, it has consistently addressed the fundamental principles of beneficence, nonmaleficence, fidelity, and veracity.

The *Code of Ethics for Nurses* establishes ethical standards for the nursing practice and provides a framework to guide nurses in ethical analysis and decision making. Its purpose is threefold (ANA, 2015a, p. viii):

1. It is a succinct statement of the ethical obligations and duties of every individual who enters the nursing profession.
2. It is the profession's nonnegotiable ethical standard.
3. It is an expression of nursing's own understanding of its commitment to society.

The current *Code of Ethics for Nurses* includes nine provisions with related interpretive statements. Provisions one through three address the fundamental values and commitments of the nurse, including dignity and respect for patients; patient rights such as self-determination, safety, privacy, and confidentiality; and acting on questionable practice. Provisions four through six describe the nurse's boundaries of duty and loyalty, such as appropriate delegation, accountability, responsibility, maintaining competence, ethical obligations, and integrity. The last three provisions describe the aspects of the nurse's duties beyond individual patient encounters and include the nurse's role in the advancement of the profession, responsibilities to the public, and maintaining the integrity of the nursing profession (ANA, 2015a). The nine provisions are presented in Box 4-2. The entire *Code of Ethics With Interpretive Statements* can be viewed online (https://www.nursing-world.org/practice-policy/nursing-excellence/ethics/code-of-ethics-for-nurses/).

The values and obligations addressed in the ANA *Code of Ethics for Nurses* apply to all nurses in all roles and in all settings (ANA, 2015a). The ethical standards outlined are nonnegotiable, and therefore all nurses are obligated to uphold and adhere to the code (ANA, 2015a).

BOX 4-2   American Nurses Association Provisions of the *Code of Ethics for Nurses With Interpretive Statements*

1. The nurse practices with compassion and respect for the inherent dignity, worth, and unique attributes of every person.
2. The nurse's primary commitment is to the patient, whether an individual, family, group, community, or population.
3. The nurse promotes, advocates for, and protects the rights, health, and safety of the patient.
4. The nurse has authority, accountability, and responsibility for nursing practice; makes decisions; and takes action consistent with the obligation to promote health and to provide optimal care.
5. The nurse owes the same duties to self as to others, including the responsibility to promote health and safety, preserve wholeness of character and integrity, maintain competence, and continue personal and professional growth.
6. The nurse, through individual and collective effort, establishes, maintains, and improves the ethical environment of the work setting and conditions of employment that are conducive to safe, quality health care.
7. The nurse, in all roles and settings, advances the profession through research and scholarly inquiry, professional standards development, and the generation of both nursing and health policy.
8. The nurse collaborates with other health professionals and the public to protect human rights, promote health diplomacy, and reduce health disparities.
9. The profession of nursing, collectively through its professional organizations, must articulate nursing values, maintain the integrity of the profession, and integrate principles of social justice into nursing and health policy.

From ANA, 2015a, p. v.

✪ Advocacy

Advocacy is briefly discussed in Chapter 1 as one of the philosophical underpinnings of nursing. Nursing advocacy encompasses caring, respect for an individual's autonomy, and empowerment. Nurse leaders and managers advocate for patients and families, staff, the profession, and themselves on a daily basis. They must commit to integrating advocacy into the design, implementation, and evaluation of policies, services, and systems (ANA, 2016a, p. 11).

Advocating for Patients and Families

The role of an advocate is to safeguard patients and their families against abuse, unsafe practice, and violations of their rights (Bandman & Bandman, 2002). Nurses have more contact with patients and their families than any other health-care professional and often develop an understanding of the values, desires, and needs of patients and their families. Therefore, nurses are in the best position to protect those interests (Bandman & Bandman, 2002).

To provide patient-centered care, nurses must advocate for patients and their families on an ongoing basis, even if they disagree with a patient's decision. Nurses must view health care "through patients' eyes" (Cronenwett et al., 2007). To be an effective patient advocate, nurses must ensure that their patients are informed, respect their patient's autonomy, and respect their patient's health-care decisions. Provision three of the ANA *Code of Ethics for Nurses With Interpretive Statements* states that "the nurse promotes, advocates for, and protects health and safety, rights of the patient" (ANA, 2015a, p. 9). Nurse leaders and managers are responsible for ensuring that nursing care is delivered with respect for the individual rights and preferences of patients (ANA, 2016a). Nurse leaders and managers must ensure that systems are in compliance with regulatory agencies and promote communication that supports the well-being of patients. Further, they must ensure that education about patient advocacy is provided to all health-care professionals and employees (ANA, 2016a).

Advocating for Employees

Nurse leaders and managers function as employee advocates by ensuring appropriate resource allocation, promoting a positive work environment (Tomajan, 2012), and creating and fostering an ethical work climate for all staff. Provision six of the ANA *Code of Ethics* states, "The nurse, through individual and collective effort, establishes, maintains, and improves ethical environment of the work setting and conditions of employment that are conducive to safe, quality health care" (ANA, 2015a, p. 23). Ideally, nurse leaders and managers collaborate with staff on issues related to workplace conditions and patient care policies to ensure satisfactory outcomes (Olson, 2010). Nurse leaders and managers should "establish, maintain, and promote conditions of employment that enable nurses to practice according to accepted standards" (ANA, 2015a, p. 28). In addition, they have a responsibility to provide a safe work environment that facilitates appropriate assignments, delegation, open communication, and promote nursing autonomy and accountability (ANA, 2016a). Nurse leaders and managers must also foster an environment that encourages self-care for nursing staff. Creating a culture of self-renewal will help nurses rediscover or maintain their caring values (Turkel & Ray, 2004).

Advocating for the Profession

Advocating for the profession is addressed by provision seven of the ANA (2015a) *Code of Ethics:* "The nurse in all roles and settings, advances the profession through research and scholarly inquiry, professional standards development, and the generation of both nursing and health policy" (p. 27). Nurse leaders and managers advocate for staff and peers in the promotion of health policies that reflect best practice and improve access to care. In addition, Nurse leaders and managers can further advocate for the nursing profession by participating in professional nursing organizations and through professional publications and presentations (ANA, 2016a).

Advocating for Self

Provision five of the *Code of Ethics* states, "The nurse owes the same duties to self as to others, including the responsibility to promote health and safety, preserve wholeness of character, and integrity, maintain competence, and continue personal and professional growth" (ANA, 2015a, p. 19). Nurses in all roles should seek to balance personal and work activities to promote and maintain their own health and well-being. It is important for nurse leaders and managers to practice self-care, manage stress, and connect with those they manage (ANA, 2016a). Nurse leaders and managers must "demonstrate a commitment to self-reflection and self-care" (ANA, 2016a, p. 46). Practicing self-care is essential to create a caring harmonious work environment (Turkel & Ray, 2004). Modeling self-care will also influence staff members in their self-renewal.

How Can the Nurse Advocate for the Patient?

Mr. H. is very spiritual. He developed cancer of the throat and was admitted for surgical removal of a tumor. After the surgical procedure, Mr. H. developed severe inflammation requiring a tracheostomy. His family approaches the surgeon to ask whether Mr. H. could wear an amulet that has healing properties around his neck. The surgeon responds angrily, "No, absolutely not! He is to have nothing around his neck!" The family is very upset and tells Mr. H.'s nurse about the interaction. How can the nurse advocate for Mr. H. and his family?

Ethical Dilemmas

An **ethical dilemma** occurs when obligations, principles, rights, values, or beliefs are in conflict. There is not always a clear-cut right or wrong solution when ethical dilemmas arise. When faced with an ethical dilemma, a nurse must make a choice between or among two or more equally undesirable alternatives. Once a choice has been made, the nurse may continue to believe that neither choice was morally preferable. **Moral uncertainty** results when a nurse senses there is a moral problem but they are not sure of the morally correct action or what moral principles apply (Jameton, 1984). When a nurse experiences moral uncertainty, they are uncomfortable about the situation but cannot explain why.

Moral distress results when a nurse knows the right action to take to solve a moral problem but cannot follow their moral beliefs because of organizational constraints. Nurses in all roles and at all levels experience moral distress. It can restrict a nurse's ability to provide optimal care and experience job satisfaction. Three elements are present in moral distress: (1) There is an ethical problem; (2) the nurse has an obligation to do something to address the ethical problem; and (3) the nurse considers the most ethically correct action (Rushton & Kurtz, 2015, p. 3).

Moral distress involves a threat to one's moral integrity (Epstein & Delgado, 2010). Factors contributing to moral distress stem from a nurse's personal traits and experiences, the work environment, and external influences such as third-party expectations (Burston & Tuckett, 2012). Further, the research supports that moral distress can contribute to a decreased quality of care, patient satisfaction, and nurse satisfaction. (See Exploring the Evidence 4-1.)

When a nurse experiences moral distress, they may consider speaking out. Overcoming the fear associated with speaking up takes courage, specifically moral courage. **Moral courage** requires a steadfast commitment to fundamental moral principles despite potential risks (Murray, 2010). A morally courageous nurse is prepared to confront unethical situations despite the negative consequences, such as emotional anxiety, shame, threats to reputation, horizontal violence, and even job loss (LaSala & Bjarnason, 2010; Murray, 2010). Examples of nurses using moral courage include reporting a colleague who is diverting drugs, questioning a health-care provider about an order that is not within a reasonable standard of care, confronting a manager about inadequate staffing, and reporting a peer for posting patient information on a social media site (Butts & Rich, 2020). Nurse leaders and managers should do their best to create and sustain work environments that promote moral courage.

Research suggests that supportive nurse leaders and managers can help nurses deal with moral distress (de Veer et al., 2013). Coaching nurses on how to deal with ethical conflicts while preserving ethical integrity is one way to support staff.

Nurse leaders and managers must be vigilant to identify situations that may result in ethical dilemmas and be prepared to advocate for staff experiencing moral distress. Additionally, nurse leaders and managers must be proactive and seek to implement programs to address moral distress, build moral resilience, and promote creating healthy work environments.

EXPLORING THE EVIDENCE 4-1

Burston, A. S., & Tuckett, A. G. (2012). Moral distress in nursing: Contributing factors, outcomes and interventions. *Nursing Ethics, 20*(3), 312–324.

Aim
The initial aim was to identify literature on moral distress in terms of contributing factors, interventions, and outcomes within the aged care environment. However, because of limited findings, the researchers expanded their search to include other care environments.

Methods
The investigators searched the literature published from 1980 through 2011 related to moral distress in the following electronic databases: CINAHL, PsycINFO, MEDLINE, Social Sciences Citation Index, and Arts and Humanities Citation Index. The keywords used were *moral distress, moral distress scale, nursing home,* and *long-term care.*

Key Findings
Three core themes emerged related to moral distress: (1) specialist critical nursing, (2) specialist nursing, and (3) specialist nonnursing. The findings related to the second theme, specialist nursing, were discussed:

1. Contributing factors to moral distress originate from three primary sources: (1) the individual nurse and factors about the nurse, character traits, and personal worldview; (2) site-specific systems, including factors such as staffing levels, staffing mix, and type of care or lack of care; and (3) external influences or what researches referred to as the "world of work," which describes the practice setting and can involve feelings of danger or patient and role boundary issues.
2. Outcomes describe the impact or consequences of moral distress. Outcomes are related to the following: (1) the nurse's personal feelings (self) and tension between what is done and what ought to be done, resulting in guilt, remorse, regret, feeling of failure, and a sense of personal grief, all of which erode the

nurse's personal integrity and values; (2) the nurse's feelings toward others, including feeling powerless toward others in a given situation and possibly putting the nurse at risk for becoming cynical, calloused, and frustrated; and (3) the nurse's feelings toward the system (e.g., the nurse knowing the morally correct action to take but finding it impossible to pursue because of system constraints, leading nurses to choose to take no action at all). Consequences related to the outcomes of moral distress lead to issues with quality of patient care and patient satisfaction.

3. Interventions identified as appropriate to rectify nurses' moral distress include those that focus on the individual nurse and interventions that are more collaborative: (1) The individual approach recommends education focused on improved understanding of moral distress and development of effective coping strategies; and (2) the collaborative approach uses education and fosters participation in an interprofessional environment where health-care professionals can develop understandings of other health-care professionals and decision-making processes and can participate in forums to discuss patient goals.

Implications for Nurse Leaders and Managers

Nurse leaders and managers can help nurses by focusing on managing factors that contribute to moral distress and employ strategies to help thwart moral distress by (1) providing an environment where nurses feel safe to discuss ethical issues, share their frustrations, and discuss situations that feel unsafe; (2) assisting nurses with understanding the contributing factors and identifying the signs of moral distress; and (3) fostering an environment that supports intraprofessional and interprofessional teamwork.

Moral resilience is the capacity to sustain, restore, or deepen one's integrity in response to moral complexity, confusion, distress, or setbacks (Rushton, 2016, p. 1). Moral resilience is rooted in a person's awareness of and commitment to their values (Rushton & Kurtz, 2015).

Rushton et al. (2017) suggest that moral resilience is an evolving concept that can mitigate the detrimental effects of moral distress. Resilient nurses use transformational coping strategies of understanding and contextualizing the situation with a healthy sense of commitment, control, and challenge. In fact, nurses who are morally resilient have the ability to deal with ethical situations without moral distress (Lachman, 2016). Nurses at all levels can cultivate moral resilience by adopting the following strategies (Rushton, 2016, pp. 2–4):

- **Foster self-awareness** by exploring one's thoughts and feelings that accompany moral distress and acknowledging that they may be biased, incorrect, or congruent with one's values.
- **Develop self-regulation capacities** by cultivating one's ability to make and uphold moral commitments despite fear or uncertainty.

- **Develop ethical competence** living one's values and align inner character with outward behaviors.
- **Speak up with clarity and confidence** by stating one's concerns in interprofessional encounters using a clear, compelling, and ethically robust vocabulary.
- **Find meaning in the midst of despair** by stabilizing emotions to neutralize reactivity using strategies such as journaling, debriefing, and reflection to release moral residue.
- **Engage with others** by leveraging connections with others to support one's integrity and well-being.
- **Participate in transformational learning** by using the opportunity to learn from moral crisis and situations that result in moral distress.
- **Contribute to the culture of ethical practice** by contributing to and leveraging interprofessional efforts to develop structures that increase moral resilience.
- **Commitment to moral resilience** through dedication, discipline, and compassion toward our limitations and inevitable setbacks.

There is evidence that nurse resilience is higher in older nurses, nurses with higher education, and nurses who have been employed over 20 years (see Exploring the Evidence 4-2). Nurse leaders and managers can foster moral resilience by promoting and modeling the strategies outlined earlier. Lachman (2016) suggests that the resilience of nurse leaders and managers influences the resilience of their staff.

Ethical Decision Making

A nurse's values and beliefs influence the way they approach and solve ethical dilemmas. There are numerous ethical decision-making models in the nursing literature, many of which have similar elements. Regardless of the framework or model, ethical decision making should be holistic and begin with gathering all the facts. It is critical to think through the issue, feel empathetic toward all persons involved, and avoid knee-jerk reactions. There are four key aspects of ethical decision making (Cooper, 2012, p. 608):

1. Identifying an ethical problem and gathering relevant facts
2. Considering all involved in terms of impact, views, and opinions
3. Identifying possible options, and choosing and justifying an option
4. Implementing the decision

Nurses at all levels often encounter situations in practice that require them to make decisions in collaboration with others involved in the situation, such as patients, families, other nurses, and other health-care professionals. Nurse leaders and managers are charged with advocating "for the establishment and maintenance of an ethical environment that is conducive to safe, accessible, equitable, and quality health care" (ANA, 2016a, p. 46). Nurse leaders and managers are often involved with ethical decision making that include issues related to patient care, personnel management, and material and fiscal resources. The ANA has published numerous position statements and guidelines to assist nurses dealing with ethical decisions in everyday practice.

EXPLORING THE EVIDENCE 4-2

Leng, M., Xiu, H., Yu, P., Feng, J., Wei, Y., Cui, Y., Zhang, M., Zhou, Y., & Wei, H. (2020). Current state and influencing factors of nurse resilience and perceived job-related stressors. *Journal of Continuing Education in Nursing, 51*(3), 132–137. doi:10.3928/00220124-20200216-08

Aim

The aim of this study was to examine the state and influencing factors of nurse resilience and perceived job-related stressors, and identify strategies to promote resilience.

Methods

The investigators used a cross-sectional design using a demographic question-naire, the Connor-Davidson Resilience Scale, and a questionnaire developed by the authors to measure nurses' perceptions of stressors. The sample was a convenience sample of 2,981 full-time registered nurses in a university-affiliated hospital in China.

Key Findings

There were significant relationships between nurse resilience and age, education, clinical rank, and years of employment ($P < 0.05$).

- Nurses older than 45 years had the highest resilience scores and nurses between ages 26 and 35 years had the lowest resilience scores.
- Nurses with a master's degree or higher had the highest resilience scores and nurses with an associate degree had the lowest scores.
- Nurses who worked for more than 20 years had the highest resilience scores and nurses who worked between 6 and 10 years had the lowest scores.
- Nine major job stressors were identified: monthly supervisor inspections, monthly nursing knowledge and skill examinations, heavy workload, low wages, conflict with patients, mandatory overtime and shift changes, few promotion opportunities, research requirement, and work/life imbalance.

Implications for Nurse Leaders and Managers

Although this study was conducted in China, the findings may apply globally. The investigators suggested that nurse leaders can have a significant impact on improving nurses' professional growth and promoting a caring environment, and that both strategies can help build nurse resilience. Nurse leaders and managers can further help nurses by (1) providing opportunities for nurses to develop professionally; (2) offering classes to help nurses prepare to move up the clinical ladder; (3) collaborating with resilience trainers to provide resilience skill training; and (4) encouraging nurses to perform physical and emotional hygiene to reduce stress, get adequate sleep, exercise, eat healthy, and seek social support.

Ethics Committees

In the early 1990s, The Joint Commission (TJC) recognized the need for a mechanism to address ethical issues in health-care organizations and established a standard for accreditation. Since then, health-care organizations seeking accreditation or maintaining accreditation must address ethical issues through an ethics consultation service. Typically, interprofessional committees or teams provide ethics consultation services when ethical dilemmas arise during the delivery of care. The goals of ethics committees include promotion of patient rights; shared decision making between patients and health care providers; and fair and equitable policies and procedures that enhance the quality of patient-centered care (Guido, 2014).

Ethics committees in organizations have three interrelated functions: (1) institutional policy review and development, (2) ethics education, and (3) case consultation (Lachman, 2010). Most ethics committees are responsible for developing and reviewing policies and procedures, such as those relating to informed consent, advance directives, and withholding or withdrawing life support measures. Ethics education is an ongoing process among committee members and throughout an organization. Education for committee members is accomplished through invitation of expert guest speakers, sharing of article and case reviews, and sharing of knowledge by other members that was gleaned from ethics workshops/conferences (Lachman, 2010). Organization-wide education occurs through ethics workshops and conferences. The nature of ethics committees is interprofessional; nurse leaders and managers frequently participate on ethics committees.

A common service provided by an ethics committee is consultation to address ethical issues related to current clinical situations. The goals of consultation include intervening to protect patient rights, making recommendations to resolve ethical conflicts, providing moral support for those involved in an ethical situation, and reducing the risk of legal liability. The bedside nurse, health-care provider, family member, health-care surrogate, or patient can request an ethics consultation. In fact, anyone can refer a situation to the ethics committee for review. As part of patient-centered care, nurses must understand that conflict can arise between the patient's wishes and professional care. In some cases, requesting an ethics consultation can require a nurse to be morally courageous. Nurse leaders and managers must empower patients and nurses to foster a patient-centered approach to ethical decision making.

▶ ETHICAL ISSUES

Technological advances, economic constraints, increased complexity of health care, social demands, aging population, and limited resources can result in challenges for nurses at all levels. Ethical issues emerge in the health-care setting when conflict arises and/or individuals cannot assert their own rights.

Conscientious Objection

Conscientiousness is when an individual is "motivated to do what is right because it is right, has worked with due diligence to determine what is right, intends to do what is right, and exerts appropriate effort to do so" (Beauchamp & Childress, 2019, p. 42). Conscientious objection occurs when a nurse refuses to participate in a situation or the care of a patient because they believe the action would violate a deeply held moral or ethical value about right and wrong and threaten their integrity (Beauchamp & Childress, 2019; Lachman, 2014). Nurses have a right to conscientious objection based on maintaining moral integrity (Lachman, 2014). According to the ANA Code for Nurses (2015a, pp. 20–21), "nurses have a right and a duty to act according to their personal and professional values and to accept compromise only if reaching a compromise preserves the nurse's moral integrity and does not jeopardize the dignity or well-being of the nurse or others." Respecting conscientious objections is an important value and should be accommodated (Beauchamp & Childress, 2019). However, acts of conscientious objection cannot be arbitrary or based on personal preferences, prejudice, bias, or convenience (ANA, 2015a).

When an activity is morally objectionable to a nurse, the nurse must notify their supervisor in advance, if possible, so that arrangements can be made for patient care. If it is not realistic to give advance notice, the nurse must ensure that the patient is provided for until alternate arrangements can be made to avoid patient abandonment. The nurse may leave only when assured that the patient will be cared for safely.

Nurse leaders and managers must ensure that policies address conscientious objection. In a case where the integrity of nurses is compromised due to organizational behavior or the erosion of an ethical environment, nurse leaders and managers must respond to nurses' concerns and work to resolve the issues in a manner that preserves integrity. In addition, they must seek to change activities or expectations in the work environment that are morally objectionable (ANA, 2015a).

Disruptive Behavior, Incivility, and Bullying

In 2008, TJC published a Sentinel Event Alert describing behaviors that undermine a culture of safety. Disruptive behavior includes "overt actions such as verbal outbursts and physical threats, as well as passive activities such as refusing to perform assigned tasks or quietly exhibiting uncooperative attitudes during routine activities" (TJC, 2008, para. 2). Such behavior threatens patient safety and a healthy work environment because of a breakdown in communication and collaboration.

Lateral violence, incivility, and bullying are examples of disruptive behaviors often seen on the nursing unit. Lateral violence refers to acts that occur between nurses. Incivility consists of rude and discourteous actions and includes gossiping and spreading rumors. Bullying is described as unwanted harmful actions intended to humiliate, offend, and cause distress (ANA, 2015c). Bullying can include negative acts perpetrated by one in a higher level of authority, a misuse of power (ANA, 2015c). Lateral violence, incivility, and bullying have a major impact on nursing, including low staff morale; increased absenteeism; attrition; unmanaged anger leading to insomnia, hypertension, depression, and gastrointestinal disorders; and threatened patient care quality (ANA, 2015c). Nurses must treat all individuals with whom they interact with respect and compassion.

The ANA *Code of Ethics for Nurses* asserts that nurses must create an ethical environment and culture of civility and kindness and treat colleagues, coworkers, employees, students, and others with dignity and respect. Further, "disregard for the effects of one's actions on others, bullying, harassment, intimidation, manipulation, threats, or violence are always morally unacceptable behaviors" (ANA, 2015c, p. 4).

Nurses can help combat disruptive behavior by being mindful of their own behavior and stepping in when they see disruptive behavior (ANA, 2015c). Nurse leaders and managers must promote workplace respect and develop and maintain policies and procedures to address disruptive behavior. Disruptive behavior, incivility, and bullying are discussed further in Chapter 12.

End-of-Life Issues

Nurses "actively participate in assuring the responsible and appropriate use of interventions to optimize the health and well-being of those in their care. This includes acting to minimize unwarranted, unwanted, or unnecessary medical treatment and patient suffering" (ANA, 2015a, p. 2). Patients have the ethical and legal right to self-determination and nurses are called to always work in the best interest of the patient. Situations arise where the patient's wishes are known but they are in conflict with the family's wishes and, sometimes, even the healthcare provider's. In such cases, the nurse must respect patient autonomy while supporting the family during the impending death of their loved one. Nurses are obligated help resolve such conflicts, and if the conflict persists, the nurse's commitment is always to the patient (ANA, 2015a). Provisions one, two, and four of the *ANA Code of Ethics for Nurses* address the nurse's primary commitment to the patient and responsibility to respect and honor the patient's right to self-determination, including the right to accept, refuse, and terminate treatment (ANA, 2015a). Common end-of-life issues arise related to advance directives, specifically living wills and do-not-resuscitate (DNR) orders, which are discussed further in Chapter 5.

LEARNING ACTIVITY 4-3

Case Scenario

You are beginning the day shift. The night nurse gives you report on Mr. Hernandez, who is 78 years old and arrived to the emergency department yesterday with shortness of breath. He was admitted to a medical-surgical unit with a diagnosis of pneumonia. Mr. Hernandez's condition deteriorated during the night and he was transferred to the intensive care unit, intubated, and placed on mechanical ventilation. The nurse informs you that Mr. Hernandez requested to complete a living will before he was intubated. At this time, Mr. Hernandez is not responsive. Mrs. Hernandez is at the bedside and tells you that she wants everything done for her husband.

1. How would you respond to Mrs. Hernandez?
2. What ethical principles apply to this situation?

Euthanasia

Euthanasia comes from the Greek words *eu,* which means well, and *thanatos,* which means death, together meaning "a good death." Active euthanasia is the intentional act of causing the immediate death of another, whether the person requested to die or not; passive euthanasia is the intentional act of withholding or withdrawing life-sustaining care (Butts & Rich, 2020).

Active euthanasia is not legal in the United States; however, some confuse it with medical aid in dying or physician-assisted suicide, which is legal in some states. Medical aid in dying is when an individual with a terminal illness and the ability to make decisions is administered oral or enteral medication (self-administer or administered by health professional, family, or friend) that will result in death (ANA, 2019). Medical aid in dying is legal in six states (Washington, Oregon, California, Colorado, Vermont, and Hawaii) and the District of Columbia (Butts & Rich, 2020).

Nurses are obligated "to provide comprehensive and compassionate end-of-life care," which involves establishing individualized care (ANA, 2016b, p. 1). According to the ANA (2019), nurses are called to prevent and alleviate suffering and they must support patients with end-of-life conversations and advocating optimized palliative and hospice care services; however, they are ethically prohibited from administering medical aid in dying (p. 2).

Unsafe or Questionable Practice

The ANA *Code of Ethics for Nurses* directs nurses to intervene when unsafe or questionable practice is witnessed. "Nurses must be alert to and must take appropriate action in all instances of incompetent, unethical, illegal, or impaired practice, or actions that place the rights or best interests of the patient in jeopardy" (ANA, 2015a, p. 12). Examples of unsafe or questionable practice include providing substandard nursing care, neglecting to follow hand washing procedures, failure to follow institutional policy and procedures, and practicing while under the influence of alcohol or drugs. A nurse leader or manager who observes a nurse performing unsafe practice should confront the nurse in an effort to change the practice. After speaking to the nurse, if care continues to be unsafe, a nurse leader or manager must take action (disciplinary action is further discussed in Chapter 11). Nurse leaders and managers must also support staff members who report unsafe practice by listening and acting on the information provided. In some cases, the unsafe practitioner is reprimanded for violating policy and procedure. However, nurse leaders and managers may be required to report the nurse to the state board of nursing if the state's Nurse Practice Act is violated.

Impaired Practice

Impaired practice can result in unsafe practice, and nurses are obligated to protect patients from potential harm if a health-care professional appears to be impaired. "The nurse's duty is to take action to protect patients and to ensure that the impaired individual receives assistance" (ANA, 2015a, p. 13). Nurse leaders and managers have an obligation to ensure policies are in place that support nurses who report impaired practice against retaliation, as well as support the impaired individual by providing access to due legal process and guidance from professional organizations, employee assistance programs, or similar resources (ANA, 2015a).

▶ SUMMARY

There are many ethical aspects of professional nursing. Nurses should use the ANA *Code of Ethics for Nurses* as a guide to everyday clinical practice. In addition, the ANA has numerous position statements that can guide nurses in ethical decision making. Nurses at all levels are obligated to practice with compassion and respect for the dignity and unique attributes of all individuals. Nurse leaders and managers must advocate for policies and systems to preserve patient and employee dignity, values, beliefs, and rights.

NCLEX®-STYLE REVIEW QUESTIONS

Multiple Choice

1. The director of nurses has implemented a new salary scale that does not take into account the educational level of the nurse. The director of nurses may have violated which ethical principle?
   1. Beneficence
   2. Justice
   3. Fidelity
   4. Veracity

2. The director of nursing at the county health department is aware that which ethical theory is most commonly used by nurses in public health agencies?
   1. Deontology
   2. Principlism
   3. Utilitarianism
   4. Principle of duty

3. A staff nurse has been caring for a patient with chronic obstructive pulmonary disease (COPD) through repeated hospitalizations, and his condition continues to get worse despite multiple treatments. The patient states that he is "ready to die" and wants the doctor to "make him a DNR" (do not resuscitate). The doctor refuses to write the order and instead insists that there is a chance the patient will improve and have some quality of life. The nurse notifies the chair of the hospital ethics committee about the situation and knows the doctor will most likely be very upset by this development. What has the nurse displayed by doing this?
   1. Moral distress
   2. Moral courage
   3. Moral uncertainty
   4. Moral trepidation

4. The nurse manager of a medical-surgical unit is discussing conscientious objection at a monthly staff meeting. Which of the following statements by a nurse indicates additional education is needed?
   1. "Acts of conscientious objection cannot be based on personal preferences or bias."
   2. "I must notify my supervisor, in advance if possible, if an assignment is morally objectionable to me."
   3. "I can refuse to care for a patient anytime I feel my moral integrity is in jeopardy."
   4. "I must ensure another nurse can care for my patient to avoid abandonment."

5. A nursing student shares with the clinical instructor that a patient refused to take his blood pressure medication, saying that he normally takes his medication before bedtime. The student asks the instructor if she can make the patient take the medication. The instructor explains to the student that forcing the patient to take his medication in the morning rather than at bedtime would violate which ethical principle?
   1. Fidelity
   2. Justice
   3. Autonomy
   4. Beneficence

6. Which of the following statements best describes beneficence?
   1. Self-determination
   2. To do no harm
   3. One's actions should promote good
   4. Keeping promises to others

7. A patient with terminal pancreatic cancer says to the nurse, "I have decided to stop treatment." Which is the best response by the nurse?
   1. "Are you sure that is the best decision?"
   2. "I will support whatever decision you make."
   3. "You need to discuss this with your doctor first."
   4. "Why don't I call you a chaplain so you can discuss this with him?"

Multiple Response

8. The nurse educator is preparing a group of registered nursing students for graduation and licensure and completes a discussion of the professional values. The students identify which values as part of the five core professional values for nurses? *Select all that apply.*
   1. Integrity
   2. Beneficence
   3. Human dignity
   4. Altruism
   5. Veracity

9. Ethical dilemmas can arise anytime in the clinical setting. When there is an ethical dilemma related to care delivery, who can refer the situation to the ethics committee for consultation? *Select all that apply.*
   1. The nurse assigned to the patient
   2. A family member
   3. A chaplain
   4. The physician caring for the patient
   5. A physical therapist

10. The nurse manager is acting as a staff advocate in which of the following situations? *Select all that apply.*
    1. Assigning a rigid schedule for staff lunch breaks
    2. Implementing a self-scheduling model for staff
    3. Promoting a positive work environment
    4. Reprimanding a nurse for refusing to administer an unsafe dosage of an ordered medication
    5. Encouraging staff to engage in self-care.

REFERENCES

American Association of Colleges of Nursing (AACN). (2008). *The essentials of baccalaureate education for professional nursing practice.* Author. www.aacn.nche.edu/education-resources/baccessentials08.pdf

American Association of Colleges of Nursing. (2021). *The essentials: Core competencies for professional nursing education.* Author. https://www.aacnnursing.org/Portals/42/AcademicNursing/pdf/Essentials-2021.pdf

American Nurses Association (ANA). (2010). *Nursing's social policy statement: The essence of the profession.* Author.

American Nurses Association (ANA). (2015a). *Code of ethics for nurses with interpretive statements.* Author.

American Nurses Association (ANA). (2015b). *Position statement: Risk and responsibility.* Author.

American Nurses Association (ANA). (2015c). *Incivility, bullying, and workplace violence.* https://www.nursingworld.org/practice-policy/nursing-excellence/official-position-statements/id/incivility-bullying-and-workplace-violence/

American Nurses Association (ANA). (2016a). *Nursing administration: Scope and standards of practice* (2nd ed.). Author.

American Nurses Association (ANA). (2016b). *Nurses' roles and responsibilities in providing care and support at the end of life.* https://www.nursingworld.org/practice-policy/nursing-excellence/official-position-statements/

American Nurses Association (ANA). (2019). *The nurse's role when a patient requests medical aid in dying.* https://www.nursingworld.org/practice-policy/nursing-excellence/official-position-statements/

American Organization for Nursing Leadership (AONL). (2015a). *AONL nurse manager competencies.* Author.

American Organization for Nursing Leadership (AONL). (2015b). *AONL nurse executive competencies.* Author.

Bandman, E., & Bandman, B. (2002). *Nursing ethics through the life span* (4th ed.). Prentice Hall.

Beauchamp, T. L., & Childress, J. F. (2019). *Principles of biomedical ethics* (7th ed.). Oxford University Press.

Black, B. P. (2014). *Professional nursing concepts and challenges* (7th ed.). Elsevier.

Burkhardt, M. A., & Nathaniel, A. K. (2014). *Ethics and issues in contemporary nursing* (4th ed.). Thompson Delmar Learning.

Burston, A. S., & Tuckett, A. G. (2012). Moral distress in nursing: Contributing factors, outcomes and interventions. *Nursing Ethics, 20*(3), 312–324.

Butts, J. B., & Rich, K. L. (2020). *Nursing ethics: Across the curriculum and into practice* (5th ed.). Burlington, MA: Jones & Bartlett Learning.

Canadian Nurses Association (CNA). (2017). *2017 edition: Code of ethics for registered nurses.* Author. https://www.cna-aiic.ca/en/search#q=code%20of%20ethics&f:cna-website-facet=[cna]

Cooper, R. J. (2012). Making the case for ethical decision-making models. *Nurse Prescribing, 10*(12), 607–611.

Cronenwett, L., Sherwood, G., Barnsteiner, J., Disch, J., Johnson, J., Mitchell, P., Sullivan, D. T., & Warren, J. (2007). Quality and safety education for nurses. *Nursing Outlook, 55*(3), 122–131.

Davis, A. J., Fowler, M., & Aroskar, M. (2010). *Ethical dilemmas and nursing practice* (5th ed.). Pearson.

de Veer A. J., Francke, A. L. , Struijs, A., Willems, D. L. (2013). Determinants of moral distress in daily nursing practice: a cross sectional correlational questionnaire survey. *International Journal of Nursing Studies, 50*(1), 100-108.

Epstein, E. G., & Delgado, S. (2010). Understanding and addressing moral distress. *OJIN: The Online Journal of Issues in Nursing, 15*(3), 1.

Guido, G. W. (2014). *Legal and ethical issues in nursing* (6th ed.). Pearson.

Greiner, A. C., & Knebel, E. (Ed.) (2003). *Health professions education: A bridge to quality.* National Academies Press.

International Council of Nurses (ICN). (2012). *The ICN code of ethics for nurses.* www.icn.ch/images/stories/documents/about/icncode_english.pdf

Jameton, A. J. (1984). *Nursing practice: The ethical issues.* Prentice-Hall.

Joel, L. A. (2006). *The nursing experience: Trends, challenges, and transitions* (5th ed.). McGraw-Hill.

Johnstone, M.-J. (2016). *Bioethics: A nursing perspective* (6th ed.). Churchill Livingstone Elsevier.

Laabs, C. (2011). Perceptions of moral integrity: Contradictions in need of explanation. *Nursing Ethics, 18*(3), 431–440.

Lachman, V. D. (2010). Clinical ethics committees: Organizational support for ethical practice. *Medsurg Nursing, 19*(6), 351–353.

Lachman, V. D. (2014). Conscientious objection in nursing: Definition and criteria for acceptance. *Medsurg Nursing, 23*(3), 196–198.

Lachman, V. D. (2016). Moral resilience: Managing and preventing moral distress and moral residue. *Medsurg Nursing, 25*(2), 121–124.

LaSala, C. A., & Bjarnason, D. (2010). Creating workplace environments that support moral courage. *OJIN: The Online Journal of Issues in Nursing, 15*(3), 4.

Leng, M., Xiu, H., Yu, P., Feng, J., Wei, Y., Cui, Y., Zhang, M., Zhou, Y., & Wei, H. (2020). Current state and influencing factors of nurse resilience and perceived job-related stressors. *Journal of Continuing Education in Nursing, 51*(3), 132–137.

Murray, E. J. (2003). *Struggling for dignity and respect: Patients' beliefs of their rights while hospitalized in an acute care facility* (Unpublished dissertation). University of Miami.

Murray, J. S. (2010). Moral courage in health care: Acting ethically even in the presence of risk. *OJIN: The Online Journal of Issues in Nursing, 15*(3), 2.

Olson, L. L. (2010). Provision six. In M. D. M. Fowler (Ed.), *Guide to the code of ethics for nurses: Interpretation and application.* American Nurses Association.

Reinhart, R. J. (2020). *Nurses continue to rate highest in honesty, ethics.* Gallup. https://news.gallup.com/poll/274673/nurses-continue-rate-highest-honesty-ethics.aspx

Rushton, C. (2016). Building moral resilience to neutralize moral distress. *American Nurse Today, 11*(10), 1–6. https://www.americannursetoday.com/building-moral-resilience-neutralize-moral-distress/

Rushton, C. H., & Kurtz, M. J. (2015). *Moral distress and you.* American Nurses Association.

Rushton, C. H., Schoonover-Shoffner, K., & Kennedy, M. S. (2017). Executive summary: Transforming moral distress into moral resilience in nursing. *Journal of Christian Nursing, 34*(2), 82-86.

Sakellariouv, A. M. (2015). Virtue ethics and its potential as the leading moral theory. *Discussions, 12*(1). http://www.inquireisjournal.com/a?id=1385

Stievano, A., & Tschudin, V. (2019, May). The ICN code of ethics for nurses: A time for revision. *International Nursing Review.* doi:10.1111/inr.12525

The Joint Commission (TJC). (2008, July 9). Behaviors that undermine a culture of safety. *Sentinel Event Alert, 40.* www.jointcommission.org/assets/1/18/SEA_40.PDF

Tomajan, K. (2012). Advocating for nurses and nurses. *OJIN: The Online Journal of Issues in Nursing, 17*(1), 4.

Turkel, M. C., & Ray, M. A. (2004). Creating a caring practice environment through self-renewal. *Nursing Administration Quarterly, 28*(4), 249–254.

Volbrecht, R. M. (2002). *Nursing ethics: Communities in dialogue.* Prentice-Hall.

To explore learning resources for this chapter, go to FADavis.com

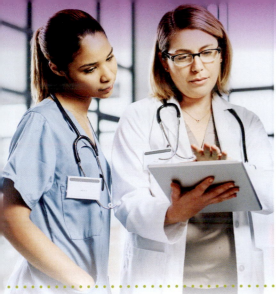

Chapter 5

Legal Aspects of Nursing Practice

Elizabeth J. Murray, PhD, RN, CNE

LEARNING OUTCOMES

- Understand the federal and state regulations that affect health care and nursing.
- Describe federal and state employment laws that nurse leaders and managers must know.
- Describe the five elements of malpractice.
- Discuss areas of potential liability related to the nurse leader and manager's role.
- Analyze the types of legal issues nurse leaders and managers may face.

KEY TERMS

Accountability
Advance directive
Civil law
Confidentiality
Contract law
Criminal law
Informed consent
Liability
Licensure
Malpractice
Negligence
Nursing
Privacy
Respondeat superior
Standard of care
Tort

The Knowledge, Skills, and Attitudes Related to the Following Are Addressed in This Chapter:

Core Competencies
- Patient-Centered Care
- Safety
- Quality Improvement
- Informatics

The Essentials: Core Competencies for Professional Nursing Education (AACN, 2021)

Domain 8: Information and Healthcare Technologies
8.5 Use information and communication technologies in accordance with ethical, legal, professional, and regulatory standards, and workplace policies in the delivery of care (p. 51).
Domain 9: Professionalism
9.4 Comply with relevant laws, policies, and regulations (p. 54).

Code of Ethics with Interpretive Statements (ANA, 2015)

Provision 1.4: The right to self-determination (pp. 2–3)
Provision 3.1: Protection of the rights of privacy and confidentiality (pp. 9–10)
Provision 3.3: Performance standards and review mechanisms (p. 11)
Provision 4.1: Authority, accountability, and responsibility (p. 15)
Provision 4.2: Accountability for nursing judgments, decisions, and actions (pp. 15–16)
Provision 4.3: Responsibility for nursing judgments, decisions, and actions (pp. 16–17)

Nurse Manager (NMC) Competencies (AONL, 2015a) and Nurse Executive (NEC) Competencies (AONL, 2015b

NMC: Human Resource Management (p. 4)
- Scope of practice
  - Develop role definitions for staff consistent with the scope of practice
  - Implement changes in role consistent with scope of practice
NMC: Appropriate Clinical Practice Knowledge (p. 5)
- Each role and institution has expectations regarding the clinical knowledge and skill required of the role.
NMC: Personal and Professional Accountability (p. 7)
- Achieve certification in an appropriate field/specialty
NEC: Knowledge of the Health Care Environment (p. 6)
- Clinical practice knowledge
  - Communicate patient care standards as established by accreditation, regulatory and quality agencies
  - Ensure compliance with the State Nurse Practice Act, State Board of Nursing regulations, state and federal regulatory agency standards, federal labor standards, and policies of the organization

The Knowledge, Skills, and Attitudes Related to the Following Are Addressed in This Chapter:—cont'd

- Adhere to professional association standards of nursing practice
- Integrate bioethical and legal dimensions into clinical and management decision-making
- Health-care economics and policy
  - Use knowledge of federal and state laws and regulations that affect the provision of patient care (e.g., tort reform, malpractice/negligence, reimbursement
- Risk management
  - Identify areas of risk/liability
  - Facilitate staff education on risk management and compliance issues
  - Develop systems that result in prompt reporting of potential liability by staff at all levels
  - Correct areas of potential liability
  - Ensure compliance by staff with all required standards

NEC: Professionalism (p. 9)
- Personal and professional accountability
  - Hold self and other accountable for mutual professional expectations and outcomes
  - Achieve and maintain professional certification for self
  - Role model standards for professional practice (clinical, educational, and leadership) for colleagues and constituents

NEC: Business Skills (p. 11)
- Information management and technology
  - Participate in evaluation of enabling technology in practice settings
  - Identify technological trends, issues, and new developments as they apply to patient care

Nursing Administration Scope and Standards of Practice (ANA, 2016)	**Standard 1: Assessment** The nurse administrator collects pertinent data and information relative to the situation, issue, problem, or trend (pp. 35–36). **Standard 4: Planning** The nurse administrator develops a plan that defines, articulates, and establishes strategies and alternatives to attain expected, measurable outcomes (p. 39). **Standard 9: Communication** The nurse administrator communicates effectively in all areas of practice (p. 49). **Standard 11: Leadership** The nurse administrator leads within professional practice setting, profession, healthcare industry, and society (pp. 51–52). **Standard 12: Education** The nurse administrator attains knowledge and competence that reflect current nursing practice and promotes futuristic thinking (p. 53).

Continued

The Knowledge, Skills, and Attitudes Related to the Following Are Addressed in This Chapter:—cont'd

Standard 14: Quality of Practice The nurse administrator contributes to quality nursing practice (p. 55).

Standard 15: Professional Practice Evaluation The nurse administrator evaluates one's own and others' nursing practice (p. 56).

Source: American Association of Colleges of Nursing. (2021). *The essentials: Core competencies for professional nursing education.* Author; American Nurses Association (ANA). (2015). *Code of ethics for nurses with interpretive statements.* Author; American Nurses Association (ANA). (2016). *Nursing administration: Scope and standards of practice* (2nd ed.). Author; American Organization for Nursing Leadership (AONL). (2015a). *AONL nurse manager competencies.* Author; American Organization for Nursing Leadership (AONL). (2015b). *AONL nurse executive competencies.* Author; Cronenwett, L., Sherwood, G., Barnsteiner, J., Disch, J., Johnson, J., Mitchell, P., Sullivan, D. T., & Warren, J. (2007). Quality and safety education for nurses. *Nursing Outlook, 55*(3), 122–131; and Greiner, A. C., & Knebel, E. (Eds.) (2003). *Health professions education: A bridge to quality.* National Academies Press.

Nurses at all levels must engage in responsible, accountable, and competent nursing practice. In fact, society has a right to expect nurses to consistently demonstrate accountability and competence. Further, nurses have authority, accountability, and responsibility to make decisions that result in safe, quality, and evidence-based nursing practice (American Nurses Association [ANA], 2015a, 2015b). Nurses are licensed and authorized by state nurse practice acts to practice nursing. Therefore, nurses are legally accountable for their own actions and for the actions of those to whom they delegate care. Nurse leaders and managers are responsible and accountable for ensuring that staff members maintain competence and practice within legal and regulatory boundaries. In today's complex health-care system, ethical and legal issues very often become entwined.

In this chapter, nurse leaders and managers learn the legal aspects of nursing practice, including their essential roles in developing, maintaining, and/or monitoring standards, licensure, and regulation of professional nursing practice to ensure safe care and quality outcomes. Additionally, the elements and categories of malpractice along with common legal issues nurse leaders and managers may face are presented.

▶ LEGAL ASPECTS

Nurses are required to demonstrate professional standards of ethical and legal conduct, assume accountability for personal and professional behavior, and adhere to the registered nurse scope and standards of practice (American Association of Colleges of Nursing [AACN], 2021, p.54). **Accountability** is "to be answerable to oneself and others for one's own choices, decisions and actions as measured against a standard" (ANA, 2015a, p. 41), such as those established by the ANA *Code of Ethics for Nurses With Interpretive Standards,* the ANA *Nursing Scope and Standards* *of Practice,* and state nurse practice acts (ANA, 2015a, 2015b). To be accountable, nurses at all levels must embrace an approach to nursing practice that includes application of ethical principles; respect for the dignity, worth, and autonomy of patients; adherence to the scope and standards of nursing practice and legal and regulatory agencies; and fulfillment of society's need for conscientious and qualified nurses (ANA, 2010, 2015b).

Nurse leaders and managers must have a complete understanding of the minimum standards of clinical practice, the requirements of licensure, regulations that affect nursing, federal and/or state legislation in place to protect both health-care workers and their patients, classifications of law that relate to nursing practice, and malpractice. Additionally, nurse leaders and managers are responsible and accountable for ensuring their nursing staff members have the knowledge, skills, and attitudes necessary to perform their professional responsibilities.

Standards of Care for Clinical Practice

All nurses must be aware of the minimum standards of care for nursing practice. **Standards of care** are the degree of quality considered adequate for nursing and include the minimum knowledge, skills, and attitudes required to deliver an acceptable level of nursing care. There are four foundational resources that provide registered nurses in the United States with the critical knowledge needed to inform clinical decision making and guide professional nursing practice:

1. The ANA *Code of Ethics for Nurses With Interpretive Statement* (2015a), which was discussed in Chapter 4, details the ethical standards for nurses in all roles and in all settings.
2. *Nursing's Social Policy Statement: The Essence of the Profession* (ANA, 2010) describes nursing's commitment to society and provides a definition of nursing.
3. *Nursing: Scope and Standards of Practice* (ANA, 2015b) presents the standards of professional nursing practice and accompanying competencies.
4. The nurse practice act (NPA) of the state in which a nurse practices is discussed in greater detail in the next section, "Licensure and Regulation of Nursing Practice."

Nursing's Social Policy Statement: The Essence of the Profession

Nursing's Social Policy Statement defines nursing, describes the role of professional nursing in society and health care, and provides an overview of the essence of nursing practice (ANA, 2010). **Nursing** is defined as "the protection, promotion, and optimization of health and abilities, prevention of illness and injury, alleviation of suffering through the diagnosis and treatment of human response, and advocacy in the care of individuals, families, communities, and populations" (ANA, 2010,

p. 10). The profession of nursing has a contract with society that grants the profession authority and reflects nursing's core values and strong code of ethics. This social contract identifies the profession's active leadership role related to the following six social concerns (ANA, 2010, p. 4–5):

1. Organization, delivery, and financing of quality health care
2. Provision for the public's health
3. Expansion of nursing and health-care knowledge and appropriate application of technology
4. Expansion of health-care resources and health policy
5. Definitive planning for health policy and regulation
6. Duties under extreme conditions

Nurse leaders and managers can use *Nursing's Social Policy Statement* as a foundational resource to reinforce with nursing staff on a regular basis the concepts of autonomy and competence, the scope and standards of nursing practice, and the nursing process. In addition, this resource can provide a basis for developing a unit vision, mission, and philosophy, as well as strategic planning.

Nursing: Scope and Standards of Practice

To provide a complete picture of the dynamic and complex nature of nursing practice, the "who, what, when, where, why, and how" of nursing practice must be detailed (ANA, 2015b). *Nursing: Scope and Standards of Practice* answers each of these questions and "describes a competent level of nursing practice and professional performance common to all registered nurses" (ANA, 2015b, p. 1). This document delineates the professional scope and standards of practice and responsibilities of all registered nurses in all settings and serves as a basis for the following (ANA, 2015b, pp. 49–50):

- Quality improvement systems
- Health-care reimbursement and financing methodologies
- Development and evaluation of nursing service delivery systems and organizational structures
- Certification activities
- Position descriptions and performance appraisals
- Agency policies, procedures, and protocols
- Educational offerings
- Regulatory systems
- Establishing the legal standard of care

As nurses have evolved from novice to expert clinicians, specialized education and certifications in various clinical specialties have emerged (ANA, 2015b). All nurses are educated in the art and science of nursing, but some may also develop expertise in a specialty area. ANA works with specialty nursing organizations to outline the components of professional nursing practice essential for any particular specialty (ANA, 2010). The competencies identified for an individual specialty area of practice may be defined by separate specialty scope and standard documents (ANA, 2010). Nurses who seek specialization must ensure they are familiar with the specific scope and standards related to their specialty. Nurse leaders and managers rely on the *Scope and Standards of Practice* to ensure that staff members provide safe and competent care.

Licensure and Regulation of Nursing Practice

Health care in the United States is a highly regulated industry. Nursing care can pose a risk of harm to the public if practiced by professionals who are unprepared or incompetent. Federal and state governments have a responsibility to protect those receiving health care through licensure of individuals and regulation of health-care organizations.

Licensure

Licensure is the process by which boards of nursing grant permission to an individual to engage in nursing practice after determining that the applicant has the necessary competencies (National Council of State Boards of Nursing [NCSBN], 2020). In the United States and Canada, nursing licensure is mandatory. In the United States, the basic requirements for a nursing license are graduating from an approved nursing program and successfully passing the National Council Licensing Examination for Registered Nurses (NCLEX-RN®), developed by the NCSBN. Nursing licensure assures the public that those calling themselves nurses have met regulatory standards specific to the nursing profession. Licensure is a way to hold nurses who violate nurse practice acts and standards of practice accountable for their actions and ensures that foreign-educated nurses have met U.S. standards (NCSBN, 2011a). Nurse leaders and managers must verify and monitor licensure of all nursing staff.

Regulation

The nursing profession ensures that members act in the public's best interest when providing nursing care through professional regulation, self-regulation, and legal regulation (ANA, 2010). Professional regulation consists of the oversight, monitoring, and controlling of members based on principles, guidelines, and rules deemed standard in the profession. Self-regulation is personal accountability for one's professional nursing practice based on those same principles, guidelines, and rules; nurses regulate their own practice by maintaining current knowledge, skills, and attitudes through academic and continuing education. Legal regulation consists of oversight and monitoring based on applicable statutes and regulations such as licensure, nurse practice acts, civil law, and criminal law (ANA, 2010). Federal and state regulations are overseen by administrative agencies; two of the most important are the NCSBN and the state boards of nursing.

State Nurse Practice Acts

All states and territories of the United States have enacted a nurse practice act (NPA) through state legislature. Each NPA establishes a board of nursing that has the authority to develop rules and regulations to clarify the law. The rules and regulations must be consistent with the NPA and undergo a process of public review before enacted (Russell, 2017). All NPAs include the following (Russell, 2017 p, 19):

- Definitions
- Authority, power, and composite of a state board of nursing
- Education program standards
- Requirements for licensure
- Types of titles and licenses
- Protection of titles
- Scope and standards of nursing practice
- Grounds for disciplinary action, other violations, and possible remedies

Nurses are accountable for the rules and regulations that govern nursing practice in any state in which they work. Therefore, it is nurses' responsibility to ensure that they have a good understanding of their state's NPA. Nurse leaders and managers have a responsibility to ensure that nursing staff members comply with the state NPA.

LEARNING ACTIVITY 5-1	**Check Your State Nurse Practice Act**

Review your state's nurse practice act. You can find your state's NPA here: https://www.ncsbn.org/npa.htm

1. Can you identify the key elements recommended by the NCSBN?
2. How does it reflect the *ANA Nursing Scope and Standards of Practice*?

National Council of State Boards of Nursing

Besides developing the NCLEX-RN®, the NCSBN is responsible for promoting uniformity of nursing regulation. The NCSBN is a not-for-profit organization whose membership consists of a board of nursing members from the United States, the District of Columbia, and the U.S. territories of American Samoa, Guam, Northern Mariana Islands, Puerto Rico, and the Virgin Islands. The purpose of the NCSBN is to provide an organization that empowers and supports nursing regulators in their mandate to protect the public (NCSBN, 2020, para. 1). The NCSBN also maintains a national database on disciplinary action taken against nurses, the National Practitioner Data Bank. Important information about NCSBN, licensure, and the NCLEX-RN® can be found at www.ncsbn.org.

State Boards of Nursing

State boards of nursing protect the public by enforcing the NPA to promote safe, competent nursing care. The role of the state board of nursing varies by state but typically includes the following (NCSBN, 2011a):

- Enforcing the state's NPA and nurse licensure
- Accrediting or approving nursing education programs

- Developing practice standards, policies, and administrative rules and regulations
- Addressing violations of the NPA

Unsafe or incompetent nursing practice should be reported to the state board of nursing. Violations of the NPA or unsafe nursing practice is taken seriously. The state board of nursing reviews each case to determine whether misconduct or unsafe practice has occurred and what actions should be taken. Examples of serious reportable behaviors that violate the NPA include the following (NCSBN, 2018a, p. 4):

- Being impaired by drugs or alcohol while working
- Stealing from a patient, including medications
- Practicing out of the scope of practice, such as providing treatment that should be provided only by a physician or advanced practice registered nurse
- Falsifying records
- Boundary issues, including physically or sexually abusing a patient
- Not following accepted standards of care while caring for patients
- Participating in criminal conduct

Nurse leaders and managers are responsible for understanding the state board of nursing regulations and the state NPA.

Federal and/or State Legislation

Many federal and state laws have been implemented to improve health care and, in turn, affect nursing practice.

Health Insurance Portability and Accountability Act

The Health Insurance Portability and Accountability Act (HIPAA) was enacted in 1996 to improve portability and continuity of health insurance coverage; combat waste, fraud, and abuse in health insurance and health-care delivery; promote the use of medical savings accounts; improve access to long-term care coverage and services; simplify the administration of health insurance; and protect individuals from wrongful disclosure of identifiable health information (HIPAA, 1996).

The privacy regulations extend coverage to all forms of personal records, require consent for routine use and disclosure of health records, protect against unauthorized use of medical records for employment purposes, and ensure that health-care providers have necessary information to treat their patients. The privacy and confidentiality regulations went into effect in 2003, with the primary purpose to improve efficiency and effectiveness of health-care systems by standardizing the electronic exchange of administrative and financial data (United States Department of Health and Human Services [USDHHS], 2003).

The HIPAA Privacy, Security, and Breach Notification Rules protect the privacy of health information and provide individuals with rights to their health information. The Privacy Rule protects all identifiable health information or protected health information (PHI). PHI includes information that relates to an individual's past, present, or future physical or mental health or condition; the provision of health care to the individual; or the past, present, or future payment for the provision of health care to the individual (USDHHS, 2018, pp. 1–2). Common examples of PHI are patient identifiers such as name, address, Social Security number, birthdate, gender, insurance company name, and medical diagnosis. The Security Rule outlines specific safeguards that covered entities and associates must implement to protect confidentiality, integrity, and availability of electronic protected health information (ePHI) (USDHHS, 2018, pp. 1–3). When a breach of HIPAA occurs, the Breach Notification Rule requires entities to notify the affected individuals; USDHHS; and, in some cases, the media of the breach of unsecured PHI (USDHHS, 2018, pp. 1, 3-4). Basic information for health-care providers is available at https://www.cms.gov/Outreach-and-Education/Medicare-Learning-Network-MLN/MLNProducts/Downloads/HIPAAPrivacyandSecurity.pdf.

A HIPAA violation occurs when PHI is inappropriately used or is disclosed to a person not involved in the patient's care, to a person who does not require the information to provide care, or in a situation in which disclosure is not in the patient's best interest (McGowan, 2012). Violations of HIPAA can result in substantial fines and prison sentences. Nurse leaders and managers must ensure that patient information remains private and confidential.

Patient Self-Determination Act

Congress passed the Patient Self-Determination Act (PSDA) in 1990 to ensure that health-care organizations inform patients about their rights and institutional policies to accept or refuse treatment and to prepare advance directives (Beauchamp & Childress, 2019). The basic premise of the PSDA is to promote patients as active participants in health-care decisions, thus increasing patient autonomy. The PSDA requires hospitals and other health-care agencies serving Medicare and Medicaid patients to develop and maintain written policies and procedures and to provide written information to adults receiving health care. Materials must describe the following:

- The individual's right under the law to make decisions about medical care, including the right to accept or refuse medical and surgical treatment.
- The individual's right under state law to dictate advance directives such as living wills or durable power of attorney for health care.
- The policies and procedures that the institution has developed to honor these rights. Institutions must specify how the advance directives are to be identified, recorded, and retrieved when needed.

The legislation requires institutions to provide educational programs on advance directives for their staff and communities. The PSDA prohibits staff from conditioning the provision of care or discriminating against individuals in other ways because they do or do not have advance directives. Hospitals and nursing homes must provide all newly admitted patients with written information detailing these policies and procedures, and home health and hospice agencies must provide information when the individual begins to receive care from the agency (PSDA, 1990).

Safe Medical Devices Act

The Safe Medical Devices Act (SMDA) was enacted in 1990 and amended in 1992 to require health-care agencies to report to the Food and Drug Administration (FDA) serious injuries, illness, or death resulting from the use of a medical device (SMDA, 1990). A medical device is any medical product that is not absorbed in the body. When a serious injury, illness, or death occurs, the SMDA requires health-care agencies to report to the FDA within 10 days of the event the following information: name, serial number, and model of the device; name and address of the manufacturer; and a brief description of the event. A nurse's responsibility related to an incident involving a medical device covered under the SMDA includes the following (Brent, 2001):

- Discontinue the use of the device immediately.
- Follow your agency's policies related to equipment use.
- Document the incident accurately in the medical record, on an incident report, and on any agency-specific forms.
- Record the identification number of the device in the medical record and other forms on a regular basis.

Nurse leaders and managers are responsible for making certain that policies and procedures related to equipment use are in place. Further, should equipment malfunction, nurse leaders and managers must facilitate processes to sequester the equipment to ensure patient safety.

Good Samaritan Laws

All states have enacted Good Samaritan laws to encourage health-care professionals to render care in emergencies. Good Samaritan laws protect anyone who renders care during an emergency or disaster or at the scene of an accident as long as care is provided at the scene of the emergency, care is not grossly negligent, appropriate standards of care are used, and care is rendered without pay (Aiken, 2004; Guido, 2014). Good Samaritan protection is necessary because, although many may feel a moral duty, health-care professionals are not legally obligated to render care to a stranger in an emergency. Good Samaritan laws vary from state to state, so nurses must become familiar with the law in their state.

Disclosure Statutes

Federal and state laws require disclosure of health-related information to appropriate government agencies to protect the public (Guido, 2014). Nurses as well as other health-care professionals must report suspected child neglect and suspected child abuse to the state-designated officials. Health-care providers are protected from liability if they report suspected child abuse or neglect in good faith but an investigation determines the report is groundless (Guido, 2014). Conversely, failure to report suspected child abuse or neglect could result in liability. Some states also require mandatory reporting of suspected abuse of dependent adults and older adults. Nurses should check their state laws to know the mandatory disclosure requirements.

Additionally, some communicable diseases and sexually transmitted diseases must be reported to local or state public health officials. Health-care workers should follow their agency's policies and reporting procedures. In a community setting, it is critical that information is reported to the proper agency. An example of the importance of reporting communicable diseases occurred during the Coronavirus Disease 2019 (COVID-19) pandemic in 2019–2021. The Centers for Disease Control and Prevention (CDC) worked with local, regional, national, and global agencies to attempt to protect society from the threat COVID-19 presented. The process of case surveillance was implemented, which is critically important with new diseases to understand the similarities and differences among cases, including the following (CDC, 2020, para. 1):

- Demographic, clinical, and epidemiological characteristics
- Exposure and contact history
- Course of clinical illness and care received

Under mandatory disclosure laws, frontline nurses collect the information and must report to the state or local health department. Whereas case reporting is mandatory by the state, reporting to the CDC includes "de-identifying" data and is voluntary (CDC, 2020, para. 4).

A list of reportable diseases is updated annually and is available through the Centers for Disease Control National Notifiable Diseases Surveillance System at https://wwwn.cdc.gov/nndss/conditions/notifiable/2020/.

Employment Laws

Federal and state governments are responsible to enact laws that protect employees from unfair treatment, discrimination, and unsafe work conditions. Because nurses make up the largest labor force in the health-care industry, nurse leaders and managers must keep up to date concerning the laws and regulations that are aimed at protecting the nursing workforce. Table 5-1 is a summary of important federal employment laws of which nurse leaders and managers must be aware.

Classifications of Law That Relate to Nursing Practice

In the United States, the major classifications of law that apply to nursing practice are contract law, criminal law, and civil law.

A voluntary agreement between or among two or more competent people is the basis for **contract law**. The contract creates an obligation for a person to do or not to do something and creates enforceable rights or legal duties (e.g., an employer-employee agreement) (Brent, 2001).

Criminal law relates to conduct that is harmful to society as a whole as well as to an individual victim. Crimes are classified as either a misdemeanor, which is punishable by fines or imprisonment for less than 1 year, or a felony, a more

Table 5-1	Common Federal Employment Legislation Nurse Managers and Leaders Must Know
Federal Legislation	**Protection**
Age Discrimination in Employment Act (ADEA) of 1967, P.L. 90-202	Prohibits discrimination against a person 40 years or older when forming an employment relationship or promotion
Americans With Disabilities Act (ADA) of 1990, P.L. 101-336; Amendments Act, 2008, P.L. 110-325	Prohibits discrimination against a person with mental or physical impairment in the workplace and requires the employer to make reasonable accommodations to allow employees to perform essential job functions
Civil Rights Act of 1964, 1991 P.L. 82-352	Prohibits discrimination on the basis of race, national origin, or lineage when forming an employment relationship; amended in 1991 to define sexual harassment and the employer's responsibility related to it
Consolidated Omnibus Budget Reconciliation Act (COBRA) of 1985, P.L. 99-272	Ensures employees and their families have health-care coverage for a specified time after employment is terminated, hours are reduced, or an employee becomes eligible for Medicare
Emergency Medical Treatment and Labor Act (EMTALA) of 1986, 2003, P.L. 95-452	Establishes a right of access to emergency medical care regardless of a person's citizenship, age, or ability to pay; amended in 2003 to expand the definition of an emergency patient to include persons a reasonably prudent person would believe had an emergency medical condition and to include the rule that if a person refuses medical treatment, every effort must be made to obtain the refusal in writing
Family and Medical Leave Act (FMLA) of 1993, P.L. 103-3	Maintains job protection for an individual for up to 12 weeks of unpaid leave per year for an employee to care for an ill family member, after adoption, or for their own health
False Claims Amendments Act of 1986, P.L. 99-562	Also called the "Whistleblower Law," protects employees from retaliation and threats against discharge when the employee, in good faith, reports a violation of federal or state laws or rules
Occupational Safety and Health Act of 1970, P.L. 91-595	Ensures safe and healthy work conditions for employees and protects employees from workplace hazards such as blood and body fluid exposure, hazardous materials, and fires

serious offense punishable by imprisonment for more than 1 year or death. Examples of misdemeanors in health care include a nurse failing to report suspected child abuse or dependent adult abuse (Allen, 2013) or an individual using the title "nurse" or "registered nurse" without being duly licensed or certified. Examples of felonies in health care include some HIPAA violations and diversion of controlled substances from a health-care facility. In addition, some violations of the state NPA can be charged as a felony (e.g., using or attempting to use a nursing license that has been suspended or revoked).

Civil law pertains to the rights and duties of private citizens and is enforced through the courts as damages or monetary compensation. Tort law is the foundation of civil law and is the most common type of law that affects health-care professionals (Guido, 2014). A **tort** is a civil wrong committed against another person or a person's property and includes personal injury inflicted on another through actions of commission or omission. The law allows the injured person to seek monetary compensation for injuries at the expense of the wrongdoer (Brent, 2001). The three types of torts are as follows:

1. *Intentional torts:* Willful acts that are intentional and cause injury. An intentional tort is a direct violation of a person's legal rights and includes assault, battery, false imprisonment, and fraud.
2. *Quasi-intentional torts:* Willful acts that cause injury but are unintentional torts. A quasi-intentional tort typically involves communication issues that result in defamation of character, violation of personal privacy, or breach of confidentiality (Aiken, 2004).
3. *Unintentional torts:* Careless acts or accidents that cause injury. Negligence and malpractice are examples of unintentional torts.

Table 5-2 summarizes the three types of torts as they relate to nursing practice.

Negligence and Malpractice

As mentioned, torts are the most frequent causes of legal action taken against health-care professionals, and, of those, the unintentional torts of negligence and

Table 5-2   Three Types of Torts and How They Relate to Nursing Practice

Torts	Description	Examples in Nursing Practice
Intentional Torts		
Assault	Intentionally threatening a patient with physical harm	Threatening to restrain a patient if they get out of bed
Battery	Physically harming a patient	Holding down a patient to insert a catheter against the patient's wishes
False imprisonment	Intentional confinement of a patient	Restraining a competent patient against their wishes
Fraud	Intentional misrepresentation that results in an illegal benefit to self or others	Billing a patient for services not rendered
Quasi-Intentional Torts		
Defamation of character	Intentional written defamation (libel) or oral defamation (slander) of a patient	Charting that a patient is acting crazy (libel); telling another nurse you think a patient is crazy (slander)
Violation of privacy	Intentional intrusion into a patient's privacy	Looking up your neighbor's blood work on the hospital computer system
Breach of confidentiality	Intentional sharing of a patient's private health-care information they have shared with you	Posting information about a patient's medical status on Facebook
Unintentional Torts		
Negligence	Failing to perform an action that a reasonably prudent nurse would do in a similar situation	Failure to assess a patient's IV site according to standard of care
Malpractice (professional negligence)	Unintentional injury to a patient as the result of a breach of duty	Failure to prevent injury to a patient because the IV became infiltrated

malpractice are the most common. **Negligence** is a deviation from the standard behavior or actions that an average, prudent person would use in a similar situation. Although often used interchangeably with *negligence,* **malpractice** is a more specific term and addresses a professional standard of care. Malpractice, also known as *professional negligence,* is a deviation from the standard of care that a reasonably prudent health-care professional would use in a similar situation. In other words, when a nurse is charged with professional negligence, the nurse's action or lack of action is compared with what another ordinary, reasonable, and prudent nurse would do under the same or similar circumstances.

Elements of Malpractice

Five essential elements must be present for malpractice to be charged (Reisling, 2012):

1. Duty owed the patient
2. Breach of the duty owed the patient
3. Foreseeability of harm
4. Causation
5. Injury or harm

If one of these elements is missing, the malpractice claim will not be successful.

Duty Owed the Patient

The basis of the duty owed is the nurse–patient relationship, which implies that the patient is dependent on the nurse for safe and quality nursing care. Nurses are obligated to deliver care according to established standards based on the nursing process and that represent the minimum requirement for acceptable nursing practice. For example, a standard of care related to medication administration is to check the patient's medical record for allergies. When administering medications to patients, nurses have a duty to follow this standard and always check for allergies.

Breach of the Duty Owed the Patient

Nurses must deliver care according to a standard of care that a reasonably prudent nurse under similar circumstances would use. A breach of duty results when care deviates from the standard. Using the previous scenario, if a patient is allergic to penicillin and a nurse did not check the patient's medical record for allergies before administering penicillin, the nurse breached the standard of care and thus the duty owed to the patient.

Foreseeability of Harm

Certain actions can be expected to have specific consequences. A nurse must have knowledge about the standard of care and understand that failure to meet the standard may result in harm or injury. For example, all nurses learn safe medication administration in foundational nursing courses. All nurses know that neglecting to check the medical record for allergies before administering a medication could result in harm to a patient.

Causation

Any injury that occurs is directly a result of the breach of duty owed to the patient. In other words, the failure to meet the standard of care by action or lack of action caused harm or injury to the patient. If the patient in the scenario develops an allergic reaction after the nurse administers the penicillin, there is a cause-and-effect relationship between failure to check allergies on the medical record and the resultant allergic reaction.

Injury or Harm

Some type of physical injury must result from the breach of duty. Administration by the nurse of penicillin to the patient who is allergic could have several sequelae:

1. Nothing happens, and therefore the five elements of malpractice are not present.
2. The patient develops a mild allergic reaction that is not severe and recovers without incident. Again, the five elements of malpractice are not present.
3. The patient develops anaphylactic shock and dies. In this case, all elements of malpractice are present, and the nurse is liable for malpractice.

LEARNING ACTIVITY 5-2   **A Legal Situation**

Lisa is a registered nurse assisting Bethany, also a registered nurse, insert an intravenous (IV) catheter. Lisa observes Bethany stick herself with the sterile IV catheter, thus contaminating the IV catheter. Lisa mentions her observation to Bethany and offers to get another IV catheter. Bethany says, "It's no big deal," and inserts the IV catheter anyway.

1. How should Lisa advocate for the patient?
2. Are the elements of malpractice present in this situation?
3. Who is at fault if the patient develops an infection at the IV site?
4. What actions should the nurse leader and manager take in this situation?
5. Is there also an ethical issue in this situation? What provision of the *ANA Code of Ethics* could apply to this situation?

Major Categories of Malpractice

Malpractice suits against nurses have increased since 2000 and continue to rise (Guido, 2014; Reisling, 2012). Research indicates that six common categories of nursing practice have the potential for negligence and possible malpractice (Croke, 2003; Reisling, 2012):

1. Failure to assess and monitor
2. Failure to follow standards of care
3. Failure to communicate
4. Failure to document
5. Failure to act as a patient advocate
6. Failure to use equipment in a responsible manner

(See Exploring the Evidence 5-1.) Failing to perform these actions can constitute negligence if the required elements are present.

Failure to Assess and Monitor

The ANA resource, *Nursing: Scope and Standards of Practice,* describes a competent level of nursing practice and professional performance common to all registered nurses in all settings regardless of role—in other words, the minimum requirement for acceptable nursing practice. According to these standards, "The registered nurse collects pertinent data and information relative to the health-care consumer's health or situation" (ANA, 2015b, p. 53). Nurses must be accurate in assessing, monitoring, and reporting changes in health status. Failure to complete a shift assessment, implement a plan of care, observe a patient's progress, or accurately interpret a patient's signs and symptoms can be considered negligence.

Failure to Follow Standards of Care

The ANA standards are "authoritative statements of the duties that all registered nurses, regardless of role, population, or specialty are expected to perform competently" (ANA, 2015b, p. 51). Nurses must be knowledgeable about their state's NPA and standards of care, hospital policies and procedures, and institution's standardized protocols. Failure to follow standards of care or hospital policies can be considered negligence. Violating the state NPA can also have legal implications.

Failure to Communicate

According to the ANA (2015b) standards, "The registered nurse communicates effectively in all areas of practice" (p. 71). Nurses must communicate effectively the nature and degree of any changes in a patient's progress. Failure to listen to a patient and act on their concerns or failure to ensure effective teaching of self-care or discharge instructions to a patient can be considered negligence.

Failure to Document

Documentation is a critical competency for quality and safe nursing practice and is related to all ANA standards of practice (ANA, 2015b). Documentation must accurately reflect the nursing process. Failure to document pertinent assessment information or a patient's response to nursing interventions can be considered negligence.

Failure to Act as a Patient Advocate

Advocacy is a fundamental aspect of professional nursing practice and is related to all ANA standards of practice (ANA, 2015b). Nurses at all levels are patient advocates, and as such they must support and promote patient rights. Failure to act on incompetent practice, question illegible medical orders, or provide a safe environment for patients can be considered negligence. Similarly, the nurse leaders and managers must support and promote nurses' rights. Failure to advocate for their staff members to ensure they have adequate resources, a culture of safety, and a healthy workplace to provide safe and quality care can be considered negligence.

Failure to Use Equipment in a Responsible Manner

Patient safety is a priority in health care today. Nurses are responsible for coordinating and implementing plans of care in accordance with patient safety goals. Nurses must know how equipment functions, follow manufacturer's guidelines for operation, check the equipment for safety before use, and place equipment properly during treatment. There is no substitute for nursing knowledge and skill. Therefore, nurses remain "accountable for their practice even in instances of system of equipment technology failures" (ANA, 2015a, p. 16). Failure to handle equipment in a safe manner can be considered negligence.

EXPLORING THE EVIDENCE 5-1

Croke, E. M. (2003). Nurses, negligence, and malpractice: An analysis based on more than 250 cases against nurses. *American Journal of Nursing, 103*(9), 54–63.

Aim

This article aimed to identify the actions and issues that led to charges of professional negligence against nurses and to identify areas of nursing practice most frequently cited.

Methods

A total of 253 cases that involved charges of negligence and malpractice against nurses from 1998 through 2001 were analyzed to identify the actions that prompted the legal charges and the areas of nursing practice most frequently identified in the complaints.

Key Findings

The six areas of negligence that most frequently resulted in professional negligence were as follows:

1. Failure to assess and monitor
2. Failure to follow standards of care
3. Failure to communicate
4. Failure to document
5. Failure to act as a patient advocate
6. Failure to use equipment in a responsible manner

Implications for Nurse Leaders and Managers

Nurse leaders and managers must ensure that they, as well as their staff, are aware of current standards of practice, rules and regulation, ethical guidelines, and organizational policies and procedures. In addition, they must ensure that nurses provide safe competent care that follows the nursing process. Nurse leaders and managers must promote effective intraprofessional and interprofessional communication, which includes accurate documentation of nursing care. Finally, nurse leaders and managers are responsible to verify that staff members are properly educated and competent to use all equipment in a responsible manner.

Expert Witnesses

In nursing negligence cases, the federal court and all state courts in the United States require expert nurse witnesses designated by the prosecution and the defense to establish the standard of care (Myers & Boutier, 2011). The role of the nurse expert witness is to help educate the jury regarding the nurse's actions in the particular case and the applicable standard of care (Brent, 2001; Guido, 2014). Three factors are critical to selecting the best nurse expert witness: The nurse expert must have the necessary qualifications, must have experience testifying in the role, and must be able to testify accurately and with confidence. It is also important to note that the expert nurse witness has no relationship with the defendant or the defendant's institution (Guido, 2014).

Liability

In the case of nursing negligence, **liability** refers to the nurse's responsibility for a possible or actual loss, penalty, burden, or expense that the law requires the nurse to compensate the victim (Brent, 2001). Personal liability defines a nurse's accountability for professional actions to patients and families, peers, themselves, and ultimately, society (ANA, 2010). In other words, a nurse is accountable for their behavior, including negligent behavior.

The doctrine of **respondeat superior**, Latin for "let the master answer," holds employers accountable for the negligent actions of their employees, or vicarious liability (Guido, 2014). Nurse leaders and managers can avoid issues of vicarious liability by ensuring that staff members are qualified and competent to perform their assigned duties and that they consistently follow policies and procedures. Nurses are accountable for actions delegated to others assisting in providing nursing care. Therefore, nurses may also have vicarious liability related to delegation. Chapter 14 examines delegation in more detail. Nurse leaders and managers can be considered negligent when they do not fulfill specific responsibilities such as the following (Guido, 2014):

- *Failure to orient, educate, and evaluate:* Nurse leaders and managers have an ongoing duty to ensure that nurses are performing safe and competent care. This duty requires nurse leaders and managers to respond promptly to any concerns about unsafe or questionable nursing care. They must act immediately to investigate a situation, correct the situation, and evaluate the nurses involved. On a thorough investigation, nurse leaders and managers must follow up and document in the nurses' employment records as evidence that the nurse is competent to practice in the clinical setting.
- *Inappropriate assigning of staff and failure to supervise:* Major responsibilities of nurse leaders and managers include delegation, assignments, and supervision of staff. Nurse leaders and managers retain liability when making assignments and delegating tasks; therefore, they must be knowledgeable about staff education, qualifications, and experiences.
- *Unsafe staffing:* Many state and federal legislation as well as regulatory agencies mandate adequate and safe staffing in health-care institutions. Nurse leaders and managers must address any unsafe staffing issues.

- *Negligent retention practices:* Nurse leaders and managers have a duty not to allow staff members to continue to work if they consistently function below the acceptable standard of care.
- *Failure to warn:* Nurse leaders and managers must provide factual and objective information to subsequent employers. Failure to warn potential employers of employee incompetence or substance misuse can lead to potential liability.

The challenges for nurse leaders and managers include determining and providing for educational needs, assessing competency, providing appropriate evaluations essential to enhance patient safety, and minimizing organizational liability.

Professional Liability Insurance

All nurses are vulnerable to malpractice claims. A malpractice suit can have a significant negative impact on a nurse's life, both emotionally and financially. Professional liability insurance protects nurses against lawsuits related to alleged errors that occur while delivering nursing care. Professional liability insurance benefits include payment for the cost of legal advice and representation, payment for court costs, settlement, and reimbursement for lost wages incurred during a malpractice trial. Nurses can be covered by an individual insurance policy, under an employer-sponsored institutional policy, or as a member of a group such as a nurse-owned corporation (Aiken, 2004; Guido, 2014). Health-care institutions typically carry employer-sponsored insurance and cover nurses with representation should the need arise. However, insurance provided by a health-care institution limits protection of the nurse to only activities performed within the scope of employment. In addition, if a nurse is sued for malpractice and as a result the employer pays for damages caused by the nurse's action or inaction, the employer can sue the nurse to be paid back (Aiken, 2004). Therefore, it is in a nurse's best interest to carry their own malpractice insurance. "An individual policy provides the nurse with 24-hour protection regardless of job description and setting" (Aiken, 2004, p. 406). The nurse would be protected when engaging in nursing activities such as volunteer work, consulting, private duty, and administering care to a neighbor (Aiken, 2004).

There are numerous arguments against nurses' having professional liability insurance. A common argument is that if a nurse is found liable and has their own insurance policy, the monetary award will be higher. This is a fallacy because, to avoid prejudice and ensure justice, neither judge nor jury can be informed about insurance coverage (Guido, 2014). Another common argument is that the patient will more likely bring a lawsuit if they know that a nurse has insurance. However, a patient would know whether a nurse has their own insurance policy only if the nurse tells the patient. Whether a nurse has insurance coverage has no bearing on whether or not a patient will sue. The bottom line is that having professional liability insurance will not protect a nurse from a lawsuit, but it will help the nurse with attorney fees, court costs, and the financial obligations if a nurse is found negligent (Guido, 2014).

▶ PRACTICE ISSUES

Some issues nurse leaders and managers face may be viewed from both an ethical and a legal perspective. In these cases, nurse leaders and managers must have a good understanding of the ethical principles that guide nursing practice as well as the laws and regulations that govern health care, nursing practice, and employment.

Advance Directives

According to the ANA *Code of Ethics for Nurses,* nurses have an obligation to be knowledgeable about the moral and legal rights of their patients regarding self-determination (ANA, 2015a). The PSDA, discussed earlier, mandates that all patients have the opportunity to initiate an **advance directive**, which is a document that provides information about a person's desires should they become unable to make health-care decisions. In other words, an advance directive provides directions to family and health-care professionals by a person in advance of becoming ill and incapacitated. Nurses and other health-care professionals have an ethical and legal duty to respect a patient's advance directive. Nurses can be held liable for violating a patient's advance directive and could be charged with battery and malpractice. A nurse's responsibilities related to advance directives include the following:

- Initiating discussion with a patient about advance directives
- Providing a patient with written information about advance directives
- Communicating the presence of an advance directive to all members of the health-care team
- Ensuring that advance directives are current and accurately reflect the patient's wishes

Establishing an advance directive or having discussions with families about life-sustaining care can reduce the burden of decision making for loved ones (Hickman & Pinto, 2013). In addition, advance directives can assist with the delivery of patient-centered care. (See Exploring the Evidence 5-2.) There are three types of advance directives:

- A living will
- A do not resuscitate (DNR) order
- A durable power of attorney for health care

Nurse leaders and managers may find themselves advocating for patients and families regarding advance directives. They must ensure that information about advance directives is clear, accessible, and adequate. Further, nurse leaders and managers must provide support for nursing staff when situations arise that may affect a patient's right to self-determination.

Living Will

A living will is a legal document that details a person's wishes regarding health-care treatments and procedures in the event the person becomes incapacitated and is facing end of life. Living wills are legal in all states, but elements or what is allowed may vary. Nurses must be familiar with the statutes related to living wills in the state and organization in which they practice.

Do Not Resuscitate

A DNR order indicates the life-sustaining measures that should be withheld in the event of impending death. In some instances, an allow natural death (AND) order is initiated, which means that only comfort measures will be provided. As patient advocates, nurses play an active role in initiating discussions about DNR and AND orders with patients, families, and members of the health-care team (ANA, 2020). There are ethical issues related to DNR that were discussed in Chapter 4.

Durable Power of Attorney for Health Care

A durable power of attorney for health care is a legal document that identifies a health-care surrogate. The surrogate is a person designated to make health-care decisions for another person, should that person become incapacitated. The health-care surrogate should have a clear understanding of the person's wishes regarding health care and be willing to respect those wishes even if they do not agree. By participating in discussions with surrogates, providing guidance and referrals, and identifying problems in the decision-making process, nurses will support patient self-determination (ANA, 2015a).

Nurse leaders and managers must ensure that policies and procedures support the appropriate use of interventions to minimize patient suffering and optimize end-of-life nursing care. They must advocate for compassionate systems of care delivery that preserve and protect patient and family dignity, rights, values, beliefs, and autonomy (ANA, 2016, p. 45).

Confidentiality and Information Security

Every patient has an ethical and legal right to privacy and confidentiality. Nurses are bound by their code of ethics to respect patients' privacy and confidentiality, which includes ensuring patient information is secure at all times.

Privacy

The principle of **privacy** refers to a person's right to have control over access to their personal information. Privacy is not just an ethical principle but also a legal right and is protected by HIPAA (discussed earlier). Patients confide in nurses and trust them with personal information. Nurses, in turn, must respect patients' privacy and discuss patient information only with other health-care professionals and only on a need-to-know basis. Nurse leaders and managers promote patient privacy when they create an environment that allows for physical and auditory privacy for discussion of patient information and establish policies and

EXPLORING THE EVIDENCE 5-2

Hickman, R. L., & Pinto, M. D. (2013). Advance directives lessen the decisional burden of surrogate decision-making for the chronically ill. *Journal of Clinical Nursing, 23,* 756–765.

Aim

This article aims to identify the relationships among advance directive status, demographics, and decisional burden of surrogate decision makers of patients with chronic critical illness.

Methods

The investigators conducted a secondary analysis of cross-sectional data obtained from 489 surrogate decision makers of patients with chronic critical illness. They used questionnaires to collect demographic and role stress data. The Center for Epidemiological Studies Depression Scale was used to determine the surrogate's decisional burden.

Key Findings

The presence of advance directives diminishes the decisional burden of surrogates by reducing their role stress and lessens the severity of depressive symptoms. Participants who were nonwhite and had low socioeconomic status and low educational levels were less likely to have documentation of an advance directive. The presence of advance directives promotes patient-centered care by improving the quality of shared decision making.

Implications for Nurse Leaders and Managers

Nurse leaders and managers can ensure that nursing staff members are aware of their responsibilities related to advance directives. Further, they can provide education to ensure that nurses understand the positive benefits of advance directives in reducing surrogate role stress and decisional burden as well as promoting patient-centered care.

procedures that protect patient privacy (ANA, 2015a). Nurse leaders and managers show respect for employee privacy by keeping an employee's religious beliefs and lifestyle choices private.

Confidentiality

Patients have little or no choice to share private information with nurses and other members of the health-care team. The principle of **confidentiality** means preventing disclosure of private information shared between a patient and the health-care team. Once a patient shares personal information, the nurse can use that information only as authorized by the patient. Nurses are required to maintain confidentiality of all patient information. Nurses at all levels have a duty to maintain confidentiality of all patient information, both personal and clinical, in the work setting and off duty in all venues, including social media or any other means of communication (ANA, 2015a, p. 9). Nurse leaders and managers provide employees confidentiality by securing their personal information such as Social Security numbers and medical information. Only staff members who have a legitimate need within the performance of their job duties should have access to employee personal information.

The HIPAA, discussed earlier in this chapter, requires that nurses protect all verbal and written communication about patients, including medical records, electronic records, and verbal exchange of patient information such as patient teaching and change-of-shift report. The HIPAA requires health-care agencies to monitor staff adherence to related policies and procedures, computer privacy, and data security. Nurses must be aware of institutional policies and procedures related to patient privacy and confidentiality.

A new area of concern internationally is the use of social media and other electronic communication. Although social networks such as Facebook, Twitter, Snapchat, Instagram, YouTube, and LinkedIn offer opportunities for knowledge exchange and dissemination among local, national, and global communities, they also pose substantial risks. All nurses have an obligation to understand the nature, benefits, and consequences of participating in social networking (ANA, 2011).

Misusing social media can have severe consequences, such as disciplinary action by state boards of nursing that range from cautionary letters to licensure suspension. Violation of federal and state laws can result in civil or criminal penalties, including fines and imprisonment (Spector & Kappel, 2012). Nurses can also face liability for defamation, invasion of privacy, and harassment, depending on the type of postings and social media (NCSBN, 2011b, 2018b).

Nurse leaders and managers are obligated to enforce organizational policies and procedures related to social media and networking and to address any breach of confidentiality and privacy immediately. As long as nurses remain aware of their professional obligations, using social networking will not be an issue. The ANA's Principles for Social Networking are listed in Box 5-1.

LEARNING ACTIVITY 5-3

Is This a Breach of Privacy?

Susan is a registered nurse caring for Mr. Jones, who was just admitted for possible pancreatic cancer. Bill, a nurse from a different unit, stops by to visit and tells Susan that Mr. Jones is his neighbor. Later, Susan observes Bill at the computer looking at Mr. Jones's electronic health record.

1. Do Bill's actions violate HIPAA rules?
2. What action should Susan take?
3. What action should the nurse leader and manager take?
4. Is there also an ethical issue in this situation? What provision of the *ANA Code of Ethics* could apply to this situation?

BOX 5-1 American Nurses Association Principles for Social Networking

1. Nurses must recognize they have an ethical and legal obligation to maintain patient privacy and confidentiality at all times.
2. Nurses are strictly prohibited from transmitting by way of any electronic media a patient-related image.
3. Nurses are restricted from transmitting any information that violates a patient's right to privacy and confidentiality, or otherwise degrades or embarrasses a patient.
4. Nurses must not transmit or place online individually identifiable patient information.
5. Nurses must not refer to patients in a disparaging manner.
6. Nurses must observe ethically prescribed professional patient–nurse boundaries in the use of electronic media.
7. Nurses must not take photos or videos of patients on personal devices, including cell phones.
8. Nurses must promptly report any breach of confidentiality or privacy.
9. Nurses must be aware of and comply with employer policies regarding the use of work computers, cameras, and other electronic devices, and use of personal devices in the workplace.
10. Nurses must not make disparaging remarks about employers or coworkers.
11. Nurses must not make threatening, harassing, profane, obscene, sexually explicit, racially derogatory, homophobic, or other offensive comments.
12. Nurses must not post content or otherwise speak on behalf of the employer unless authorized to do so.
13. Nurses should understand that patients, colleagues, institutions, and employers may view postings.
14. Nurses should bring to the attention of appropriate authorities content that could harm a patient's privacy, rights, or welfare.
15. Nurses should participate in developing institutional policies governing online conduct.

Adapted from ANA, 2011, pp. 6–7; NCSBN, 2018b, pp. 12–13.

Informed Consent

Informed consent is a legal process by which a patient or legal representative voluntarily gives permission for a treatment or procedure. There are two required components to informed consent: "The patient must be fully informed and there must be voluntary consent" (Guido, 2014, p. 119). Informed consent mandates that the patient must be given information in terms they understand, alternatives to the planned procedure, and the related risks and benefits of all options. This information allows the patient to make an informed decision. Informed consent also represents the ethical principle of autonomy and reflects the patient's autonomous decision to accept or refuse health care.

Nurses must obtain informed consent from their patients for all procedures, treatments, and interventions they perform. This type of informed consent is not necessarily a written document but must be a verbal consent or an implied consent based on the patient's actions (Guido, 2014). This requires the nurse to continually communicate with patients about all procedures (e.g., injections, dressing changes, medication administration, etc.) and obtain their permission. In addition, nurses must also respect the patient's right to refuse any procedures, treatments, and interventions.

Accountability for obtaining informed consent for medical procedures lies with the healthcare provider (Guido, 2014). However, some institutions allow nurses to obtain the signature on the informed consent form for medical procedures being performed by another provider. In that case, the nurse's role in obtaining informed consent includes the following (Guido, 2014):

- Verifying that the health-care provider gave the patient the necessary information to make an "informed" consent
- Ensuring that the patient understands the information and procedure or treatment
- Validating that the patient is competent to give consent
- Witnessing that the patient signs the consent form
- Notifying the health-care provider if the patient does not understand the procedure or treatment
- Documenting the informed consent process

The consent is considered valid until withdrawn by the patient (verbal or written) or until the patient's condition changes significantly (Guido, 2014).

▶ SUMMARY

Nurses must use the ANA *Code of Ethics for Nurses, Nursing's Social Policy Statement, Scope and Standards of Practice,* and their state NPA to guide their nursing practice daily. Nurses at all levels and in all settings are accountable and responsible for their decisions, judgments, and actions. There are many legal aspects of professional nursing. Nurse leaders and managers play a major role in establishing, maintaining, and monitoring standards of nursing care; ensuring that nursing staff are competent; and ensuring that regulatory and legal standards are in place and followed. Nurse leaders and managers are charged with determining and providing for educational needs of their staff and with assessing and evaluating staff competency to optimize patient safety and minimize organizational liability.

NCLEX®-STYLE REVIEW QUESTIONS

Multiple Choice

1. A patient dies as the result of a wound infection. When the family sues the hospital and the nurses involved in this patient's care, it is discovered that wound care was only charted three times despite a twice-daily order from the health-care provider. What category of nursing practice will be the focus of the resulting lawsuit?
   1. Failure to act as a patient advocate
   2. Failure to assess and monitor
   3. Failure to document
   4. Failure to communicate

2. The nurse leader is responsible for patients on six different units in the acute care facility, including the newborn nursery and the intensive care unit. In which nursing unit would the nurse leader face potential liability?
   1. The newborn nursery has to admit 10 babies from labor and delivery and only 7 cribs have been cleaned completely and released back to the nursery. The nurse leader tells the nurses to clean the necessary number of cribs themselves and the housekeeping staff will finish the cleaning in the morning.
   2. The medical-surgical unit experiences a patient fall related to a patient neglecting to use the call button to ask for assistance.
   3. The intensive care unit experienced a patient injury after an experienced nurse administered the incorrect medication.
   4. The orthopedic unit had a patient who became septic and had to be moved to the intensive care unit because a nursing assistant, employed by the facility for 15 years, forgot to check the patient's vital signs as ordered.
3. The nurse leader is supervising the entire acute care facility and is notified that many employees have called in sick related to an outbreak of influenza. The nurse leader sends a registered nurse who works on a transitional care unit to the emergency department to provide care. In what area could this nurse potentially experience liability?
   1. Failure to warn
   2. Inappropriate assigning of staff and failure to supervise
   3. Negligent retention practices
   4. Unsafe staffing
4. The nurse manager of a busy medical-surgical unit has received an anonymous note that one of the unit's LPNs has routinely been documenting care that has not been given. What is the best action of this nurse manager concerning this situation?
   1. Immediately report the LPN to the state board of nursing.
   2. Question each RN about the anonymous note.
   3. Ask the LPN if the anonymous note is true.
   4. Check the LPN's documentation after observing the LPN.
5. Who is accountable for obtaining informed consent?
   1. The patient's nurse
   2. The health-care professional performing the procedure
   3. The nurse assisting the health-care professional performing the procedure
   4. The health-care agency's attorney
6. A nurse approaches another nurse and says, "I can't remember my password for the computer, can I use yours?" Which of the following is the best response by the nurse?
   1. "Sure, let me write it down for you."
   2. "No, you need to contact the nursing supervisor for the general password."
   3. "I am sorry, but I cannot share my password because it violates policy."
   4. "I'm too busy, go ask another nurse."

7. In each state, who/what defines the legal boundaries of nursing?
   1. The legal counsel of the state
   2. The Nurse Practice Act
   3. The ANA Standards of Practice
   4. The ANA Code of Ethics

8. The question of whether a nurse's actions reflect what a reasonable and prudent nurse should do under the same circumstances can be proven by which of the following:
   1. The defendant's explanation of what the nurse did
   2. The testimony of an expert medical witness
   3. The trial judge based on prior similar court cases
   4. The testimony of an expert nurse witness

Multiple Response

9. A lawsuit pertaining to professional negligence must include which of the following? *Select all that apply.*
   1. Duty owed the patient
   2. Foreseeability of harm
   3. Intent and risk
   4. Breach of duty owed the patient
   5. Causation

10. Good Samaritan Laws protect people who render care at the scene of an accident under which of the following conditions? *Select all that apply.*
    1. Care is provided by a licensed health-care professional
    2. Care is not grossly negligent
    3. Care is provided at the scene of the accident
    4. Care is rendered without pay
    5. Care is provided according to appropriate standards

REFERENCES

Aiken, T. D. (2004). *Legal, ethical, and political issues in nursing* (2nd ed.). F. A. Davis.

Allen, J. F., Jr. (2013). *Health law and medical ethics for health care professionals.* Pearson.

American Association of Colleges of Nursing (AACN). (2008). *The essentials of baccalaureate education for professional nursing practice.* Author. www.aacn.nche.edu/education-resources/baccessentials08.pdf

American Association of Colleges of Nursing. (2021). *The essentials: Core competencies for professional nursing education.* Author. https://www.aacnnursing.org/Portals/42/AcademicNursing/pdf/Essentials-2021.pdf

American Nurses Association (ANA). (2010). *Nursing's social policy statement: The essence of the profession.* Author.

American Nurses Association (ANA). (2011). *Fact sheet: Navigating the world of social media.* AboutANA/Social-Media/Social-Networking-Principles-Toolkit/Fact-Sheet-Navigating-the-World-of-Social-Media.pdf

American Nurses Association (ANA). (2015a). *Code of ethics for nurses with interpretive statements.* Author.

American Nurses Association (ANA). (2015b). *Nursing: Scope and standards of practice* (3rd ed.). Author.

American Nurses Association (ANA). (2016). *Nursing administration: Scope and standards of practice* (2nd ed.). Author.

American Nurses Association (ANA). (2020). Position statement: Nursing care and do-not-resuscitate (DNR) decisions. *OJIN: The Online Journal of Issues in Nursing, 25*(3). doi: 10.3912/OJIN.Vol25No03 PoSCol02

American Organization for Nursing Leadership (AONL). (2015a). *AONL nurse manager competencies.* Author.

American Organization for Nursing Leadership (AONL). (2015b). *AONL nurse executive competencies.* Author.

Beauchamp, T. L., & Childress, J. F. (2019). *Principles of biomedical ethics* (8th ed.). Oxford University Press.

Brent, N. J. (2001). *Nurses and the law: A guide to principles and applications* (2nd ed.). Saunders.

Centers for Disease Control and Prevention (CDC). (2020). *FAQ: COVID-19 data and surveillance.* https://www.cdc.gov/coronavirus/2019-ncov/covid-data/faq-surveillance.html

Croke, E. M. (2003). Nurses, negligence, and malpractice: An analysis based on more than 250 cases against nurses. *American Journal of Nursing, 103*(9), 54–63.

Cronenwett, L., Sherwood, G., Barnsteiner, J., Disch, J., Johnson, J., Mitchell, P., Sullivan, D. T., & Warren, J. (2007). Quality and safety education for nurses. *Nursing Outlook, 55*(3), 122–131.

Greiner, A. C., & Knebel, E. (Ed.) (2003). *Health professions education: A bridge to quality.* National Academies Press.

Guido, G. W. (2014). *Legal and ethical issues in nursing* (6th ed.). Boston: Pearson.

Health Insurance Portability and Accountability Act of 1996 (HIPAA). P.L. No. 104-191, 110 Stat. 1938 (1996).

Hickman, R. L., & Pinto, M. D. (2013). Advance directives lessen the decisional burden of surrogate decision-making for the chronically ill. *Journal of Clinical Nursing, 23*, 756–765.

McGowan, C. (2012). Patients' confidentiality. *Critical Care Nurse, 32*(5), 61–65.

Myers, W., & Boutier, B. P. (2011). Preparing a nursing negligence expert report in six paragraphs. *Journal of Legal Nursing Consulting, 22*(2), 13–15.

National Council of State Boards of Nursing (NCSBN). (2011a). *Fact sheet: Licensure of nurses and state board of nursing.* Author. www.ncsbn.org/Fact_Sheet_Licensure_of_Nurses_and_State_Boards_of_Nursing.pdf

National Council of State Boards of Nursing (NCSBN). (2011b). *White paper: A nurse's guide to the use of social media.* Author. www.ncsbn.org/Social_Media.pdf

National Council of State Boards of Nursing (NCSBN). (2018a). *State and territorial boards of nursing: What every nurse should know.* Author. https://www.ncsbn.org/3748.htm

National Council of State Boards of Nursing (NCSBN). (2018b). *A nurse's guide to the use of social media.* Author. https://www.ncsbn.org/3739.htm

National Council of State Boards of Nursing (NCSBN). (2020). *About NCSBN.* www.ncsbn.org/about.htm

Patient Self-Determination Act of 1990 (PSDA). P.L. No. 101-508, §§4206 and 4751 of the Omnibus Budget Reconciliation Act (1991).

Reisling, D. L. (2012). Make your nursing care malpractice-proof. *American Nurse Today, 7*(1), 24–29.

Russell, K. A. (2017). *Nurse practice acts guide and govern: Update 2017. Journal of Nursing Regulation, 8*(3), 18–23.

Safe Medical Devices Act of 1990 (SMDA). P.L. No. 101-629, 101st Congress. (1990).

Spector, N., & Kappel, D. M. (2012). Guidelines for using electronic and social media: The regulatory perspective. *OJIN: The Online Journal of Issues in Nursing, 17*(3), 1.

United States Department of Health and Human Services (USDHHS). (2003). Summary of the HIPAA privacy rule. www.hhs.gov/hipaa/for-professionals/privacy/laws-regulations/index.html

United States Department of Health and Human Services (USDHHS). (2018). *HIPAA basics for providers: Privacy, security, and breach notification rules.* https://www.cms.gov/Outreach-and-Education/Medicare-Learning-Network-MLN/MLNProducts/Downloads/HIPAAPrivacyandSecurity.pdf

 To explore learning resources for this chapter, go to FADavis.com

Chapter 6

Critical Thinking, Decision Making, and Clinical Reasoning

Elizabeth J. Murray, PhD, RN, CNE

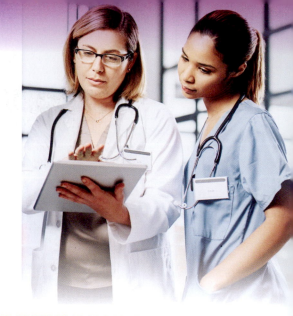

KEY TERMS

Appreciative inquiry
Clinical judgment
Clinical reasoning
Critical thinking
Decision making
Intuitive thinking
Problem-solving
Reactive thinking
Reflective thinking
Shared decision making

LEARNING OUTCOMES

- Explain the importance of critical thinking and clinical reasoning in the provision of safe and quality care.
- Describe elements of critical thinking and the cognitive skills necessary to think critically.
- Examine how nurse leaders and managers can foster critical thinking among staff members.
- Discuss the relationship between the nursing process and decision making.
- Describe the benefits of shared decision making.
- Describe the four steps of appreciative inquiry.

The Knowledge, Skills, and Attitudes Related to the Following Are Addressed in This Chapter:

Core Competencies	• Patient-Centered Care • Teamwork and Collaboration • Safety • Evidence-Based Practice
The Essentials: Core Competencies for Professional Nursing Education (AACN, 2021)	**Domain 1: Knowledge for Nursing Practice** 1.3 Demonstrate clinical judgment founded on a broad knowledge base (p. 27).
Code of Ethics with Interpretive Statements (ANA, 2015)	**Provision 4.2:** Accountability for nursing judgments, decisions, and actions (pp. 15–16) **Provision 4.3:** Responsibility for nursing judgments, decisions, and actions (pp. 16–17)

Nurse Manager (NMC) Competencies (AONL, 2015a) and Nurse Executive (NEC) Competencies (AONL, 2015b)	**NMC: Foundational Thinking Skills (p. 4)**
	• Apply systems thinking knowledge as an approach to analysis and decision making
	NMC: Strategic Management (p. 5)
	• Shared decision making
	NMC: Relationship Management and Influencing Behaviors (p. 6)
	• Influence others
	  • Assist others in developing problem-solving skills
	NMC: Personal Journey Disciplines (p. 7)
	• Apply action learning
	• Engage in reflective practice
	NEC: Communication and Relationship Building (p. 4)
	• Influencing behaviors
	  • Promote decisions that are patient-centered
	NEC: Leadership (p. 8)
	• Foundational thinking skills
	  • Recognize one's own method of decision making and the role of beliefs, values, and inferences
	• Systems thinking
	  • Use knowledge of classic and contemporary systems thinking in problem-solving and decision making
	  • Consider the impact of nursing decisions on the healthcare organization as a whole

Continued

The Knowledge, Skills, and Attitudes Related to the Following Are Addressed in This Chapter:—cont'd

Nursing Administration Scope and Standards of Practice (ANA, 2016)	**Standard 5: Implementation** The nurse administrator implements the identified plan (p. 40).
	Standard 5A: Coordination The nurse administrator coordinates implementation of the plan and associated processes (p. 41).
	Standard 10: Collaboration The nurse administrator collaborates with healthcare consumers, colleagues, community leaders, and other stakeholders to advance nursing practice and healthcare transformation (p. 50).

Source: American Association of Colleges of Nursing. (2021). *The essentials: Core competencies for professional nursing education.* Author; American Nurses Association (ANA). (2015). *Code of ethics for nurses with interpretive statements.* Author; American Nurses Association (ANA). (2016). *Nursing administration: Scope and standards of practice* (2nd ed.). Author; American Organization for Nursing Leadership (AONL). (2015a). *AONL nurse manager competencies.* Author; American Organization for Nursing Leadership (AONL). (2015b). *AONL nurse executive competencies.* Author; Cronenwett, L., Sherwood, G., Barnsteiner, J., Disch, J., Johnson, J., Mitchell, P., Sullivan, D. T., & Warren, J. (2007). Quality and safety education for nurses. *Nursing Outlook, 55*(3), 122–131; and Greiner, A. C., & Knebel, E. (Eds.) (2003). *Health professions education: A bridge to quality.* National Academies Press.

In response to advances in health care since the 1960s, the responsibilities of professional nurses have evolved to accommodate the complexity of health care, advanced technology, changing demographics of the patient population, and the acuity of patients. Nurses must be able to process an ever-increasing amount of information to make complex decisions and solve complicated problems in the delivery of patient care (Facione et al., 1994). Nurses must master effective critical thinking, clinical judgment, clinical reasoning, communication, and assessment skills (American Association of Colleges of Nursing [AACN], 2008). In other words, "think like a nurse."

Nurse leaders and managers must not only practice critical thinking and effective decision making but also be role models to their staff. They must develop the intellectual capacities and skills necessary to become disciplined, self-directed, critical thinkers (Heaslip, 2008, para. 1). In addition, they must be experts in decision making and problem-solving at various levels of the organization. This chapter breaks down the processes of critical thinking and decision making, relates them to the nursing process, and describes effective tools nurse leaders and managers can use when engaged in these processes.

▶ CRITICAL THINKING

Critical thinking is a complicated process that involves skillfully directing the thinking process and imposing intellectual standards on the elements of thought. A more formal definition is as follows: "the intellectually disciplined process of actively and skillfully conceptualizing, applying, analyzing, synthesizing, and/ or evaluating information gathered from or generated by, observation, experience, reflection, reasoning, or communication, as a guide to belief and action" (Scriven

& Paul, n.d., para. 1). Nursing organizations and accrediting agencies identify critical thinking as an important skill for professional nursing practice (AACN, 2008; American Nurses Association [ANA], 2015a; National Council of State Boards of Nursing [NCSBN], 2013).

Critical thinking in nursing "includes adherence to intellectual standards, proficiency in using reasoning, a commitment to develop and maintain intellectual traits of the mind and habits of thought and the competent use of thinking skills and abilities for sound clinical judgments and safe decision-making" (Heaslip, 2008, para. 2). Table 6-1 displays various definitions of critical thinking found in the nursing literature. Critical thinking is an important component of professional nursing because it is an essential skill for processing patient data

Table 6-1 Definitions of Critical Thinking in Nursing

Source	Definition
Rushing & Masters, 2020	Critical thinking for clinical decision making is the ability to think in a systematic and logical manner, with openness to question and reflect on the reasoning process used to ensure safe nursing practice and quality care (p. 130).
Porter-O'Grady & Malloch, 2013	[Critical thinking is] active, purposeful, organized thinking that takes into consideration focus, language, frame of reference, attitudes, assumptions, evidence, reasoning, conclusions, implications, and context when deciding what to believe or do (pp. 432–433).
AACN, 2008	Critical thinking underlies decision making and involves the process of questioning, analyzing, synthesizing, interpreting, inferring, using inductive and deductive reasoning, using intuition, and creativity (p. 36)
Benner et al., 2008	Critical thinking involves the application of knowledge and experience to identify patient problems and to direct clinical judgment and actions that result in positive patient outcomes (p. 2)
Heaslip, 2008	[Critical thinking is] the ability to think in a systematic and logical manner with openness to question and reflect on the reasoning process used to ensure safe nursing practice and quality care (para. 2).
Alfaro-LeFevre, 2006	Critical thinking is deliberate, purposeful, and informed outcome-focused thinking that requires careful identification of key problems, issues, and risks involved. Further, critical thinking requires specific knowledge, skills, and experience (p. 30).
Ignatavicius, 2001	Purposeful, outcome-directed thinking is based on a body of scientific knowledge derived from research and other courses of evidence (p. 31)
Scheffer & Rubenfeld, 2000	[Critical thinking is] an essential component of professional accountability and quality nursing care and includes the cognitive skills of analyzing, applying standards, discriminating, information seeking, logical reasoning, predicting, and transforming knowledge (p. 357).
Bittner & Tobin, 1998	[Critical thinking is] a process influenced by knowledge and experience using strategies such as reflective thinking as a part of learning to identify the issues and opportunities and holistically synthesize the information in nursing practice (p. 268).
Facione et al., 1994	[Critical thinking is] purposive, self-regulatory judgment (p. 349).

and is inherent in making sound clinical judgments and safe patient care decisions. Critical thinking plays an integral role in clinical practice as well as in nursing leadership and management. It is a critical process that systematically frames the nurse leader and manager's thoughts, decisions, and actions (Porter-O'Grady et al., 2005).

Elements of and Cognitive Skills for Critical Thinking

Critical thinking involves eight elements of thought (Heaslip, 2008, para. 5):

1. The problem, question, concern, or issue being thought about by the thinker (i.e., what the thinker is attempting to figure out)
2. The purpose or goal of the thinking (i.e., what does the thinker hope to accomplish?)
3. The frame of reference, point of view, or worldview the thinker holds about the issue or problem
4. The assumptions the thinker holds true about the issue or problem
5. The central concepts, ideas, principles, and theories the thinker uses in reasoning about the issue or problem
6. The evidence, data, or information provided to support the claims the thinker makes about the issue or problem
7. The interpretations, inferences, reasoning, and lines of formulated thought that lead to the thinker's conclusions
8. The implications and consequences that follow from the positions the thinker holds on the issue or problem

Critical thinking is a skill that requires practice and that must be nurtured and reinforced over time (Ignatavicius, 2001). It is more than seeking a solution to an issue or problem—it involves examining and analyzing situations, considering all points of view, and identifying options. To think critically and make sound decisions, nurse leaders and managers must engage in the processes of reflection, judgment, evaluation, and criticism (Zori & Morrison, 2009). There are six essential cognitive skills necessary to becoming an expert critical thinker (Porter-O'Grady et al., 2005):

1. *Interpretation* involves clarifying data and circumstances to determine meaning and significance. For nurse leaders and managers, interpretation reflects their ability to comprehend the significance of a wide variety of circumstances, establish priorities, categorize data, and clarify the related impact on people and systems.
2. *Analysis* is determining a problem or issue based on assessment data. Nurse leaders and managers engage in analysis to identify relationships among structures, processes, outcomes, and other frameworks of thought with the goals of examining various arguments, issues, and themes and determining elements and origins of the argument.
3. *Inference* is about drawing conclusions. Nurse leaders and managers draw conclusions about situations after careful analysis and begin to form a foundation on which an action will be based.

4. *Evaluation* is determining whether expected outcomes have or have not been met. If outcomes have not been met, evaluation also involves examining why. Nurse leaders and managers engage in evaluation to assess the reliability and credibility of the descriptions, perceptions, experiences, situations, and relationships of these elements to determine their value in the overall process. The nurse leader and manager gains confidence in the evaluation of the outcome, which will direct decisions and actions.

5. *Explanation* is the ability to justify actions with evidence. Nurse leaders and managers establish a viable explanation about the conclusions drawn during the evaluation process. The role of the nurse leader and manager is to provide systematic and organized reasoning behind the conclusion so that it can be translated into a level of understanding for others.

6. *Self-regulation* is the process of examining one's practice for strengths and weaknesses in critical thinking and promoting continuous improvement. Nurse leaders and managers engage in self-regulation to become more informed and refine their skills in problem identification, analysis, and inference and to develop expert critical thinking skills.

Reactive, Reflective, and Intuitive Thinking

Nurses use critical thinking to explore, understand, analyze, and apply knowledge in various practice situations. Not engaging in critical thinking when caring for patients, making decisions, or dealing with challenging situations can result in the use of reactive thinking. **Reactive thinking** is an automatic or kneejerk reaction to situations that has consequences leading to vague or inaccurate reasoning, sloppy and superficial thinking, and poor nursing practice (Heaslip, 2008; Zori & Morrison, 2009). Nurse leaders and managers who engage in reactive thinking use automatic, thoughtless responses to solve problems that often result in errors or ineffective decision making. Consider the following scenario: Several nurses are going back to school to advance their education, and they approach the nurse manager about implementing a different scheduling method that would allow nurses to work every weekend with extra days off during the week, rather than the current practice of scheduling all nurses to work every other weekend. The nurse manager does not believe that the proposed scheduling method would be fair to all nurses and refuses to consider any changes. In this example, the nurse manager does not consider input from the staff, makes an assumption without taking any time to think about the decision critically, and does not give staff the opportunity to engage in shared decision making, thus possibly resulting in nurse dissatisfaction. The nursing staff members will probably not challenge the nurse manager's decision because they may not feel comfortable discussing the topic further. Reactive thinking restricts innovation and maintains status quo (Zori & Morrison, 2009).

Rather, critical thinking should involve some reflection on previous experiences to analyze a situation, make judgments, and draw conclusions. **Reflective thinking** consists of deliberate thinking and understanding using one's own personal experiences and knowledge, and it involves assessing what is known, what needs to be known, and how to bridge the gap between the two (Rushing & Masters, 2020). Reflective thinking requires thoughtful personal self-assessment, analysis, and synthesis of strengths, all of which can help nurses develop the skill of self-improvement. Using reflective thinking, nurses must examine and question underlying assumptions and their validity (Benner et al., 2008).

When engaged in reflective thinking, nurses do all of the following (Rushing & Masters, 2020, p. 133):

- Determine what information is needed for understanding the issue.
- Examine what has already been experienced related to an issue.
- Gather available information.
- Synthesize the information and opinions.
- Consider the synthesis from different perspectives and frames of reference.
- Create some meaning from the relevant information and opinions.

Using reflective thinking in complex situations is beneficial for nurse leaders and managers because it forces them to step back, assess the situation, and think about how to solve the problem. Reflective thinking can result in fewer errors and more effective decision making. Considering the situation just discussed, using reflecting thinking when the staff members make their request, the nurse manager tells the staff members that she will consider alternative scheduling methods. She reviews the organization's staffing policies and determines that a change is feasible. The nurse leader and manager creates a team and asks for nurses from all shifts to volunteer to be part of the team. At the first meeting, she outlines the current policies and charges the team to determine the number of nurses willing to work weekends and to identify a feasible schedule to ensure safe staffing. After input from all staff members, the team finalizes a feasible schedule, which is then implemented. By engaging in reflective thinking, the nurse manager promotes shared decision making among the staff members, who then feel empowered and satisfied with the scheduling process.

There are instances in which nurses claim to use intuition or "gut feelings" when providing patient care. **Intuitive thinking** is an instant understanding of knowledge without supporting evidence. It has also been described as an intuitive grasp or a clear understanding of a situation based on a background of similar situations (Benner, 1984). Some reject intuition as an element of critical thinking because it is abstract and seems irrational. However, intuition is a cognitive skill used by nurses to assist assessment of situations and can lead the nurse to take quick action in the delivery of safe, effective patient care (Robert et al., 2014). Intuitive thinking is a nonconscious state of knowing that integrates memory and pattern recognition without cognitive direction (Payne, 2015). Expert nurses do not rely on critical thinking alone; rather, they form an intuitive understanding of a patient's situation based on previous knowledge, experiences, and pattern recognition (Benner, 1984; Payne, 2015). Nurse leaders and managers use intuitive thinking as they deal with day-to-day unit-level situations. Intuition is based on previous knowledge and experience and triggers a response or reflection to resolve an issue.

Modeling Critical Thinking

Nurses use critical thinking continually while caring for patients, coordinating care, collaborating with others, advocating for patients, problem-solving, resolving issues, and ensuring that safe and quality patient care is provided. One's ability to think critically can be affected by many factors, such as age, education, experience, and work environment. Nurse leaders and managers play a pivotal role in helping staff members enhance their critical thinking skills (Ignatavicius, 2001). A major function of nurse leaders and managers is to be a role model for staff by being critical thinkers themselves. In addition, staff members rely on nurse leaders and managers to help solve clinical, interpersonal, and unit-related problems. Nurse leaders and managers who use reflective thinking and provide guidance to staff in a credible manner will create a sense of trust and safety on the unit (Zori et al., 2010). In contrast, nurse leaders and managers who engage in reactive thinking may miss opportunities for self-growth, to role model critical thinking for staff, and to create changes that are long-lasting and goal driven (Zori & Morrison, 2009). In an evidence-based practice world, it is becoming increasingly important that nurse leaders and managers articulate to staff the value and application of critical thinking as a normal expectation of professional nursing practice (Porter-O'Grady et al., 2005). Nurse leaders and managers must encourage staff to analyze situations, challenge assumptions, explore alternative options, and embrace continuous improvement. Enforcing the expectation of using critical thinking with rewards and recognition can result in a positive work environment. The encouragement of critical thinking by nurse leaders and managers creates a legitimate foundation for accurate and effective decision making on the unit (Porter-O'Grady et al., 2005).

▶ DECISION MAKING

People, in general, make many decisions in an average day. Some decisions are small and are made with little effort (i.e., deciding what to eat for breakfast), whereas others may be more involved and take several days (i.e., purchasing a new car). Regardless of how complex a decision may be, the basic elements of the decision-making process are present. **Decision making** "is a process of choosing the best alternatives to achieve individual and organizational objectives" (Guo, 2008, p. 118). Nurses at the bedside typically make two types of decisions: (1) patient care decisions, or those that affect direct patient care; and (2) condition-of-work decisions, or those that affect the work environment (Krairiksh & Anthony, 2001). Decisions made by nurse leaders and managers have a broader scope, in that they can affect many people and can have a greater impact on the overall unit or organization.

Decision making consists of the following steps (McConnell, 2000):

1. *Gathering information* involves collecting information that will direct the decision-making process. Often, gathering information involves observations. The focus during this step is to gather data that are worthwhile and pertinent to the decision to be made. One shortcoming for most people is the tendency to move from observation to conclusion without enough information.
2. *Analyzing information and creating alternatives* often overlap with gathering information because, in this step, information is logically arranged and put into context for evaluation. As information is being organized, alternatives emerge. The amount of time spent analyzing and creating alternatives is directly related to the weight of the decision to be made.

3. *Selecting a preferred alternative* comes about during analysis, when often the best alternative emerges. During this step, it is important to consider what is a realistic and feasible alternative, keeping in mind factors such as time, money, quality, personalities, and policies.

4. *Implementation* consists of taking the selected alternative and putting it into action.

5. *Follow-up on implementation* includes communication and clarification to ensure that staff members know what is expected of them; checking on the timing and ensuring that the change is not overwhelming to staff because of other factors; performing ongoing analysis and monitoring of any circumstances that may require adjustments to the implementation plan; evaluating suggestions from others; withdrawing a poor choice, if necessary; admitting mistakes; and, in the end, sticking with the right decision.

Decision making is a dynamic process and must include evidence-based research. All nurses have the authority, accountability, and responsibility to make decisions and take action consistent with the obligation to promote health and to provide optimal patient care (ANA, 2015a). Nurse leaders and managers must make autonomous operational decisions with the same considerations.

Decision Making and the Nursing Process

The ANA (2015a) *Nursing Scope and Standards of Practice* delineates the competent level of nursing practice and uses the nursing process as a critical-thinking framework to guide nursing practice. The nursing process is cyclical and dynamic, interpersonal and collaborative, and universally applicable. It is fundamental to nursing practice and provides a clinical reasoning approach to patient care that uses six interrelated steps (ANA, 2015a). Nurse leaders and managers integrate the nursing process with leadership and management competencies to effectively make decisions that guide nursing practice, set strategic goals, create and sustain healthy work environments, influence organizational and public policy, resource management (human, material, financial), population health management, legal and regulatory compliance, and promote safe quality patient outcomes (ANA, 2016). Nurse leaders and managers apply the steps of the nursing process when making decisions at the unit and organizational levels:

- *Assessment* involves continually collecting data in a systematic manner relative to an issue, situation, the work environment, or trends. Nurse leaders and managers use data collected to problem solve, make decisions, identify gaps in care, and identify patterns and variances related to the situation.
- *Diagnosis (analysis)* includes identifying issues, problems, or trends and validating them with stakeholders when possible. Nurse leaders and managers use data to support and enhance decision making and document issues, problems, or trends to help determine an individualized plan.
- *Outcomes identification* includes identifying expected outcomes for an individualized plan of care. Nurse leaders and managers identify expected outcomes for a plan developed to address issues, problems, or trends.
- *Planning* is the development of an individualized plan in partnership with members of the health-care team and the appropriate stakeholders. The plan

is prioritized and includes a timeline. Nurse leaders and managers design the plan by considering the current statutes, rules, regulations, and standards and by integrating best practices.

- *Implementation* of the plan involves coordinating the implementation of a plan and associated processes in collaboration with the health-care team in a safe and timely manner using evidence-based interventions specific to the issue, problem, or trend (ANA, 2016). Nurse leaders and managers incorporate principles of systems management, new knowledge, and strategies to initiate change, achieve desired outcomes, and establish strategies to promote health, education, and a safe environment (ANA, 2016).
- *Evaluation* involves ongoing evaluation of the outcomes in relation to structures, processes, nurse-sensitive indicators, and stakeholder responses. Nurse leaders and managers use the results of evaluation analysis to make or recommend changes to policies and procedures as needed.

The nursing process encompasses all actions taken by nurses at every level, provides a framework for critical thinking, and forms the foundation of decision making with the goal of safe, quality, and evidence-based nursing care (ANA, 2015a, 2016). Table 6-2 shows the relationship between the nursing process and decision making for nurse leaders and managers.

Table 6-2   Comparison of Nursing Process and Decision Making for Nurse Leaders and Managers

Nursing Process	Decision Making	Example Related to Short Staffing
Assessment	D = Define the problem	• The nurse leader and manager gathers data related to the issue and trends. • Data to consider would be unit census, patient acuity, the number of discharges and admissions, and staff mix.
Diagnosis	E = Establish the criteria	• The nurse leader and manager identifies the problem, explores possible causes, considers alternative strategies for staffing, and identifies the expected outcome.
Identification of outcomes	C = Consider alternatives I = Identify the best alternatives	• Alternatives to consider may include altering current staffing methods and increasing staff levels during peak admission and discharge times. • The expected outcome is safe staffing.
Planning	D = Develop and implement a plan of action	• The nurse leader and manager develops a staffing plan that identifies strategies to achieve the expected outcome of safe staffing. • The nurse leader and manager implements the staffing plan in a timely and efficient manner.
Implementation		• The nurse leader and manager coordinates the material and the interprofessional and intraprofessional resources needed to implement the plan.
Evaluation	E = Evaluate and monitor the solution and feedback if necessary	• The nurse leader and manager evaluates the progress of the staffing plan and whether the expected outcome of safe staffing is met. • If safe staffing is not met, the cycle begins again with assessment.

Compiled from ANA, 2016, ANA, 2015a, and Guo, 2008.

Tools for Decision Making

Tools for decision making provide nurse leaders and managers a systematic way to collect and manage necessary data and assist in visualizing alternatives. There are numerous tools and techniques available that can be used to ensure effective decision making. By using a tool for decision making, nurse leaders and managers can approach decision making in an organized and systematic manner.

DECIDE Model

Using a decision-making model can help ensure that all steps of decision making are addressed, thereby avoiding jumping to a conclusion before all information is collected and analyzed. A model for decision making identified by Guo (2008) uses the acronym DECIDE to represent the steps in the decision-making process. The steps of the DECIDE model are listed in Box 6-1.

Decision-Making Grid Analysis

Decision-making grid analysis is one of the simplest tools a nurse leader and manager can use, especially if the decision involves more than one feasible alternative. This technique involves listing options and factors on a table or grid. The possible options or alternatives are listed on the rows of the table, and factors affecting the decision are listed on the columns. Next, a numerical score (e.g., in a range of 0 to 3) is assigned to each option to indicate poor to very good or not likely to very likely; it is acceptable to use the same score more than once. For example, a nurse manager is determining which shift would be best for a particular unit. Options or alternatives include 12-hour shifts, 10-hour shifts, and 8-hour shifts. Next, factors to consider are determined by the nurse manager with staff input and are based on evidence. Factors to be considered in this case are nurse satisfaction, nurse fatigue, patient satisfaction, and potential for adverse events. Then, the nurse manager assigns weights first to each option and then to each factor based on importance, with 0 being the least important and 3 being the most important. The weights for each option are multiplied by the weights assigned to the factors for a total. The option with the highest total becomes the most feasible option. In the example shown in Table 6-3, 10-hour shifts have the highest total, and this shift length is the final outcome of this decision-making process.

BOX 6-1 Steps of the DECIDE Model

D = Define the problem, if necessary
E = Establish criteria
C = Consider the alternatives
I = Identify the best alternative

D = Develop and implement a plan of action
E = Evaluate and monitor the solution, seek feedback
   if necessary

Adapted from Guo, 2008.

Table 6-3 Decision-Making Grid for Determining Shifts					
	High Nurse Satisfaction	**Low Nurse Fatigue**	**High Patient Satisfaction**	**Few Adverse Events**	**Totals**
Weight	2×	3×	2×	3×	
12 hours	3 (6)	1 (3)	2 (4)	1 (3)	16
10 hours	3 (6)	2 (6)	2 (4)	2 (6)	22
8 hours	0 (0)	2 (6)	2 (4)	3 (9)	19

LEARNING ACTIVITY 6-1

Using a Decision-Making Grid

Think about an important personal decision you need to make. Use a decision-making grid to analyze this decision.

SWOT Analysis

A SWOT analysis is a tool frequently used in marketing and organizational strategic planning. However, it can also be very useful in decision making for nurses. SWOT stands for **S**trengths, **W**eaknesses, **O**pportunities, and **T**hreats. Strengths and weaknesses are internal factors, or those within the organization or the unit, whereas opportunities and threats are seen as external factors, or those outside the organization or unit (Pearce, 2007). Nurse leaders and managers who make decisions using a SWOT analysis can improve outcomes for both patients and nurses by identifying the strengths and weaknesses of the staff, areas for improvement, and opportunities for facilitating positive change. SWOT analysis is discussed further in Chapter 7.

Shared Decision Making

The role of the nurse leader and manager is shifting from making all unit-related decisions to designing effective shared decision-making processes. **Shared decision making** is the inclusion of staff nurses in decision making related to patient care and work methods at the unit and organizational levels. Shared decision making requires nurse leaders and managers to involve staff nurses in decisions about hiring, scheduling, and performance evaluations (appraisals), as well as include them in general unit discussions (Graham-Dickerson et al., 2013). Nurses engaged in shared decision making are empowered to provide effective, efficient, safe, and compassionate quality care and have opportunities for ongoing professional growth and development (ANA, 2015b). Unit cultures with shared decision making foster a healthy work environment and promote safe and quality patient care. Moreover, shared decision making is a positive factor in job satisfaction and nurse recruitment and retention (Houser et al., 2012; Scherb et al., 2011; Shiparski, 2005).

Although not yet the norm in all organizations, shared decision making is a standard in Magnet-recognized organizations and has been shown to have a positive impact on nurse satisfaction, nurse recruitment and retention, patient satisfaction, and reduction of adverse events (Houser et al., 2012). The ANA's *Code of Ethics for Nurses With Interpretive Statements* suggests that nurse leaders and managers are responsible to ensure that nurses are included on teams at the unit and organizational level and in decision-making processes that affect the quality and safety of patient care (ANA, 2015b). According to the ANA's *Nursing Administration: Scope and Standards of Practice,* nurse leaders and managers are encouraged to develop skills in shared decision making (ANA, 2016).

Appreciative Inquiry

In many cases, part of the decision-making process involves problem-solving. **Problem-solving** consists of the act of identifying a problem and implementing an

---

EXPLORING THE EVIDENCE 6-1

Graham-Dickerson, P., Houser, J., Thomas, E., Casper, C., Erkenbrack, L., Wenzel, M., & Siegrist, M. (2013). The value of staff nurse involvement in decision making. *Journal of Nursing Administration, 43*(5), 286–292.

Aim
The aims of this study were to explore the perceptions of hospital-based nurses regarding their involvement in decision making and to gain an understanding of the ways nurses would like to be involved in decision making.

Methods
The investigators used a qualitative descriptive design and conducted focus groups with registered nurses and individual interviews with chief nursing officers from 10 rural and suburban hospitals in Colorado.

Key Findings
Data were analyzed using components of grounded theory. Seven themes emerged: collaboration, increased involvement, problem identification, formal or informal communication, accountability, autonomy in decision making, and empowerment. Involvement in decision making was perceived by all in the study as having a positive impact on the work environment and nurse satisfaction at work. Nurses indicated that being involved in decision-making made them feel more confident and valued by the organization. Further, they described involvement as an investment and a sense of personal ownership of the organization.

Implications for Nurse Leaders and Managers
Nurse leaders and managers can use the findings of this study to inform their management styles. The authors suggest that nurse leaders and managers should listen to their staff when they make recommendations and provide feedback on how the recommendations will be implemented or modified. Further, including staff nurses in unit-level decision making can improve patient outcomes and nurse satisfaction.

active systematic process to solve that problem. Problem-solving requires looking closely at problems, failures, and negative outcomes and then finding a solution.

One possible approach to problem-solving is appreciative inquiry. **Appreciative inquiry** is a problem-solving strategy that capitalizes on the positive characteristics of an outcome by valuing and building on them. The end product of appreciative inquiry is a culture change or the development of a vision or plan (Manion, 2011). Appreciative inquiry is based on the belief that there is something similar in the organization somewhere that is already working, and it focuses on recognizing and finding a positive attribute and studying that element to gain insight into handling the current issue (Manion, 2011; Meline & Brehm, 2015). Appreciative inquiry is a collaborative process that engages staff in a healthy exchange of knowledge to solve problems and innovate change. It avoids focusing on the negatives by shifting the perspective to what works best in the organization.

There are four stages of appreciate inquiry, commonly referred to as the four Ds. Stage one is discovery, or the discovery phase, and it involves storytelling. The question answered in this phase is "What gives life?" The goal in this first phase is to identify what works best. The next stage is dreaming, or the envisioning phase, during which the question to be answered is "What might be?" Staff members think ahead and imagine a future based on the positives identified during the discovery phase. Stage three is design, or the co-constructing phase, because the focus during this stage is to design the ideal and to identify the structures and processes necessary to make the dream a reality. The question asked at this stage is "What should be?" The final stage is destiny, or the sustaining phase. The goal of the last phase is to determine how to actualize, sustain, or create the identified characteristics. During the last stage, the focus is on the positive and on empowering everyone to sustain the vision. For an example of using appreciative inquiry in shared decision making, see Exploring the Evidence 6-2.

EXPLORING THE EVIDENCE 6-2

Meline, D. L., & Brehm, S. N. (2015). Sustaining shared decision making: A biennial task force process. *American Nurse Today, 10*(3), 52–54.

Aim
The authors share their experience of using appreciative inquiry to enhance shared decision making. The nursing division of a hospital in Ohio established a shared decision-making task force that convenes biennially to critically review current suggestions, structures, and processes to improve patient care and professional nursing practice.

Process
At the first meeting of the task force each year, a current purpose is defined. In the example provided by the authors, the purpose was to influence and enhance the future of professional nursing practice through evaluation of their shared

Continued

governance structure and function (p. 53). Once the focus of the appreciative in-quiry process is identified, the task force proceeds with discovery, dream, design, and destiny:

Discovery: The task force asks the following questions:
- What is working now?
- What do we not want to lose?
- What are our shared decision-making strengths?

The task force then focuses on the strengths, to shift the process from problem-solving to appreciating and improving the positive qualities.

Dream: The goal in this step is to start a creative process. The team begins this step asking the members to draw a picture to symbolize their dream for the nursing division. During this step, they also engage in brainstorming.

Design: The task force identifies the top ideas for improvement from the brain-storming session. Communication, mentoring, and accountability were identi-fied in the example the authors presented. The team then identified a list of specific desires related to each topic. Next, to merge the dream with reality, the task force asks the following questions:
- What is the benefit?
- What actions are needed to make the change?
- Who will the change affect?
- Who should be involved?

Destiny: The task force envisions their destiny by writing recommendations with detailed rationales and submits them to the leadership council.

Outcomes
The authors conclude that using appreciative inquiry in their shared decision-making process has enhanced their process and guided the task force in making their dream a reality.

Implications for Nurse Leaders and Managers
This article provides nurse leaders and managers with an example of the real-life application of shared decision making and appreciative inquiry in nursing. The processes can be used at both the unit and organizational levels.

▶ THINKING LIKE A NURSE

Thinking like a nurse is complex and involves critical thinking, problem-solving, clinical reasoning, and clinical judgment. In 2010, Benner et al. called for a trans-formational "shift from an emphasis on critical thinking to an emphasis on clinical reasoning and multiple ways of thinking that include critical thinking" (p. 84).

Clinical reasoning is "the process by which nurses and other clinicians make their judgments, and includes both the deliberate process of generating alternatives, weighing them against the evidence, and choosing the most appropriate, and those patterns that might be characterized as engaged, practical reasoning" (Tanner, 2006, pp. 204–205). Clinical reasoning is a systematic process that involves the following cyclical process (Theobald & Ramsbotham, 2019):

- Considering the patient and context
- Collecting cues and information
- Processing information
- Identifying problems/issues
- Establishing goals
- Taking acting/intervening
- Evaluating outcomes
- Reflecting on process and new learning

Clinical judgment is a complex process that includes "an interpretation or conclusion about a patient's needs, concerns, or health problems, and/or the decision to take action (or not), use or modify standard approaches, or improvise new ones as deemed appropriate by the patient's response" (Tanner, 2006, p. 204). Manetti (2019) suggests that "sound clinical judgment is a cognitive process in which the nurse forms a holistic assessment of a patient situation" (p. 106). Clinical judgment is a key attribute of professional nursing and provides a basis for sound clinical reasoning (AACN, 2019).

Tanner developed a model of clinical judgment that still applies today (Caputi & Kavanaugh, 2018). The clinical judgment model encompasses the following four aspects (Tanner, 2006, p. 208):

1. *Noticing:* a perceptual grasp of the situation
2. *Interpreting:* developing a sufficient understanding of the situation to respond
3. *Responding:* deciding on an appropriate course of action appropriate for the situation
4. *Reflecting:* attending to the patient's response to the action while reviewing outcomes of the action and the appropriateness of all preceding aspects

Good clinical judgment requires an understanding of the pathophysiological and diagnostic aspects of a patient's condition as well as the health-care experience of both the patient and the patient's family (Tanner, 2006). Nurses make many decisions every day that require critical thinking, clinical reasoning, and sound clinical judgment.

▶ SUMMARY

All nurses, regardless of their role, must develop critical thinking and decision-making skills. Providing safe and quality patient care involves effective critical thinking skills, and nurse leaders and managers must encourage staff members to be critical thinkers. Critical thinking involves thinking in a systematic and logical way and generating, implementing, and evaluating approaches to promoting positive patient and nurse outcomes. Reflective thinking and intuitive thinking are elements of critical thinking, and they are based on well-established experiences and provide valuable insight into decision making. Critical thinking is interrelated with decision making, the nursing process, clinical reasoning, and clinical judgment. Nurse leaders and managers achieve outcomes by building on the nursing process when making patient care and unit decisions. Effective nurse leaders and managers model sound critical thinking and decision-making skills as well as foster open communication and give voice to staff by encouraging shared decision making. Nurses at all levels must develop effective clinical reasoning and sound clinical judgment to be able to *think like a nurse.*

NCLEX®-STYLE REVIEW QUESTIONS

Multiple Choice

1. The nurse leaders of a large acute care facility have decided to implement shared decision making on each nursing unit and expect to see what result?
   1. Improved retention of nurses
   2. More nurses applying for leadership positions
   3. Decreased nurse-to-patient ratio
   4. Elimination of medication errors

2. The staff nurses from an orthopedic surgery unit are dissatisfied with the admission process of a patient following surgery. The nurses state that there may be four to five admissions within a 1-hour period as they are discharged from the postanesthesia recovery unit. With many patients arriving at the same time, the staff does not feel able to give the patients the close assessment they deserve and complete the admission process. The director of nursing suggests that these nurses observe the system that the women's health unit uses for the multiple admissions that happen at the same time due to deliveries and female surgeries. What problem-solving technique is the director of nursing using?
   1. Critical thinking
   2. Shared decision making
   3. DECIDE model
   4. Appreciative inquiry

3. The nurse manager knows that which of the following is the first step in the critical thinking process?
   1. Reflection
   2. Judgment
   3. Evaluation
   4. Criticism

4. The nurse manager has been evaluating the nursing unit's strengths and weaknesses in an effort to ensure that the unit continues to improve its safety practices and is using what cognitive skill of the critical thinking process in this exercise?
   1. Interpretation
   2. Self-regulation
   3. Analysis
   4. Evaluation

5. The nurse manager knows that which nurse on the medical-surgical unit will be the best at using intuitive thinking?
   1. The nurse who graduated from nursing school 6 months ago and has worked on the unit for 3 months.
   2. The nurse who just started working on the unit but has worked on a pediatric unit for 2 years.
   3. The nurse who worked in the intensive care unit for 1 year and has worked on this unit for 4 months.
   4. The nurse who worked in a long-term care facility for 6 years and has worked on this unit for 6 months.

6. The nurse leader manages a nursing unit that has a preponderance of nurses who have graduated from nursing school within the last 12 months and knows that what type of thinking will provide the best guidance to the nursing staff?
   1. Reactive
   2. Intuitive
   3. Reflective
   4. Automatic

7. The nurse manager has determined that the nursing unit should see a reduction in medication errors by 50% and knows that this decision equates to what part of the nursing process?
   1. Assessment
   2. Diagnosis
   3. Outcomes identification
   4. Planning

8. The nurse manager has determined that patient care on the nursing unit would be more efficient if a different nursing model was used and plans to use what tool for decision making that gives the manager the opportunity to look at more than one feasible alternative?
   1. Decision-making grid
   2. DECIDE model
   3. SWOT analysis
   4. Shared decision making

9. The nurse manager has decided to begin a shared decision-making model on the nursing unit and knows that individual staff nurses will receive what benefit from this decision?
   1. Sense of entitlement
   2. Sense of empowerment
   3. Sense of inquiry
   4. Sense of intellect

10. The nurse manager is holding a unit meeting and asks each staff member to share one thing that the individual believes works best on the unit. What technique is the nurse manager using in this meeting?
    1. Critical thinking
    2. Shared decision making
    3. Appreciative inquiry
    4. Reflective thinking

Multiple Response

11. A nurse leader is explaining the process of appreciative inquiry to a group of nurses who hope to use this process in bringing change to their nursing unit. The leader shares that what are stages of appreciative inquiry? *Select all that apply.*
    1. Discovery
    2. Dreaming
    3. Dramatics
    4. Design
    5. Destiny

12. The nurse manager is planning to use the DECIDE model to assist in improving nursing staff self-scheduling and is explaining the use of this tool by comparing it to the nursing process and knows that the ECI of the model corresponds to what parts of the nursing process? *Select all that apply.*
    1. Assessment
    2. Diagnosis
    3. Identification of outcomes
    4. Planning
    5. Evaluation

REFERENCES

Alfaro-LeFevre, R. (2006). *Applying nursing process: A tool for critical thinking* (6th ed.). Lippincott Williams & Wilkins.

American Association of Colleges of Nursing (AACN). (2008). *The essentials of baccalaureate education for professional nursing practice.* Author. www.aacn.nche.edu/education-resources/baccessentials08.pdf

American Association of Colleges of Nursing. (2021). *The essentials: Core competencies for professional nursing education.* Author. https://www.aacnnursing.org/Portals/42/AcademicNursing/pdf/Essentials-2021.pdf

American Nurses Association (ANA). (2015a). *Nursing: Scope and standards of practice* (3rd ed.). Author.

American Nurses Association (ANA). (2015b). *Code of ethics for nurses with interpretive statements.* Author.

American Nurses Association (ANA). (2016). *Nursing administration: Scope and standards of practice* (2nd ed.). Author.

American Organization for Nursing Leadership (AONL). (2015a). *AONL nurse manager competencies.* Author.

American Organization for Nursing Leadership (AONL). (2015b). *AONL nurse executive competencies.* Author.

Benner, P. (1984). *From novice to expert: Excellence and power in clinical nursing practice.* Addison-Wesley.

Benner, P., Hughes, R., & Sutphen, M. (2008). Clinical reasoning, decision making, and action: Thinking critically and clinically. In R. Hughes (Ed.), *Patient safety and quality: An evidence-based handbook for nurses.* Agency for Healthcare Research and Quality.

Benner, P., Sutphen, M., Leonard, V., & Day, L. (2010). *Educating nurses: A call for radical transformation.* Jossey-Bass.

Bittner, N., & Tobin, E. (1998). Critical thinking: Strategies for clinical practice. *Journal of Nursing Staff Development, 14*(6), 267–272.

Caputi, L. J., & Kavanagh, J. M. (2018). Want your graduates to succeed? Teach them to think! *Nursing Education Perspectives, 39*(1), 2–3. doi: 10.1097/01.NEP.0000000000000271

Cronenwett, L., Sherwood, G., Barnsteiner, J., Disch, J., Johnson, J., Mitchell, P., Sullivan, D. T., & Warren, J. (2007). Quality and safety education for nurses. *Nursing Outlook, 55*(3), 122–131.

Facione, N. C., Facione, P. A., & Sanchez, C. A. (1994). Critical thinking disposition as a measure of competent clinical judgment: The development of the California Critical Thinking Disposition Inventory. *Nursing Education, 33*(8), 345–350.

Graham-Dickerson, P., Houser, J., Thomas, E., Casper, C., Erkenbrack, L., Wenzel, M., & Siegrist, M. (2013). The value of staff nurse involvement in decision making. *Journal of Nursing Administration, 43*(5), 286–292.

Greiner, A. C., & Knebel, E. (Ed.) (2003). *Health professions education: A bridge to quality.* National Academies Press.

Guo, K. L. (2008). DECIDE: A decision-making model for more effective decision making by health care managers. *Health Care Manager, 27*(2), 118–127.

Heaslip, P. (2008). *Critical thinking and nursing.* Foundation for Critical Thinking. www.criticalthinking.org/pages/critical-thinking-and-nursing/834

Houser, J., ErkenBrack, L., Handberry, L., Ricker, F., & Stroup, L. (2012). Involving nurses in decisions: Improving both nurse and patient outcomes. *Journal of Nursing Administration, 42*(7/8), 375–382.

Ignatavicius, D. (2001). Six critical thinking skills for at-the-bedside success. *Dimensions of Critical Care Nursing, 20*(2), 30–33.

Krairiksh, M., & Anthony, M. K. (2001). Benefits and outcomes of staff nurses' participation in decision making. *Journal of Nursing Administration, 31*(1), 16–23.

Manetti, W. (2019). Sound clinical judgment in nursing: A concept analysis. *Nursing Forum, 54*(1), 102–110. doi: 10.1111/nuf.12303

Manion, J. (2011). *From management to leadership: Strategies for transforming health care* (3rd ed.). Jossey-Bass.

McConnell, C. R. (2000). The anatomy of a decision. *Health Care Manager, 18*(4), 63–74.

Meline, D. L., & Brehm, S. N. (2015). Sustaining shared decision making: A biennial task force process. *American Nurse Today, 10*(3), 52–54.

National Council of State Boards of Nursing (NCSBN). (2013). *NCLEX-RN examination: Detailed test plan for the National Council licensure examinations for registered nurses: Item writer/item reviewer/nursing educator version.* Author. www.ncsbn.org/2013_NCLEX_RN_Detailed_Test_Plan_Educator.pdf

Payne, L. K. (2015). Intuitive decision making as the culmination of continuing education: A theoretical framework. *Journal of Continuing Education in Nursing, 46*(7), 326–332.

Pearce, C. (2007). Ten steps to carrying out a SWOT analysis. *Nursing Management, 14*(2), 25.

Porter-O'Grady, T., Igein, G., Alexander, D., Blaylock, J., McComb, D., & Williams, S. (2005). Critical thinking for nursing leadership. *Nurse Leader, 3*(4), 28–31.

Porter-O'Grady, T., & Malloch, K. (2013). *Leadership in nursing practice: Changing the landscape of health care.* Jones & Bartlett Learning.

Robert, R. R., Tilley, D.S., & Petersen, S. (2014). A power in clinical nursing practice: Concept analysis on nursing intuition. *Medsurg Nursing, 23*(5), 343–349.

Rushing, J., & Masters, K. (2020). Competencies for professional nursing practice. In Masters, K. (Ed), *Role development in professional nursing practice* (5th ed.). Jones & Bartlett Learning.

Scheffer, B. K., & Rubenfeld, M. G. (2000). A consensus statement on critical thinking in nursing. *Journal of Nursing Education, 39*(9), 352–360.

Scherb, C. A., Specht, J. K., Loes, J. L., & Reed, D. (2011). Decisional involvement: Staff nurse and nurse manager perceptions. *Western Journal of Nursing Research, 33*(2), 161–179.

Scriven, M., & Paul, R. (n.d.). *Defining critical thinking.* Foundation for Critical Thinking. www.critical thinking.org/pages/defining-critical-thinking/410

Shiparski, L. A. (2005). Engaging in shared decision making: Leveraging staff and management expertise. *Nurse Leader, 3*(1), 36–41.

Tanner, C. (2006). Thinking like a nurse: A research-based model of clinical judgment in nursing. *Journal of Nursing Education, 45*(6), 204–211.

Theobald, K. A., & Ramsbotham, J. (2019). Inquiry-based learning and clinical reasoning scaffolds: An action research project to support undergraduate students' learning to "think like a nurse." *Nurse Education in Practice, 38*(2019), 59–65. doi: 10.1016/j.nepr.2019.05.018

Zori, S., & Morrison, B. (2009). Critical thinking in nurse managers. *Nursing Economics, 27*(2), 75–79, 98.

Zori, S., Nosek, L. J., & Musil, C. M. (2010). Critical thinking of nurse managers related to staff RNs' perceptions of the practice environment. *Journal of Nursing Scholarship, 42*(3), 305–313.

To explore learning resources for this chapter, go to FADavis.com

Part II

Promotion of Patient Safety and Quality Care

Chapter *7*

High-Reliability Health-Care Organizations

Elizabeth J. Murray, PhD, RN, CNE

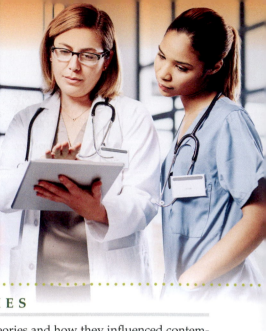

KEY TERMS

Centralized structure
Chain of command
Complexity theory
Continuum of care
Decentralized structure
For-profit
Futures thinking
General systems theory
High-reliability organization
Learning organization
Learning organization theory
Magnet
Magnet Recognition Program
Mission statement
Not-for-profit
Organizational structure
Organizational theory
Philosophy
Primary care
Secondary care
Span of control
Strategic foresight
Strategic planning
Tertiary care
Unity of command
Vision statement

LEARNING OUTCOMES

- Describe historical organizational theories and how they influenced contemporary organizational theories.
- Examine the characteristics of a high-reliability organization.
- Explain the elements of a health-care organization.
- Discuss the relationships among the mission, vision, and philosophy of an organization and nursing unit.
- Describe the purpose and steps of strategic planning.
- Explain the impact of regulation and accreditation on nursing and health-care organizations.
- Explain how nurse leaders and managers can use contemporary organizational theories to provide safe and quality care.

The Knowledge, Skills, and Attitudes Related to the Following Are Addressed in This Chapter:

Core Competencies	• Safety • Quality Improvement • Evidence-Based Practice
The Essentials: Core Competencies for Professional Nursing Education (AACN, 2021)	**Domain 7: Systems-Based Practice** 7.1 Apply knowledge of systems to work effectively across the continuum of care (p. 46).
Code of Ethics with Interpretive Statements (ANA, 2015)	**Provision 3.3:** Performance standards and review mechanisms (p. 11) **Provision 3.4:** Professional responsibility in promoting a culture of safety (pp. 11–12)

Nurse Manager (NMC) Competencies (AONL, 2015a) and Nurse Executive (NEC) Competencies (AONL, 2015b)	**NMC: Strategic Management (p. 5)**
	• Facilitate change
	• Project management
	• Contingency plans
	• Collaborate with other service lines
	• Shared decision-making
	  • Establish a vision statement
	  • Facilitate a structure of shared governance
	  • Implement structures and processes
	  • Support a just culture
	NEC: Knowledge of the Health Care Environment (pp. 6–7)
	• Governance
	  • Use knowledge of the role of the governing body of the organization in the following area: Performance management
	  • Represent patient care issues to the governing body
	  • Participate in strategic planning and quality initiatives with the governing body
	  • Interact with and educate the organization's board members regarding health care and the value of nursing care
	  • Represent nursing at the organization's board meetings
	• Patient safety
	  • Support the development of an organization-wide patient safety program

Nursing Administration Scope and Standards of Practice (ANA, 2016)	**Standard 5: Implementation** The nurse administrator implements the identified plan (p. 40). **Standard 6: Evaluation** The nurse administrator evaluates progress toward the attainment of goals and outcomes (p. 43).

Continued

The Knowledge, Skills, and Attitudes Related to the Following Are Addressed in This Chapter:—cont'd

Standard 10: Collaboration The nurse administrator collaborates with healthcare consumers, colleagues, community leaders, and other stakeholders to advance nursing practice and healthcare transformation (p. 50).

Standard 14: Quality of Practice The nurse administrator contributes to quality nursing practice (p. 55).

Standard 16: Resource Utilization The nurse administrator utilizes appropriate resources to plan, allocate, provide, and sustain evidence-based, high quality nursing services that are person, population, or community centered, culturally appropriate, safe, timely, effective, and fiscally responsible (p. 57).

Source: American Association of Colleges of Nursing. (2021). *The essentials: Core competencies for professional nursing education.* Author; American Nurses Association (ANA). (2015). *Code of ethics for nurses with interpretive statements.* Author; American Nurses Association (ANA). (2016). *Nursing administration: Scope and standards of practice* (2nd ed.). Author; American Organization for Nursing Leadership (AONL). (2015a). *AONL nurse manager competencies.* Author; American Organization for Nursing Leadership (AONL). (2015b). *AONL nurse executive competencies.* Author; Cronenwett, L., Sherwood, G., Barnsteiner, J., Disch, J., Johnson, J., Mitchell, P., Sullivan, D. T., & Warren, J. (2007). Quality and safety education for nurses. *Nursing Outlook, 55*(3), 122–131; and Greiner, A. C., & Knebel, E. (Eds.) (2003). *Health professions education: A bridge to quality.* National Academies Press.

Nurses work in many different types of health-care organizations and take on varying roles within each. Nurses at all levels must have a good understanding of how health-care systems work to be able to function effectively within an organization and deliver safe and quality nursing care. Understanding the nuances of health-care systems allows nurse leaders and managers to better navigate an organization, recognize the level of complexity, comprehend the need for change and innovation, and, in turn, see how nurses best play a role in the environment. With knowledge of how different systems work, nurse leaders and managers can better facilitate compliance with health-care regulations, identify opportunities and threats for strategic planning, and manage personnel and units and/or departments effectively.

In this chapter, organizational structures and theories that provide the frameworks for today's health-care environment are discussed. In addition, the basic elements of a health-care organization are outlined, including their role in the continuum of care.

▶ ORGANIZATIONAL THEORIES

Health-care organizations are called to deliver safe, timely, effective, equitable, evidence-based, patient-centered care. To understand how health-care organizations function in today's complicated health-care landscape, nurse leaders and managers need to be knowledgeable about some theoretical elements that shape organizations and explain organizational behavior. In general, organizations are complex, unpredictable, ambiguous, and, at times, deceptive. As a result, they can be difficult to manage (Bolman & Deal, 2008). Nurse leaders and managers who are able to see beyond the complexity and apply appropriate organizational theories can influence organizational effectiveness. **Organizational theory** can provide a framework to bring people together to accomplish work (Roussel, 2013). An organizational theory is not one size fits all. In fact, organizational administrators, leaders, and managers may vacillate among various theoretical concepts based on organizational behavior. Various schools of thought about leadership, management, and human behavior make up the various organizational theories (Mensik, 2014).

Classical Organization Theories

Organizational theories became prevalent during the industrial age, when large organizations were first developed; before this period in history, most businesses were family owned and run. Max Weber, a German sociologist, believed that a more formal approach was needed to foster success in the new organizations of the late 1800s and early 1900s. In turn, he developed the first organizational theory, the bureaucratic management theory, which focused on the structure of formal organizations, the authority of management, and rules and regulations to improve the success of an organization. He believed that a bureaucratic structure would protect employees from arbitrary decisions from supervisors and promote opportunities for employees to become specialists in their work area (Max Weber's theory of bureaucracy, 2009). A subsequent theory was the principles of management theory, developed by the engineer Henri Fayol, who is best known for identifying management functions of planning, organization, command, coordination, and control—all of which are still used today (Krenn, 2011). The scientific management theory was developed by another engineer, Frederick Taylor, who used scientific knowledge and mathematical formulas to manage the amount of work that could be accomplished in a specific time period and improve productivity. Taylor introduced the concept of using financial rewards to increase productivity (Dininni, 2011).

In the early 20th century, organizational theories began to explore the underlying differences in human behavior, characteristics, and roles of the work group. Mary Parker Follett was a theorist who embraced human relations theory and developed basic principles of participatory and humanistic management. She advocated for the principles of negotiation, conflict resolution, and power sharing (Dininni, 2010). All the classical theories were developed in an effort to improve overall organizational management and productivity, as well as define the functions of the manager and create a formal structure for solving problems in the organization.

Contemporary Organizational Theories

Contemporary organizational theories were built on the classical theories, and, in fact, elements of classical theories are present in many organizations today. However, modern organizations demand new organizational structures to survive as they discover that the linear theories of the past are not effective. Contemporary organizational theories need to reflect patterns, purposes, and processes and require a continuum-based, person- and outcome-driven system design (Porter-O'Grady & Malloch, 2013). Emerging theories are cyclical rather than linear and require organizations to react with speed and flexibility. Contemporary organizational theories that can be used to understand the complexity of health-care organizations include the general systems theory, complexity theory, learning organization theory, and high-reliability theory.

General Systems Theory

The primary premise of the **general systems theory** is that "the whole is greater than the sum of its parts" (Mensik, 2014, p. 38). The theory is based on two types of systems: an open system, which interacts with systems inside and outside; and a closed system, which has little or no interaction outside. Health-care organizations are seen as complex open systems in a dynamic state of flux. Open systems are composed of interrelated elements including inputs, throughputs, and outputs. The inputs are resources such as staff, patients, equipment, and supplies. The work of the organization is the throughput. The outcome of the work is the output. In the nursing environment, input is nursing personnel and their knowledge, skills, beliefs, and education; throughput involves the management of patient care by nurses; and output consists of patient care outcomes (Roussel, 2013). The system is a constant cycle of input, throughput, and output.

For example, a hospital is an open system, and within the hospital are departments or units, the subsystems (the laboratory, pharmacy, radiology, various nursing units, and so on). The overall effectiveness of the organization relies on the interdependent functioning of the subsystems. Open subsystems have permeable boundaries and are in constant interaction with other subsystems. In contrast, closed subsystems do not interact with other subsystems.

Nurse leaders and managers need to be flexible and open to new ideas to maintain the nursing unit as part of the open system. A nurse leader or manager who works in a closed-system unit is overly focused on internal functions and does not recognize that the unit is part of the larger system. This thinking can have a negative impact on the overall functioning of the organization. By being open to the system, nurse leaders and managers can maximize the functioning of the unit and enhance patient outcomes (Mensik, 2014).

Complexity Theory

Complexity theory is derived from the general systems theory, as well as physics, and it suggests that relationships are the key to everything (Mensik, 2014). Some key concepts of complexity theory are attractors, simple rules, independent agents, fractals, distributed leadership, butterfly effect, nonlinearity, self-organization, and emergence. Attractors are points of attraction that describe behavior in a complex system in which patterns of energy attract more energy (Crowell, 2020, pp. 20–25). As attractors interrelate in many different nonlinear ways, self-organization occurs, and unexpected new ideas or structures emerge. Hierarchical structures with top-down management approaches are no longer effective in the complexity of health care today. Patient care involves numerous processes with multiple factors that influence outcomes in various ways. At any given time, it is impossible to predict patient outcomes with 100% accuracy because many of the factors that influence patients' responses are unknown.

Nurse leaders and managers need to abandon linear, controlling, orderly, and predictable approaches to management. Instead, they must embrace the complexity of health care, patients, staff, and the work environment to promote a relationship-oriented structure that is adaptable, self-organizing, and self-renewing. Nurse leaders and managers face situations daily in which stability and instability are present at the same time (Crowell, 2020). In this paradox, nurse leaders and managers must balance three areas of tension in their roles. First, the nurse leader and manager must be efficient and effective, which involves managing the relationship between resource inputs and clinical outputs. Nurse leaders and managers are called to do more with less and manage staffing, skill mix, and patient care process while ensuring that safe, effective, evidence-based nursing care is delivered, all in compliance with regulations and professional standards. Second, nurse leaders and managers are ultimately accountable for the knowledge and competency of nursing staff and for the relational aspects of nursing care. Finally, nurse leaders and managers are responsible for stability and change, by balancing the need to ensure that patient care activities are on track and predictable with the drive for innovation and change needed for safe nursing practice (Crowell, 2020, p. 64). Nurse leaders and managers must constantly monitor the balance between stability and complete chaos to maximize variety and creativity within the system (Porter-O'Grady & Malloch, 2010). Further, nurse leaders and managers must focus on outcomes, develop fluid roles, and be able to act with speed and adaptability through chaos.

Learning Organization Theory

The **learning organization theory** was first described by Peter Senge (1990), who suggested that to excel, future organizations will need to "discover how to tap people's commitment and capacity to learn at all levels in an organization" (p. 4). He called on leaders to move away from traditional authoritarian "controlling organizations" and instead create learning organizations. Senge (1990) defined a **learning organization** as an "organization where people continually expand their capacity to create the results they truly desire, where new and expansive patterns of thinking are nurtured, where collective aspiration is set free, and where people are continually learning how to learn together" (p. 3). Senge (1990) identified five disciplines that organizations need to adopt and practice to become learning organizations:

1. *Systems thinking:* The understanding that everything is connected and interdependent
2. *Personal mastery:* The development of high-level personal proficiency, involving "the discipline of continually clarifying and deepening our personal vision, of focusing our energies, of developing patience, and of seeing reality objectively" (p. 7)
3. *Mental models:* Deeply ingrained assumptions that influence how a person understands and reacts to the world; understanding current mental models through reflection and inquiry, resulting in awareness of one's attitudes and perceptions and helping avoid jumping to conclusions and assumptions

4. *Building shared vision:* The establishment of a "mutual purpose" (p. 32) that fosters genuine commitment to the vision and organizational goals, rather than compliance
5. *Team learning:* Involving dismissal of assumptions, free-flowing exchange of meaning that allows group members to discover insights they would not attain individually, and a focus on working toward common goals

Members of a learning organization are continually practicing the five disciplines and are continually learning. Nurse leaders and managers can support a learning organization by involving staff in problem-solving and decision making, promoting interprofessional and intraprofessional teamwork, improving communication, and empowering staff. In the quest to deliver safe and quality patient care, health-care organizations must seek continuous learning and quality. A learning organization is no longer an ideal but an imperative (Glaser & Overhage, 2013).

High-Reliability Theory

High-reliability theory in health care includes principles of organizational design and leadership and management approaches that prevent patient harm and promote quality and safety (Riley, 2009). High reliability refers to consistent performance of a complex organization delivering high-risk services at high levels of safety over time (Chassin & Loeb, 2011; Weick & Sutcliffe, 2015). In this theory, reliability is the priority and it is enhanced by cultural norms. Leaders assume that risk exists and they devise strategies to anticipate and cope with risk. Emphasis is on developing a culture of mindfulness (Tamuz & Harrison, 2006).

Weick and Sutcliffe (2015) suggest that it is more than mindfulness, it is *collective mindfulness,* because high reliability is viewed through the lens of the effect people have on others' behaviors. Collective mindfulness is a mental orientation that is continuously evaluating the environment, tracking small failures, resisting oversimplification, and maintaining resilience. High-reliability theory is the foundation of high-reliability organizations.

High-Reliability Organizations

Health care organizations are challenged to consistently provide safe and reliable care. A **high-reliability organization (HRO)** is a complex organization that operates in complex, high-risk domains and consistently deliver services without serious accidents or failures (Agency for Healthcare Research and Quality [AHRQ], 2019). Further, HROs create processes, systems, and a culture that radically reduce system failures and/or effectively respond when failures do occur (AHRQ, 2019). High reliability is believed, by some, to mean effective standardization of health care processes. However, the principles go beyond standardization and involve a condition of persistent mindfulness throughout the organization. HROs use systems thinking to relentlessly prioritize safety and anticipate problems at all levels (AHRQ, 2019).

There are five key characteristics fundamental to designing processes and systems for HROs (AHRQ, 2019, p. 1):

- Sensitivity to operations
- Reluctance to simplify

- Preoccupation with failure
- Deference to expertise
- Resilience

Descriptions of each key characteristic are displayed in Box 7-1.

Becoming an HRO is a complex challenge and does not occur in a stepwise fashion. It is a transformation that must occur over time and consider numerous factors such as "including general environment issues; training and oversight of staff; processes for planning, implementing, and for measuring new initiatives; and specific work processes occurring on units" (AHRQ, 2008, p. 11). The first steps in becoming an HRO include establishing leadership commitment to zero harm; creating and sustaining a positive safety culture; and implementing a robust process for improvement (AHRQ, 2019).

Organizations become highly reliable by redesigning systems and changing processes. Everyone in the organization, from frontline providers to top-level administrators, must embrace a high-reliability mindset and strive for patient safety by committing to zero harm. Adelman (2019) contends that to become an HRO, organizations must commit to two strategic goals:

- A just culture, an environment where everyone feels safe to report errors and the focus is on correcting system issues rather than blaming the individual
- Leveraging technology and building systems that are resilient to human error

BOX 7-1 Key Characteristics for HROs		
KEY CONCEPTS	**DESCRIPTION**	**OUTCOMES**
Sensitivity to Operations	Constant awareness (situational awareness) by leaders and staff of the state of the systems and process that affect patient care.	Results in quick identification of potential and actual errors and ultimately reduce the number of errors.
Reluctance to Simplify	Simplistic explanations for why things work or fail are risky. Avoiding overly simple explanations that can place the patient at risk.	Results in all staff being encouraged to recognize the range of things that can go wrong and not assume that failures result for a single or simple cause. In turn, staff are more aware of potential errors.
Preoccupation with Failure	Near misses are viewed as evidence of systems that need improvement and opportunities to learn about systems.	Results in the constant concern that something may have been missed. Focus is on predicting and eliminating rather than reacting to failures.
Deference to Expertise	Leaders and supervisors must accept that staff may know how processes work and offer valuable insights. Deemphasizes hierarchy of the organization.	Empowers those closed to the work because they are the most knowledgeable about the work.
Resilience	There is a fundamental understanding that system failures are unpredictable. Everyone must be educated and prepared to know how to respond when system failures occur.	Everyone is prepared for failures and perform quick assessments, work effectively as a team, and rapidly respond to system failures.

Compiled from AHRQ, 2008, 2019; Weick & Sutcliffe, 2015.

Nurse leaders and managers can model a high-reliability mindset for staff and ensure that patient safety and quality are top priorities (ANA, 2016).

Framework for Safe, Reliable, and Effective Care

To help guide health-care organizations working toward achieving high reliability, a group of content experts from the Institute for Healthcare Improvement (IHI) and Safe and Reliable Healthcare (SRH) collaborated to develop the *White Paper: A Framework for Safe, Reliable, and Effective Care* (Frankel et al., 2017). The holistic framework provides direction for organizations "on key strategic, clinical, and operational components involved in achieving safe and reliable operational excellence" (Frankel et al., 2017, p. 6). The framework encompasses two overarching domains of culture and the learning system and nine interconnected components along with a core of patient and family engagement. In addition, all parts of the framework are interdependent with success in one area dependent on success in another (Frankel et al., 2017).

The components of the cultural domain include psychological safety, accountability, teamwork and collaboration, and negotiation. Transparency, reliability, improvement and measurement, and continuous learning are the components of the learning system. Leadership is a shared component of the cultural and learning system domains as it plays a critical role in supporting both. Leaders and managers must be committed to achieving safe, reliable, and effective health care, as well as fully understand, encourage, and apply the concepts of safety, reliability, improvement, and continuous learning (Frankel et al., 2017).

The engagement of patients and their families is at the core of the framework, which acknowledges their critical role as members of the health-care team. Further, effort should be focused on caring for patients and their families with emphasis on realizing the best outcomes across the continuum of care. To reach the goal of high reliability, patients and families must be engaged with the cultural and learning system domains as well as the interconnected components. Figure 7-1 illustrates the Framework for Safe, Reliable, and Effective Care. Additional information about the framework is available at http://www.ihi.org/resources/Pages/IHIWhitePapers/Framework-Safe-Reliable-Effective-Care.aspx

▶ BASIC ELEMENTS OF A HEALTH-CARE ORGANIZATION

Various types of health-care organizations providing different levels of care are needed in today's society. The variety of care and services received by patients from a variety of health-care providers in a variety of settings constitutes a continuum of care. **Continuum of care** is defined as "a concept involving a system that guides and tracks patients over time through a comprehensive array of health services spanning all levels and intensity of care" (Young et al., 2014, para. 1). The continuum of care covers the delivery of health care over a period of time, as expansive as from birth to end of life, and is important to ensure safe and quality care and to decrease fragmentation of care.

Nurses at all levels need to develop an understanding of the continuum of care and the basic elements of health-care to integrate health promotion, injury prevention, disease prevention, and disease management elements into their nursing

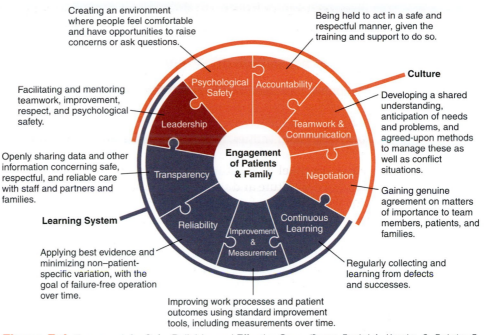

Creating an environment where people feel comfortable and have opportunities to raise concerns or ask questions.

Being held to act in a safe and respectful manner, given the training and support to do so.

Culture

Facilitating and mentoring teamwork, improvement, respect, and psychological safety.

Developing a shared understanding, anticipation of needs and problems, and agreed-upon methods to manage these as well as conflict situations.

Openly sharing data and other information concerning safe, respectful, and reliable care with staff and partners and families.

Gaining genuine agreement on matters of importance to team members, patients, and families.

Learning System

Applying best evidence and minimizing non–patient-specific variation, with the goal of failure-free operation over time.

Regularly collecting and learning from defects and successes.

Improving work processes and patient outcomes using standard improvement tools, including measurements over time.

Figure 7-1 Framework for Safe, Reliable, and Effective Care. *(Source: Frankel, A., Haraden, C., Federico, F., & Lenoci-Edwards, J. [2017]. A framework for safe, reliable, and effective care. Institute for Healthcare Improvement and Safe & Reliable Healthcare. [Available on ihi.org]. Reprinted with permission.)*

practice (American Association of Colleges of Nursing [AACN], 2008). Nurse leaders and managers must be knowledgeable and develop necessary skills to coordinate the care of patients with many other health-care providers and organizational units involved in providing care. Understanding the basic types of health-care organizations and the levels of services provided across them is the first step in achieving a continuum of care.

For-Profit Versus Not-for-Profit Organizations

Some health-care organizations are **for-profit** organizations, meaning they are owned by stockholders, shareholders, or corporate owners. Money brought in is reinvested into the organization to keep it running (e.g., in areas including maintenance, expansion, purchasing of equipment and supplies) and to develop new services. A for-profit organization must always have reserve funds to pay the corporate owners or the stockholders. As a result, funds may not always be readily available for certain purposes that can affect nurses and patient care. In contrast, **not-for-profit** organizations do not have stockholders or shareholders yet must also have funds available to run the organization. Possible sources of funding for not-for-profit organizations are public and/or government funding, grants, private donations, or a combination of these sources. A not-for-profit organization typically serves a large number of nonpaying patients. This can cause the organization to spend more money than it is bringing in. Additionally, a not-for-profit organization may have to cut services or make other changes to ensure a positive cash flow.

Types of Health-Care Organizations

Hospitals represent the largest type of health-care organization, and, in fact, more nurses work in hospitals than in any other type of health-care organization (Bureau of Labor Statistics, 2020). Other types of health-care organizations include extended care facilities, retirement and assisted living facilities, ambulatory care centers, home health care agencies, medical homes, psychiatric care facilities, and substance abuse treatment facilities. See Figure 7-2 for a breakdown of the types of health-care organizations in which nurses work.

Levels of Service

Health-care organizations are frequently categorized according to the complexity of the level of care provided throughout the continuum, which can be primary care, secondary care, or tertiary care. **Primary care** is the first line of defense and involves health promotion and illness prevention. In a primary care facility, the focus is on health education and health screening. Examples of primary care facilities include health-care provider's offices, immunization centers, and wellness centers. **Secondary care** involves emergency care and acute care. In this environment, the focus is on diagnosis, treatment, and limiting disability. Examples of secondary care facilities include hospitals, urgent care centers, ambulatory care facilities, and birthing centers. **Tertiary care** involves restoration and rehabilitation. In this environment, the focus is on maintaining and improving (if appropriate) the current state of health. Examples of tertiary care facilities are rehabilitation centers, assisted living centers, long-term care facilities, and hospices.

▶ ORGANIZATIONAL STRUCTURE AND CULTURE, AND STRATEGIC PLANNING

The structure and culture of a health-care organization need to be understood by nurse leaders and managers to ensure a safe and healthy work environment.

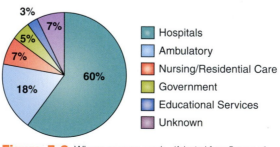

Figure 7-2 Where nurses work. *(Adapted from Bureau of Labor Statistics, U.S. Department of Labor, 2020.)*

Organizational Structure

Organizational structure outlines who is accountable and responsible for the work in an organization and subsequently helps define working relationships. Health-care organizations continue to be fairly traditional, with most having a hierarchical organizational structure and reflecting the classical principles of chain of command, unity of command, and span of control (Rundio et al., 2016). **Chain of command** refers to a formal line of authority from the top to the bottom of the organization. Each unit is connected to another, and reporting relationships are hierarchical (i.e., a unit's immediate manager reporting to the one above). **Unity of command** suggests that each individual employee is accountable to only one manager, with expectations clearly defined and well understood (Rundio et al., 2016, p. 16). **Span of control** defines a manager's scope of responsibility and reflects the number of employees who report to a given manager. Theoretically, the goal is to accomplish the work of the organization by dispersing responsibilities and duties equally so that one individual or unit is not overburdened. Organizational charts visually represent these principles, with each unit connected in a hierarchal manner. The goal of an organizational chart is to reflect formal relationships between and among units within an organization.

Organizational structures can be centralized or decentralized. A **centralized structure**, often referred to as tall (or hierarchical), is one in which the authority for decision making is held by a few individuals at the top level of management. Typically, the chief executive officer and administrators hold the highest level in the organization. They have authority to hire and fire, make financial decisions, and implement change. Depending on the levels of management, some authority may be delegated to those employees reporting to an administrator. In a centralized structure, there is minimal innovation or creativity, and problems are dealt with by a few leaders and managers; this system sometimes results in delays in decision making. Communication flows from top to bottom and is tightly controlled. Nurses may or may not participate in decision making in a centralized structure. Responsibilities of nurse leaders and managers vary depending on their position and level in the organization. Figure 7-3 illustrates a centralized organizational chart.

In a **decentralized structure**, often referred to as flat, authority and power for decision making are shared by a number of individuals across the organization. In this environment, problems can often be solved at the level where they occur. Typically, staff members are responsible for making decisions related to their areas of expertise. Communication flows from the bottom upward and between units. Nurses participate in decisions that affect their nursing practice and patient care. Nurse leaders and managers foster shared governance and teamwork and collaboration. A decentralized structure fosters autonomy at all levels. Figure 7-4 illustrates a decentralized organizational chart.

Organizational Culture

Organizational culture is an informal, yet recognizable, group philosophy or worldview that guides behaviors of the members of the organization. It is shaped

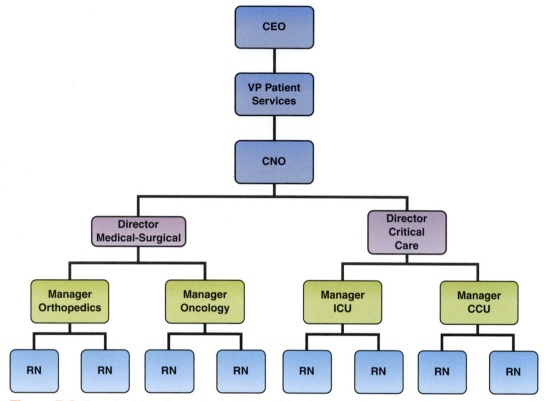

Figure 7-3 Centralized (or tall) organizational chart. *CCU,* Coronary care unit; *CEO,* chief executive officer; *CNO,* chief nursing officer; *ICU,* intensive care unit; *RN,* registered nurse; *VP,* vice president.

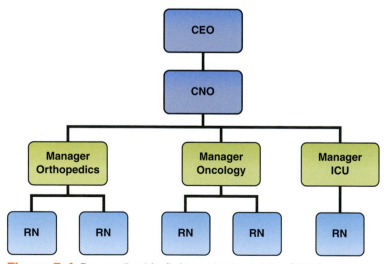

Figure 7-4 Decentralized (or flat) organizational chart. *CEO,* Chief executive officer; *CNO,* chief nursing officer; *ICU,* intensive care unit; *RN,* registered nurse.

by the mission, vision, and philosophy of the organization and reflects its values and beliefs as well.

The **mission statement** of an organization describes the organization's overall purpose. Being future oriented, the mission statement should reflect the direction toward which the organization intends to head. The **vision statement** reflects the image for the future the organization plans to create (Roussel, 2013, p. 343). Mission and vision statements often are created by top-level administration. However, when all staff members are involved in developing mission and vision statements, they will believe in their abilities and become committed to the organization (Roussel, 2013; Rundio et al., 2016). A **philosophy** is a statement of beliefs, values, concepts, and principles that reflect the ideas, convictions, and attitudes of the organization. The philosophy of an organization becomes the basis for operationalizing the mission and vision of the organization (Tuck et al., 2000).

Nurse leaders and managers have a major responsibility to model the core values of the organization and ensure that the activities of their unit or department reflect the vision, mission, and philosophy of the organization. The nursing mission, vision, and philosophy emerge from the organization's and should articulate the nature of the nurse's role, the values of nursing, what nursing should and will be, and what populations are served, as well as a purpose statement (Roussel, 2013). Additionally, the mission, vision, and philosophy of nursing should be known and understood by everyone within the organization, including health-care providers, patients and families, and the community (Roussel, 2013). The ideal culture in a health-care environment is a culture of safety, as discussed in detail in Chapter 9.

Strategic Planning

Strategic planning is how an organization defines its future. It is based on an understanding of an organizational mission and vision and aligns an organization with defined goals and can be considered a roadmap for the future of an organization (Schaffner, 2009; Thomas & Winter, 2020). **Strategic planning** is defined as "a continuous, systematic process of making risk-taking decisions today with the greatest possible knowledge of their effects on the future; organizing efforts necessary to carry out these decisions and evaluating results of these decisions against expected outcome through reliable feedback mechanisms" (Drucker, 1974, p. 125). Nurse leaders and managers participate in strategic planning at the organizational and department or unit level. Strategic planning forecasts the future success of an organization and begins by ensuring that its mission, vision, and philosophy are up to date (Conway-Morana, 2009). Steps of the strategic planning process are displayed in Box 7-2.

A primary goal of strategic planning is to maximize organizational performance. One strategy used in the planning process is evaluation of the organization's strengths, weaknesses, opportunities, and threats, known as SWOT analysis. SWOT analysis can assist nurse leaders and managers in improving care delivery by identifying the strengths of the unit and/or staff, areas for improvement, and opportunities for facilitating positive change. The first step in a SWOT analysis is to collect data, which may include staff characteristics, unit census,

---

BOX 7-2   Strategic Planning Process

1. Clearly define the purpose of the organization.
2. Establish realistic goals and objectives consistent with the mission and vision of the organization.
3. Identify the organization's external stakeholders, and determine their assessment of the organization's purposes and operation.
4. Clearly communicate the goals and objectives to the organization's stakeholders.
5. Develop a sense of ownership of the plan.
6. Develop strategies to achieve the goals.
7. Ensure effective use of organization resources.
8. Provide a benchmark to measure progress.
9. Provide a mechanism for informed change as needed.
10. Build a consensus about where the organization is going.

---

patient characteristics, and more. Next, the data are analyzed and sorted into one of the four categories: strengths, weaknesses, opportunities, and threats. Organization or unit strengths and opportunities are viewed as positive or helpful, whereas weaknesses and threats are considered negative or harmful. Additionally, strengths and weaknesses originate internally, whereas opportunities and threats originate externally. Table 7-1 displays a SWOT matrix commonly used in a SWOT analysis.

Nurse leaders and managers lead strategic planning, conduct SWOT analyses, and provide strategic direction for their staff and units (AONL, 2015b) Typically, nurse leaders and managers also contribute to organizational strategic planning. An expectation of nurse leaders and managers in upper-level positions within an organization is that they will provide leadership in the development of the organizational mission, vision, and philosophy and the strategic planning process (ANA, 2016). Further, nurse leaders and managers are accountable for communicating, implementing, and evaluating strategic plans. Employees must have the

Table 7-1   SWOT Analysis

Positive or Helpful	Negative or Harmful
Internal Origin	
STRENGTHS	WEAKNESSES
• Internal characteristics that assist an organization or unit in achieving goals	• Internal characteristics that hinder an organization or unit in achieving goals
• Result in outstanding organizational or unit performance	• Result in increased costs, decreased patient satisfaction, or decreased quality
• Examples: staff expertise, patient satisfaction, staff satisfaction	• Examples: increased cost for benefits, staffing shortages, fragmented care
External Origin	
OPPORTUNITIES	THREATS
• External influences that assist an organization or unit in achieving goals	• External influences that threaten an organization or unit in achieving goals
• Examples: new programs and services, advanced technology, increased funding	• Examples: nursing shortage, economic instability, decreased reimbursement, increased regulation

necessary skills to participate in developing and designing care delivery models that support the organization's strategic visions (ANA, 2016). Nurse leaders and managers are critical to ensuring that the nursing strategic goals are in line with the organization's goals.

LEARNING ACTIVITY 7-1

Conducting a SWOT Analysis

Think about a personal area in your life you would like to change (e.g., beginning an exercise program). Use a SWOT analysis matrix and identify the strengths, weaknesses, opportunities, and threats related to the change.

Given the current state of health care and the focus on cost containment, operational efficiencies, and safety and quality mandates, some believe that strategic planning will need to shift from a traditional business approach to a more futuristic approach. Impeding this change is the reality that many health-care stakeholders continue to be entrenched in an outdated mindset that focuses on financial rewards for providing health-care services to the sick, rather than promoting health and preventing disease (Luzinski, 2014). The enactment of the Patient Protection and Affordable Care Act of 2010 placed pressure on health-care organizations to improve their patients' experiences, the safety and quality of care, employee culture, and financial status. This change requires a more futuristic approach to planning, such as using strategic foresight (Luzinski, 2014). Although new to health care, strategic foresight has been used for years in other industries. **Strategic foresight** is seeing the relevant opportunities that could emerge from the future and strategizing how to make the most of them. Leaders must shift their focus from the current existing state of the organization to envisioning the organization 10 years into the future (Luzinski, 2014).

Futures thinking and foresight are seen as prerequisite competencies for success in the dynamic health-care system (Freed & McLaughlin, 2011; Luzinski, 2014). **Futures thinking** entails bringing vision to the planning process, seeing the relevant opportunities that are emerging, and creating a desired future. Nurse leaders and managers need to become self-aware of their current mental model and embrace changing to futures thinking. Four practices that "create a culture where the future can be assessed and leveraged" are collaborating, reflecting, envisioning, and strategizing (Emelo, 2011, p. 8). Collaboration is needed because foresight emerges from the interactive vision of people throughout the organization. Collaborating with people with differing perspectives helps leaders better reflect on the past, evaluate current data and trends, and thoughtfully consider possible future options. Foresight embraces the past and requires leaders to reflect on previous performance to identify patterns that may indicate actions for the future. Reflecting on the past allows all involved parties to envision the future. Once future opportunities are identified, leaders must strategize approaches to bring the opportunities into reality (Emelo, 2011).

Nurses have always been prepared for the future, but now nurse educators are called to help nursing students develop futures thinking. Thinking for the future will assist all nurses as well as nurse leaders and managers to "make decisions in future-oriented ways, develop increased awareness and sensitivity to multiple influences and their interactions that have bearing on the future, take responsibility to build and shape desired futures (their own futures, the profession's future, and the future of the health care system)" (Freed & McLaughlin, 2011, p. 177).

▶ REGULATION AND ACCREDITATION

Nurses at all levels must understand the complex health-care system and the impact of policy, regulations, and accreditation on these systems (AACN, 2008). Nurse leaders and managers are responsible for setting expectations for staff adherence to legislative and regulatory processes and interpret the impact on nursing and health-care organizations (AONL, 2015b; ANA, 2016).

Regulation

Health care is a highly regulated industry. Health-care regulatory policies directly and indirectly influence nursing practice and the nature and functioning of the health-care system (AACN, 2008). Regulations are developed and implemented by federal, state, and local governments, as well as private organizations, and can be very complex and difficult to understand (Mensik, 2014). Regulations and policies can affect the quality of patient care, the workplace environment, the availability of resources, and finances. Nurse leaders and managers need to stay current regarding federal and state laws and regulations that can affect patient care (AONL, 2015b; ANA, 2016).

Accreditation

Nurses must have a basic understanding of not only the legislative and regulatory processes but also the accreditation process. Accreditation ensures that health-care organizations meet certain national quality standards. When health-care organizations are accredited, it means the accrediting agency has conferred deeming status on the organization and the organization has met Medicare and Medicaid certification standards (Shi & Singh, 2008). Although accreditation is voluntary, Medicare, Medicaid, and most insurance companies require accreditation by The Joint Commission or the DNV GL through state regulatory agencies to provide funds to an organization. State governments also oversee the licensure and certification of health-care organizations. State standards address the "physical plant's compliance with building codes, fire safety, climate, control, space allocations, and sanitation" (Shi & Singh, 2008, p. 320). State departments of health certify health-care organizations through periodic inspections. Certification entitles health-care organizations to receive Medicare and Medicaid funding.

The Joint Commission

The Joint Commission (TJC) is an independent not-for-profit organization founded in 1951. The mission of the TJC is "to continuously improve health care for the public, in collaboration with other stakeholders, by evaluating health care organizations and inspiring them to excel in providing safe and effective care of the highest quality and value" (TJC, 2020, para. 2). TJC accredits more than 22,000 health-care organizations in the United States, and the international arm of TJC accredits health-care agencies in more than 100 countries. TJC accreditation can be earned by many types of health-care organizations, including hospitals, doctor's offices, nursing homes, office-based surgery centers, behavioral health treatment facilities, and providers of home care services (TJC, 2020).

DNV GL

DNV GL was created in 2013 in a merger between Det Norske Veritas (Norway) and Germanischer Lloyd (Germany). The international organization partners with National Integrated Accreditation for Healthcare Organizations (NIAHO) to provide accreditation for health-care agencies. The NIAHO standards are based on Medicare Conditions of Participation standards and the International Organization for Standardization (ISO) 9001 quality management standards. The ISO 9001 standards provide a framework for organizations to implement quality management systems that will streamline processes, maintain efficiency, and increase productivity (ACS Registrars, 2014, para. 1). More than 600 hospitals now have accreditation through DNV GL (DNV GL, 2019).

Magnet Recognition Program

In 1983, the American Academy of Nursing task force on nursing practice in hospitals conducted a study to determine what attracted nurses to hospitals (American Nurses Credentialing Center [ANCC], n.d.c). The study determined that 41 of 163 hospitals could be considered **Magnet** hospitals—in other words, they possessed qualities that attracted and retained nurses (ANCC, n.d.c). A total of 14 qualities were identified that distinguished these hospitals from others, and these qualities became known as the "Forces of Magnetism." Building on this study, the Magnet Hospital Recognition Program for Excellence in Nursing was approved by the American Nurses Association in December 1990 (ANCC, n.d.c). The University of Washington Medical Center in Seattle, Washington, became the first ANCC Magnet-designated organization, in 1994. Since then, the **Magnet Recognition Program** has expanded to include long-term care facilities and health-care organizations internationally (ANCC, n.d.c). As of 2019, about 8% of all hospitals in the United States had achieved Magnet recognition (ANCC, n.d.b).

The ANCC integrated the 14 Forces of Magnetism into the following five model components (ANCC, n.d.d):

1. *Transformational leadership:* Nursing leaders at all levels of a Magnet-recognized organization must use futures thinking and demonstrate advocacy and support on behalf of staff and patients to transform values, beliefs, and behaviors. Nurse leaders and managers must be transformational and lead staff "where they need to be in order to meet the demands of the future" (para. 6). The Forces

of Magnetism represented in this element are Quality of Nursing Leadership and Management Style.

2. *Structural empowerment:* Nurse leaders and managers at all levels of a Magnet organization are influential and participate in an innovative environment where professional practice flourishes. Nurse leaders and managers must develop, direct, and empower staff to participate in achieving organizational goals and desired outcomes. The Forces of Magnetism represented in this element are Organizational Structure; Personnel Policies and Programs; Community and the Health-Care Organization; Image of Nursing; and Professional Development (para. 7).

3. *Exemplary professional practice:* Exemplary professional practice in Magnet-recognized organizations is evidenced by a comprehensive understanding of the role of nursing, strong intraprofessional and interprofessional teamwork, and ongoing application of new knowledge evidence in practice. Nurse leaders and managers must promote interprofessional collaboration and teamwork. The Forces of Magnetism represented include Professional Models of Care, Consultation and Resources, Autonomy, Nurses as Teachers, and Interdisciplinary Relationships (para. 8).

4. *New knowledge, innovations, and improvements:* Magnet-recognized organizations embrace transformational leadership and foster professional empowerment. Nurse leaders and managers must focus on redesigning and redefining practice to be successful in the future. The Force of Magnetism represented is Quality Improvement (para. 9).

5. *Empirical quality results:* The empirical measurement of quality outcomes related to nursing leadership and clinical practice in Magnet-recognized organizations is imperative. Currently, organizations have some structure and processes in place. However, the focus in the future must shift from "What do you do?" or "How do you do it?" to "What difference have you made?" Nurse leaders and managers must participate in establishing quantitative benchmarks for measuring outcomes related to nursing, the workforce, patients, consumers, and the organization. The Force of Magnetism represented is Quality of Care (para 10).

These five model components form a framework of excellence in nursing practice and make up the Magnet Model. Overarching the Magnet Model are Global Issues in Nursing and Healthcare, which reflect the various factors and challenges facing nursing today (ANCC, n.d.d).

Achieving Magnet status benefits the organization and all stakeholders. Further, Magnet-recognized organizations are able to recruit and retain top-notch nursing talent; improve patient care, patient safety, and staff safety; increase patient satisfaction; foster a collaborative culture; advance nursing standards and professional practice; and improve business stability and financial success (ANCC, n.d.a). Magnet designation is associated with many positive outcomes for patients and nurses (Ulrich et al., 2007). Higher overall patient satisfaction, lower morbidity and mortality rates, decreased numbers of pressure ulcers, patient safety, and higher-quality care are evident in Magnet hospitals (ANCC, n.d.b). Nurses report job satisfaction, autonomy and control over nursing practice, fewer injuries, and less burnout than do nurses working in non-Magnet organizations (Ulrich et al., 2007). Health-care consumers are becoming more aware of the Magnet designation and recognize a Magnet hospital as one with high-quality nursing care.

LEARNING ACTIVITY 7-2	**Identifying the Accrediting Body and Magnet Status of an Organization**

Explore the Web site of a clinical agency where you have worked or had clinical experience during nursing school. Address the following:

1. Identify the accrediting body.
2. Does the agency have Magnet status?
3. Was it easy to find this information?

✪ Hospital Consumer Assessment of Health-Care Providers and Systems

In the past, hospitals collected data on patient satisfaction for internal use and focused on clinical outcomes as the primary measure of effectiveness and quality. Although many hospitals collected data on patient satisfaction, there was no national standard for collecting and publicly reporting the information. Health care is moving from a disease-focused model of care to patient-centered care. Along with this transition, patient satisfaction with care has become an important indicator of quality health care. The Patient Protection and Affordable Care Act of 2010 requires implementation of value-based purchasing (VBP), which bases Medicare reimbursement to hospitals on quality of care.

To measure patients' perceptions of their health-care experience, the Hospital Consumer Assessment of Healthcare Providers and Systems (HCAHPS) survey was implemented in 2006 by the Centers for Medicare & Medicaid Services (CMS, 2019). The HCAHPS allows valid comparisons across hospitals locally, regionally, and nationally, and it has three major goals (CMS, 2019, p. 1):

1. The standardized survey and implementation protocol produces data that allow objective and meaningful comparisons of hospitals on topics that are important to patients and consumers.
2. Public reporting of HCAHPS results creates new incentives for hospitals to improve quality of care.
3. Public reporting enhances accountability in health care by increasing transparency of the quality of hospital care provided in return for the public investment.

The HCAHPS is administered to a random sample of adult inpatients between 24 hours and 6 weeks after discharge (CMS, 2019, p. 2). HCAHPS scores based on four consecutive quarters of patient surveys are publicly reported annually on the Medicare Web site (www.medicare.gov/hospitalcompare).

A major incentive for hospitals to work toward high quality of care is that hospital payment from CMS through the VBP program is linked to performance on a set of quality measures related to HCAHPS scores (CMS, 2019). Hospitals are working toward identifying and implementing changes that can increase patient satisfaction outcomes. Studies indicate that quality nursing care is a predictor of higher HCAHPS scores (Chen et al., 2014; Kutney-Lee et al., 2009; Otani et al., 2010; Wolosin et al., 2012). Additionally, one study found a significant link between Magnet hospitals and higher HCAHPS scores (Chen et al., 2014).

EXPLORING THE EVIDENCE 7-1

Chen, J., Koren, M. E., Munroe, D. J., & Yao, P. (2014). Is the hospital's Magnet status linked to HCAHPS scores? *Journal of Nursing Care Quality, 29*(4), 327–335.

Aim
The aims of this study were:

1. To identify the differences in HCAHPS scores between Magnet and non-Magnet hospitals.
2. To assess the extent to which Magnet status and other variables among hospital and nursing characteristics contributed to the HCAHPS scores.

Methods
This study was a cross-sectional, secondary analysis of data from the Illinois Hospital Report Card. The database houses more than 175 indicators of quality, safety, utilization, and charges for specific procedures and medical conditions among Illinois hospitals.

   The study included all adult acute care hospitals in Illinois with 100 beds or more, available results of HCAHPS, nursing hours per patient day (NHPPD), RN nursing hours per patient day, and RN turnover rate in 2009. The sample consisted of 110 hospitals or 58.8% of total adult acute care hospitals in Illinois. The researchers analyzed data reported between January 2009 and December 2009. Data were analyzed using independent samples t test, Pearson χ^2, and linear multiple regression.

Key Findings
Magnet hospitals were significantly more likely to:

1. Be teaching hospitals.
2. Have a larger number of beds.
3. Have lower percentages of African American patients and Medicare payments.
4. Have more NHPPD and RN-NHPPD than the non-Magnet hospitals.

   Magnet hospitals received higher scores than non-Magnet hospitals in all of the seven HCAHPS measures with significant differences in all measures, except for "patients always received help as soon as they wanted."

   Magnet status of the hospital was the second important contributor to the HCAHPS scores, explaining 5% to 13% of the variance in six of the seven HCAHPS measures. Again, the only measure that it did not explain was "patients always received help as soon as they wanted."

   The positive association between Magnet status and the HCAHPS scores was most significant in the following two measures:

1. "Percentage of patients highly satisfied."
2. "Patients would definitely recommend this hospital to friends and family."

   Hospitals with higher RN-NHPPD were more likely to receive higher scores in "patients always received help as soon as they wanted." Hospitals with lower RN turnover rate were more likely to receive higher scores in "percentage of patients highly satisfied," "patients would definitely recommend this hospital to friends and family," and "staff always explained about medicines."

Implications for Nurse Leaders and Managers

The findings of this study support the need to consider RN-NHPPD and RN turnover rates as significant contributors to positive scores on some HCAHPS measures. In addition, this study suggests that other factors embedded in Magnet hospitals positively influence HCAHPS scores. The investigators suggest that an environment that supports professional practice and environmental factors such as structural empowerment and adequate access to support and resources can promote quality of care and improve patient satisfaction.

Nurse leaders and managers, even those not working in Magnet hospitals, can use these findings to create a work environment that embraces Magnet characteristics with the goals of improving the quality of nursing care and patient satisfaction outcomes.

▶ SUMMARY

Health-care organizations are complex systems that are constantly changing and that are moving away from being disease focused to patient centered. Nurses at all levels must understand the basic makeup of these systems as well as the role that organizational theories, organizational structure and culture, and regulation and accreditation play in the delivery of safe and quality evidence-based care. Overall, leaders, managers, and frontline staff must embrace a high-reliability mindset to become a high-reliability organization. High-reliability organizations foster a learning environment and promote a safety culture, evidence-based practice, and a positive work environment for nurses. In addition, they are committed to improving the safety and quality of care.

NCLEX®-STYLE REVIEW QUESTIONS

Multiple Choice

1. The nurse leader is using general systems theory to assist in implementing changes on the nursing unit and knows that what nursing activities are considered throughput?
   1. Nursing skills
   2. Nursing education
   3. Nursing management of care
   4. Nursing beliefs

2. A nurse leader has begun to look for a new position in a different health-care organization because the present organization is a closed system. The nurse leader is aware that this system has led to what issue on the nursing unit?
   1. The nurse leader has had to be open to new ideas.
   2. The nurse leader had difficulty recognizing the nursing unit was a part of the whole organization.
   3. The nurse leader did not like the flexibility required as part of this type of system.
   4. The nurse leader was not prepared for the self-renewing, self-organizing aspect of the nursing unit.

3. The nurse manager in a for-profit health-care facility explains to a new staff nurse that the profits from care are used in what capacity?
   1. Pay for a new magnetic resonance imaging (MRI) machine
   2. Increase the pay for all staff members
   3. Provide for extra services for patients
   4. Give bonuses to executives of the facility

4. The nurse manager in a not-for-profit health-care facility is aware that what issue may arise due to the funding for this type of organization?
   1. The care provided to patients is of lower quality than the care given in for-profit health-care organizations.
   2. There is a possibility that staff must be reduced because of decreased available funds.
   3. The health-care organization will move all inpatient to outpatient care.
   4. If available funds are reduced, managers will be let go and each unit will run itself.

5. Nurse managers know that what category of worker in a health-care organization is employed more than any other?
   1. Nursing
   2. Maintenance
   3. Dietary
   4. Environmental/housekeeping

6. A nurse manager is planning to take on the responsibility for a nursing unit that specializes in tertiary care. The nurse manager knows that this unit will be responsible for the care of what type of patients?
   1. Those who are giving birth
   2. Those who are being treated for pneumonia
   3. Those who are seeking treatment for a knee strain
   4. Those who had a knee replacement and are receiving rehabilitation

7. The nurse manager reports directly to the director of nursing and knows that this defines what type of command?
   1. Span of command
   2. Chain of command
   3. Unity of command
   4. Organizational structure

8. The nurse manager is conducting a SWOT analysis as a part of a strategic planning process and arranges for the new electronic health record being used on the nursing unit to be featured in the local newspaper. The nurse manager knows that this corresponds to what part of the SWOT analysis?
   1. Strengths
   2. Weaknesses
   3. Opportunities
   4. Threats

9. The nurse manager recognizes that what is fostered at all levels in a decentralized health-care organization?
   1. Authority to hire and fire
   2. Feelings of autonomy
   3. Ability to make changes at all levels
   4. Top-to-bottom communication

10. The nurse manager is involved in strategic planning and knows that what is the reason for this process to be instituted?
    1. Strategic planning defines the future of the organization.
    2. Strategic planning reflects the image of the future the organization plans to create.
    3. Strategic planning reflects the attitudes, ideas, and convictions of the organization.
    4. Strategic planning reflects the direction in which the organization intends to head.

11. The nurse manager is planning a change to the nursing unit that requires all patients to receive health promotion education but knows that this may be difficult for what reason?
    1. The regulations of the Patient Protection and Affordable Care Act of 2010
    2. The need to focus on health promotion and disease prevention
    3. Focus of financial rewards for providing health care to the sick
    4. The shift from a traditional to a futuristic planning approach

Multiple Response

12. The director of nursing is encouraging the nurse managers to begin seeking Magnet status for the facility and knows that this status is associated with what positive outcomes for both nurses and patients? *Select all that apply.*
    1. Increased patient satisfaction
    2. Decreased morbidity with static mortality rates
    3. Decreased numbers of peripheral intravenous infiltrations
    4. More nursing autonomy
    5. Decreased nurse burnout

REFERENCES

ACS Registrars. (2014). *ISO 9001 revision.* www.acsregistrars.com/2014/11/27/iso-9001-revision-due-in-2015

Adelman, J. (2019). High-reliability healthcare: Building safer systems through just culture and technology. *Journal of Healthcare Management, 64*(3), 137–141. doi:10.1097/JHM-D-19-00069

Agency for Healthcare Research and Quality (AHRQ). (2008). *Becoming a high reliability organization: Operational advice for hospital leaders.* AHRQ Publication No. 08-0022. Author.

Agency for Healthcare Research and Quality (AHRQ). (2019). Patient safety primer: High reliability. https://psnet.ahrq.gov/primer/high-reliability

American Association of Colleges of Nursing (AACN). (2008). *The essentials of baccalaureate education for professional nursing practice.* Author.

American Association of Colleges of Nursing. (2021). *The essentials: Core competencies for professional nursing education.* Author. https://www.aacnnursing.org/Portals/42/AcademicNursing/pdf/Essentials-2021.pdf

American Nurses Association (ANA). (2015). *Code of ethics for nurses with interpretive statements.* Author.

American Nurses Association (ANA). (2016). *Nursing administration: Scope and standards of practice* (2nd ed.). Author.

American Nurses Credentialing Center (ANCC). (n.d.a). *About Magnet: Benefits.* https://www.nursingworld.org/organizational-programs/magnet/about-magnet/why-become-magnet/benefits/

American Nurses Credentialing Center (ANCC). (n.d.b). *About Magnet: Growth.* https://www.nursingworld.org/organizational-programs/magnet/about-magnet/growth/

American Nurses Credentialing Center (ANCC). (n.d.c). *About Magnet: History of the magnet program.* https://www.nursingworld.org/organizational-programs/magnet/about-magnet/

American Nurses Credentialing Center (ANCC). (n.d.d). *Magnet model—Creating a magnet culture.* https://www.nursingworld.org/organizational-programs/magnet/magnet-model/

American Organization for Nursing Leadership (AONL). (2015a). *AONL nurse manager competencies.* Author.

American Organization for Nursing Leadership (AONL). (2015b). *AONL nurse executive competencies.* Author.

Bolman, L. G., & Deal, T. E. (2008). *Reframing organizations: Artistry, choice, and leadership* (4th ed.). Jossey-Bass.

Bureau of Labor Statistics, U.S. Department of Labor. (2020). Registered nurses. *Occupational Outlook Handbook, 2020.* www.bls.gov/ooh/healthcare/registered-nurses.htm

Centers for Medicare & Medicaid Services. (2019). *HCAHPS fact sheet.* https://hcahpsonline.org/en/facts/

Chassin, M. R., & Loeb, J. M. (2011). The ongoing quality improvement journey: Next stop, high reliability. *Health Affairs, 30*(4), 559–568.

Chen, J., Koren, M. E., Munroe, D. J., & Yao, P. (2014). Is the hospital's magnet status linked to HCAHPS scores? *Journal of Nursing Care Quality, 29*(4), 327–335.

Conway-Morana, P. L. (2009). Nursing strategy: What's your plan? *Nursing Management, 40*(3), 25–29.

Cronenwett, L., Sherwood, G., Barnsteiner, J., Disch, J., Johnson, J., Mitchell, P., Sullivan, D. T., & Warren, J. (2007). Quality and safety education for nurses. *Nursing Outlook, 55*(3), 122–131.

Crowell, D. M. (2020). *Complexity leadership: Nursing's role in health care delivery* (3rd ed.). F. A. Davis.

Dininni, J. (2010). Management theory of Mary Parker Follett. *Business.com.* www.business.com/management/management-theory-of-mary-parker-follett

Dininni, J. (2011). Management theory of Frederick Taylor. *Business.com.* www.business.com/management/management-theory-of-frederick-taylor

DNV GL. (2019). *Hospital accreditation.* http://dnvgl/us/assurance/healthcare/ac

Drucker, P. F. (1974). *Management tasks, responsibilities, politics.* Harper & Row.

Emelo, R. (2011). Strategic foresight: See and seize emerging opportunities. *Leadership Excellence, 28*(3), 8.

Frankel, A., Haraden, C., Federico, F., & Lenoci-Edwards, J. (2017). *White paper: A framework for safe, reliable, and effective care.* Institute for Healthcare Improvement and Safe & Reliable Healthcare.

Freed, P. E., & McLaughlin, D. E. (2011). Futures thinking: Preparing nurses to think for tomorrow. *Nursing Education Perspectives, 32*(11), 173–178.

Glaser J., & Overhage J. M. (2013). The role of healthcare IT: Becoming a learning organization. *Healthcare Financial Management, 67*(2), 56–62, 64.

Greiner, A. C., & Knebel, E. (Eds.) (2003). *Health professions education: A bridge to quality.* National Academies Press.

Krenn, J. (2011). Management theory of Henri Fayol. *Business.com.* www.business.com/management/management-theory-of-henri-fayol

Kutney-Lee, A., McHugh, M. D., Sloane, D. M., Cimiotti, J. P., Flynn, L., Felber Neff, D., & Aiken, L. H. (2009). Nursing: A key to patient satisfaction. *Health Affairs, 28*(4), w669–w677.

Luzinski, C. (2014). Identifying leadership competencies of the future: Introducing the use of strategic foresight. *Nurse Leader, 12*(4), 37–39, 47.

Max Weber's theory of bureaucracy. (2009). *Business mate.* www.businessmate.org/Article.php?ArtikelId=30

Mensik, J. (2014). *Lead, drive, & thrive in the system.* American Nurses Association.

Otani, K., Herrmann, P. A., & Kurz, R. S. (2010). Patient satisfaction integration process: Are there any racial differences? *Health Care Management Review, 35*(2), 116–123.

Porter-O'Grady, T., & Malloch, K. (2010). *Innovation leadership: Creating the landscape of health care.* Jones & Bartlett Learning.

Porter-O'Grady, T., & Malloch, K. (2013). *Leadership in nursing practice: Changing the landscape of health care.* Jones & Bartlett Learning.

Riley, W. (2009). High reliability and implications for nursing leaders. *Journal of Nursing Management, 17*(2), 238–246.

Roussel, L. (2013). *Management and leadership for nurse administrators* (6th ed.). Jones & Bartlett Learning.

Rundio, A., Wilson, V., & Maloy, F. A. (2016). *Nurse executive review and resource manual* (3rd ed.). American Nurses Credentialing Center.

Schaffner, J. (2009). Roadmap for success: The 10-step nursing strategic plan. *Journal of Nursing Administration, 39*(4),152–155.

Senge, P. (1990). *The fifth discipline: The art and practice of the learning organization.* Doubleday.

Shi, L., & Singh, D. (2008). *Delivering health care in America.* Jones & Bartlett Learning.

Tamuz, M., & Harrison, M. I. (2006). Improving patient safety in hospitals: Contributions of high-reliability theory and normal accident theory. *Health Sciences Research, 41*(4), 1654–1676. doi:10.1111/j.1475-6773.2006.00570x

The Joint Commission (TJC). (2020). *About The Joint Commission.* www.jointcommission.org/an/about-us/about_the_joint_commission_main.aspx

Thomas, P. L., & Winter, J. (2020). Strategic practices in achieving organizational effectiveness. In Roussel, L., et al. (Eds.), *Management and leadership for nurse administrators* (8th ed., pp. 135–154). Jones & Bartlett Learning.

Tuck, I., Harris, L. H., & Baliko, B. (2000). Values expressed in philosophies of nursing services. *Journal of Nursing Administration, 30*(4), 180–184.

Ulrich, B. T., Buerhaus, P. I., Donelan, K., Norman, L., & Dittus, R. (2007). Magnet status and registered nurse views of the work environment and nursing as a career. *Journal of Nursing Administration, 37*(5), 212–220.

Weick, K. E., & Sutcliffe, K. M. (2015). *Managing the unexpected: Sustained performance in a complex world* (3rd ed.). Wiley & Sons.

Wolosin, R., Ayala, L., & Fulton, B. R. (2012). Nursing care, inpatient satisfaction, and value-based purchasing: Vital connections. *Journal of Nursing Administration, 42*(6), 321–325.

Young, B., Clark, C., Kansky, J., & Pupo, E. (2014). *Continuum of care.* Healthcare Information and Management Systems Society. www.himss.org/ResourceLibrary/genResourceDetailPDF.aspx?ItemNumber=30272

To explore learning resources for this chapter, go to FADavis.com

Chapter **8**

Effective Communication

Elizabeth J. Murray, PhD, RN, CNE

LEARNING OUTCOMES

- Define verbal and nonverbal communication, and explain why both are needed for effective communication.
- Explain the importance of practicing active listening.
- Define factors that affect communication.
- Compare and contrast informal and formal communication, and identify appropriate use of each.
- Delineate among organizational communication, interprofessional communication, and intraprofessional communication.
- Discuss the importance of effective communication to safe and quality patient care.
- Identify strategies nurse leaders and managers can use to facilitate effective communication.

The Knowledge, Skills, and Attitudes Related to the Following Are Addressed in This Chapter:

Core Competencies	• Patient-Centered Care • Teamwork and Collaboration • Safety
The Essentials: Core Competencies for Professional Nursing Education (AACN, 2021)	**Domain 2: Person-Centered Care** 2.2 Communicate effectively with individuals (pp. 28–29). **Domain 6: Interprofessional Partnerships** 6.1 Communicate in a manner that facilitates a partnership approach to quality care delivery (p. 43).
Code of Ethics with Interpretive Statements (ANA, 2015a)	**Provision 2.3:** Collaboration (p. 6) **Provision 3.4:** Professional responsibility in promotion a culture of safety (pp. 11–12)

Nurse Manager (NMC) Competencies (AONL, 2015a) and Nurse Executive (NEC) Competencies (AONL, 2015b)	**NMC: Performance Improvement (p. 4)**
	• Promote intradepartmental/interdepartmental communication.
	NMC: Relationship Management and Influencing Behaviors (p. 6)
	• Relationship management
	  • Promote team dynamics
	  • Mentor and coach staff and colleagues
	  • Apply communication principles
	NEC: Communication and Relationship Building (pp. 4–5)
	• Effective communication
	• Relationship management
	• Influencing behaviors
	• Diversity
	• Medical/staff relationships
	• Academic relationships

Nursing Administration Scope and Standards of Practice (ANA, 2016)	**Standard 8: Culturally Congruent Practice** The nurse administrator practices in a safe manner that is congruent with cultural diversity and inclusion principles (pp. 47–48). **Standard 9: Communication** The nurse administrator communicates effectively in all areas of practice (p. 49).

Continued

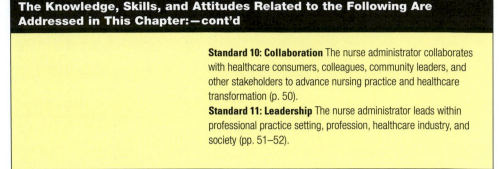

The Knowledge, Skills, and Attitudes Related to the Following Are Addressed in This Chapter:—cont'd

Standard 10: Collaboration The nurse administrator collaborates with healthcare consumers, colleagues, community leaders, and other stakeholders to advance nursing practice and healthcare transformation (p. 50).

Standard 11: Leadership The nurse administrator leads within professional practice setting, profession, healthcare industry, and society (pp. 51–52).

Source: American Association of Colleges of Nursing. (2021). *The essentials: Core competencies for professional nursing education.* Author; American Nurses Association (ANA). (2015a). *Code of ethics for nurses with interpretive statements.* Author; American Nurses Association (ANA). (2016). *Nursing administration: Scope and standards of practice* (2nd ed.). Author; American Organization for Nursing Leadership (AONL). (2015a). *AONL nurse manager competencies.* Author; American Organization for Nursing Leadership (AONL). (2015b). *AONL nurse executive competencies.* Author; Cronenwett, L., Sherwood, G., Barnsteiner, J., Disch, J., Johnson, J., Mitchell, P., Sullivan, D. T., & Warren, J. (2007). Quality and safety education for nurses. *Nursing Outlook, 55*(3), 122–131; and Greiner, A. C., & Knebel, E. (Eds.) (2003). *Health professions education: A bridge to quality.* National Academies Press.

Communication is an essential tool for nursing practice because a critical link exists between effective communication and positive patient outcomes. Nurses must communicate effectively with all members of the health-care team, including other nurses, the patient, and the patient's family (American Association of Colleges of Nursing [AACN], 2008; 2021). All nurses at all levels must be able to effectively communicate with patients and their families about treatment options, resources, and capacity for self-care (American Nurses Association [ANA], 2015a). Effective communication involves two distinct steps: first, adequately articulating ideas; and second, understanding the listening audience with whom one is communicating (Rosenblatt & Davis, 2009).

Effective communication is accurate and timely, enhances quality of care, and fosters a healthy work environment. Mastering the art of communication seems simple because communicating is something people do every day. However, the intricacies of effective communication, such as knowing when communication is blocked or ineffective and registering nonverbal cues, must be studied and practiced. This chapter illustrates communication basics, details the elements of effective communication, and describes the three most common types of communication used in nursing: organizational, interprofessional, and intraprofessional.

▶ WHY EFFECTIVE COMMUNICATION IS CRITICAL

Effective communication is necessary for the delivery of high quality, safe, individualized nursing care (AACN, 2021). Nurses must be as proficient in communication skills as they are in clinical skills (American Association of Critical-Care Nurses, 2016). In fact, **effective communication** is as critical to clinical practice as it is to building interprofessional and intraprofessional teams, and it is a key element of successful nursing leadership.

Effective communication is also vital to each Quality and Safety Education for Nurses (QSEN) core competency, particularly patient-centered care, teamwork and collaboration, and safety (Cronenwett et al., 2007). To achieve patient-centered care, nurses must effectively communicate with patients and their families to ensure that patients can make informed decisions and participate fully in their care. Teamwork and collaboration require nurses to be competent in communication skills to function productively on interprofessional and intraprofessional teams. Most important, nurses must understand that ineffective communication, in the form of miscommunication and gaps in communication, can lead to medical errors that jeopardize patient safety. In fact, The Joint Commission (TJC, 2014) cites communication errors as a leading root cause of sentinel events.

In 2004, VitalSmarts, in partnership with the American Association of Critical-Care Nurses, conducted a nationwide study to explore specific concerns of health-care professionals related to communication that may contribute to avoidable errors (Maxwell et al., 2005). The investigators identified seven crucial conversations that health-care professionals frequently fail to have that could add to unacceptable error rates. The lack of these crucial conversations lead to "medical errors, patient safety, quality of care, staff commitment, employee satisfaction, discretionary effort, and turnover" (Maxwell et al., 2005, p. 2). The researchers conducted focus groups and interviews and collected survey data from more than 1,700 participants. The areas of concern identified were broken rules, mistakes, lack of support, incompetence, poor teamwork, disrespect, and micromanagement. Although more than half of the health-care professionals surveyed witnessed colleagues cutting corners and demonstrating incompetent practice in these areas, only 1 in 10 discussed their concerns with the coworker. Further, most surveyed did not believe it was their responsibility to address these concerns.

The three primary reasons health-care professionals do not speak up regarding their concerns were identified as a person's lack of ability, belief that it was not their responsibility, and low confidence that speaking up would result in any good. Interestingly, the researchers identified a minority of 5% to 15% of health-care professionals who did speak up and noted a significant correlation that indicates that health-care professionals "who are confident in their ability to have crucial conversations achieve positive outcomes for their patients, for the hospitals, and for themselves" (Maxwell et al., 2005, p. 7). In contrast, when health-care professionals do not speak up and address their concerns, morale and productivity suffer, and patient safety is compromised (Maxwell et al., 2005). The investigators urged health-care organizations to create cultures of safety in which all employees feel comfortable approaching each other about concerns. Such an environment will improve productivity, reduce nursing turnover, and increase physician cooperation.

Nurses at all levels must communicate effectively in all areas of practice (ANA, 2015b, 2016). However, nurse leaders and managers have an obligation to promote effective communication in the workplace and, essentially, must model effective communication for staff. Characteristics of effective communicators include respecting what others have to say, having empathy, listening actively, avoiding sarcasm, asking not commanding, avoiding talking down or up to others, and encouraging input from others (Smith, 2011). Facilitating effective communication and teamwork and ensuring that nurses are competent in communication skills are the responsibilities of nurse managers and leaders (Timmins, 2011). Nurse leaders and managers can significantly influence the use of effective communication by doing the following (Huston, 2014):

- Being effective communicators and role models themselves in all settings
- Establishing and upholding administrative structures to support and require effective communication and teamwork
- Effectively confronting and managing conflicts that arise from poor communication

A nurse leader and manager who is a role model for good communication skills can provide staff nurses with informal support and leadership, which ultimately create positive work environments and improve nurses' confidence, motivation, and morale (Timmins, 2011).

▶ BASICS OF COMMUNICATION

According to the AACN (2021), communication is a core element in all areas of nursing practice. To succeed in communicating effectively, nurses must first become experts in the basics of communication. Basic communication skills cannot be overlooked. Potential for patient harm is introduced with ineffective or inaccurate communication (TJC, 2017). The following is a brief review of communication basics.

The Communication Process

The **communication process** includes the following elements (Adler & Proctor, 2014; Harkreader et al., 2007):

- *Sender:* The person who begins the transfer of information, thoughts, or ideas, and engages one or more other persons
- *Encoding:* The process the sender uses to transmit the message, including verbal language, voice inflection, and body language
- *Message:* The information or content the sender is transferring, which can be transmitted verbally, nonverbally, and in writing
- *Sensory channel:* The manner in which the message is sent, including visual (e.g., facial expressions, posture, and body language), auditory (e.g., spoken word), kinesthetic (e.g., touching and nonverbal communication), and electronic (e.g., media such as e-mail or text message)
- *Receiver:* The person or persons whom the sender intended to receive the message
- *Decoding:* The process of interpreting the message
- *Feedback:* Determines whether the message was received as intended; can be verbal and nonverbal and allows the sender to correct or clarify the message sent and verify the message was received accurately

Figure 8-1 illustrates the basic model for communication.

A fatal flaw in the communication process is overlooking the final step of **feedback**. As simply sending a message and believing it to be clear and therapeutic does not mean that the message was clear or therapeutic to the receiver. For instance, when

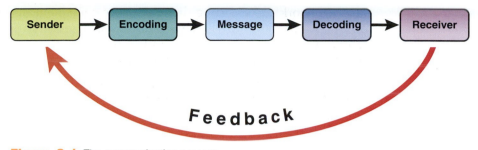

Figure 8-1 The communication process.

communicating with a patient who is hearing impaired, using the auditory channel only most likely will not result in effective communication. Because the receiver must be able to decode the information the sender is transmitting, a hearing-impaired patient would benefit more from the visual channel than from the auditory channel. Nurses should never assume that they have communicated effectively until they have verified through feedback that the receiver clearly understood the message.

Verbal and Nonverbal Communication

People communicate using a combination of verbal language, or the use of words to convey messages by speaking or writing, and nonverbal cues, such as gestures, facial expressions, eye contact, posture, and use of space. Effective communication results when verbal and nonverbal messages are congruent.

Verbal Communication

Verbal communication is a conscious method of communication (Blais & Hayes, 2011; Harkreader et al., 2007). It occurs face to face, by telephone, and through written messages such as e-mails and memos. The average person uses approximately 20,000 words in an average day to communicate with others (Schuster & Nykolyn, 2010). Unfortunately, not all words have the same meaning for everyone. To communicate effectively, selecting words that are clear and avoiding ambiguous messages are best, as is seeking feedback to ensure that the message was received with the intended meaning (Schuster & Nykolyn, 2010).

Effective communication, whether spoken or written, is essential for nurses when dealing with patients, especially when documenting nursing care and providing discharge instructions for patients and families. Precise documentation of nursing care is vital because it is used by other nurses and health-care professionals and in administrative records across an organization (ANA, 2010). Clear and understandable discharge instructions can make the difference between a patient's complete recovery and a repeat visit to the hospital.

For nurse leaders and managers, communicating verbally with staff in an effective matter is also critical. Nurse leaders and managers must convey clearly, typically in writing, information that is important for employees to know, such as policies and procedures and performance evaluations. Nurse leaders and managers must develop basic communication skills including the ability to use different techniques such as e-mail and text messaging. With written communication particularly, clarity is important because feedback is typically not immediate, and it may be some time before nurse leaders and managers are able to address questions and concerns. Regardless of the purpose, effective written communication must contain language and terminology appropriate to the party or parties being addressed; correct grammar, spelling, and punctuation; logical organization; and appropriate use and citation of references (Blais & Hayes, 2011).

Nonverbal Communication

Even in moments of silence, communication continues. **Nonverbal communication** encompasses behaviors, actions, and facial expressions that transmit messages in lieu of or in addition to verbal communication. Nonverbal communication plays a central role in human interactions and is crucial in transmitting emotional and relational information (Henry et al., 2012). Nonverbal communication can be conscious as well as subconscious and includes eye contact, facial expressions, gestures, posture, body movement, touch, and physical appearance. Facial behavior and expressions in particular (e.g., eye contact or lack of, smiling or grimacing) provide valuable clues and can indicate a person's comfort level with the topic under discussion.

Beyond paying attention to the receiver's nonverbal cues, the speaker must be aware of their own body language because it must match the verbal message being sent. Consider a staff nurse who approaches the nurse leader and manager and asks whether they have a few minutes to discuss a patient situation. The nurse leader and manager says "sure" but proceeds to continually look at their watch, and hence the verbal message sent to the staff nurse is incongruent with the nonverbal message. In addition, nonverbal communication alone can have great impact. Sometimes the mere presence of the nurse manager on the unit sends a message to staff, "I am interested in what is going on here." Never underestimate the power of nonverbal communication.

Active Listening

Effective communication requires the ability to listen actively (ANA, 2015b). Hearing and listening are two different things: Hearing is the physiological process of sound communicating with the hearing apparatus, whereas listening is more active and participatory (Rebair, 2012) and requires energy and a high level of concentration (Weaver, 2010). **Active listening** is broken down into five stages (Rebair, 2012):

1. *Receiving:* Ensuring the nurse is in a good position to hear information clearly
2. *Attending:* Engaging in the conversation by adopting positive body language, facial expressions, and gestures
3. *Understanding:* Gaining an understanding of what is being said and what may not be said
4. *Responding:* Responding to the patient in a nonjudgmental manner and being aware if anything may have upset them

5. *Remembering:* Recalling previous conversations with the patient to establish a starting point when reengaging

Active listening also requires the nurse to put aside judgment, evaluation, and approval in a concerted effort to be aware of the emotions and attitudes of others (Weaver, 2010).

Although nurses are often the senders of messages in the communication process, they also need to practice attentive listening skills to achieve effective communication. Without active listening, a nurse will not be able to determine the patient's perspective and consequently provide safe and quality nursing care. Nurses should take as many opportunities as possible to be the receiver, by focusing on adopting body language, facial expressions, and gestures that are positive and relay to the sender that they are engaged in the conversation (e.g., being eye level with the patient, positioning the body so it is squarely in front of them), as well as reducing or blocking out distractions (Rebair, 2012). Responding appropriately to the information communicated is also necessary and can be accomplished by reflecting back to the person (e.g., "I heard you say…") or requesting clarification for something that was not understood (e.g., "I'm not sure I understand…") (Beach, 2010; Rebair, 2012).

To be good communicators, nurse leaders and managers must be good listeners (Gokenbach & Thomas, 2020). Actively listening to staff as well as patients is a critical communication skill. Staff should feel that the nurse leader and manager cares about what they have to say (Gokenbach & Thomas, 2020). Another characteristic of a good communicator is self-awareness of how one is perceived by others. To have a satisfied and productive staff, nurse leaders and managers must hear what employees are saying as well as what they are not saying. Whether communicating with patients or staff, nurse leaders and managers who listen to and remember what others says gain rapport and trust for future encounters. "When trust is high, communication is easy, effortless, instantaneous, and accurate…. When trust is low, communication is extremely difficult, exhausting, and ineffective" (Covey, 1991, p. 138).

▶ FACTORS THAT AFFECT COMMUNICATION

When the message the sender transmits is what the receiver understands, clear and effective communication has taken place. However, elements that alter or affect communication can occur at any time during the process. Nurse leaders and managers must be aware of factors that can interfere with message transmission, including gender, generation, values and perceptions, personal space, environment, and roles and relationships. Further, they must pay attention to their tone of voice and ensure they are communicating with respect and avoiding accusatory, demanding, and overbearing tones which may put others on the defensive (Gokenbach & Thomas, 2020).

Gender

Gender differences exist in society and the workplace. Nurse leaders and managers can bridge the gender gap by using gender-neutral language in all communication methods and being aware of how their own gender affects their communication style. Effective nurse leaders and managers will be fair, sensitive to staff perceptions of gender differences, and handle issues appropriately and in a timely manner (Gokenbach & Thomas, 2020).

Generation

The nursing workforce is comprised of individuals spanning five different generations: veterans (1922 to 1945), baby boomers (1946 to 1964), generation X (1965 to 1981), generation Y (1982 to 1996), and generation Z (1997 to 2015) (Murray, 2013; Parker & Igielnik, 2020). Each generation comes with its own unique characteristics, values, work ethic, communication style, and expectations of a work environment (Murray, 2013; Strauss & Howe, 1991). Nurse leaders and managers must identify and implement various communication strategies to reach all generations. For example, some baby boomers may prefer personal forms of communication, whereas some from generations X, Y, and Z may be more comfortable with technology and favor electronic forms of communication.

Culture

A person's culture can influence communication in many ways, whether because of the native language of the culture or because of verbal and nonverbal behavior variations. Nurse leaders and managers must be attentive to cultural differences in employees. In one study, health-care professionals identified the ability to adjust language, whether verbal or nonverbal, to the target audience as an important communication skill, whether communicating with patients and families or working in interprofessional and intraprofessional teams (Suter et al., 2009). Nurse leaders and managers must ensure that "communication within the healthcare setting is culturally appropriate and linguistically sensitive" and includes the consistent use of medical interpreters and translators (ANA, 2016, p. 47).

Values and Perceptions

One's own values and perceptions influence how one communicates. Patients, families, and other nurses may encode, send, receive, decode, and interpret messages differently based on their own value systems, life experiences, and worldviews. Nurse leaders and managers must consider differences in values and perceptions when communicating with patients, families, health-care providers, peers, and managers to avoid miscommunication and misunderstandings.

Personal Space

Personal space, or the space between parties when communication takes place, also influences communication. What one individual considers appropriate personal space, an amount that feels comfortable and safe, can differ dramatically from another person's view (Hall, 1990; McLaughlin et al., 2008). However, there are commonly accepted parameters for distance between persons communicating, depending on the situation.

Environment

Environment plays a major role in whether communication is effective, staff is productive, and teamwork is collaborative. Nurse leaders and managers should strive to create an environment that supports communication as a two-way dialogue in which people think and make decisions together and with minimal distractions (American Association of Critical-Care Nurses, 2016). A supportive environment such as this allows patients and families to feel comfortable enough to share information, ask questions, and offer opinions. In addition, a healthy environment ensures that staff members feel more comfortable sharing ideas, asking questions, and offering solutions to problems. In contrast, a negative or unhealthy environment promotes one-way communication and a sense that staff and patients have little power.

Roles and Relationships

A nurse's role and their relationships with others influence the communication process. Roles can influence the words people choose, their tone of voice, communication channel, and body language (Blais & Hayes, 2011). For example, nurses may choose a face-to-face method when communicating with patients and families but may use the telephone to communicate with health-care providers. Nurse leaders and managers often use a face-to-face method to communicate sensitive information to staff and e-mail to communicate policy changes.

To be an effective communicator, nurse leaders and managers must also adapt their communication style based on the ability of the individual—whether a patient, family member, or staff member—to process and comprehend the interaction (Smith, 2011). Often, noise occurs during transmission (Fig. 8-2). Noise comprises the physical and/or psychological forces that can disrupt effective communication. Physical noise includes conspicuous environmental distractions, such as excessive sounds, activity, physical separation, and interruptions, that interfere

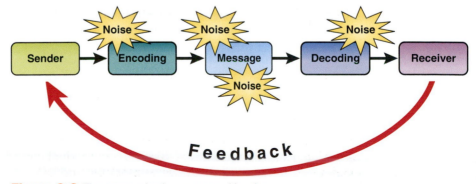

Figure 8-2 The communication process with noise.

with a person's ability to listen actively. Psychological noise includes internal distractions, such as one's values, stress and anxiety levels, emotions, and judgments, that impede their ability to send or receive a message clearly.

Nurse leaders and managers can prevent physical noise by creating a supportive environment with as few distractions as possible, as described earlier. Psychological noise can be reduced by encouraging staff to employ empathy for the patient. Physical touch and caring nonverbal cues also can help establish a calm atmosphere for a patient and their family.

LEARNING ACTIVITY 8-1

Reflect on a Recent Communication Interaction

Think about a recent interaction you had or observed that resulted in miscommunication. Consider the following:

1. Were verbal communication and nonverbal communication congruent?
2. What factors may have affected communication (e.g., gender, generations, culture, values, environment)?
3. Could there have been physiological or psychological noise?

▶ FORMAL AND INFORMAL COMMUNICATION

Communication in health care occurs along two different channels: formal and informal. **Formal communication** is described as "a type of verbal presentation or document intended to share information and which conforms to established professional rules, standards and processes and avoids using slang terminology" (Formal communication, 2014). Formal communication follows the line of authority in an organizational hierarchy, and it also reflects the culture of the organization; communication is planned rather than allowed to occur randomly (Triolo, 2012). Examples of formal communication that nurse leaders and managers may use include interviewing, counseling, dealing with complaints, managing conflict, evaluating, and disciplining (Sullivan, 2012). During the formal communication process, it is critical for nurse leaders and managers to maintain professionalism and be effective communicators by doing the following:

- Using plain, direct language and avoiding jargon
- Using familiar illustrations to get points across
- Listening objectively
- Keeping questions short
- Giving clear, concise direction or instructions
- Seeking frequent feedback
- Providing frequent feedback

On the other end of the spectrum, informal communication occurs among staff members without formal lines of authority or responsibility. **Informal communication** is a "casual form of information sharing typically used in personal conversations with friends or family members" (Informal communication, 2014). Nurse leaders and managers may use informal communication when conversing with patients about personal business, such as children or pets. Informal communication is used for nurse managers and leaders to establish open lines of communication with staff and to create a culture in the workplace that allows employees to feel connected with each other (Parboteeah et al., 2010).

One negative example of informal communication is the grapevine. **Grapevine communication** flows quickly and haphazardly at all levels of the organization and becomes more and more distorted as it moves along (Phillips, 2007). Communication on the grapevine travels in multiple directions at a rapid speed and carries both positive and negative information. Misinformation can run rampant, thus causing low morale and decreased productivity. Nurse leaders and managers must monitor the grapevine and intervene quickly to provide accurate information to avert unrest and job dissatisfaction among employees. Employees prefer regular communication from nurse leaders and managers, rather than hearing information through the grapevine (Triolo, 2012). Nurse leaders and managers must anticipate grapevine communication and keep communication with staff more focused and meaningful through proactive staff meetings, sharing as much information as possible, and answer questions openly and honestly.

▶ TYPES OF COMMUNICATION IN A HEALTH-CARE ENVIRONMENT

Three types of communication come into play in a health-care work environment: organizational, interprofessional, and intraprofessional. Nurses must understand and be able to apply all three when communicating.

Organizational Communication

Health-care systems must communicate important information, such as regulations, policies, and procedures. The goal of **organizational communication** is to convey the same message across the entire system. The ease with which communication flows through an organization has a great impact on the individual employee because it sets the tone for the climate of the working environment (Parboteeah et al., 2010). In fact, lack of effective communication at the organizational level can result in conflict and poor adherence to guidelines (Parboteeah et al., 2010; Pavlakis et al., 2011).

Various directions of communication may be used at the organizational level. **Downward communication** reflects the hierarchical nature of the organization (e.g., the sending of information by administrators to nurse leaders and managers or by nurse leaders and managers to staff). Downward communication includes directives to employees, expectations for employees, and performance feedback (Phillips, 2007; Sullivan, 2012).

Lateral communication is the sharing of information among nurse leaders and managers or other staff at the same level. Examples of lateral communication are coordination between units and services, information sharing, problem-solving, and conflict management (Phillips, 2007).

Communication with others in the organization who are not on the same level in the hierarchy is considered **diagonal communication**. This occurs, for example, when a nurse leader and manager communicates with the chief financial officer or the medical director (Phillips, 2007).

Finally, **upward communication** is the sending of information up the hierarchal chain (e.g., staff to the nurse manager or leader, or nurse leader and manager to higher-level managers and administrators). Common instances of upward communication are requests for resources, sharing ideas or suggestions for improvement, and employee grievances (Phillips, 2007; Sullivan, 2012).

Organizational communication occurs in staff meetings, group discussions, committee meetings, and in-service education. Written communication is by far the most common form of organizational communication used (Parboteeah et al., 2010). E-mail, faxes, and bulletins posted in high-traffic areas are common forms of organizational written communication.

Interprofessional Communication

According to the AACN (2021), interprofessional refers to "engagement involving two or more professions or professionals" (p. 65). Effective **interprofessional communication** fosters patient-centered care and results in quality outcomes. All nurses are expected to lead interprofessional teams and to communicate effectively (ANA, 2015b).

To communicate interprofessionally, nurse leaders and managers must communicate with all members of the health-care team, as well as with patients and their families. The Interprofessional Education Collaborative Expert Panel (2011, 2016) identified communication as one of four competencies for interprofessional collaborative practice; the specific interprofessional communication competencies are listed in Box 8-1.

Failure to effectively communicate interprofessionally has been found to be a significant contributing factor associated with many preventable medical errors (Stevens et al., 2011). In fact, evidence suggests that poor interprofessional communication affects patient safety and quality of care globally. The World Health Organization (2008) identified the lack of communication and coordination as the number one research priority in developed countries and the number three research priority in countries in transition.

Specifically, miscommunication between nurses and physicians contributes to medication errors, patient injuries, and patient deaths (Kesten, 2011). Part of the challenge in combating interprofessional miscommunication between nurses and physicians is that styles differ between the two disciplines: Nurses are taught to be more descriptive, whereas physicians are taught to communicate in a more concise manner (Thomas et al., 2009). In addition, some traditional health-care environments often support a culture in which nurses are intimidated by physicians, thus leading to delays in sharing important medical information. Communication between nurses and physicians should be timely, accurate, complete, and unambiguous for care to be safe and effective. Effective communication among all health-care professionals is a worldwide goal today (Mitchell et al., 2010).

BOX 8-1   Interprofessional Communication Competencies

GENERAL COMPETENCY STATEMENT

Communicate with patients, families, communities, and professionals in health and other fields in a responsive and responsible manner that supports a team approach to the promotion and maintenance of health and the prevention and treatment of disease. Specific interprofessional communication competencies:

1. Choose effective communication tools and techniques, including information systems and communication technologies, to facilitate discussions and interactions that enhance team function.
2. Communicate information with patients, families, community members, and health team members in a form that is understandable, and avoid discipline-specific terminology when possible.
3. Express one's knowledge and opinions to team members involved in patient care and population health improvement with confidence, clarity, and respect, working to ensure common understanding

of information, treatment, care decisions, and population health programs and policies.

4. Listen actively, and encourage ideas and opinions of other team members.
5. Give timely, sensitive, instructive feedback to others about their performance on the team, and respond respectfully as a team member to feedback from others.
6. Use respectful language appropriate for a given difficult situation, crucial conversation, or interprofessional conflict.
7. Recognize how one's own uniqueness (experience level, expertise, culture, power, and hierarchy within the health team) contributes to effective communication, conflict resolution, and positive interprofessional working relationships.
8. Communicate consistently the importance of teamwork in patient-centered and population health programs and policies.

From Interprofessional Education Collaborative, 2016 Update, p. 10, with permission.

Common strategies that enhance and promote interprofessional communication include team rounding, huddles, TeamSTEPPS, and SBAR.

Interprofessional Team Rounding

One strategy that is enhancing communication among health-care professionals, producing quality outcomes, increasing patient satisfaction, reducing error rates, and improving patient safety is **interprofessional team rounding** (Baldwin et al., 2011). As the coordinator of care, the nurse possesses the majority of information that is valuable to the health-care team. With interprofessional team rounding, key members of the interprofessional team gather at specified times to discuss the progress of the patient's plan of care. The patient and their family have the opportunity to meet with all members of the health-care team as well. Each member of the interprofessional team, including the patient and their family, contributes during team rounding to provide individual expertise to a holistic plan of care. For example, during interprofessional team rounding, the patient's bedside nurse ensures that patient information is current and available for the meeting and offers the team insight into care issues, with the goals of advocating for the patient and respectfully communicating the patient's wishes to the health-care team (Weaver, 2010). After team rounding, nurse leaders and managers are responsible for communicating the outcome of the interprofessional team round to any members not present and for communicating feedback to the team as needed.

Huddles

A **huddle** (also called a safety huddle) is a short interprofessional meeting at the beginning of the day or shift with the purpose of sharing information and highlighting concerns for follow-up (Institute for Healthcare Improvement [IHI], 2019; Shaikh, 2020). Huddles involve the interprofessional team, patient, and their family. Many high reliability organizations use huddles to enable frontline staff to proactively share safety successes, concerns, risks, and perform safety measures (Shaikh, 2020). Huddles are not used to solve problems, but rather to proactively manage quality and safety (IHI, 2019).

The huddle process is most efficient if team members are provided with an agenda that includes a review of the previous day, any current safety issues, a short discussion regarding any patients who may be at risk for safety issues, and plan to address the issues. Huddles can occur in outpatient and inpatient settings. Box 8-2 illustrates an example agenda for a huddle in inpatient and outpatient settings.

Nurse leaders and managers can empower and engage frontline staff by implementing daily huddles. Huddles help staff work collaboratively to identify problems and safety concerns, thereby building a culture of quality and safety.

TeamSTEPPS

TeamSTEPPS, or Team Strategies and Tools to Enhance Performance and Patient Safety, is an evidence-based teamwork system developed by the U.S. Department of Defense in collaboration with the Agency for Healthcare Research and Quality (AHRQ) that is aimed at optimizing patient safety outcomes by improving communication and teamwork skills among health-care professionals (AHRQ, n.d.). One of the competencies covered by TeamSTEPPS is positive and conflict-free communication as a requirement for effective teamwork. The focus of TeamSTEPPS is concise information exchange techniques, including the following (Guimond et al., 2009; Sherman & Eggenberger, 2009):

- *Two-challenge rule:* Requires the nurse to voice concerns at least twice to receive acknowledgment from another interprofessional team member. The two-challenge rule is used when a standard of care is not followed. If the team member does not acknowledge the concern being challenged, the nurse takes

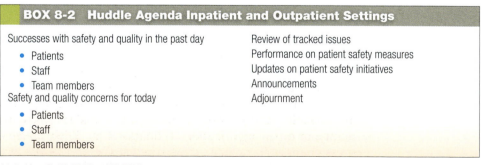

BOX 8-2   Huddle Agenda Inpatient and Outpatient Settings

Successes with safety and quality in the past day

- Patients
- Staff
- Team members

Safety and quality concerns for today

- Patients
- Staff
- Team members

Review of tracked issues
Performance on patient safety measures
Updates on patient safety initiatives
Announcements
Adjournment

Adapted from Shaikh (2020) and IHI (2019).

stronger action or follows the hospital chain of command. Nurse leaders and managers use this technique when dealing with team members who do not follow policies.

- *Call-out:* Simultaneously informs team members of important information and assigns tasks during a critical event or situation. Nurse leaders and managers use this technique when an emergency situation arises on the unit (e.g., respiratory arrest).
- *Check-back:* Requires the nurse to use closed-loop communication and verify that the information that is being received is correct. Nurse leaders and managers use this technique when assigning care to staff or when clarifying a change in treatment or medications.

SBAR

SBAR, or Situation-Background-Assessment-Recommendation, is a communication tool meant to simplify communication by framing it in the following manner (IHI, 2014):

S = Situation (a concise statement of the problem)
B = Background (pertinent and brief information related to the situation)
A = Assessment (analysis and considerations of options—what the nurse found or thinks)
R = Recommendation (action requested/recommended—what the nurse wants)

The SBAR communication tool is an effective method for improving communication within the interdisciplinary health-care team because it assists team members in organizing and prioritizing their thoughts before communicating with other health-care professionals. It fosters improved critical thinking and professional communication skills by developing a brief synopsis of the reason for the contact between providers through an organized and predictable format. When used properly, SBAR allows for an assertive dialogue, the precise relay of crucial information, and an increased situational awareness that can greatly enhance safe delivery of patient care by setting expectations for the information communicated and for how information is delivered (Stevens et al., 2011). Table 8-1 illustrates the SBAR tool and examples of statements nurses can use to relay information and recommendations to the health-care provider.

By enabling the continuous and collaborative exchange of information pertaining to patient care throughout the care environment, the SBAR tool increases the satisfaction level of nurses, physicians, and patients while improving the safety of the care being delivered. In fact, SBAR can effectively decrease the rate and frequency of medical errors associated with miscommunication among health-care providers. Teamwork is crucial to the delivery of safe and effective high-quality patient care, and SBAR has been shown to build teamwork and strengthen working relationships among health-care providers. Moreover, it can facilitate proficient communication and continuity during the transfer of care among nurses, levels of acuity, or other organizations (Thomas et al., 2009). It also allows the nurse to express changes in patient status successfully and leaves little room for missed or inaccurate information being relayed, thereby leading to an increased level

Table 8-1	SBAR Tool	
S = Situation	The nurse describes the problem and why they are calling.	Specifics to report: • Identify self, unit, patient, room number • Briefly state problem, when it happened, how severe • "I am concerned about..."
B = Background	The nurse provides pertinent information related to the situation (i.e., the clinical facts).	Specifics to report could include the following: • Current medications, allergies • Recent laboratory results • Most recent vital signs • Code status • Other clinical information
A = Assessment	The nurse provides an analysis of the situation (i.e., what they think the problem is).	Possible phrases: • "I think the problem is..." • "I am not sure what the problem is, but the patient is getting worse..."

R = Recommendation	The nurse makes recommendation(s) (i.e., what they believe will resolve the situation or problem).	Recommendations could include the following:
		• "I request that you [say what you want done]:
		  • Come in to see the patient
		  • Talk to the patient's family about code status
		  • Transfer the patient to the intensive care unit (ICU)
		• If change in treatment, be sure to ask:
		  • How often do you want vital signs?
		  • When do you want me to call again?

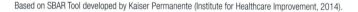

Based on SBAR Tool developed by Kaiser Permanente (Institute for Healthcare Improvement, 2014).

of safety and the quality of care given. Research has shown that when SBAR is used, patients have reported an enriched atmosphere of patient protection within the hospital setting (Beckett & Kipnis, 2009). Nurses use SBAR during patient care and shift reports and to communicate an unexpected change in a patient's condition. SBAR has been applied in many settings, including high-risk departments such as intensive care, emergency departments, and operating rooms, and has yielded improved satisfaction of patients and care providers, enhanced quality of clinical outcomes, improved communication among inter-professional team members, and an increase in the safety of the delivery of patient care (Kesten, 2011).

The SBAR technique can also be used to address nonclinical, management issues, such as workload and staffing levels. In one example, staff nurses on a rehabilitation unit used the technique to present poor staffing and workload issues to management. The tool provided them with a mechanism to present the issues along with recommendations for improvement in a professional manner (Boaro et al., 2010).

EXPLORING THE EVIDENCE 8-1

Donahue, M., Miller, M., Smith, L., Dykes, D., & Fitzpatrick, J. J. (2013). A leadership initiative to improve communication and enhance safety. *American Journal of Medical Quality, 26*(3), 206–211.

Aim

This study had three goals: (1) translation of SBAR for paraprofessionals, (2) reduction of cultural and educational barriers to interprofessional communication, and (3) examination of the Educating and Mentoring Paraprofessionals on Ways to Enhance Reporting (EMPOWER) intervention on barriers to interpersonal communication practices and perceptions of a safety culture using SBAR.

Methods

The project was implemented in two phases. The first phase focused on surveying paraprofessional staff members to establish baseline measures related to patient safety culture. The second phase focused on validation, testing of the EMPOWER training module, and recommendations for improving the safety culture by using SBAR.

Key Findings

The evaluation of the EMPOWER project focused on effectiveness of the SBAR training for paraprofessionals and reinforcement of SBAR training among all staff members. Initial surveys were conducted among 280 paraprofessionals, and 182 completed the survey. As part of the project, the leadership team began making rounds throughout the hospital to ensure that staff members understood their commitment to a culture of safety. After implementation of the EMPOWER project, surveys were conducted again and were compared with the first survey. The following key changes were revealed:

- In the first survey, 33% of the paraprofessionals indicated that when a patient safety event was reported, it felt as if the person was being written up rather than the problem; in the second survey, this percentage dropped to 21.7%.
- In the first survey, 78% of the paraprofessionals indicated that hospital management felt that patient safety was a top priority; in the second survey, this percentage increased to 86%.
- The use of SBAR by paraprofessionals increased from 74% at the end of the EMPOWER project to 90% after 1 year.

Implications for Nurse Leaders and Managers

Nurse leaders and managers can learn from this project the importance of recognizing paraprofessionals as members of the interprofessional team. The results of this study further promote the value of SBAR as an effective tool for increasing team communication and a standard for enhancing a culture of safety.

> ### LEARNING ACTIVITY 8-2
>
> ### Case Study Using SBAR
>
> Tracey is a registered nurse caring for a 70-year-old female patient who returned from recovery after abdominal surgery approximately 4 hours ago. On admission to Tracey's unit, the patient's blood pressure was 128/80 and pulse was 86. One hour after admission, the patient complained of pain and indicated that her pain was 8 on a scale of zero to 10. At that time, her abdomen was firm and tender without bowel sounds, and her blood pressure was 110/68 with a pulse of 98. Tracey medicated the patient for pain. Two hours after admission, the patient continues to complain of abdominal pain and says "It's the worse pain I've ever had." Her abdomen continues to be firm and tender without bowel sounds. Her blood pressure is now 90/60, and her pulse is 110. Tracey decides to contact the health-care provider. Using the SBAR tool in Table 8-1, indicate what Tracey should communicate to the health-care provider.
>
> S = Situation:
> B = Background:
> A = Assessment:
> R = Recommendation:

Intraprofessional Communication

Intraprofessional means "working with healthcare team members within the profession to ensure that care is continuous and reliable" (AACN, 2008, p. 38). For nurses, **intraprofessional communication** means working with other nursing staff to deliver safe and quality patient care. In the *Principles for Collaborative Relationships Between Clinical Nurses and Nurse Managers* developed by the ANA and the American Organization of Nurse Executives (AONE) (ANA & AONE, 2012), one focus is effective communication. The principles of effective communication can bridge the "us versus them" divide often prevalent between nursing management and staff (ANA & AONE, 2012). The principles related to effective intraprofessional communication are listed in Box 8-3.

Nurse-to-Nurse Transitions in Care

Health-care organizations have found how important it is to standardize nurse-to-nurse transitions in care. At one time commonly referred to as a **handoff** and

---

> **BOX 8-3   American Nurses Association and American Organization of Nurse Executives Principles of Collaborative Relationships: Effective Communication**
>
> 1. Engage in active listening to fully understand and contemplate what is being relayed.
> 2. Know the intent of a message, as well as the purpose and expectations of that message.
> 3. Foster an open, safe environment.
> 4. Whether giving or receiving information, be sure it is accurate.
> 5. Have people speak to the person they need to speak to, so the right person gets the right information.
>
> From ANA and AONE, 2012, p. 2.

more recently termed a **handover** to reflect more accurately the two-sided process (Barnsteiner, 2017), these transitions in care occur when a patient is transferred from one unit to another, when a nurse must accompany one patient to a procedure and leave other patients under the care of another nurse, when a nurse takes a break for lunch, and when there is a change of shift (Chen et al., 2011; Griffin, 2010). The purpose of the nurse-to-nurse handover is to acquaint a nurse who has not cared for the patient with the patient's needs and condition; to provide an opportunity for education on unfamiliar medications, equipment, and the care process; and to acquaint the nurse with the patient and not just the tasks (Griffin, 2010). The handover of patient care from one nurse to another requires effective communication to avoid negative consequences for patients (Barnsteiner, 2017). Handovers also transfer accountability and responsibility from one nurse to another (Griffin, 2010). According to The Joint Commission (TJC) Sentinel Alert Event, Issue 58, potential for patient harm can occur during handoffs. The problem is related to communication being out of balance between the sender and the receiver. During handoffs, the sender is responsible for patient data and relinquishing care of the patient to the receiver, who will receive patient data and accept care of the patient (TJC, 2017, para. 3). Numerous sentinel events result from inadequate handoffs, including "wrong site surgery, delays in treatment, falls, and medication errors" (TJC, 2017, para. 6). The high frequency of handoffs is identified as a major contributor to errors. It is estimated that more than 4,000 handoffs can occur daily in a typical teaching hospital (TJC, 2017).

Nurse-to-nurse handovers vary with each facility. For example, handovers in the acute care setting look very different from those in an outpatient care environment. Handovers may also vary from unit to unit in inpatient settings, although inpatient care facilities have begun standardizing handovers to reduce errors (Chen et al., 2011; Griffin, 2010). Reports on handovers may be verbal or written and given in an individual or group format. Many health-care institutions are deciding to "bring report to the bedside" in an effort to improve patient satisfaction and reduce medical errors because studies show that increasing patient involvement reduces errors in communication and the continuum of care (Griffin, 2010). To promote patient safety, many organizations are including the patient and their family in the handover process. This allows the patient and family to "contribute, ask questions, and verify information" (Barnsteiner, 2017, p. 162). The TJC (2017) calls all health-care facilities to use a process to identify causes of handoff communication failures and implement solutions that improve performance. Further, TJC suggest the following actions (pp. 3–5):

1. Demonstrate leadership's commitment to successful handoffs and other aspects of safety culture.
2. Standardize critical content to be communicated by the sender to the receiver during handoffs.
3. Conduct face-to-face handoff communication between senders and receivers in a location free of interruptions and include interprofessional team members and the patient and family.
4. Standardize training on how to conduct a successful handoff.

5. Use electronic health record capabilities and other technologies to enhance communication between senders and receivers.
6. Monitor the success of interventions to improve handoff communication.
7. Sustain and spread best practices in handoffs making high-quality handoffs a priority.

EXPLORING THE EVIDENCE 8-2

Staggers, N., & Blaz, J. W. (2013). Research on nursing handoffs for medical and surgical settings: An integrative review. *Journal of Advanced Nursing, 69*(2), 247–262.

Aim

The aim of this integrated review was to synthesize outcomes from research of nursing handoffs on medical surgical units to guide future computerization of the handoff process.

Methods

The investigators conducted an integrated literature review of studies published in peer-reviewed nursing journals between 1980 and March 2011. Studies about nurses' perceptions and informal reports were excluded from the review. The search yielded 247 references, of which 62 were duplicates. The references were reviewed and rated for relevance. The studies were classified as relevant, not relevant, or questionable. A total of 81 studies were retrieved by the investigators for additional review and classification. The final sample included 30 research studies (20 qualitative, 4 experimental, and 6 descriptive).

Key Findings

All studies examined handoffs from the nursing perspective except two, which traced patient-centered handoffs across hospitalizations. One-third of the studies reviewed found issues with information effectiveness, accuracy, and efficiency. All studies revealed that handoffs are complex processes. Researchers found that structured formats tailored to individual medical and surgical units improved information completeness. The investigators noted that most studies did not address the context of handoffs, even though context is critical to the computerization of the handoff process. The investigators found that the current trend of bedside face-to-face handoffs in medical and surgical units was not supported in the studies reviewed. In addition, no findings reflected the patient's perspective, which can have implications for the accuracy of information being relayed across units and settings.

Implications for Nurse Leaders and Managers

Nurse leaders and managers should be aware of these findings to assist in more effective relay of information during handoffs. In addition, the process of bedside handoffs that is common practice today in medical and surgical units is not supported by the available evidence.

Patient care handovers can result in important information gaps, omissions, errors, and harm to the patient (Staggers & Blaz, 2013). Potential causes of errors during handovers include the following (Chen et al., 2011, p. 380):

- Environmental distractions
- Simultaneous transfer of equipment and knowledge
- No previous information for the receiving nurse on the patient's history or condition, thereby creating a situation in which vast amounts of information are shared in a limited time
- Clinically unstable patients who require attention during handovers, thus resulting in a limited time for reviewing medical history

It is not possible to eliminate all of these causes for error during the handover process; for instance, if a patient requires care immediately, it must be given. However, standardizing handovers may help to decrease confusion and errors. When the receiving nurse is given information in a format that is familiar, such as SBAR, the information will not seem overwhelming. In addition, this approach provides a standard of care for what information is shared and reminds the nurse who is giving report to furnish complete information on each point before moving onto the next (Chen et al., 2011).

LEARNING ACTIVITY 8-3

Maria is an RN who works the night shift on an oncology unit. She approaches Elena, the day shift nurse, for report. Elena immediately begins to complain about the patient in room 345. She says, "That patient thinks she knows everything because she is a nurse! She questions everything and wants to know why the medication was ordered and why she had to go to x-ray. I have had the worst time getting anything done! Have fun with her tonight!"

1. How should Maria respond to Elena?
2. What are some barriers that may hinder effective communication with the patient?
3. What communication skills should Maria use when interacting with the patient?

▶ SUMMARY

Communication is one of the knowledge, skills, and attitudes that nurse leaders and managers—and in fact all nurses—must use with extreme proficiency. Communicating across the organization, among professionals, and among nurses is critical for safe and quality patient-centered care. Miscommunication is a source for error that could be potentially harmful to patients, so nurse leaders and managers must genuinely try to understand what others are saying, listen carefully, and maintain composure in difficult situations (Batcheller, 2007). Lack of effective communication can affect the health-care work environment and result in misinformation, misunderstanding, fear, suspicion, insecurity, and job dissatisfaction, as well as compromise patient safety and quality of nursing care. Nurse leaders and managers who are role models for good communication skills can provide staff nurses with informal support and leadership, which ultimately create a positive work environment and improve nurses' confidence, motivation, and morale (Timmins, 2011).

NCLEX®-STYLE REVIEW QUESTIONS

Multiple Choice

1. The nurse manager is aware that preventable medical errors are associated with what communication failure?
   1. Lack of interprofessional communication
   2. Lack of upward communication
   3. Lack of intraprofessional communication
   4. Lack of downward communication
2. The nurse manager plans to implement which communication strategy that has been found to reduce errors and improve patient safety while increasing patient satisfaction?
   1. TeamSTEPPS
   2. Interprofessional team rounding
   3. Diagonal communication
   4. Oral report in the conference room
3. The nurse from the postanesthesia care unit (PACU) is giving report to the unit nurse at the bedside of a patient who just had surgery for a total hip replacement. Approximately 20 minutes after the patient's admission to the unit, the patient experiences a period of respiratory depression that was later attributed to medication received in the PACU. What error that occurred during the nurse-to-nurse handover may have contributed to this patient's problem?
   1. The PACU nurse was giving report while helping to transfer the patient into bed.
   2. The PACU nurse arrived with the patient 15 minutes later than was expected.
   3. The unit nurse was not available for the nurse-to-nurse handover for 5 minutes after the PACU nurse arrives.
   4. The unit nurse was familiar with the patient from previous hospitalizations.
4. The nurse leader is working to improve communication on the nursing unit and knows that effective communication requires an articulate sharing of ideas and what other important element?
   1. The nurse manager must understand the audience for which the message is intended.
   2. The staff on the nursing unit must agree with the ideas of the nurse manager.
   3. The nurse manager must ensure that the ideas presented are important to the staff of the nursing unit.
   4. The staff on the nursing unit must have person-to-person contact for the communication to be received.

5. The nurse manager recognizes that communication that is congruent is more likely to be received. Which statement by the nurse manager to a staff nurse is an example of congruent communication?
   1. The nurse manager is smiling. "This latest episode of tardiness may cause you to be terminated from this job."
   2. The nurse manager is standing with arms crossed. "You have been 10 minutes late three times this month."
   3. The nurse manager is shaking her head sideways. "It's good to see that you have finally decided to come to work."
   4. The nurse manager stares down at the floor. "You are making a habit of being late. You can feel free to talk to me anytime."

6. The nurse manager is aware that what element of communication is essential to the transmission of relational information?
   1. Feedback
   2. Nonverbal communication
   3. Responding
   4. Receiving

7. The nurse manager would suggest what communication tool to assist staff nurses in organizing and prioritizing information before communicating with the health-care provider?
   1. Interprofessional team rounding
   2. TeamSTEPPS
   3. SBAR
   4. Call-out

8. The nurse manager is aware that SBAR may be used in what nonclinical issues?
   1. Staffing levels
   2. Nursing pay levels
   3. Nursing clinical ladder issues
   4. Required continuing education

9. The nurse is communicating to the health-care provider the patient's current medications, allergies, vital signs, and current laboratory values and is using which section of SBAR in giving this information?
   1. Situation
   2. Background
   3. Assessment
   4. Recommendation

Multiple Response

10. The nurse manager is aware that what communication is considered verbal? *Select all that apply.*
    1. E-mail message
    2. Facebook post
    3. Facial grimace
    4. Telephone message
    5. Arms and legs crossed

11. The nurse manager is preparing to institute the use of SBAR for interprofessional communication. The nurse manager has based this decision on what benefits to this tool? *Select all that apply.*
    1. Assertive dialogue between professionals
    2. Most essential information delivery
    3. Safer delivery of patient care
    4. Decreased continuity of patient care
    5. Increased time spent in interprofessional communication

12. The nurse manager is using the Principles of Collaborative Relationships: Effective Communication by the American Nurses Association (ANA) to improve communication on the nursing unit and knows that these principles require the staff nurses to use what communication practices? *Select all that apply.*
    1. Speak to multiple persons about the issue.
    2. Use active listening techniques.
    3. Keep the environment closed and private.
    4. Ensure accuracy in the information transmitted.
    5. Know the purpose of the message transmitted.

REFERENCES

Adler, R. B., & Proctor, R. F., II. (2014). *Looking out, looking in* (14th ed.). Wadsworth.

Agency for Healthcare Research and Quality (AHRQ). (n.d.). TeamSTEPPS: *Team strategies and tools to enhance performance and patient safety.* teamstepps.ahrq.gov/about-2cl_3.htm

American Association of Colleges of Nursing (AACN). (2008). *The essentials of baccalaureate education for professional nursing practice.* Author. www.aacn.nche.edu/education-resources/baccessentials08.pdf

American Association of Colleges of Nursing. (2021). *The essentials: Core competencies for professional nursing education.* Author. https://www.aacnnursing.org/Portals/42/AcademicNursing/pdf/Essentials-2021.pdf

American Association of Critical-Care Nurses. (2016). *AACN standards for establishing and sustaining healthy work environments: A journey to excellence* (2nd ed.). Author. www.aacn.org/wd/hwe/docs/hwestandards.pdf

American Nurses Association (ANA). (2010). *ANA's principles for nursing documentation: Guidance for registered nurses.* Author.

American Nurses Association (ANA). (2015a). *Code of ethics for nurses with interpretive statements.* Author.

American Nurses Association (ANA). (2015b). *Nursing: Scope and standards of practice* (3rd ed.). Author.

American Nurses Association (ANA). (2016). *Nursing administration: Scope and standards of practice* (2nd ed.). Author.

American Nurses Association (ANA) & American Organization of Nurse Executives (AONE). (2012). *ANA/AONE principles for collaborative relationships between clinical nurses and nurse managers.* www.nursingworld.org/MainMenuCategories/ThePracticeofProfessionalNursing/NursingStandards/ANAPrinciples/Principles-of-Collaborative-Relationships.pdf

American Organization for Nursing Leadership (AONL). (2015a). *AONL nurse manager competencies.* Author.

American Organization for Nursing Leadership (AONL). (2015b). *AONL nurse executive competencies.* Author.

Baldwin, P. K., Wittenberg-Lyles, E., Oliver, D. P., & Demiris, G. (2011). An evaluation of interdisciplinary team training in hospice care. *Journal of Hospice and Palliative Nursing, 13*(3), 172–182.

Barnsteiner, J. (2017). Safety. In G. Sherwood & J. Barnsteiner (Eds.), *Quality and safety in nursing: A competency approach to improving outcomes* (2nd ed., pp. 153–171). Wiley Blackwell.

Batcheller, J. (2007). Maximize your impact with leadership domains. *Nursing Management, 38*(8), 52–53.

Beach, M. (2010). Enhancing communications for better patient outcomes. *Johns Hopkins Advanced Studies in Medicine, 10*(2), 49–52.

Beckett, C. D., & Kipnis, G. (2009). Collaborative communication: Integrating SBAR to improve quality/patient safety outcomes. *Journal for Healthcare Quality, 31*(5), 19–28.

Blais, K., & Hayes, J. S. (2011). *Professional nursing practice: Concepts and perspectives* (6th ed.). Pearson.

Boaro, N., Fancott, C., Baker, R., Velji, K., & Andreoli, A. (2010). Using SBAR to improve communication in interprofessional rehabilitation teams. *Journal of Interprofessional Care, 24*(1), 111–114.

Chen, J. G., Wright, M. C., Smith, P. B., Jaggers, J., & Mistry, K. P. (2011). Adaptation of a postoperative handoff communication process for children with heart disease: A quantitative study. *American Journal of Medical Quality, 26*(5), 380–386.

Covey, S. R. (1991). *Principle-centered leadership.* Fireside Press.

Cronenwett, L., Sherwood, G., Barnsteiner, J., Disch, J., Johnson, J., Mitchell, P., Sullivan, D. T., & Warren, J. (2007). Quality and safety education for nurses. *Nursing Outlook, 55*(3), 122–131.

Donahue, M., Miller, M., Smith, L., Dykes, P., & Fitzpatrick, J. J. (2013). A leadership initiative to improve communication and enhance safety. *American Journal of Medical Quality, 26*(3), 206–211.

Formal communication. (2014). In *BusinessDictionary.com.* www.businessdictionary.com/definition/formal-communication.html

Gokenbach, V., & Thomas, P. (2020). Maximizing human capital. In Roussel, L., et al. (Eds.), *Management and leadership for nurse administrators* (8th ed., pp. 189–226). Jones & Bartlett Learning.

Greiner, A. C., & Knebel, E. (Eds.) (2003). *Health professions education: A bridge to quality.* National Academies Press.

Griffin, T. (2010). Bringing change-of-shift report to the bedside: A patient- and family-centered approach. *Journal of Perinatal and Neonatal Nursing, 24*(4), 348–353.

Guimond, M. E., Sole, M. L., & Salas, E. (2009). TeamSTEPPS. *American Journal of Nursing, 109*(11), 66–68.

Hall, E. T. (1990). *The hidden dimension.* Anchor Books.

Harkreader, H., Hogan, M. A., & Thobaben, M. (2007). *Fundamentals of nursing: Caring and clinical judgment* (3rd ed.). Elsevier Science.

Henry, S. G., Fuhrel-Forbis, A., Rogers, M. A., & Eggly, S. (2012). Association between nonverbal communication during clinical interactions and outcomes: A systematic review and meta-analysis. *Patient Education and Counseling, 86*(3), 297–315.

Huston, C. J. (2014). *Professional issues in nursing: Challenges and opportunities* (3rd ed.). Wolters Kluwer Lippincott Williams & Wilkins.

Informal communication. (2014). In *BusinessDictionary.com.* www.businessdictionary.comdefinition/informal-communication.html

Institute for Healthcare Improvement (IHI). (2014). *SBAR toolkit.* www.ihi.org/knowledge/Pages/Tools/SBARToolkit.aspx

Institute for Healthcare Improvement (IHI). (2019). *Patient safety essentials toolkit: Huddles.* http://www.ihi.org/resources/Pages/Tools/Huddles.aspx

Interprofessional Education Collaborative Expert Panel. (2011). *Core competencies for interprofessional collaborative practice: Report of an expert panel.* Interprofessional Education Collaborative. www.aacn.nche.edu/education-resources/ipecreport.pdf

Interprofessional Education Collaborative. (2016). *Core competencies for interprofessional collaborative practice: 2016 update.* Interprofessional Education Collaborative. https://www.ipecollaborative.org/core-competencies.html

Kesten, K. S. (2011). Role-play using SBAR technique to improve observed communication skills in senior nursing students. *Journal of Nursing Education, 50*(2), 79–87.

Maxwell, D., Grenny, J., McMillan, R., Patterson, K., & Switzler, A. (2005). *Silence kills: The seven crucial conversations in healthcare.* www.silenttreatmentstudy.com/silencekills

McLaughlin, C., Olson, R., & White, M. J. (2008). Environmental issues in patient care management: Proxemics, personal space, and territoriality. *Rehabilitation Nursing, 33*(4), 143–147, 177.

Mitchell, M., Groves, M., Mitchell, C., & Batkin, J. (2010). Innovation in learning: An interprofessional approach to improving communication. *Nurse Education in Practice, 10*(6), 379–384.

Murray, E. J. (2013). Generational differences: Uniting the four-way divide. *Nursing Management, 44*(12), 36–41.

Parboteeah, K. P., Chen, H. C., Lin, Y.-T., Chen, I.-H., Lee, A. Y.-P., & Chung, A. (2010). Establishing organizational ethical climates: How do managerial practices work? *Journal of Business Ethics, 97*(4), 599–611.

Parker, K., & Igielnik, R. (2020). *On the cusp of adulthood and facing an uncertain future: What we know about Gen Z so far.* Pew Research Center. https://www.pewsocialtrends.org/essay/on-the-cusp-of-adulthood-and-facing-an-uncertain-future-what-we-know-about-gen-z-so-far/

Pavlakis, A., Kaitelidou, D., Theodorou, M., Galanis, P., Sourtzi, P., & Siskou, O. (2011). Conflict management in public hospitals: The Cyprus case. *International Nursing Review, 58*(2), 242–248.

Phillips, C. G. (2007). Organizational communication. In R. P. Jones (Ed.), *Nursing leadership and management: Theories, processes and practice* (pp. 113–130). F. A. Davis.

Rebair, A. (2012). Lend an ear with care. *Nursing Standard, 27*(10), 64.

Rosenblatt, C. L., & Davis, M. S. (2009). Effective communication techniques for nurse managers. *Nursing Management, 40*(6), 52–54.

Schuster, P. M., & Nykolyn, L. (2010). *Communication for nurses: How to prevent harmful events and promote patient safety.* F. A. Davis.

Shaikh, U. (2020). *AHRQ patient safety primer: Improving patient safety and team communication through daily huddles.* https://psnet.ahrq.gov/primer/improving-patient-safety-and-team-communication-through-daily-huddles

Sherman, R., & Eggenberger, T. (2009). Taking charge: What every charge nurse needs to know. *Nurses First, 2*(4), 6–10.

Smith, M. A. (2011). Are you a transformational leader? *Nursing Management, 42*(9), 44–50.

Staggers, N., & Blaz, J. W. (2013). Research on nursing handoffs for medical and surgical settings: An integrative review. *Journal of Advanced Nursing, 69*(2), 247–262.

Stevens, J. D., Bader, M. K., Luna, M. A., & Johnson, L. M. (2011). Cultivating quality: Implementing standardized reporting and safety checklists. *American Journal of Nursing, 111*(5), 48–53.

Strauss, W., & Howe, N. (1991). *Generations: The history of America's future, 1584–2069.* William Morrow.

Sullivan, E. J. (2012). *Effective leadership and management in nursing* (8th ed.). Pearson.

Suter, E., Arndt, J., Arthur, N., Parboosingh, J., Taylor, E., & Deutschlander, S. (2009). Role understanding and effective communication as core competencies for collaborative practice. *Journal of Interprofessional Care, 23*(1), 41–51.

The Joint Commission (TJC). (2014). *Sentinel event data: Root causes by event type, 2004-Q2 2014.* www.jointcommission.org/assets/1/18/root_causes_by_event_type_2004-2014.pdf

The Joint Commission (TJC). (2017). Inadequate hand-off communication. *Sentinel Event Alert, 58.* https://www.jointcommission.org/-/media/tjc/documents/resources/patient-safety-topics/sentinel-event/sea_58_hand_off_comms_9_6_17_final_(1).pdf

Thomas, C. M., Bertram, E., & Johnson, D. (2009). The SBAR communication technique: Teaching nursing students professional communication skills. *Nurse Educator, 34*(4), 176–180.

Timmins, F. (2011). Managers' duty to maintain good workplace communications skills. *Nursing Management, 18*(3), 30–34.

Triolo, P. K. (2012). Creating cultures of excellence: Transforming organizations. In G. Sherwood & J. Barnsteiner (Eds.), *Quality and safety in nursing: A competency approach to improving outcomes* (pp. 305–322). Wiley-Blackwell.

Weaver, D. (2010). Communication and language needs. *Nursing and Residential Care, 12*(2), 60–63.

World Health Organization. (2008). *Global priorities for research in patient safety.* Author. www.who.int/patientsafety/research/priorities/global_priorities_patient_safety_research.pdf?ua=1

To explore learning resources for this chapter, go to FADavis.com

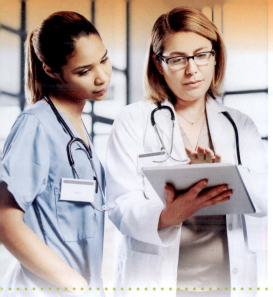

Chapter 9

Improving and Managing Safe and Quality Care

Elizabeth J. Murray, PhD, RN, CNE

LEARNING OUTCOMES

- Discuss the nurse leader and manager's role in ensuring safe and quality patient care.
- Discuss the prevalence of medical errors in today's health-care environment, and identify types of medical errors.
- Describe a culture of safety and strategies to promote a culture of safety.
- Describe initiatives to promote patient safety and how nurse leaders and managers can use these initiatives to improve patient care.
- Identify the principles of quality improvement and quality management.
- List common tools used in quality improvement.

KEY TERMS

Adverse event
Bar chart
Culture of safety
Donabedian Model
Error of commission
Error of omission
Fishbone diagram
Flow chart
Histogram
Incident report
Just culture
Lean Model
Medical error
Near miss
Nursing-sensitive quality
  indicators
Outcome indicators
Pareto chart
Patient safety event
Plan-do-study-act (PDSA)
Process indicators
Quality improvement
Root cause analysis
Run chart
Sentinel event
Six Sigma Model
Standardization
Structure indicators

The Knowledge, Skills, and Attitudes Related to the Following Are Addressed in This Chapter:

Core Competencies	• Patient-Centered Care • Teamwork and Collaboration • Quality Improvement • Safety • Informatics
The Essentials: Core Competencies for Professional Nursing Education (AACN, 2021)	**Domain 5: Quality and Safety** 5.1 Apply quality improvement principles in care delivery (pp. 40–41). 5.2 Contribute to a culture of patient safety (pp. 41–42). **Domain 7: Systems-Based Practice** 7.3 Optimize system effectiveness through application of innovation and evidence-based practice (p. 47). **Domain 8: Information and Healthcare Technologies** 8.3 Use information and communication technologies and informatics processes to deliver safe nursing care to diverse populations in a variety of settings (pp. 49–50).
Code of Ethics with Interpretive Statements (ANA, 2015a)	**Provision 2.3:** Collaboration (p. 6) **Provision 3.3:** Performance standards and review mechanisms (p. 11) **Provision 3.4:** Professional responsibility in promoting a culture of safety (pp. 11–12) **Provision 3.5:** Protection of patient health and safety by acting on questionable practice (pp. 12–13). **Provision 3.6:** Patient protection and impaired practice (p. 13). **Provision 5.2:** Promotion of personal health, safety, and well-being (p. 19)

Nurse Manager (NMC) Competencies (AONL, 2015a) and Nurse Executive (NEC) Competencies (AONL, 2015b)	**NMC: Performance Improvement (p. 4)**
	• Performance improvement
	  • Identify key performance indicators
	  • Establish data collection methodology
	  • Evaluate performance data
	  • Respond to outcome measurement findings
	• Patient safety
	  • Monitor and report sentinel events
	  • Participate in root cause analysis
	  • Promote evidence-based practices
	  • Manage incident reporting
	• Maintain survey and regulatory readiness

The Knowledge, Skills, and Attitudes Related to the Following Are Addressed in This Chapter:—cont'd

NEC: Knowledge of the Health Care Environment (p. 7)
- Evidence-based practice/outcome measurement and research
  - Design and interpret outcome measures
  - Monitor and address nurse sensitive outcomes and satisfaction indicators
- Patient safety
  - Support the development of an organization-wide patient safety program
  - Use knowledge of patient safety science (e.g., human factors, complex adaptive systems, LEAN and Six Sigma)
  - Monitor clinical activities to identify both expected and unexpected risks
  - Support a Just Culture (nonpunitive) reporting environment, supporting a reward system for identifying unsafe practices
  - Support safety surveys, responding and acting on safety recommendations
  - Lead/facilitate performance improvement teams to improve systems/processes that enhance patient safety
- Performance improvement/metrics
  - Articulate the organization's performance improvement program and goals
  - Use evidence-based metrics to align patient outcomes with the organization's goals and objectives
  - Apply high reliability concepts for the organization
  - Establish quality metrics by
    - Identifying the problem/process
    - Measuring success at improving specific areas of patient care
    - Analyzing the root causes or variation from quality standards
    - Improving the process with the evidence
    - Controlling solutions and sustaining success
- Risk management
  - Identify early warning predictability indications for errors
  - Ensure compliance by staff with all required standards

Nursing Administration Scope and Standards of Practice (ANA, 2016)	**Standard 2: Identification of Problems, Issues, and Trends** The nurse administrator analyses the assessment data to identify problems, issues, and trends (p. 37). **Standard 3: Outcomes Identification** The nurse administrator identifies expected outcomes for a plan tailored to the system, organization, or population problem, issue, or trend (p. 38).

Continued

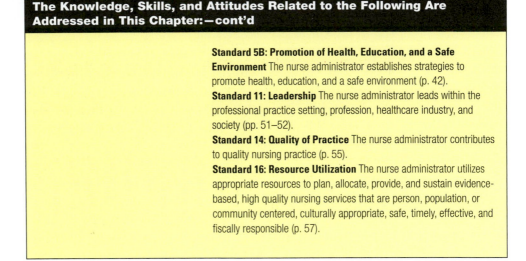

The Knowledge, Skills, and Attitudes Related to the Following Are Addressed in This Chapter:—cont'd

Standard 5B: Promotion of Health, Education, and a Safe Environment The nurse administrator establishes strategies to promote health, education, and a safe environment (p. 42).

Standard 11: Leadership The nurse administrator leads within the professional practice setting, profession, healthcare industry, and society (pp. 51–52).

Standard 14: Quality of Practice The nurse administrator contributes to quality nursing practice (p. 55).

Standard 16: Resource Utilization The nurse administrator utilizes appropriate resources to plan, allocate, provide, and sustain evidence-based, high quality nursing services that are person, population, or community centered, culturally appropriate, safe, timely, effective, and fiscally responsible (p. 57).

Source: American Association of Colleges of Nursing. (2021). *The essentials: Core competencies for professional nursing education.* Author; American Nurses Association (ANA). (2015a). *Code of ethics for nurses with interpretive statements.* Author; American Nurses Association (ANA). (2016). *Nursing administration: Scope and standards of practice* (2nd ed.). Author; American Organization for Nursing Leadership (AONL). (2015a). *AONL nurse manager competencies.* Author; American Organization for Nursing Leadership (AONL). (2015b). *AONL nurse executive competencies.* Author; Cronenwett, L., Sherwood, G., Barnsteiner, J., Disch, J., Johnson, J., Mitchell, P., Sullivan, D. T., & Warren, J. (2007). Quality and safety education for nurses. *Nursing Outlook, 55*(3), 122–131; and Greiner, A. C., & Knebel, E. (Eds.) (2003). *Health professions education: A bridge to quality.* National Academies Press.

Patient safety and quality care are concepts on a continuum: Although safe nursing care results in the lowest potential to do harm to patients, high-quality nursing care results in the greatest potential to achieve the best possible patient outcomes (Galt, Paschal, et al., 2011). Since the Institute of Medicine's (IOM's) groundbreaking report *To Err Is Human: Building a Safer Health System* was released in 2000, there has been tremendous movement toward decreasing errors and improving the safety and quality of health care (Kohn et al., 2000). Two additional IOM reports in 2004, *Patient Safety: Achieving a New Standard for Care* (Aspden et al., 2004) and *Keeping Patients Safe: Transforming the Work Environment of Nurses* (Page, 2004), also brought significant attention to the need to improve the safety and quality of the care delivered.

However, patient safety issues present an ongoing threat to achieving quality health care, and despite significant achievements since the IOM reports were published, patients remain at risk of serious harm (Robert Wood Johnson Foundation, 2014). In 2010, the U.S. Department of Health and Human Services reported that in a study of 780 Medicare beneficiaries, 13.5% experienced adverse events and 13.5% experienced temporary harm events during hospitalization (U.S. Department of Health and Human Services Office of Inspector General, 2010). Further investigation revealed that at least 44% of the events were preventable. The IOM's estimate of 44,000 to 98,000 preventable medical errors per year has been challenged by a newer report that reviewed contemporary literature (published between 2006 and 2012) to identify types and numbers of preventable adverse events in hospitals (James, 2013). The report's findings suggest that 210,000 to 400,000 deaths each year in hospitals in the United States are associated with preventable adverse events.

Improving safety and quality in health care is not just an issue in the United States; it is a global public health concern. Close to 10% of patients hospitalized in developed countries will fall victim to preventable errors or adverse events (World Health Organization [WHO], 2019). In fact, patients are at higher risk of injury while hospitalized (1 in 300) than when flying on an airplane (1 in 1,000,000) (WHO, 2019).

As the largest group of health-care professionals—as of 2019, there were 2,982,280 registered nurses in the workforce in the United States (Bureau of Labor Statistics, 2020)—nurses are in the key position to improve patient safety and quality care, and in fact they have an ethical obligation to promote safe and quality care. This obligation is reflected in Provision 3 of the ANA *Code of Ethics for Nurses with Interpretive Statements:* "The nurse promotes, advocates for, and protects the rights, health, and safety of the patient" (American Nurses Association [ANA], 2015a, p. 9). Further, Provision 4 states that "nurses have vested authority, and are accountable and responsible for the quality of their practice" (p. 15). In addition, it is the mission of the International Council of Nurses (ICN) "to ensure quality nursing care for all and sound health policies globally" (2014, para. 1). The ICN also believes that nurses must ensure patient safety in all aspects of care delivery. According to the ICN, promoting patient safety "involves a wide range of actions in the recruitment, training and retention of health care professionals, performance improvement, environmental safety and risk management, including infection control, safe use of medicines, equipment safety, safe clinical practice, safe environment of care, and accumulating an integrated body of scientific knowledge focused on patient safety and the infrastructure to support its development" (ICN, 2012, para. 1).

This chapter presents an overview of the prevalence and types of medical errors in health care today and patient safety initiatives underway to address them. Further, it discusses the roles of nurses at all levels in ensuring patient safety, from developing a culture of safety to standardizing processes, and improving patient safety, including using safety initiatives and incorporating tools for quality improvement (QI).

▶ MEDICAL ERRORS

Health care is becoming more complex, and along with increased complexity comes the growing problem of medical errors. The IOM defines a **medical error** as "the failure of a planned action to be completed as intended (i.e., error of execution) or the use of a wrong plan to achieve an aim (i.e., error in planning)" (Kohn et al., 2000, p. 28). An injury to a patient caused by medical management rather than the patient's underlying condition is called an **adverse event** or a **patient safety event** (The Joint Commission [TJC], 2020a), and most of these events are preventable. Several highly publicized cases of preventable medical errors spurred numerous initiatives to promote patient safety and improvement of quality of care. Table 9-1 illustrates some of these incidents related to preventable errors and the policy outcomes that resulted.

Table 9-1   Medical Error Incidents and Policy Outcomes

Year	Incident	Outcome
1984	Libby Zion was an 18-year-old college student with a history of depression who went to the emergency department with complaints of fever, agitation, jerking body movements, and disorientation. She was admitted for hydration and observation but died several hours later from a possible drug-drug interaction. Of note, an intern and a resident assigned to Libby's care were working 36-hour shifts, which are believed to have contributed to the error that caused her death (Lerner, 2006).	Public discussion came about regarding the excessive work hours and lack of supervision of residents in training. In 2003, the Accreditation Council for Graduate Medical Education (ACGME) established standards dictating a maximum of 80 work hours/week and no more than 30 hours/shift.
1994	Betsy Lehman was a 39-year-old award-winning health columnist for the *Boston Globe* who died after a massive overdose of chemotherapy medications (Altman, 1995).	This case was the one of the catalysts for the modern patient safety movement. It resulted in a new focus on medication errors and an impetus for computerized prescribing (Wachter & Gupta, 2018).
1995	Willie King was a 51-year-old man with diabetes who had the wrong foot amputated (Leisner, 1995).	TJC established the Universal Protocol for Preventing Wrong Site, Wrong Procedure, and Wrong Person Surgery that became effective July 1, 2004. The three components of the Universal Protocol are a preprocedure verification, site marking, and a time-out (TJC, n.d.).
2001	Josie King was an 18-month-old little girl admitted with second-degree burns over 60% of her body after falling into a bathtub full of hot water. After 2 weeks in the intensive care unit, Josie was transferred to a general unit, and her family was making plans for her discharge. Josie died 1 week later of severe dehydration that had gone unnoticed and as a result of an administration of methadone that should not have been given (Niedowski, 2003).	Josie's mother, Sorrel King, has used her experience to become an advocate for patient safety. She established the Josie King Foundation to "prevent others from dying or being harmed by medical errors" (Niedowski, 2003).
2002	Lewis Blackman was a 15-year-old boy admitted for a routine surgical procedure for pectus excavatum. Four days later, Lewis bled to death from an undetected perforated ulcer (Monk, 2002).	Helen Haskell, Lewis's mother, has worked diligently to ensure that patients and families have access to physicians and rapid response teams (Acquaviva et al., 2013).
2006	Julie Thao was a registered nurse who unintentionally administered an epidural anesthetic intravenously, instead of an antibiotic. The patient died, and Thao was arrested on felony charges ("Nurse charged," 2007).	Thao has become a spokesperson for patient safety and second victims (Quaid et al., 2010).
2007	Dennis Quaid's twins were hospitalized in the neonatal intensive care unit and received heparin overdoses twice. The twins were administered 10,000 units/mL for a catheter flush instead of 10 units/mL (Ornstein, 2008).	The Quaids renewed attention to dangerous medical errors and started a patient safety foundation (Quaid et al., 2010).

There are two types of errors: an error of omission and an error of commission. An **error of omission** results when an action is not taken, or *omitted,* such as when a nurse does not assess a patient after surgery or does not administer a medication; in both situations, the nurse omitted an action that is a standard of care. An **error of commission** results when the wrong action is taken, or *committed.* Examples of errors of commission include a nurse giving a medication to the wrong patient or performing a procedure incorrectly (e.g., a nurse breaking sterile technique when inserting a Foley catheter).

When an error occurs in the presence of a potential hazard, it is an unsafe act (Reason, 1990). Some unsafe acts do not result from errors but from violations. A violation is a deliberate deviation from safe practices as identified by designers, managers, and regulatory agencies to maintain a safe system (Reason, 1990). For example, a common standard of care is that nurses must check a patient's name band before medication administration; neglecting to check a patient's name band before administering medications is a violation. Errors and violations do not always result in harm or accidents. However, they have the potential to do so.

Further, errors can be classified as slips, lapses, and mistakes (Reason, 1990). Slips and lapses are execution failures—in other words, they occur from actions that do not result in the intended outcome. Slips are observable by others (e.g., a nurse documenting that she gave a medication on the wrong patient's chart), whereas lapses usually involve memory failure and may be apparent only to the person experiencing the failure (e.g., a nurse forgetting to administer a medication but not documenting it anywhere). Mistakes are errors that occur when an action goes as planned but the action is incorrect. Mistakes are subtler and more complex than slips or lapses. As a result, mistakes are often difficult to detect and pose a greater danger to patients than slips or lapses (Reason, 1990). For example, a nurse is told by unlicensed assistive personnel (UAP) that a patient's temperature is elevated. The nurse checks the patient's chart for an order and administers medication for the fever. Later, the nurse realizes that the UAP told her that the wrong patient had the elevated temperature, and so the nurse gave the medication to a patient who had an order but did not have an elevated temperature. This constitutes a mistake because the action was taken with the incorrect patient, and therefore the action was incorrect.

To truly ensure safety, any **near miss**, or a potential error that was discovered before it was carried out, must be monitored. For example, a nurse enters a patient's room to administer a medication and realizes that it is the wrong patient. She immediately leaves the room with the medication and avoids the commission of an error. In this situation, a near miss occurred and should be investigated to avoid an actual error in the future.

A **sentinel event** is a patient safety event that results in any of the following: death, permanent harm, and severe temporary harm and intervention required to sustain life (TJC, 2020a, para. 2). A sentinel event signals "the need for immediate investigation and response" (TJC, 2020a, para. 4). Sentinel events are tracked by TJC. However, reporting a sentinel event is voluntary.

Human errors can be viewed from two perspectives: the person approach and the systems approach (Reason, 2000). The person approach focuses on unsafe acts of health-care professionals and errors as the result of human behaviors, such as inattention, forgetfulness, negligence, and incompetence. Organizations that focus on the person approach often attempt to correct human behavior through naming, blaming, shaming, and retraining. The systems approach, however, acknowledges that errors happen because humans are not perfect. With this approach, the focus is less on the individual making the error and more on system processes that led to the error. In fact, errors are expected, and many defenses are in place to safeguard against them. Organizations that focus on the systems approach concentrate on changing the work environment by establishing barriers and safeguards against the errors (Reason, 2000). Highly educated and competent nurses make errors; human factors can provide explanations for these errors.

Unintentional human errors and system errors account for most preventable adverse events (Denham, 2007). Although most errors have multiple causes, the most common are related to human factors, communication, and leadership (Shepard, 2011):

- *Human factors* include staffing levels, staff education and competency, and staffing shortages. When staffing is inadequate or nurses lack experience, patient safety is jeopardized.
- *Communication* includes intraprofessional and interprofessional communication as well as interactions with patients and their families. Optimal patient outcomes rely on effective communication.
- *Leadership* includes leadership and management at all levels, organizational structure, policies and procedures, and practice guidelines. When leadership factors are inadequate, nurses may make decisions that can result in adverse events or near misses.

Preventing errors and adverse events relies on a systems approach that reduces the likelihood of patient safety events. Nurse leaders and managers must be able to follow through with the following activities to ensure patient safety (Galt, Paschal, et al., 2011, pp. 8–9):

- Develop a culture that is founded on the concept of safety for both patients and staff.
- Standardize as many processes as possible while simultaneously allowing staff the independent authority to solve problems in a creative manner as well as avoiding automatic action.
- Implement initiatives created by health-care organizations to improve safety and quality.
- Analyze complex processes by using appropriate tools.
- Collect data on errors and incidents within the unit to identify opportunities for improvement and track progress.

Nurse leaders and managers can encourage staff to report incidents to facilitate quality improvement and safety. One of the most common ways to report and monitor incidents is through an incident report.

Reporting Incidents, Events, and Unusual Occurrences

An **incident report** is a report of an incident, event, or unusual occurrence, most often a self-report of an error by a health-care professional (Wachter & Gupta,

2018). Other incidents such as patient falls, visitor injuries, employee injuries, dangerous situations, and medical errors, to name a few, are also documented using an incident report. Federal and state regulations require health-care organizations to establish incident reporting systems (Guido, 2014). Incident reports are used to review and evaluate patient care situations and to augment and improve quality of care. In situations involving patient care, health-care professionals should follow specific guidelines (Guido, 2014, p. 175):

- The incident report should be initiated by the person who observed the incident or who first arrived on the scene.
- Incorporate the patient's account of the incident in the report.
- Document only facts in the report—avoid assumptions.
- Have other health-care professionals who witness the event contribute to the report and cosign.
- Have the injured patient or individual seen by a health-care provider, if appropriate.
- Do not indicate in the health-care record that an incident report was completed.
- Forward the incident report to departments as required by organizational policies.
- Minimize the number of copies of the incident report to maintain confidentiality.

As technology has evolved, health-care organizations have adopted computerized incident reporting systems (IR systems). Incident reports are entered into IR systems to facilitate aggregation and management of data, follow-up, and identification of themes (Wachter & Gupta, 2018).

IR systems are passive forms of safety surveillance and rely on involved parties to submit reports. Historically, health-care professionals completed paper reports whenever there was an incident, event, or irregular occurrence, most often an error of some type. The reports were sent to the risk manager whose role was to limit the organization's legal liability. Routinely, the focus was on identifying the person or persons responsible for the error and applying some punitive sanction with minimal attention given to systems causes or improvement. This process fostered a culture of blame and resulted in many errors going unreported. There are times when an error occurs due to reckless behavior and breaking rules and the individual responsible should be held accountable. However, an overly punitive system decreases the trust and open dialogue needed for a just culture or a culture of safety (Wachter & Gupta, 2018).

▶ CREATING A CULTURE OF SAFETY

A **culture of safety** is a blame-free environment in which staff members feel comfortable reporting errors and near misses. Until the early 2000s, when an error was made by a nurse, the approach by management was punitive and involved identifying the individual who made the error and requiring that they be named in an incident report and complete a medication review course. This approach did not seek the root cause of the error and was not effective in reducing errors. Sadly, this approach still occurs today. A culture of safety supports nurses in that it is nonpunitive and emphasizes account-ability, excellence, honesty, integrity, and mutual respect (Barnsteiner, 2017; Johnson, 2017).

In a culture of safety, patient and employee safety is the priority, and organi-zational leadership is committed to providing safe and quality care as well as creating a safe work environment. A culture of safety develops over time and includes three stages (Page, 2004, pp. 296–298):

Stage 1. Safety management is based on rules and regulations: The organization sees safety as an external requirement imposed by regulatory bodies, and mere compliance with rules and regulations is considered adequate.

Stage 2. Good safety performance becomes an organizational goal: Safety is per-ceived by leadership and management as important, but safety performance is addressed in terms of goals rather than as part of the strategic plan and culture of the organization.

Stage 3. Safety performance is seen as dynamic and continuously improving: Safety performance is viewed by everyone in the organization as dynamic and in need of continuous improvement in this stage. There is a strong emphasis on communication, training, management style, and improving efficiency and effectiveness.

A culture of safety promotes staff engagement and empowerment and focuses on *why* an error was made rather than *who* made the error. Embed-ded within a culture of safety is a **just culture**, or a culture that is fair to those who make an error. A just culture improves patient safety because it encour-ages nurses to learn from each other's mistakes and to report all errors and near misses without fear of repercussion. Nurses are responsible for their own actions and are expected to provide constructive feedback to their peers (ANA, 2016; Shepard, 2011).

Nurse leaders and managers are responsible for promoting a culture of safety and creating an environment where nursing care is delivered safely and effec-tively (ANA, 2015b). Creating a culture of safety is hard work; however, once a culture of safety is established, "it is easy to identify its presence, as well as its absence" (Wachter & Gupta, 2018, p. 301).

Part of creating a culture of safety is encouraging staff members to voice their concerns when they feel that a situation is a safety risk. This can be done through a communication technique called "CUS," a three-step process that assists staff members in stopping an activity when they sense or discover a safety breach. CUS stands for the following (TJC, 2012, p. 52):

1. I am **Concerned**.
2. I am **Uncomfortable**.
3. This is a **Safety issue**.

Further, nurse leaders and managers can "promote a process of mistake or error mitigation that recognizes that errors may be the result of system breakdowns or failures to build a good system, as opposed to putting the total blame on individu-als" (ANA, 2015b, p. 6).

<table>
<tr><td>

LEARNING ACTIVITY 9-1

</td><td>

Culture of Blame Versus Culture of Safety

Compare and contrast a culture of blame with a culture

</td></tr>
</table>

of safety related to the following:

- Medication errors
- Near misses
- Sentinel events

A culture of safety relies on a systems approach that reduces the likelihood of patient safety events. A key aspect of preventing errors and adverse events is to avoid automatic actions. As nurses become experienced with a specific task, cognitive adaptive mechanisms kick in and allow for nurses to go on "autopilot" (Galt, Fuji, et al., 2011). Unfortunately, this ability to take complex skills and make them routine can have a negative impact on patient safety. As tasks and skills become automatic, nurses pay less attention to details, and this deficit can result in variations in care and the possibility of a patient safety event or error. Evidence shows that varying patterns of care lead to poor clinical outcomes. In contrast, standardizing care can improve clinical outcomes, reduce inefficiencies, and decrease costs (Leotsakos et al., 2014). Nurse leaders and managers can intervene by ensuring that nurses use standardized procedures and checklists rather than relying on memory and automatic approaches to patient care. When there are variations in processes and procedures, confusion, delays in care, and varying levels of nursing care quality can result. Standardizing processes and procedures can help reduce errors and improve quality care. **Standardization** is the process of developing, agreeing on, and implementing uniform criteria, methods, processes, designs, or practices that can improve patient safety and quality of care (Leotsakos et al., 2014). Standardized processes benefit health care by doing the following:

- Providing nurse leaders and managers and nursing staff with a method for comparing outcomes resulting from standardized processes across the organization
- Enabling nurse leaders and managers to compare data and interpret relevance and efficacy of a specific intervention or process
- Allowing for a way for nurses at all levels (as well as other health-care professionals) to communicate with one another in meaningful ways (i.e., use of standardized terms)
- Increasing the likelihood of user familiarity with technology and equipment that can reduce risk of human errors
- Allowing nurses at all levels as well as other health-care professionals to learn from each other's experiences

Standardization can take many forms including using checklists, approved abbreviations and practice guidelines, electronic health records, and computerized physician order entry; storing equipment and supplies in the same location on units; and designing units using the same floor plan within a facility. Although a challenge, nurse leaders and managers must standardize as many processes as possible while simultaneously allowing staff the independent authority to solve problems in a creative manner.

▶ PATIENT SAFETY INITIATIVES

Patient safety advocacy groups have emerged since the 1980s in response to concerns about the less than stellar quality of the American health-care system and the prevalence of patient safety concerns. The leaders of many of these groups are

---

✿ Second Victim

The primary victim of any medical error is the patient, as well as their family. However, there is always a second victim: the nurse or health-care professional involved in an error that injures a patient (Smetzer, 2012). Fatal errors and those that cause major injury or disability can result in stress-related psychological and physiological reactions for the nurse involved. Often, second victims experience a medical emergency equivalent to post-traumatic stress disorder (PTSD). Many second victims feel abandoned, isolated, and a loss of security, and the traumatic event changes their self-perception (Denham, 2007; Smetzer, 2012). The second victim needs compassion, caring, and respect. Provision 1.5 of the ANA Code of Ethics states, "Respect for persons extends to all individuals with whom the nurse interacts. Nurses maintain professional, respectful, and caring relationships with colleagues and are committed to fair treatment, transparency, integrity-preserving compromise, and the best resolution of conflict" (ANA, 2015a, p. 4).

Five rights for second victims have been identified using the acronym TRUST (Table 9-2; Denham, 2007):

1. Treatment that is just
2. Respect
3. Understanding and compassion
4. Supportive care
5. Transparency and the opportunity to contribute

Health-care leaders must address the rights of all health-care professionals involved in unintentional harm to patients through systems failures and human errors. Nurse leaders and managers must promote respect for nurse's rights and responsibilities, maintain empathetic and caring relationships, and establish a supportive and healthy work environment (ANA, 2015b).

Table 9-2	TRUST
Treatment that is just	Nurses who make an error cannot be held 100% accountable when system failures predispose them to human errors.
Respect	All health-care professionals are susceptible to making an error and deserve to be treated with respect should an error occur. Health-care organizations must avoid the name-blame-shame cycle.
Understanding and compassion	Nurses who make an error need to be allowed to progress through the stages of grief.
Supportive care	Nurses who make an error can experience the signs and symptoms of post-traumatic stress disorder and need psychological support.
Transparency and the opportunity to contribute	Improving patient safety requires all health-care professionals to be more honest and transparent about errors by identifying, disclosing, and reporting medical errors.

Adapted from Denham, 2007.

people who have had personal experiences with medical errors, thus putting a human face on patient safety issues (Wachter & Gupta, 2018). The modern patient safety movement does not call for perfection from health-care professionals; rather, it acknowledges that humans make errors and replaces the blame-and-shame game with systems thinking (Wachter & Gupta, 2018). Systems thinking acknowledges that humans make errors and "safety depends on creating systems that anticipate errors and either prevent or catch them before they cause harm" (Wachter & Gupta, 2018, p. 21).

The following are organizations that have put in place safety initiatives that can be used by nurse leaders and managers to promote safe and quality care. All of these patient safety initiatives can have a positive impact on the overall quality of health care.

Agency for Healthcare Research and Quality

Established in 1989 as the Agency for Health Care Policy and Research within the Department of Health and Human Services, the Agency for Healthcare Research and Quality (or AHRQ, which it became in 1999) has always had the mission "to make health care safer, higher quality, more accessible, equitable, and affordable" (AHRQ, 2018, para. 1). In response to the IOM sentinel report *To Err Is Human,* the AHRQ set out to build a foundation to better understand patient safety. In 2005, the AHRQ established the Patient Safety Network (PSNet), a Web site featuring essential resources relevant to the patient safety community. Materials are selected for inclusion on the site according to the following criteria (AHRQ, n.d., para. 4):

- Support multidisciplinary, "systems" approach to minimizing errors in health care
- Come from a wide range of disciplines and sources
- Have been written and/or sponsored by credible sources
- Are of interest to the patient safety community at large, both expert and novice
- Are of value for gaining insight into and supporting patient safety

Nurses at all levels can use PSNet to find tips for preventing medical errors and promoting patient safety. Nurse leaders and managers can use PSNet for suggestions about measuring health-care quality as well as accessing consumer assessment of health plans, evaluation software, report tools, and case studies.

American Nurses Association

In 1994, the ANA launched an initiative to investigate the impact of health-care restructuring on the safety and quality of patient care and the nursing profession (Montalvo, 2007). The Patient Safety and Quality Initiative focused on educating registered nurses about quality measurement, informing the public about safe and quality health care, and investigating methods to evaluate the safety and quality of patient care empirically. Through this initiative, strong links between nursing actions and patient outcomes were identified (Montalvo, 2007).

In 1998, the ANA established the National Database of Nursing Quality Indicators (NDNQI), which collects data from participating facilities on nursing-sensitive quality indicators. The NDNQI is used by 2,000 hospitals nationwide and reports national comparison information related to nursing-sensitive quality indicators and unit performance. Until recently, the NDNQI was managed by the University of Kansas School of Nursing. In 2014, Press Ganey acquired NDNQI to offer more specific insights into nursing performance to improve patient experiences and outcomes (Press Ganey, 2014). Nurse leaders and managers should use these nursing-sensitive quality indicators as part of a comprehensive approach to measuring and evaluating quality of care and assist in improving patient safety. These indicators reflect the characteristics of the nursing workforce, nursing processes, and patient outcomes, which vary according to the characteristics or processes of nursing (Montalvo & Dunton, 2007, p. 1). In addition, the NDNQI also measures characteristics of the nursing workforce that affect the quality of patient care and the patient's experience, such as staffing levels, nurse turnover, and nurse education and certification (Press Ganey, 2019).

Nursing-sensitive quality indicators are indicators that reflect elements of patient care that are directly affected by the quality and quantity of nursing care and include the following:

- **Structure indicators** relate to the care environment and include staffing levels, hours of nursing care per patient day, nursing skill levels, and education of staff.
- **Process indicators** relate to how nursing care is provided and include elements falling under the nursing process (i.e., assessment, diagnosis, planning, intervention, and evaluation of nursing care) and job satisfaction.
- **Outcome indicators** relate to the results of nursing care and include changes in a patient's health status related to nursing care, such as pressure ulcers and patient falls. Outcome indicators improve when there is greater quality and quantity of nursing care.

Box 9-1 provides a list of nursing-sensitive quality indicators currently being collected.

National Quality Forum

The National Quality Forum (NQF) is a nonprofit organization established in 1999 in response to the recommendations from the Advisory Commission on Consumer Protection and Quality in the Health Care Industry (NQF, 2020a). The NQF is committed to helping the United States achieve better and affordable care and, ultimately, improving the overall health of Americans (NQF, 2020b). The NQF is involved in the following activities to meet this goal (NQF, 2020b):

- Setting standards for health-care measurements
- Recommending measures for use in payment and public reporting programs
- Identifying and accelerating QI priorities
- Advancing electronic measurement to capture necessary data needed to measure performance
- Providing information and tools to help health-care decision makers

---

BOX 9-1 Current Nursing-Sensitive Quality Indicators

STRUCTURE QUALITY INDICATORS

- Admissions, discharges, and transfers
- Emergency department throughput
- Nurse turnover
- Patient contacts
- Patient volume and flow
- RN education and specialty certification
- Staffing and skill mix*
- Workforce characteristics

PROCESS QUALITY INDICATORS

- Care coordination
- Device utilization
- Pain impairing function
- Patient falls*
- Pediatric pain, assessment, intervention, reassessment (AIR) cycle
- Pressure injuries
- Restraints

OUTCOME QUALITY INDICATORS

- Assaults on nursing personnel
- Assaults by psychiatric patients
- Catheter-associated urinary tract infections (CAUTIs)
- Central line catheter–associated bloodstream infections (CLABSIs)
- *C. difficile* infections
- Hospital readmissions
- Methicillin-resistant *Staphylococcus aureus* (MRSA) infections
- Multidrug-resistant organisms (MDROs)
- Pain
- Patient burns
- Patient falls*
- Pediatric peripheral intravenous infiltrations
- Perioperative clinical measure set
- Surgical errors
- Unplanned postoperative transfers/admissions
- Pressure injuries
- Ventilator-associated events (VAEs)
- Ventilator-associated pneumonia (VAP)

STRUCTURE, PROCESS, AND OUTCOME QUALITY INDICATORS

- RN survey with job satisfaction scales
- RN survey with practice environment scale (PES)*

*National Quality Forum–endorsed indicators.
From Press Ganey, 2019, pp. 2–3; NDNQI, 2020; NQF, 2020b.

One national priority the NQF is focusing on is patient safety. The NQF identifies the following three goals as critical in making health care safer for Americans (NQF, 2020c, para. 2):

1. Reduce preventable hospital admissions and readmissions.
2. Reduce the incidence of adverse health-care–associated conditions.
3. Reduce harm from inappropriate or unnecessary care.

The NQF has endorsed a set of nursing-sensitive quality indicators that have been pivotal to understanding nursing's influence on patient outcomes as well as promoting a measure for QI. The nursing-sensitive quality indicators endorsed by the NQF are indicated by an asterisk in Box 9-1. Nurse leaders and managers should consider monitoring and measuring these quality indicators as they strive to create an environment of safe and quality care.

Institute for Healthcare Improvement

The Institute for Healthcare Improvement (IHI) was founded in the late 1980s and is currently a leading innovator in health and health-care improvement in the United States and globally (IHI, 2020a). The IHI collaborates with the health-care improvement community to remove improvement roadblocks and launch innovations that dramatically improve patient care (IHI, 2020b).

The IHI has been responsible for two nationwide initiatives, the 100,000 Lives Campaign and the 5 Million Lives Campaign, which spread best practice changes to thousands of hospitals in the United States. The 100,000 Lives Campaign ran from January 2005 through June 2006, with the goal to reduce morbidity and mortality significantly in the American health-care system. The IHI called on hospitals and health-care providers to implement the following interventions to reduce harm and death from medical error (IHI, 2020c, para. 3):

- Deploy rapid response teams to patients at risk of cardiac or respiratory arrest.
- Deliver reliable, evidence-based care to patients with myocardial infarctions to prevent deaths from heart attacks.
- Prevent adverse drug events through medication reconciliation, a process of comparing the patient's list of medications with those ordered by health-care providers on admission, transfer, and/or discharge.
- Prevent central line infections by implementing a series of evidence-based steps called the "Central Line Bundle."
- Prevent surgical site infections by administering the appropriate preoperative antibiotics and at the proper time.
- Prevent ventilator-associated pneumonia by implementing a series of evidence-based steps called the "Ventilator Bundle."

The IHI estimated that more than 2,000 hospitals made a commitment to implement the interventions to reduce harm, and 122,300 lives were saved during the 18-month campaign (IHI, 2020c; Saver, 2006).

The 5 Million Lives Campaign ran from December 2006 through December 2009. The goal was to reduce illness or medical harm, such as adverse events and surgical complications, and patient mortality significantly. The IHI encouraged hospitals and health-care providers to continue the efforts begun in the 100,000 Lives Campaign, which nurse leaders and managers should do, as well as employ the following additional strategies to reduce harm and death from medical errors (IHI, 2020c, para. 2):

- Prevent pressure ulcers by using evidence-based guidelines.
- Reduce methicillin-resistant *Staphylococcus aureus* (MRSA) through basic changes in infection control processes throughout hospitals.
- Prevent harm from high-alert medications with a focus on anticoagulants, sedatives, narcotics, and insulin.
- Reduce surgical complications by reliably implementing changes in care identified by the Surgical Care Improvement Project.
- Deliver evidence-based care to patients with congestive heart failure to reduce readmissions.
- Get hospital boards on board by defining and spreading new processes to encourage boards of directors to be more effective in the improvement of care.

At the close of the campaign, 4,050 hospitals were enrolled, reflecting an unprecedented commitment to patient safety and quality. The IHI believes that the campaign resulted in a massive reduction of patient injuries and tremendous improvement in patient outcomes, "with more than 2,000 facilities pursuing each of the Campaign's 12 interventions to reduce infection, surgical complication, medication errors, and other forms of unreliable care in facilities. Eight states enrolled 100% of their hospitals in the Campaign, and 18 states enrolled over 90% of their hospitals in the Campaign" (IHI, 2020c, para. 10). The IHI emphasizes that a national study is needed to determine whether 5 million instances of harm were prevented as a result of the campaign (IHI, 2020c).

The Joint Commission

TJC, a nonprofit organization founded in 1951, accredits and certifies approximately 22,000 health-care organizations in the United States based on established standards (TJC, 2020b). TJC is involved in numerous activities to "help organizations across the continuum of care lead the way to zero harm" (TJC, 2020c, para. 1). Its mission is to "continuously improve health care for the public, in collaboration with other stakeholders, by evaluating health-care organizations and inspiring them to excel in providing safe and effective care of the highest quality and value" (TJC, 2020c, para. 2). In support of its mission, TJC reviews agency activities in response to sentinel events.

TJC is committed to patient safety through initiatives such as its Speak Up programs. TJC worked with the Centers for Medicare and Medicaid Services to launch the Speak Up programs in 2002 with the goal of urging patients to take an active role in preventing medical errors by becoming informed participants in their care. Speak Up encourages health-care consumers to do the following (TJC, 2020d):

- **S**peak up if you have questions or concerns. If you still do not understand, ask again. It is your body, and you have a right to know.
- **P**ay attention to the care you get. Always make sure you are getting the right treatments and medicines by the right health-care professionals. Do not assume anything.
- **E**ducate yourself about your illness: Learn about the medical tests you have and your treatment plan.
- **A**sk a trusted family member or friend to be your advocate (advisor or supporter).
- **K**now what medicines you take and why you take them. Medicine errors are the most common health-care mistake.
- **U**se a hospital, clinic, surgery center, or other type of health-care organization that has been carefully checked out.
- **P**articipate in all decisions about your treatment: You are the center of the health-care team.

The Speak Up programs include free brochures, posters, and videos available at www.jointcommission.org/facts_about_speak_up. The Speak Up programs are very successful at promoting increased communication with both patients and staff about safety. Nurse leaders and managers should promote the Speak Up programs by including information about them in unit meetings and staff orientation. As advocates, nurse leaders and managers should assist patients and their families with obtaining information about Speak Up programs.

TJC also established the National Patient Safety Goals (NPSGs) program in 2002 to assist health-care organizations address patient safety concerns. A panel of patient safety experts works with TJC to identify emerging patient safety issues and strategies to best address these issues. The first set of NPSGs became effective in January 2003 and are still updated annually (TJC, 2020e). Nurse leaders and managers can keep up with the NPSGs, which address specific clinical areas such as ambulatory health care, behavioral health care, critical access hospitals, home care, hospitals, laboratory services, long-term care, and office-based surgery, at https://www.jointcommission.org/standards/national-patient-safety-goals/.

World Health Organization

WHO member states agreed on a resolution on patient safety in 2002 and recognized patient safety as a global health-care issue in 2004. Believing that every patient should receive "safe health care, every time, everywhere," the WHO launched the Patient Safety Programme in 2004. The WHO defines patient safety as "the absence of preventable harm to a patient during the process of health care" (WHO, 2020, para. 3). The WHO identified patient safety as a global problem and established 10 facts about patient safety to shed light on the enormous importance of patient safety as a serious public health issue (WHO, 2019):

1. One in every 10 patients is harmed while receiving hospital care.
2. The occurrence of adverse events due to unsafe care is likely one of the 10 leading causes of death and disability across the world.
3. Four out of every 10 patients are harmed in primary and outpatient health care.
4. At least 1 out of every 7 Canadian dollars is spent treating the effects of patient harm in hospital care.
5. Investment in patient safety can lead to significant financial savings.
6. Unsafe medication practices and medication errors harm millions of patients and cost billions of U.S. dollars every year.
7. Inaccurate or delayed diagnosis is one of the most common causes of patient harm and affects millions of patients.
8. Hospital infections affect up to 10 out of every 100 hospitalized patients.
9. More than 1 million patients die annually from complications due to surgery.
10. Medical exposure to radiation is a public health and patient safety concern.

In 2007, the WHO launched the High 5s Project to address major concerns about patient safety globally. The project derived its name from the WHO's goals to reduce the frequency of five patient safety problems in five countries over 5 years (WHO, 2014, p. 9). The goals of the High 5s Project were to use standardization across multicountry settings and to use a multipronged approach to evaluating the standard operating protocols (WHO, 2014).

Five standard operating protocols and associated evaluation instruments were developed between 2007 and 2014 to address the following issues (WHO, 2014, p. 17):

1. Medication accuracy at transitions in care
2. Correct procedure at the correct body site
3. Use of concentrated injectable medicines

4. Communication during patient care handovers
5. Health-care–associated infections

The first two standard operating protocols have been implemented by all countries participating in the High 5s Project, including the United States. Nurses at all levels should be aware of these patient safety initiatives and their impact on best practices and safe, quality nursing care. Nurse leaders and managers must embrace patient safety initiatives as they establish a work environment that fosters safe, quality care delivery.

▶ PRINCIPLES OF QUALITY IMPROVEMENT

Florence Nightingale was concerned about quality 150 years ago. She has been called "the woman who discovered quality" (Meyer & Bishop, 2007, p. 240), and she could also be considered an evangelist for performance improvement. When working in the British Military hospital system, she worked tirelessly to change the conditions for patients. She collected data, developed tables to display the data, and reported statistics to British leaders. Initially, Nightingale's work was related to mortality rates in hospitals. However, she soon informed those she reported to that "hospital mortality statistics have hitherto given little information on the efficiency of the hospital, i.e., the extent to which it fulfils the purpose it was established for, because there are elements of existence of which such statistics have hitherto taken no cognizance" (Nightingale, 1859, p. 5). She went on to discuss the need for better sanitary conditions in hospitals and that surgical operations and their results should be monitored. In essence, what Nightingale was referring to is what we know today as quality improvement.

Quality improvement (QI) as it is used in health care today was first used in industry in the early 1900s. In the 1920s at the Bell Telephone company, a young engineer by the name of Walter Shewhart explored using statistical methods to identify issues and establish strategies to improve them. His main premise was that statistical control would allow identification of causes of variations in a process. Further, by maintaining control over processes, future outputs could be predicted and allow processes to be managed economically (Smith, 2009). His quality methods were used in American industry in the 1930s. He developed various tools such as charts and graphs and principles of statistical control that resulted in the basic principles of quality control still used today. Shewhart is known as the modern father of quality control (Tague, 2005).

A student of Shewhart's, W. Edwards Deming, worked for the U.S. Census Bureau in the 1940s and also taught quality control methods to engineers and statisticians. He became disillusioned with many engineers and statisticians because they did not understand or value the benefits of the methods he taught. After World War II, he went to Japan, where he lectured on quality control and statistical and managerial concepts for quality to Japanese engineers and scientists (Tague, 2005). He believed if the Japanese manufacturers applied the principles, they could improve the quality of their products, and those products would be desired worldwide (Tague, 2005). He is known for 14 key principles for management that are used by managers and leaders to improve business and organizational effectiveness. Deming was a visionary whose belief in continuous improvement led to many theories and teachings that influence quality, management, and leadership today (W. Edwards Deming Institute, 2016).

Joseph Juran was another engineer interested in statistical control and quality. Like Shewhart, he also worked for Bell and was involved in conducting statistical quality control. He is often called the "father of quality." Juran developed the Pareto principle, which is one of the most useful tools used in management today (Juran Global, 2016). He described quality from the customer's perspective and suggested that higher quality means that more features will meet customer needs, and higher quality will also include fewer defects. Juran visited Japan and worked with Deming to further teach and help industrial managers understand their responsibilities for quality production.

In the 1970s and 1980s, the American auto and electronics industries experienced the influx of high-quality products from Japanese competition. The U.S. companies requested assistance from Deming and Juran to begin quality management and quality control programs or total quality management (TQM) (Tague, 2005). TQM is "any quality management program that addresses all areas of an organization, emphasizes customer satisfaction, and uses continuous improvement methods and tools" (Tague, 2005, p. 14).

Health-care organizations are called to use TQM by implementing QI programs aimed at monitoring, assessing, and improving the quality of health care delivered and to continuously seek higher levels of performance to optimize care. QI entails a systematic and continuous series of actions that leads to measurable improvement in health care and the health status of specific patient groups (U.S. Department of Health and Human Services [HHS] Health Resources and Services Administration [HRSA], 2011). All QI programs incorporate four key principles (HHS HRSA, 2011):

1. QI works as systems and processes.
2. There is a focus on patients.
3. There is a focus on being part of the team.
4. There is a focus on the use of data.

Successful QI also requires the following elements: "fostering and sustaining a culture of change and safety, developing and clarifying an understanding of the problem, involving key stakeholders, testing change strategies, and continuous monitoring of performance and reporting of findings to sustain the change" (Hughes, 2008, p. 18). In addition, effective QI programs require committed management, an established QI model and processes, and a set of QI tools.

There are many frameworks for QI, and most have steps that assist in asking questions, gathering appropriate data, and taking effective and efficient action to address the issue (Tague, 2005). The QI process is similar to the nursing process in that, once a plan is in place to address an issue or problem, it is reevaluated. The QI process is cyclical and involves setting standards of care, taking measures according to standards of care, evaluating care, recommending improvements, ensuring that improvements are implemented, and evaluating the improvements. Nurse leaders and managers are integral in the QI process because they are responsible for ensuring the safety and quality of nursing care. Nurse leaders and managers can improve patient safety by applying the QI principles and by using a patient-centered approach (ANA, 2016; Galt, Paschal, et al., 2011).

The QI process begins with monitoring specific measures that are part of a care process to identify variations in care and compare findings with performance levels or benchmarks established. If a measure is outside the expected performance level, a problem is identified, and an investigation ensues to determine the root cause of the problem. The following steps (illustrated in Fig. 9-1) can be used to monitor and improve performance (Donabedian, 2003):

1. *Determining what to monitor:* Some activities are directed by government agencies that provide care, pay for care, and assume responsibility for its quality to be monitored. All activities that fall below an expected level of performance must be monitored.

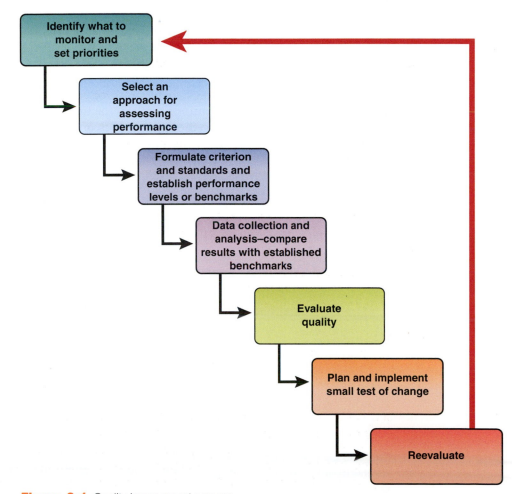

Figure 9-1 Quality improvement process.

2. *Determining priorities in monitoring:* All activities that could jeopardize patient safety should be monitored. Four characteristics guide determining the priority of a problem: the problem is believed to occur frequently; error or failure in performance is known or believed to occur frequently; when it occurs, such error or failure in performance is believed or known to have serious consequences to health and is costly; and the error or failure in question can be rather easily corrected (p. 40).

3. *Selecting approaches for assessing performance:* This step requires the nurse leader or manager to determine the type of information needed (structure, process, or outcome) to make an inference about quality. It is important to avoid focusing only on outcome measurements and to recognize that there can be weaknesses in the structure and process that lead to failures or poor performance. A combination of approaches is needed for a more comprehensive assessment of quality. By using a combination of approaches, the cause of poor performance or outcome can be attributed to structure and/or process, and this attribution helps direct the improvement process.

4. *Formulating criteria and standards:* A criterion is "an attribute of structure, process, or outcome that is used to draw an inference about quality" (p. 60), whereas a standard is "a specified quantitative measure of magnitude or frequency that specifies what is good or less so" (p. 60).

5. *Obtaining the necessary information:* Data can be collected from medical records, surveys, financial records, statistical reports, databases, and direct observations.

6. *Choosing how to monitor:* Monitoring can be prospective (or anticipatory), occurring before the event; concurrent, conducted during the course of patient care; and retrospective, occurring after the event. The most frequent type is retrospective.

7. *Constructing monitoring systems:* Monitoring of activities for improvement should be an organizational endeavor with a specific department or unit responsible to plan, coordinate, direct, and implement the process as a whole. In addition, there should be coordinated efforts at the unit level including all personnel involved in the activity under investigation.

8. *Bringing about behavior change:* Change is implemented with the goal of changing the structure and/or process and, ultimately, improving the outcome or level of performance.

Once a QI activity is identified, nurse leaders and managers form an interprofessional team to implement the QI process. Nurses at all levels may be part of an intraprofessional or interprofessional team to explore the problem identified. The team should be made up of members representing those involved with the problem. Nurse leaders and managers may lead the team or designate a nurse or other health-care professional to facilitate the QI team. For the QI process to be effective and successful, nurse leaders and managers must promote teamwork and collaboration in the workplace environment.

As members of the interprofessional team, nurses should be able to understand and use QI principles and processes as well as outcome measures. Nurses at all levels must be concerned about what they are responsible for, what is the most in need of improvement, and what they can improve (Donabedian, 2003). Moreover, nurses at all levels have an obligation to collaborate with others to provide quality health-care services safely (ANA, 2015a). Nurse leaders and managers must foster staff involvement in safety initiatives and QI processes to begin changing the processes, attitudes, and behaviors of staff (Newhouse & Poe, 2005). They must help staff members understand that patient safety and QI are not interchangeable but should be implemented simultaneously and continuously to make the most impact (McFadden et al., 2014).

▶ MODELS FOR QUALITY IMPROVEMENT

Donabedian Model

One of the most popular frameworks for assessing quality in health care is the **Donabedian Model**. This model provides a framework for examining and evaluating the quality of health care by looking at three categories of information that can be collected to draw inferences about the quality of health care: (1) structure, the conditions under which care is provided; (2) process, the activities that encompass health care; and (3) outcomes, the desirable or undesirable changes in individuals as a result of health care (Donabedian, 2003) (Table 9-3). The model has been used in health care as well as other industries. Figure 9-2 illustrates the Donabedian Model as it relates to nursing practice.

The Donabedian Model provides a starting point for any QI activity, and other QI models can be used to further define and assess safety and quality problems in health care. Typically, a health-care agency selects a model or a combination of models that will best fit their organization's mission, vision, and philosophy as well as the goals and objectives of the improvement activity. Everyone in an organization is part of continuous QI, and nurse leaders and managers often oversee QI initiatives.

Lean Model

The **Lean Model** assumes that all processes contain waste and involves the thought process of doing more with less. The model, originated at Toyota and also known

Table 9-3	Comparison of Criterion and Standard for Structure, Process, and Outcome Indicators	
Indicator	**Criterion**	**Standard**
Structure	Staffing levels in a critical care unit	Staffing levels will be maintained at a ratio of one nurse for two patients (1:2) on all shifts 7 days/week.
Process	Administration of a blood transfusion during abdominal surgery	Between 5% and 20% of all patients undergoing abdominal surgery over a 12-month period will receive blood transfusions.
Outcome	Patient's death after abdominal surgery	Less than 1% of all patients undergoing abdominal surgery over a 12-month period will die of surgical complications.

Adapted from Donabedian, 2003.

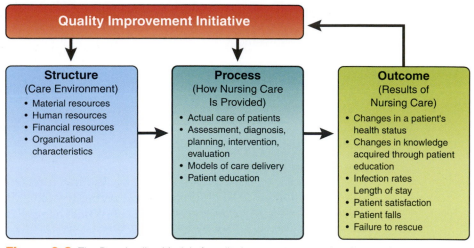

Figure 9-2 The Donabedian Model of quality improvement as related to nursing care.

as the Toyota Production System (TPS), is built on four basic principles: (1) all work processes are highly specified; (2) all customer and supplier relationships are clear; (3) pathways between people and process steps are specific and consistent; and (4) improvements are made based on scientific methods and at the lowest level of the organization (Spear & Bowen, 1999). Factors involved in the successful application of TPS in health care include eliminating non–value-added activities associated with complex processes, workarounds, and rework; involving frontline nurses throughout the QI process; and tracking issues that arise during the process (Hughes, 2008). A major advantage of the TPS is that frontline workers are empowered to identify problems and make improvements at the point of care. In this model, nurse leaders and managers provide direction and function as coaches. Lean focuses on waste reduction and achieves its goals through workplace organization, visual controls, and by using few technical tools (American Society for Quality [ASQ], 2020). Often, organizations begin with the Lean Model making the workplace as efficient and effective as possible and reducing waste. If process problems continue, the more technical Six Sigma statistical tools may be applied (ASQ, 2020).

Six Sigma Model

Originally designed as a business strategy, the **Six Sigma Model** is a rigorous method that encompasses five steps: (1) define, (2) measure, (3) analyze, (4) improve, and (5) control (DMAIC; Table 9-4). Sigma is a letter from the Greek alphabet (σ) used in statistics, and measures variation or spread. Six Sigma refers to six standard deviations from the mean (Tague, 2005). It is used in QI to define the number of acceptable errors produced by a process. Six Sigma involves improving, designing, and monitoring processes to minimize or reduce waste (Hughes, 2008). Six Sigma emphasizes variation reduction and uses statistical data analysis, design of experiments, and hypothesis testing.

Table 9-4	Six Sigma DMAIC Principles
Define	Define the process and outcome to be improved.
Measure	Track performance through data collection.
Analyze	Analyze data to verify poor performance.
Improve	Use data analysis to inform a plan for improvement.
Control	Use ongoing monitoring and improvement as needed.

Adapted from Tague, 2005.

Institute for Healthcare Improvement Model of Improvement

The IHI Model of Improvement has two parts. First, three fundamental questions are asked, in any order: (1) What are we trying to accomplish? (2) How will we know that a change is an improvement? (3) What changes can we make that will result in improvement? Second, the **plan-do-study-act (PDSA)** cycle (or rapid cycle testing) is implemented: *Plan* involves developing a plan to initiate a small change, *do* is implementing the plan and collecting data about the process, *study* includes studying and summarizing the results of the change, and *act* encompasses three possible actions—adopt the change, adapt the change, or abandon the change. Once the cycle is complete, the process starts over again (IHI, 2020d). Using the PDSA promotes continuous QI. The PDSA cycle is used to identify issues and improve care (Fig. 9-3). PDSA includes implementing small tests of change to improve care; therefore, it can be integrated with any of the QI models to implement and evaluate small tests of change. Nurse leaders and managers may use

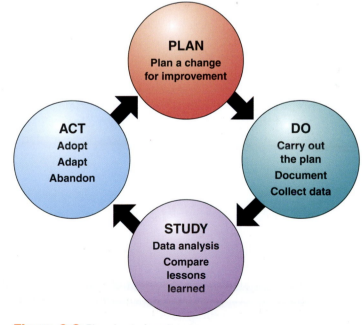

Figure 9-3 Plan-do-study-act.

PDSA when implementing any change in procedures and when planning data collection and analysis to verify root causes of a problem or error.

Failure Modes and Effects Analysis

Failure modes and effects analysis (FMEA) is useful in determining what aspect of a process needs to change. The goals of FMEA are to prevent patient safety events by identifying all possible ways a process could result in failure, estimate the probability of failure, estimate the consequences of failure, and establish an action plan to prevent potential failures from occurring.

The steps in the FMEA process include failure modes, or what could go wrong; failure causes, or why would the failure happen; and failure effects, or what would be the consequences of each failure (Nolan et al., 2004, p. 9). FMEA is a systematic approach to evaluate a process. Potential failures are prioritized according to their consequences, with most serious first. Nurse leaders and managers may use FMEA before developing plans to modify a process or analyzing failures in a current process (Tague, 2005).

Root Cause Analysis

Root cause analysis (RCA) is a "formalized investigation and problem-solving approach focused on identifying and understanding the underlying causes of an event as well as potential events that were intercepted . . . used with the understanding that system, rather than individual factors, are likely the root cause of most problems" (Hughes, 2008, pp. 6–7). Should a sentinel event occur, an RCA is required and must be followed by a realistic action plan to address and eliminate risks (TJC, 2012).

An RCA is completed after a patient safety event and includes the sequence of events that led up to the event, possible causal factors and root cause, and an action plan that identifies specific strategies to reduce the risk of a similar incident occurring in the future. A typical action plan should address the following: responsibility for implementing and overseeing the plan, pilot testing or a small test of change, timelines, and an appropriate approach for measuring the effectiveness of the plan. Nurse leaders and managers use RCA to investigate any medical error that occurs on their unit. Often, nurse leaders and managers use RCA to find the root cause of an error and use PDSA to implement a change aimed at improving or alleviating the cause.

▶ QUALITY IMPROVEMENT TOOLS

There are many tools available to use in the QI process for different purposes, whether it is to communicate information, determine whether a problem exists, or help in decision making (Boxer & Goldfarb, 2011). QI tools also help to guide data collection, identify trends and possible problems, and provide a way to display data collected. All nurses participating in the QI process should be able to use basic QI tools, such as run charts, histograms, fishbone diagrams, flow charts, and Pareto charts, to collect, analyze, and display data. Selection of an appropriate tool to

EXPLORING THE EVIDENCE 9-1

Walker, L. J., O'Connell, M. E., and Giesler, A. L. (2015). Keeping a grasp on patient safety. *American Nurse Today, 10*(1), 49–50.

Aim

The aim of this quality improvement project was to remove barriers to gait belt use by providing a visual cue to remind staff to use a gait belt when ambulating patients.

Methods

The PDSA framework was used to determine whether hanging gait belts on hooks in patients' rooms would increase their use:

1. Plan
   - A target unit was selected to implement the "test of change."
   - Staff was educated about the upcoming change.
   - Project goals were established.
   - Hooks were installed in patients' rooms.
2. Do
   - Audit tools were developed, and preaudit data were collected for 2 weeks to provide a baseline.
   - Six audits were completed over a 4-month period.
3. Study
   - The QI team used a risk-for-injury screening tool and reviewed patient fall risk scores, risk for injury scores, mental health status, mobility status, and use of assistive devices
   - The team also looked at missed opportunities where patients could have benefited from a gait belt but one was not used.
4. Act
   - The QI team reported ongoing results and collaborated with staff to foster engagement.
   - Data analysis showed that nurses were identifying patients at risk for falls accurately, and there was an overall increase of 38% in placing gait belts in patients' rooms.

Implications for Nurse Leaders and Managers

This QI project offers an example of a nurse-driven quality improvement activity that encouraged patient ambulation and promoted patient safety. Nurse leaders and managers can involve staff in QI initiatives to assist them in identifying areas for improvement, foster engagement and accountability, and provide consistent support for staff during the process.

---

analyze and display data is based on the goal of the QI project. When determining how to display data, it is important to consider the type of data and the time period during which the data is collected. For example, monthly data are best collected over a 13-month period. This provides trends over an entire year and compares the current month with the same month the previous year (Boxer & Goldfarb, 2011).

Run Chart

A **run chart** communicates data, shows trends over time, and reflects how a process is operating (Boxer & Goldfarb, 2011). In a run chart, the vertical axis (y) represents the process variable and the horizontal axis (x) represents time. The mean or median of data is displayed as a horizontal line and allows nurses and the QI team to see changes in measurements without having to compute statistics. Data points above the median indicate an improvement in a process, whereas data points below the median reflect a deterioration in the process. Run charts are among the most important tools for determining whether a change was effective (IHI, 2020e). QI teams would use run charts to display trends over time and changes in quality over time. For example, nurse leaders and managers would use a run chart to determine whether there was a change in the number of central line infections after a new dressing change protocol was implemented. Figure 9-4 displays an example of a run chart for the number of falls on a unit over a 5-month period. Looking at the chart, falls on the unit were above the median line in February and April, thus indicating a problem with the fall precaution protocols during that time. Nurse leaders and managers would use this data to investigate possible causes for the increase in falls during those months.

Bar Chart

A **bar chart** is the most common method used to display categorical data, and the scale must start at zero. When using a bar chart, categories are listed along the horizontal axis, and frequencies or percentages are listed on the vertical axis (Tague, 2005). Nurse leaders and managers would use a bar chart to illustrate categorical data. For example, in looking at the increase in the number of falls on the unit, the nurse leader and manager may investigate the staff mix (i.e., number of registered nurses, licensed practical nurses, technicians) on the unit during those time periods. Figure 9-5 displays an example of a bar chart for the educational level and gender of registered nurses employed in a hospital.

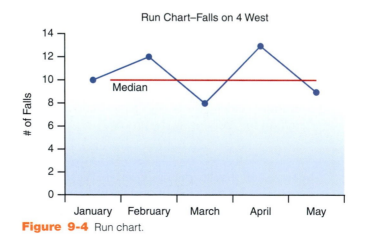

Figure 9-4 Run chart.

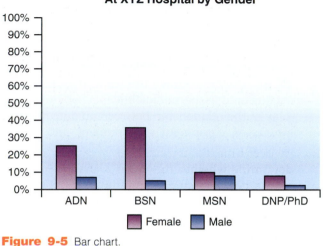

Figure 9-5 Bar chart.

Histogram

A **histogram** is a type of bar chart used to display frequency distributions and is useful when the time sequence of events is not available. For QI, histograms assist the team in recognizing and analyzing patterns in numerical data that may not be apparent by looking at data in a table or finding the mean or median of data (IHI, 2020f). Nurse leaders and managers could use a histogram to illustrate the average length of stay of surgical patients on the unit. Figure 9-6 displays an example of a histogram for student grades on a dosage calculation test.

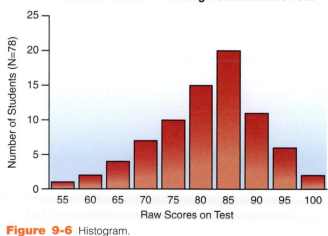

Figure 9-6 Histogram.

Fishbone Diagram

The **fishbone diagram**, also known as an Ishikawa diagram or a cause-and-effect diagram, is used to identify the many possible causes of a problem and any relationships among the causes (Phillips & Simmonds, 2013). It provides a retrospective review of events and can help nurse leaders and managers determine the root causes of a problem. Fishbone diagrams are key tools used to conduct RCAs. They encourage the team to look at all possible causes and contributing factors of an issue, not just the most obvious. The fishbone provides a graphic display of the relationship between an outcome and possible factors, such as people, processes, equipment, environment, and management. For example, a fishbone diagram would be used by nurse leaders and managers if they wanted to investigate a medication error or a sentinel event such as a patient's suicide. The fishbone allows the QI team to consider all possible causes of the event. Categories of factors that could cause a problem vary depending on the incident. The components of a fishbone diagram typically include people, processes, equipment, environment, management, and materials, but these components are not set in stone. Figure 9-7 illustrates a fishbone diagram for a medication error. In this example, the medication error is the head of the fish, the large bones represent the categories of possible causes of the medication error, and the small bones represent possible contributing factors to the causes.

LEARNING ACTIVITY 9-2

Using a Fishbone Diagram for Central Line Infections

Over the past 6 months, patients in the intensive care unit have experienced an increase in central line infections. The nurse leader and manager suspects that the increase is related to more central lines being inserted in the emergency department. A QI team is being formed to identify the root causes of central line infections. Discuss the following with classmates:

- Who should be on the QI team?
- Outline the steps in the QI process to use in this situation.
- What type of QI tools would be used to:
  - Track central line infections
  - Investigate possible causes of infections
  - Identify areas for improvement
- How would the QI team implement an activity to improve the infection rate, and how will the team know the activity worked?

Flow Chart

A **flow chart** helps clarify complex processes, shows blocks in activity in the process, and serves as a basis for designing new processes (IHI, 2020g). Flow charts provide a picture of the various steps in a sequential process and allow QI teams to understand an existing process, identify complexity in a process, identify

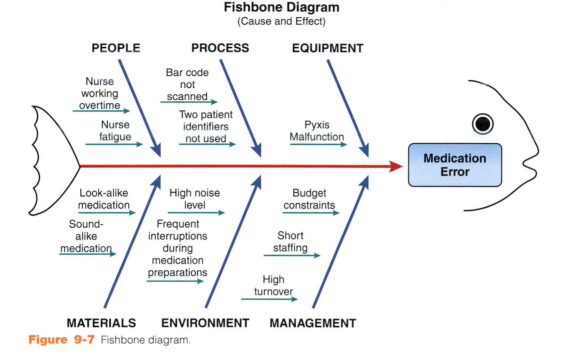

Figure 9-7 Fishbone diagram.

non–value-added steps in a process, and develop ideas about how to improve a process. Nurse leaders and managers would use a flow chart to identify problematic areas in the process of admitting a patient. Figure 9-8 displays a flow chart related to the patient admission process.

Pareto Chart

The **Pareto chart** resembles a bar chart in which the height of the bars represents frequency, and the bars are arranged on the horizontal axis in order from highest to lowest. The Pareto chart is designed to look at various causes of a specific problem. Based on the 80/20 principle, the Pareto chart is a tool to help determine the "small portion of causes that account for a large amount of the variance" in a process (Boxer & Goldfarb, 2011, p. 151). Joseph Juran developed the Pareto chart to help managers determine where to focus improvement activities because it separates the "vital few" from the "useful many." The Pareto chart visually shows areas that are most significant and provides information to help identify where to focus improvement for the greatest impact. Nurse leaders and managers would use a Pareto chart when there are many causes of an issue, such as breaks in isolation procedures, but the QI team wants to focus on the most significant cause. Figure 9-9 illustrates a Pareto chart for identifying possible causes of medication errors on a unit during a specific period of time. Based on this chart, the "vital few" categories are being short staffed, high number

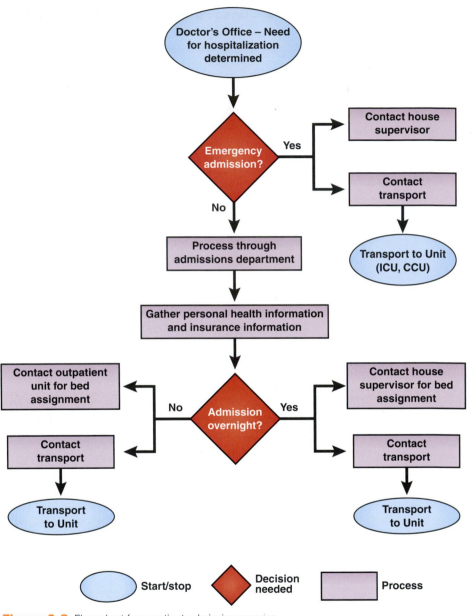

Figure 9-8 Flow chart for a patient admission process.

of admissions, high number of float nurses, and staff mix. These are the areas where QI should be focused.

The QI tools presented can assist nurses at all levels with measuring processes and outcomes of care. Additional information about QI tools can be found on the ASQ Web site (www.asq.org/learn-about-quality/quality-tools.html) and the IHI Web site (http://www.ihi.org/resources/Pages/Tools/default.aspx).

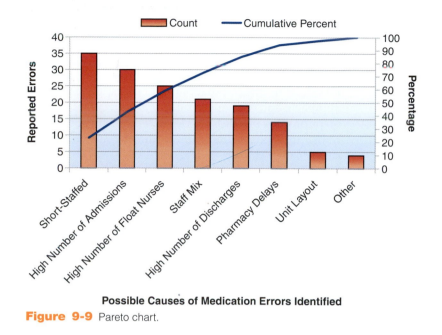

Possible Causes of Medication Errors January–October 20XX

Possible Causes of Medication Errors Identified

Figure 9-9 Pareto chart.

EXPLORING THE EVIDENCE 9-2

McFadden, K. L., Stock, G. N., & Gowen, C. R. (2014). Leadership, safety climate, and continuous quality improvement: Impact on process quality and patient safety. *Journal of Nursing Administration, 44*(10), S27–S37.

Aim

The aim of this study was to investigate how transformational leadership, safety culture, and continuous QI initiatives are related to objective quality and patient safety outcome measures.

Methods

Using a survey methodology, the investigators collected and compared data from 204 hospitals in 48 states. They used a questionnaire that measured transformational leadership, safety climate, and continuous QI and compared findings with hospital-acquired infections and process quality scores from the Hospital Compare Web site. To test four hypotheses, they used Structural Equation Modeling.

Key Findings

Research findings supported three of the four hypotheses. Transformational leadership was positively associated with patient safety climate, process quality scores were positively associated with continuous quality improvement initiatives,

Continued

and continuous quality initiatives were positively associated with process quality scores. However, continuous quality improvement was associated with an increase in hospital-acquired infections, rather than the lower rates hypothesized. The investigators suggest that preventing hospital-acquired infections requires a broad approach, and continuous quality improvement in many hospitals may be focused on improving business processes rather than patient safety. They also found that transformational leadership was directly related to employees' perceptions of a strong safety climate.

Implications for Nurse Leaders and Managers

Transformational leadership is important to creating and sustaining a positive patient safety climate. Nurse leaders and managers can use the findings of this study to promote broad continuous quality initiatives and to foster a positive patient safety climate on their units and throughout the health-care organization. Nurse leaders and managers at all levels of an organization must play an active role in creating a climate where staff members feel comfortable to voice safety concerns.

▶ SUMMARY

Safety is a basic component of health-care quality. Quality and safety are considered core values for nursing practice (AACN, 2021). Because nurses are at the frontline of care, have the most contact with patients, and are the last line of defense against medical errors, they have an integral role in discovering and correcting processes that can result in an adverse event. In addition, nurses can significantly influence the quality of care provided and are essential members of the QI team. Nurse leaders and managers must promote a culture that focuses on patient and staff safety by encouraging error reporting, error reduction, and patient safety (ANA, 2016). Nurse leaders and managers are responsible for evaluating the quality and appropriateness of nursing care (ANA, 2016), and to do so, they must engage nurses in the QI process.

NCLEX®-STYLE REVIEW QUESTIONS

Multiple Choice

1. The director of nursing is implementing a quality improvement project for the emergency department and knows that what is the first step in this process?
   1. Construction of a monitoring system
   2. Formulation of criteria and standards
   3. Determination of what activity to monitor
   4. Data collection

2. The nurse leader is beginning a quality improvement (QI) project on the nursing unit and is aware that what is most important to the ultimate success of the project?
   1. All members of the nursing unit are involved in the project.
   2. Registered nurses implement the project.
   3. Nursing assistants are used to collect data.
   4. The nurse leader is ultimately responsible for the success of the project.
3. The nurse leader is using the plan-do-study-act (PDSA) cycle for the unit's quality improvement project and knows that this comes from what quality improvement model?
   1. Six Sigma Model
   2. Lean Model
   3. Institute for Healthcare Improvement (IHI) Model
   4. Donabedian Model
4. The director of nursing at an acute care facility is aware that safety issues must be continually addressed because what percentage of patients globally experience a preventable adverse event?
   1. 5%
   2. 10%
   3. 15%
   4. 20%
5. The nurse manager has just been informed that a patient received a medication intravenously that should have only been administered as an intramuscular injection. The patient suffered a respiratory arrest and is being transferred to the intensive care unit. The nurse manager is aware that this is known as what type of error?
   1. Near miss
   2. Error of omission
   3. Sentinel event
   4. Lapse
6. The nurse manager is working with a staff nurse who committed a medication error that led to the patient requiring surgery. The nurse manager expects this staff nurse to experience what type of reaction?
   1. Termination of employment
   2. No noticeable reaction
   3. Extreme joking
   4. Avoidance of other staff
7. The nurse manager is working to establish a culture of safety and has encouraged the staff to use the CUS communication system. Which statement by a staff nurse indicates the proper use of this system?
   1. "I know that this procedure has resulted in an error before but I believe that I can complete it without making any mistakes."
   2. "I don't feel comfortable beginning this procedure. An event occurred the last time it was completed."
   3. "I think this procedure should become the focus of a study, but I believe it can still be used while it is being reviewed."
   4. "All procedures are safe as long as the nurse performing the procedure knows exactly what to do."

8. The nurse manager is preparing to discuss safety improvement at a unit meeting and will stress that what is a key aspect to error prevention?
   1. Avoiding automatic actions
   2. Asking a nurse with many years of experience to complete the procedure
   3. Having the charge nurse confirm procedure policy before completing any procedure
   4. Making each staff member an expert in a different procedure

9. The nurse manager has implemented a series of changes in the nursing unit that are intended to improve safety and will use which tool to determine whether the change has been effective?
   1. Fishbone diagram
   2. Histogram
   3. Pareto chart
   4. Run chart

Multiple Response

10. The nurse leader has implemented a quality improvement (QI) project and realizes what elements are required for the project to be successful? *Select all that apply.*
    1. Reliable quality improvement tools
    2. Object of the project kept confidential
    3. Clarification of the scope of the problem
    4. Continuous evaluation of performance
    5. Nursing unit development of its own QI model

11. The nurse leader is developing a quality improvement (QI) project for the nursing unit and knows that what characteristics are necessary to determine the priority of the issue to be investigated? *Select all that apply.*
    1. Failure in performance is known to occur infrequently.
    2. The problem itself occurs frequently.
    3. The problem has at some time caused serious consequences to health.
    4. The problem has caused issues that are costly.
    5. The problem may be very difficult to fix.

REFERENCES

Acquaviva, K., Haskell, H., & Johnson, J. (2013). Human cognition and the dynamics of failure to rescue: The Lewis Blackman case. *Journal of Professional Nursing, 29*(2), 95–101.

Agency for Healthcare Research and Quality. (2018). *Agency for Healthcare Research and Quality: A profile.* www.ahrq.gov/cpi/about/profile/index.html

Agency for Healthcare Research and Quality. (n.d.). *AHRQ PSNet: About.* https://www.psnet.ahrq.gov/information

Altman, L. K. (1995). Big doses of chemotherapy drug killed patient, hurt 2d. *The New York Times,* March 24. www.nytimes.com/1995/03/24/us/big-doses-of-chemotherapy-drug-killed-patient-hurt-2d.html?src=pm&pagewanted=2&pagewanted=all&pagewanted=print

American Association of Colleges of Nursing (AACN). (2008). *The essentials of baccalaureate education for professional nursing practice.* Author.

American Association of Colleges of Nursing. (2021). *The essentials: Core competencies for professional nursing education.* Author. https://www.aacnnursing.org/Portals/42/AcademicNursing/pdf/Essentials-2021.pdf

American Nurses Association (ANA). (2015a). *Code of ethics for nurses with interpretive statements.* Author.

American Nurses Association (ANA). (2015b). *Nursing: Scope and standards of practice* (3rd ed.). Author.

American Nurses Association (ANA). (2016). *Nursing administration: Scope and standards of practice* (2nd ed.). Author.

American Organization for Nursing Leadership (AONL). (2015a). *AONL nurse manager competencies.* Author.

American Organization for Nursing Leadership (AONL). (2015b). *AONL nurse executive competencies.* Author.

American Society for Quality (ASQ). (2020). What is six sigma? https://asq.org/quality-resources/six-sigma

Aspden, P., Corrigan, J. M., Wolcott, J., & Erickson, S. M. (Eds.). (2004). *Patient safety: Achieving a new standard for care.* National Academies Press.

Barnsteiner, J. (2017). Safety. In G. Sherwood & J. Barnsteiner (Eds.), *Quality and safety in nursing: A competency approach to improving outcomes* (2nd ed., pp. 153–171). Wiley Blackwell.

Boxer, B. A., & Goldfarb, E. B. (2011). *Creative solutions to enhance nursing quality.* Jones & Bartlett Learning.

Bureau of Labor Statistics. (2020). *Occupational employment and wages news release.* www.bls.gov/news.release/ocwage.htm

Cronenwett, L., Sherwood, G., Barnsteiner, J., Disch, J., Johnson, J., Mitchell, P., Sullivan, D. T., & Warren, J. (2007). Quality and safety education for nurses. *Nursing Outlook, 55*(3), 122–131.

Denham, C. R. (2007). TRUST: The 5 rights of the second victim. *Journal of Patient Safety, 3*(2), 107–119.

Donabedian, A. (2003). *An introduction to quality assurance in health care.* Oxford University Press.

Galt, K. A., Fuji, K. T., Gleason, J. M., & McQuillan, R. J. (2011). Why things go wrong. In K. A. Galt & K. A. Paschal (Eds.), *Foundations in patient safety for health professionals.* Jones & Bartlett.

Galt, K. A., Paschal, K. A., & Gleason, J. M. (2011). Key concepts in patient safety. In K. A. Galt & K. A. Paschal (Eds.), *Foundations in patient safety for health professionals.* Jones & Bartlett.

Greiner, A. C., & Knebel, E. (Ed.) (2003). *Health professions education: A bridge to quality.* National Academies Press.

Guido, G. W. (2014). *Legal and ethical issues in nursing* (6th ed.). Pearson.

Hughes, R. G. (Ed.). (2008). *Patient safety and quality: An evidence-based handbook for nurses.* AHRQ Publication No. 08-0043. Agency for Healthcare Research and Quality. http://archive.ahrq.gov/professionals/clinicians-providers/resources/nursing/resources/nurseshdbk/nurseshdbk.pdf

Institute for Healthcare Improvement (IHI). (2020a). *About us: History.* www.ihi.org/about/Pages/History.aspx

Institute for Healthcare Improvement (IHI). (2020b). *About us: Innovations.* www.ihi.org/about/Pages/InnovationsContributions.aspx

Institute for Healthcare Improvement (IHI). (2020c). *Overview of the 5 Million Lives Campaign.* www.ihi.org/engage/initiatives/completed/5MillionLivesCampaign/Pages/default.aspx

Institute for Healthcare Improvement (IHI). (2020d). *Science of improvement: How to improve.* www.ihi.org/resources/Pages/HowtoImprove/ScienceofImprovementHowtoImprove.aspx

Institute of Healthcare Improvement (IHI). (2020e). *Run chart tool.* www.ihi.org/resources/pages/tools/runchart.aspx

Institute of Healthcare Improvement (IHI). (2020f). *Histogram.* www.ihi.org/resources/Pages/Tools/Histogram.aspx

Institute of Healthcare Improvement (IHI). (2020g). *Flow chart.* www.ihi.org/resources/pages/tools/flowchart.aspx

International Council of Nurses (ICN). (2012). *Patient safety [position statement].* https://www.icn.ch/sites/default/files/inline-files/D05_Patient_Safety.pdf

International Council of Nurses (ICN). (2014). *Who we are.* https://www.icn.ch/who-we-are

James, J. T. (2013). A new, evidence-based estimate of patient harms associated with hospital care. *Journal of Patient Safety, 9*(3), 122–128.

Johnson, J. (2017). Quality improvement. In G. Sherwood & J. Barnsteiner (Eds.), *Quality and safety in nursing: A competency approach to improving outcomes* (2nd ed., pp. 109–130). Wiley Blackwell.

Juran Global. (2016). *Our legacy: Joseph Juran.* https://www.juran.com/about-us/dr-jurans-history/

Kohn, L. T., Corrigan, J. M., & Donaldson, M. S. (Eds.). (2000). *To err is human: Building a safer health system.* National Academies Press.

Leisner, P. (1995). Surgeon says it was too late to stop amputation on wrong leg. *Associated Press,* September 14. www.apnewsarchive.com/1995/Surgeon-Says-It-Was-Too-Late-to-Stop-Amputation-on-Wrong-Leg/id-a9b3238f7dbca20e0edf82bba7da0ab5

Leotsakos, A., Zheng, H., Croteau, R., Loeb, J. M., Sherman, H., Hoffman, C., Morganstein, L., O'Leary, D., Bruneau, C., Lee, P., Duguid, M., Thomeczek, C., van der Schrieck–De Loos, E., & Munier, B. (2014). Standardization in patient safety: The WHO High 5s Project. *International Journal for Quality in Health Care, 26*(2), 109–116.

Lerner, B. H. (2006). A case that shook medicine. *Washington Post,* November 28. www.washingtonpost.com/wp-dyn/content/article/2006/11/24/AR2006112400985.html

McFadden, K. L., Stock, G. N., & Gowen, C. R. (2014). Leadership, safety climate, and continuous quality improvement: Impact on process quality and patient safety. *Journal of Nursing Administration, 44*(10), S27–S37.

Meyer, B. C., & Bishop, D. S. (2007). Florence Nightingale: Nineteenth century apostle of quality. *Journal of Management History, 13*(3), 240–254.

Monk, J. (2002). How a hospital failed a boy who didn't have to die. *The State,* June 16, pp. A1, A8–A9. http://www.lewisblackman.net/

Montalvo, I. (2007). The National Database of Nursing Quality Indicators® (NDNQI®). *The Online Journal of Issues in Nursing, 12*(3), Manuscript 2.

Montalvo, I., & Dunton, N. (2007). *Transforming nursing data into quality care: Profiles of quality improvement in U.S. healthcare facilities.* American Nurses Association.

National Database of Nursing Quality Indicators. (2020). *NDNQI nursing-sensitive indicators.* https://nursingandndnqi.weebly.com/ndnqi-indicators.html

National Quality Forum (NQF). (2020a). *NQF's history.* www.qualityforum.org/about_nqf/history/

National Quality Forum (NQF). (2020b). *What we do.* www.qualityforum.org/what_we_do.aspx

National Quality Forum (NQF). (2020c). *Patient safety.* www.qualityforum.org/Topics/Patient_Safety.aspx

Newhouse, R., & Poe, S. (Eds.). (2005). *Measuring patient safety.* Jones & Bartlett.

Niedowski, E. (2003). How medical errors took a little girl's life. *Baltimore Sun,* December 14. www.baltimoresun.com/bal-te.sorrel14dec14-story.html#page=2

Nightingale, F. (1859). *Notes on hospitals.* Parker and Son.

Nolan, T., Resar, R., Haraden, C., & Griffin, F. A. (2004). *Improving the reliability of health care* [Innovation Series white paper]. www.ihi.org/resources/pages/ihiwhitepapers/improvingthereliabilityofhealthcare.aspx

Nurse charged with felony in fatal medical error. (2007). *Medical Ethics Advisor,* February 2. https://www.reliasmedia.com/articles/101137-nurse-charged-with-felony-in-fatal-medical-error

Ornstein, C. (2008). Quaids recall twins' drug overdose. *Los Angeles Times,* January 15. www.latimes.com/local/la-me-quaid15jan15-story.html#page=1

Page, A. (Ed.). (2004). *Keeping patients safe: Transforming the work environment of nurses.* Washington, DC: National Academies Press.

Phillips, J., & Simmonds, L. (2013). Using fishbone analysis to investigate problems. *Nursing Times, 109*(15), 18–20.

Press Ganey. (2014). *Press Ganey acquires National Database of Nursing Quality Indicators (NDNQI).* https://www.pressganey.com/resources/reports/press-ganey-acquires-national-database-of-nursing-quality-indicators-(ndnqi-)

Press Ganey. (2019). *Turn nursing quality insights into improved patient experiences.* https://www.pressganey.com/docs/default-source/default-document-library/clinicalexcellence_ndnqi_solution-summary.pdf?sfvrsn=0

Quaid, D., Thao, J., & Denham, C. R. (2010). Story power: The secret weapon. *Journal of Patient Safety, 6*(1), 5–14.

Reason, J. T. (1990). *Human error.* Cambridge University Press.

Reason, J. T. (2000). Human error: Models and management. *BMJ, 321,* 768–770.

Robert Wood Johnson Foundation. (2014, March). Ten years after keeping patients safe: Have nurses' work environments been transformed? *Charting Nursing's Future, 1.* https://www.rwjf.org/en/library/research/2014/03/cnf-ten-years-after-keeping-patients-safe.html

Saver, A. (2006). Beyond expectations: Part 1. *Nursing Management, 37*(10), 36–42.

Shepard, L. H. (2011). Creating a foundation for a just culture workplace. *Nursing, 41*(8), 46–48.

Smetzer, J. (2012). Don't abandon the "second victims" of medical errors. *Nursing, 42*(2), 54–58.

Smith, J. L. (2009). Remembering Walter A. Shewhart's contribution to the quality world. *Quality Magazine,* March 2. www.qualitymag.com/articles/85973-remembering-walter-a-shewhart-s-contribution-to-the-quality-world

Spear, S., & Bowen, H. K. (1999). Decoding the DNA of the Toyota Production System. *Harvard Business Review, 77*(5), 96–106.

Tague, N. R. (2005). *The quality toolbox* (2nd ed.). American Society for Quality.

The Joint Commission (TJC). (2012). *Improving patient and worker safety: Opportunities for synergy, collaboration, and innovation.* The Joint Commission. www.jointcommission.org/assets/1/18/tjc-improving patientandworkersafety-monograph.pdf

The Joint Commission (TJC). (2020a). *Sentinel event policy and procedures.* www.jointcommission.org/sentinel_event_policy_and_procedures

The Joint Commission (TJC). (2020b). *Facts about The Joint Commission.* www.jointcommission.org/facts_about_the_joint_commission

The Joint Commission (TJC). (2020c). *The Joint Commission: About us.* https://www.jointcommission.org/about-us/

The Joint Commission (TJC). (2020d). *Facts about Speak Up.* www.jointcommission.org/facts_about_speak_up

The Joint Commission (TJC). (2020e). *The National Patient Safety Goals.* https://www.jointcommission.org/standards/national-patient-safety-goals/

The Joint Commission (TJC). (n.d.). *The universal protocol for preventing wrong site, wrong procedure, and wrong person surgery.* www.jointcommission.org/assets/1/18/UP_Poster1.PDF

U.S. Department of Health and Human Services Health Resources and Services Administration. (2011). *Quality improvement.* www.hrsa.gov/quality/toolbox/508pdfs/qualityimprovement.pdf

U.S. Department of Health and Human Services Office of Inspector General (HHS HRSA). (2010). *Adverse events in hospitals: National incidence among Medicare beneficiaries* (OEI-06-09-00090). Government Printing Office.

W. Edwards Deming Institute. (2016). *W. Edwards Deming was truly a remarkable man.* https://deming.org/theman/overview

Wachter, R. M., & Gupta, K. (2018). *Understanding patient safety* (3rd ed.). McGraw-Hill Medical.

World Health Organization (WHO). (2014). *The high 5s project interim report.* Author. www.who.int/patientsafety/implementation/solutions/high5s/High5_InterimReport.pdf?ua=1

World Health Organization (WHO). (2019). *10 facts on patient safety.* https://www.who.int/news-room/photo-story/photo-story-detail/10-facts-on-patient-safety

World Health Organization (WHO). (2020). *Patient safety: About us.* www.who.int/patientsafety/about/en

To explore learning resources for this chapter, go to FADavis.com

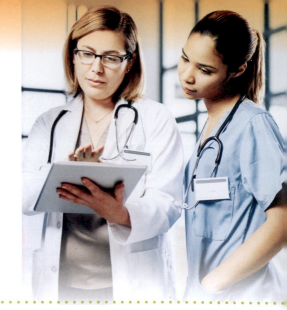

Chapter **10**

Information Technology for Safe and Quality Patient Care

Brett L. Andreasen, MS, RN-BC
Linda K. Hays-Gallego, MN, RN

KEY TERMS

Application
Artificial intelligence
Barcode medication
    administration
Coding
Computerized provider order entry
Data
Data mining
Data set
Database
Decision support systems
Electronic health record
Electronic medical record
Electronic medication
    administration record
Information systems
Information technology
Interfaces
Meaningful Use program
Network
Nursing informatics
Personal health record
Robotics
Standardized languages
Superusers
Telehealth

LEARNING OUTCOMES

- Define nursing informatics.
- Identify legislation and regulations that have advanced information technology and informatics.
- Explain the roles of information technology and informatics in ensuring safe and quality patient care.
- Describe several common information systems used in health care.
- Describe the nurse leaders and managers' role in using information technology and informatics.

The Knowledge, Skills, and Attitudes Related to the Following Are Addressed in This Chapter:

Core Competencies	• Teamwork and Collaboration • Informatics • Safety
The Essentials: Core Competencies for Professional Nursing Education (AACN, 2021)	**Domain 8: Information and Healthcare Technologies** 8.1 Describe the various information and communication technology tools used in the care of patients, communities, and populations (pp. 48–49). 8.2 Use information and communication technology to gather data, create information, and generate knowledge (p. 48). 8.3 Use information and communication technologies and informatics processes to deliver safe nursing care to diverse populations in a variety of settings (pp. 49–50). 8.4 Use information and communication technology to support documentation of care and communication among providers, patients, and all system levels (pp. 50–51).
Code of Ethics with Interpretive Statements (ANA, 2015)	**Provision 3.1:** Protection of the rights of privacy and confidentiality (pp. 9–10) **Provision 3.4:** Professional responsibility in promoting the culture of safety (pp. 11–12) **Provision 4.2:** Accountability for nursing judgments, decisions, and action (pp. 15–16)

Nurse Manager (NMC) Competencies (AONL, 2015a) and Nurse Executive (NEC) Competencies (AONL, 2015b)	**NMC: Information Technology (p. 5)**
	• Understand the effect of IT on patient care and delivery systems to reduce workload
	• Ability to integrate technology into patient care processes
	• Use information systems to support business decisions
	NEC: Business Skills (p. 11)
	• Information management and technology
	  • Use technology to support improvement of clinical and financial performance
	  • Collaborate to prioritize for the establishment of information technology resources
	  • Participate in evaluation of enabling technology in practice settings
	  • Use data management systems for decision making
	  • Identify technological trends, issues, and new developments as they apply to patient care
	  • Demonstrate skills in assessing data integrity and quality
	  • Provide leadership for the adoption and implementation of information systems

Nursing Administration Scope and Standards of Practice (ANA, 2016)	**Standard 1: Assessment** The nurse administrator collects pertinent data and information relative to the situation, issue, problem, or trend (pp. 35–36). **Standard 2: Identification of Problems, Issues, and Trends** The nurse administrator analyses the assessment data to identify problems, issues, and trends (p. 37). **Standard 4: Planning** The nurse administrator develops a plan that defines, articulates, and establishes strategies and alternatives to attain expected, measurable outcomes (p. 39).

Continued

The Knowledge, Skills, and Attitudes Related to the Following Are Addressed in This Chapter:—cont'd

Standard 5A: Coordination The nurse administrator coordinates implementation of the plan and associated processes (p. 41).

Standard 6: Evaluation The nurse administrator evaluates progress toward the attainment of goals and outcomes (p. 43).

Standard 14: Quality of Practice The nurse administrator contributes to quality nursing practice (p. 55).

Source: American Association of Colleges of Nursing. (2021). *The essentials: Core competencies for professional nursing education.* Author; American Nurses Association (ANA). (2015). *Code of ethics for nurses with interpretive statements.* Author; American Nurses Association (ANA). (2016). *Nursing administration: Scope and standards of practice* (2nd ed.). Author; American Organization for Nursing Leadership (AONL). (2015a). *AONL nurse manager competencies.* Author; American Organization for Nursing Leadership (AONL). (2015b). *AONL nurse executive competencies.* Author; Cronenwett, L., Sherwood, G., Barnsteiner, J., Disch, J., Johnson, J., Mitchell, P., Sullivan, D. T., & Warren, J. (2007). Quality and safety education for nurses. *Nursing Outlook, 55*(3), 122–131; and Greiner, A. C., & Knebel, E. (Eds.) (2003). *Health professions education: A bridge to quality.* National Academies Press.

The Institute of Medicine has identified utilizing informatics as critical to ensure patient safety and quality care (Greiner & Knebel, 2003). Nurses deal with volumes of information daily. Safe and quality nursing care relies on a nurse's ability to obtain adequate and appropriate information for effective decision making. Part of this includes development of basic computer literacy and information management skills to support all aspects of nursing practice.

Nurse leaders and managers must understand how to integrate nursing informatics and health information technology (IT) to ensure the delivery of safe and quality nursing care. They must recognize the importance of nursing data in improving practice, monitoring health-care and patient outcome trends, making judgments based on those trends, evaluating and revising patient care processes, and collaborating with others in the development, adoption, and implementation of information systems (American Nurses Association [ANA], 2015a; American Organization for Nursing Leadership [AONL], 2015b).

Nursing informatics (NI) integrates nursing science with various analytic and informational sciences—"to identify, define, manage, and communicate data, information, knowledge and wisdom in nursing practice" (ANA, 2015a, pp. 2–3). These analytical and informational sciences include computer science, information science, and many more (ANA, 2015a). With the ever-growing focus on information systems driving improvements in patient safety and operational efficiency, nursing informatics is essential to improving patient care and ensure success.

This chapter describes the basic elements of informatics and IT and provides a brief overview of some of the more technical aspects. Various legislative and regulatory requirements related to the advancement of informatics and the critical role informatics plays in the delivery of safe and quality patient care are discussed. Also presented are common information systems employed in health care and the secure use of electronic health records and information systems. How nurse leaders and managers facilitate the use of IT by staff to improve work efficiency, reduce costs, foster effective communication, and enhance the quality and safety of patient care are discussed.

► UNDERSTANDING NURSING INFORMATICS

To discuss nursing informatics, an understanding of common elements in the specialty is important, as is an at least cursory understanding of the more technical aspects.

Basic Elements of Informatics

Information systems are any systems, technology-based or otherwise, that store, process, and manage information at both the individual level and the organizational level. The two major types of information systems are administrative and clinical. Administrative systems encompass both administrative and financial systems. Vendors provide either a suite of applications within a single system to satisfy the organization's patient care needs or best-of-breed systems, which are designed for a specific specialty and do not tend to integrate well with other systems (Wager et al., 2017).

Although most information systems are purchased from a vendor, an information system may be a homegrown system as well. Most organizations use a vendor-developed system because of the time required to develop a homegrown system. Vendor systems do allow for varying degrees of customization.

System acquisition is the process of obtaining an information system. The document that initiates this process with the vendor is a request for information (RFI) form from the vendor or a request for proposal (RFP) form, depending on the organization. The vendor provides details about the information system in both these processes. The format varies. The selection process extends until the contract is signed for the purchase of the system. Activities that take place during this phase include establishing the steering committee, developing goals and objectives for the system, determining system requirements, evaluating vendor proposals, conducting a cost-benefit analysis, holding vendor demonstrations, and conducting contract negotiations (Wager et al., 2017).

An information system provides an infrastructure for the organization and requires resources for development, maintenance, and eventual retirement. The purchase of the information system should be well integrated into the strategic plan for the organization. Because it is such a large investment, the selection of the information system should be a thoughtful decision, and it is essential that the process includes input from the members of the organization, including nurses.

Once the system is delivered, the life of the system begins. The system development life cycle (SDLC) refers to the life of the system. The phases of the SDLC are planning and analysis, design, implementation, and support and evaluation (Wager et al., 2017), as described in Table 10-1. This cycle will repeat throughout the life of the system.

Nurse leaders and managers must be involved in all aspects of the process. They must be included from the beginning and have active roles in the acquisition of information systems, as well as all phases of the SDLC.

Table 10-1 Phases of the System Development Lifecycle	
Phase of the System Development Lifecycle	**Activities**
Planning and analysis	The planning phase focuses on the business need and issues. Technology will be analyzed to see how it can address the need/issues. This phase includes project planning and analysis of current state.
Design	Deciding what the system will look like (future state); requires user input, with many decisions required. This includes analysis of workflows and processes, configuration of the system, testing, and training.
Implementation	Deciding how the system will be implemented; requires use of superusers and support staff.
Support and evaluation	Maintenance and modification of the system after implementation; in all, 80% of budget resources are invested in this phase.

From Wager et al., 2017.

Information technology (IT) combines computer technology with data and telecommunications technologies to provide solutions to the health-care industry. Some examples of the way IT supports safe and quality patient care are through (1) providing cues in the tools that are used for documentation that align with nursing best practice; (2) providing data elements for data collection; and (3) real-time display of pertinent patient information.

Nursing informatics facilitates decision making in all nursing roles through the use of information systems and technology. An essential part of nursing informatics is the computerized patient record. Patient records are needed for communication, legal documentation, and billing and reimbursement (Wager et al., 2017). Electronic records improve research and quality management, metrics, data quality, and access to data that support population health. The three most common types of electronic records are the electronic medical record (EMR), the electronic health record (EHR), and the personal health record (PHR). All of these electronic records contain medical information and details about the care provided to the patient. Many people use the terms *electronic medical record* and *electronic health record* interchangeably; however, there is a difference between these technologies. The **electronic medical record** (EMR) is the electronic record of a patient that is used by a single organization. The **electronic health record** (EHR) is used by more than one organization, provides information throughout the continuum of care, and can be shared by other organizations. The EHR also provides interoperability among systems or locations (Sewell, 2016). This means that EHR information can be accessed from more than one location or organization. The **personal health record** (PHR) is an electronic form of a patient's medical record that the patient can take with them or send to a health-care provider (Hebda & Czar, 2009). The patient manages the PHR, including setting up, accessing, and updating the record (Wager et al., 2017). The content may be housed in a variety of different apps such as fitness apps.

The Institute of Medicine (IOM; 2003) describes eight core functions of an EHR: (1) health and information data, (2) result management, (3) order management, (4) decision support, (5) electronic communications and connectivity, (6) patient support, (7) administrative processes and reporting, and (8) reporting and population health. The strength of the data in an EHR can be augmented through the use of tools for financials and clinical decision support. These tools provide the ability to compare or combine data from clinical, financial, and administrative sources, thus supplying an added benefit to the organization. Depending on the health-care organization, the specialty systems with these tools may be bought from the same vendor or from multiple different vendors; this has a bearing on how difficult it will be to integrate patient information across systems or into one central data repository. Integration of clinical and financial information is becoming increasingly important in today's health-care environment because of regulatory quality and financial integration. Many EHR vendors are focusing on interoperability, which allows seamless patient care as the patient moves between medical systems.

Another benefit of electronic records is that multiple clinicians are able simultaneously to access the patient's electronic chart, and this eliminates the risk of loss that often results from tracking paper documentation.

EXPLORING THE EVIDENCE 10-1

Gold, R., Bunce, A., Cowburn, S., Dambrun, K., Dearing, M., Middendorf, M., Mossman, N., Hollombe, C., Mahr, P., Melgar, G., Davis, J., Gottlieb, L., & Cottrell, E. (2018). Adoption of social determinants of health EHR tools by community health centers. *Annals of Family Medicine, 16*(5), 399–407. doi:10.1370/afm.2275

Aim

To assess the feasibility of implementing EHR tools for addressing a patient's social determinants of health (SDH). Use of SDH in the EHR allows us to address the patient's social needs documentation and intervention, which shape the health of the patient. This study focused on SDH in community health centers (CHCs).

Methods

This was a pilot study to develop SDH tools for the EHR for both documentation and summarizing the SDH screening results. These tools were built on the Protocol for Responding to and Assessing Patient Assets, Risks, and Experiences (PRAPARE). Tools were developed in Epic (Epic Systems Corporation). This study tracks adoption of these tools at three different CHCs. Documentation tools were implemented at all OCHIN (Portland, Oregon) CHCs, but referral tools were only implemented in three CHCs that were part of the pilot.

The researchers conducted a concurrent mixed-methods analysis of the pilot clinic's adoption of the SDH data tools from June 2016 through 2017 (implementation and enhancement time period). Quantitative and qualitative data were collected.

Quantitative data included patient demographics and visit characteristics for patients older than 18 years of age, who had SDH documented in the EHR and who had more than one clinic visit during the study period. These data were used to provide prevalence of potential SDH and to quantify both related referrals and problem list diagnoses.

Continued

EXPLORING THE EVIDENCE 10 - 1—cont'd

Qualitative data included workflow observations for 6 days and interviews with team members involved in the pilot. According to the researchers, analysis utilized deductive and inductive coding. A priori codes (conceptual categories) were created for staff role, tool type, and workflow step.

Each clinic screened a limited population, then scaled up:

- Clinic A started with a few randomly chosen patients per day, then added new patients.
- Clinic B started with large management programs, then added new patients.
- Clinic C started with new patients seen by a single provider, addressed issues, and then added new patients.

Each clinic modified workflows, used a paper-based screening questionnaire requiring reentry of data into the EHR, and sought to minimize provider impact. Total patients in the study was 1,130, which was 4% to 18% of adult patients in the clinic.

Key Findings

Need to assess SDH tools for how they integrate into clinic workflow, ensure adequate training on the SDH tools for the EHR, and consider how the timing of data entry affects how and when SDH data can be used.

Facilitators of the process of documentation utilizing EHR tools to document SDH included a clinic champion who was EHR-savvy, could customize EHR views to support workflows, and was willing to use adoption data to support workflows. Sharing the collection of SDH data that could help to meet reporting requirements was helpful.

Barriers included the following: (1) tools caused a fragmented view of the patient with relevant data in multiple places and did not support the narrative of the clinic visit; (2) this style of documentation adds a layer of complexity to collecting and responding appropriately to SDH; and (3) the necessity of a data entry step if SDH was collected on a paper form. Referral processes were too time consuming.

Implications for Nurse Leaders and Managers

Even though many professional and financial organizations endorse use of SDH data due to the profound impact that SDH issues can have on a patient's health, substantial barriers to adoption exist. Because most patient data is in the EHR, it makes sense for the SDH data to be there as well.

Nurse leaders and managers may consider a staged rollout to lessen the implementation impact. It is important to ensure adequate training that includes workflow integration. It is also important to ensure that appropriate security is in place before implementation. Encourage data entry directly into the EHR rather than recording information on paper first. Investigate the potential of having the patient enter some of this information via a patient portal or a computer stationed physically in the clinic waiting room.

Technical Aspects of Informatics

As a nurse leader and manager or an informatics nurse, it is extremely beneficial to have some technical level of understanding of an information system. The IT personnel who maintain the system and the clinical specialists who actually use the systems may have entirely different educational backgrounds and may think and communicate differently. Understanding these differences will help to improve communication between these groups, and that, in turn, promotes safe and quality patient care.

Network

A **network** is the fundamental framework of an information system that allows electronic devices to transfer information to each other. The Internet is the most common example of a public network. Most health-care organizations have their own networks within the confines of their system, called intranets (Hebda & Czar, 2009). With the advancement of mobile computing in the health-care industry, most organizations also offer access to their network through wireless technology.

Data

Data comprise a collection of information, facts, or numbers. Nurses collect and manage data constantly when caring for patients. Nurse leaders and managers gather, manage, analyze, and interpret data to ensure effective operation of the unit as well as safe and effective delivery of nursing care.

Development of the concept of data along a continuum was created and enhanced by Blum et al., and Nelson and Joos (Ronquillo et al., 2016). These nursing informatics theorists describe the components of the Data, Information, Knowledge, Wisdom (DIKW) continuum as follows (Ronquillo et al., 2016):

- Data—discrete elements that lack interpretation
- Information—data that has been interpreted, organized, or structured
- Knowledge—information that has been synthesized so that interrelationships have been identified
- Wisdom—appropriate use of knowledge in managing or solving human problems

The DIKW framework is an important part of nursing informatics theory.

Database

The central place that stores data is referred to as a **database**. Databases provide a key location for data to be stored and retrieved for analysis when needed. This is where the importance of discrete data, discussed in more detail later in this chapter, comes into play because these data can be stored in the same place within the database and easily compared. (For example, when a nurse documents "yes" as a discrete response to the question "Does the patient have a history of falls in the last 6 months?" it is much easier to find and compare this value in the database.) A clinical data repository is a database in which data from all information systems within an organization are kept and controlled (Hebda & Czar, 2009). Organizations may extract information from the database and use it to create new knowledge, establish best practice, or predict outcomes; this extraction is a form of data mining, discussed next (Connolly & Begg, 2005; Sewell, 2016).

Data Mining

EHRs contain an enormous amount of data. To collect data from these records manually is an unrealistic undertaking. **Data mining** is the process of extracting specific data or knowledge that was previously unknown (Sewell, 2016). This process can be used to understand patients' symptoms, predict diseases, and identify possible interventions (Sewell, 2016). All nurses should have a basic understanding of data mining. Nurse leaders and managers use data mining to extract, predict, evaluate, and apply knowledge to develop best practices in patient care, delivery, staffing and scheduling, error reporting, incident reporting, budgeting, and forecasting and planning.

Interfaces

The health-care setting is brimming with technological devices that are capable of gathering and/or analyzing electronic data. Unfortunately, these devices are not all designed and built by the same manufacturer or with the same purpose in mind, so they often do not communicate with other devices or systems. **Interfaces** are used to match data points from one system to the other so that this information can be communicated among systems or sent to a main information system for collective use and analysis. These interfaces can send information as it is gathered (real-time processing) or can function with a delay (batch processing) to save system resources (Hebda & Czar, 2009). Interfaces can also allow devices to communicate directly with an information system, thereby reducing the time nurses spend manually entering the information, as well as eliminating data entry errors. For example, a health-care organization can use a device to gather vital sign data and transmit it through an interface into a patient's medical record.

Decision Support Systems

With the use of an information system, a health-care organization may choose to use tools called **decision support systems**, which provide warnings or other decision support methods to help health-care professionals become more aware of certain clinical information (i.e., infection precaution) or use evidence-based practices (Hebda & Czar, 2009).

Rules and Alerts

Health-care organizations may also use rules and alerts to provide decision support. Rules require an action within the system to trigger or "fire" them, such as

EXPLORING THE EVIDENCE 10-2

Luo, Y., Thompson, W. K., Herr, T. M., Zeng, Z., Berendsen, M. A., Jonnalagadda, S. R., Carson, M. B., & Starren, J. (2017). Natural language processing for EHR-based pharmacovigilance: A structured review. *Drug Safety, 40*(11), 1075–1089. doi:10.1007/s40264-017-0558-6

Aim

Utilizing the EHR to assist in the monitoring process of pharmacovigilance to proactively prevent adverse drug events (ADEs). Pharmacovigilance is accomplished by paying attention to cues in the EHR to identify ADEs. This can improve care for the individual patient and contribute to documentation of ADEs related to a drug.

Methods

A structural review to identify pharmacovigilance studies in the English language that have utilized natural language processing (NLP) for data mining of ADEs from EHR notes. Literature review was completed on available research since 2000.

A total of 1,442 records were identified. Duplicates were removed. Title and abstract review dropped the total even further. A total of 243 full-text articles were assessed to ensure they focused on NLP and pharmacovigilance. This further decreased the total number of articles to be included to 48. They used a keyword and trigger phrase–based process for general ADE detection to detection of ADEs associated with specific diseases and pharmaceutical targets.

Key Findings

- NLP is an effective method to detect ADEs in the EHR because many notes focus on the topics of ADEs and medication.
- Dramatic improvements have been made in the ability to use NLP to detect ADEs. This includes statistical analysis and machine-learning–based method development and data integration.
- Despite the advances that have been made with NLP, there are still challenges with NLP methodology development and application of ADE detection from EHRs. This is especially true for off-label drug use and polypharmacy.

Implications for Nurse Leaders and Managers

Although NLP is highly useful in the detection of ADEs, the notes from different disciplines are highly variable. The areas of remaining challenges in utilizing NLP for pharmacovigilance include both generic drugs and use of multiple drugs simultaneously. Both scenarios are common.

This information is important to nurse leaders for a couple of reasons. First, from a clinical perspective, being able to detect potential ADEs early can decrease patient impact and length of stay. In addition, education of staff in composing narrative notes in a more standard format could strengthen the ability to detect ADEs early and prevent significant patient events.

a patient being admitted with certain criteria, a laboratory result, or information documented by a health-care professional. For example, during influenza season an organization may have a rule that is triggered by all patients admitted with an inpatient status from October through April that reminds the health-care provider to perform influenza screening.

A more obtrusive decision support tool is an alert. An alert could be straightforward, such as a warning that a patient has tested positive for a resistant organism (e.g., methicillin-resistant *Staphylococcus aureus* [MRSA]) and to implement precautions per institutional policy. Alerts could also be used to require the nurse to acknowledge the warning or select a reason for override (if clinically appropriate). For example, health-care providers may receive an alert when ordering a medication that is contraindicated for the patient. They may acknowledge the warning and remove the order, or they may override it for a valid reason. The risk with alerting is that it can lead to "alert fatigue" among clinicians, in which they become used to the warnings and start to ignore them, often not realizing what the warnings said. Rules and alerts should be used on a limited basis and focus on the most crucial patient care issues.

Artificial Intelligence/Machine-Learning

With the widespread implementation and use of electronic data in health care, technologies are emerging that use this data to predict outcomes and improve patient care. This can be done through processes including, but not limited to, machine-learning and **artificial intelligence** (AI). Machine learning is "a computer science theory that often uses statistical techniques to give a computer, or artificial intelligence (AI), the ability to progressively improve performance on a given task based on the significant amount of data without any explicit program" (Lee et al., 2019, p. 220). This AI can be combined with decision support for practitioners and/or patients. As an example, AI was used to help researchers during the coronavirus (COVID-19) pandemic by assisting with finding relevant research articles and proposing factors for a potential vaccine (Etzioni & DeCario, 2020). Nurse leaders and managers can promote safe and effective use of AI by increasing awareness of the concept, reinforce involvement of nursing informatics, and advance informatics understanding among nurses and nursing students (Risling & Low, 2019).

Robotics

Robotics have been used in the health care setting for decades, from packing and handling inpatient medications to assistance with surgical operative procedures. With the advancements of machine-learning and AI, this may open more avenues for application of increasingly autonomous robotics. In fact, robotics could replace activities in health care such as "precision (e.g., surgical robots), logistic and mechanical tasks (e.g., service robots), and complex cognitive tasks (e.g., rehabilitation robots)" (Cresswell et al., 2018, p. 408).

Standardized Languages

Standardized languages are used in information systems to enable understanding among disciplines and across information systems. This common language allows for streamlined sharing of information because the same terms are used by everyone to describe the same condition. Standardized language is important for effective data mining and is required for nursing documentation in EHRs (ANA, 2015b). There are various terminologies in use at this time with none emerging as the gold standard. Using standardized language ensures that medical information as well as nursing actions and outcomes are included in EHRs and provides data that may need to be analyzed.

▶ HOW INFORMATICS CONTRIBUTES TO PATIENT SAFETY

Patient safety is a priority in health care and the most important directive for EHR design. The IOM published multiple reports on quality and patient safety that affect patients in this country, including the following: *To Err Is Human: Building a Safer Health System* (Kohn et al., 2000); *Crossing the Quality Chasm: A New Health System for the 21st Century* (IOM, 2001); *Health Professions Education: A Bridge to Quality* (Greiner & Knebel, 2003); *The Future of Nursing: Leading Change, Advancing Health* (IOM, 2011); and *Health IT and Patient Safety: Building Safer Systems for Better Care* (IOM, 2012).

These reports reflect the important safety and quality issues in our health-care system. The use of evidence-based practice cues within the information system, decision support (rules and alerts), and reminders or tasks that decrease memory-based care all contribute to improved patient outcomes. All nurses are called to assume more of a leadership role in the integration of informatics in health care (IOM, 2011, 2012). In 2010, the IOM completed a Future of Nursing Report. It advocated for the following:

- Improving access to care
- Fostering interprofessional collaboration
- Promoting nursing leadership
- Transforming nursing education
- Increasing diversity in nursing
- Collecting workforce data

This has been restudied multiple times since 2010. The IOM found that nursing has made improvement working toward these goals but has not achieved the Future of Nursing goals (IOM, 2019).

All nurses must be able to locate pertinent information and best practices to be able to provide safe and effective nursing care (Wahoush & Banfield, 2014). Further, nurses must have specific informatics competencies to be able to assist in designing user-friendly technologies that ensure patient safety and improve care delivery and patient outcomes (Sewell, 2016). Nurse leaders and managers must be active in the assimilation of information systems and evaluate and revise patient care processes and systems to facilitate safe and effective patient care (AONL, 2015b).

EXPLORING THE EVIDENCE 10-3

Wahoush, O., & Banfield, L. (2014). Information literacy during entry to practice: Information-seeking behaviors in student nurses and recent nurse graduates. *Nurse Education Today, 34*(2014), 208–213.

Aim

The aim of this study was to describe information-seeking behaviors of student nurses and registered nurses (RNs) within their clinical settings.

Methods

This pilot study used a two-phase descriptive cross-sectional design. Participants included senior nursing students, new graduate RNs, nurse leaders, and library staff. Senior nursing students and new graduate RNs were surveyed to identify the information sources and resources they used in clinical practice. Qualitative interviews were conducted with nurse leaders and library staff to understand the extent of resources available for nurses and how new RNs learned about available resources.

In phase I, 62 undergraduate senior nursing students completed the Nurses Informative Sources Survey. In phase II, 18 new graduate RNs completed the Nurses Informative Sources Survey, and six nurse leaders and library staff members were interviewed. Senior nursing students and new graduate RNs responses were grouped into three categories of information sources: electronic, print, and interpersonal.

Key Findings

Senior nursing students and new graduate RNs reported accessing at least one example from each category for information to inform their practice. Both groups reported that electronic sources of information were mostly used. Nursing students reported using print resources more than interpersonal resources, whereas new graduate RNs reported using interpersonal resources more than print resources. In all, 11% of new graduate RNs reported using personal handheld devices for clinical information, whereas no nursing students used such devices. Both groups indicated they had limited access to hospital library resources.

All nurse leaders and library staff indicated that their organization provided orientation and mentoring for new staff. Library staff reported that they welcome opportunities to assist new RN staff better access information. However, they also reported that when hospitals encountered financial challenges, services not directly linked to patient care may be reduced. In one example, the library was moved outside of the hospital, thus making it difficult for staff to use the resources.

Implications for Nurse Leaders and Managers

The findings of this pilot study support that senior nursing students and new graduate RNs use various information sources to inform their practice, including personal information devices. Nurse leaders and managers must be aware of current practices and consider needed policies and practice guidelines to ensure information security. In addition, nurse leaders and managers should be advocates for information access by nurses through new library services that provide on-demand information in the clinical setting.

▶ LEGISLATIVE AND REGULATORY EFFECTS ON INFORMATICS

Federal and state governments as well as independent institutions are establishing standards and accreditation guidelines to encourage further implementation of information systems within the health-care setting.

Health Insurance Portability and Accountability Act

The Health Insurance Portability and Accountability Act of 1996 (HIPAA), discussed in depth in Chapter 5, introduced three rules to protect health information: privacy, security, and breach notification. The HIPAA Privacy Rule was designed to safeguard an individual's health information. The HIPAA Security Rule established a set of national standards to protect electronic health information. Finally, the Breach Notification Rule requires all health-care organizations to report any data breaches (U.S. Department of Health and Human Services, n.d.). The electronic age introduced a means to minimize patient data loss, but it also introduced a platform for making patient information easier to copy and transfer. Health-care organizations must be vigilant with enforcing data protection policies and/or use software such as data encryption to minimize data breaches.

American Recovery and Reinvestment Act of 2009

The American Recovery and Reinvestment Act of 2009 (ARRA) helped to advance the field of informatics. The health-care component of this bill is known as the Health Information Technology for Economic and Clinical Health Act, or HITECH Act. The requirements include metrics to improve patient care, quality, and public health.

The ARRA initially provides incentives when metrics are met by both physician practices and hospitals to move toward electronic documentation and processes to improve patient care. In time, penalties will be assessed if these standards are not achieved. The standards for eligible hospitals and eligible providers are similar.

Regulatory Requirements

The Joint Commission, the Centers for Medicare and Medicaid Services (CMS), and the U.S. Department of Health and Human Services are all regulatory bodies that have standards that must be met. The EHR assists in meeting these requirements. Data are collected from the EHR to improve health-care and patient outcomes. The number and topics of required data vary from year to year as regulatory requirements are updated. There are many additional national quality organizations that provide recommendations for organizations, including Leap Frog, IOM, Agency for Healthcare Research and Quality, National Quality Forum, and Quality and Safety Education for Nurses (Newbold, 2013).

Many regulatory requirements also have financial implications. One of these is the **Meaningful Use program**, part of CMS Quality Incentive Programs. Meaningful Use is a CMS program that requires use of the electronic record to improve patient care. The purpose of this program was to move health care to electronic records and it ensures that certain required components will be available, thus providing meaningful use of the EHR. Meaningful Use consists of three stages (CMS, 2016):

Stage 1: Data capture and sharing
Stage 2: Advanced clinical processes
Stage 3: Improved outcomes

Reporting must be done directly from a certified EHR and must be from discrete data elements. Specific guidelines were established for both eligible professionals and eligible hospitals. Many of the criteria for these two groups aligned. Some of the components of these criteria were required; other components could be selected off the list.

In April 2018, CMS renamed the EHR Incentive Programs to Promoting Interoperability. The program has evolved over the years and is now focused on interoperability and improving patient access to health information (CMS, 2019). In 2019, the program switched to performance-based scoring with fewer required measures (CMS, 2019).

Interoperability requirements include (1) electronic prescribing with a focus on opioid treatment and monitoring, and (2) Health Information Exchange (HIE) to promote the sharing of health information. The patient access to health data is now called Provider to Patient Exchange. It focuses on providing patients electronic access to their health information (CMS, 2019). Public Health and Clinical Data Exchange remains a priority, as does the security risk analysis. The attestation reporting period continues to be a consecutive 90-day period.

▶ INFORMATICS DEPARTMENTS

Nurse leaders and managers will work with many types of IT professionals. Table 10-2 outlines some of the roles and responsibilities of this group.

Table 10-2 Roles and Responsibilities of Informatics Departments

Role	Responsibilities
Chief information officer	Strategically plans for technology and computer systems in an organization
Chief medical information officer	Physician who integrates the field of medicine and IT; participates in design and interfaces with providers
Chief nursing information officer	Integrates nursing and IT; is in charge of strategic planning for the information system
Project manager	Responsible for planning, monitoring, and execution of an informatics project; reports status to nursing leadership and other stakeholders
Network engineer	Technical expert who develops and maintains the computer network
Clinical analyst	Focuses on design, testing, and implementation of an information system; works with clinical experts from the organization
Clinical systems educator	Analyzes education needs of clinical staff members who will use the information system; develops educational materials, provides instruction, and supports users of the system

IT, Information technology.

▶ USE OF DATA IN INFORMATICS

Maintaining a high level of data quality is essential in informatics. Data quality must be reliable and effective. Standardizing data can help to provide a higher level of data quality. Data quality should be kept in mind during design of electronic records so that discrete data elements are available. Discrete data elements are much easier to pull from the system's data repository than are narrative entry (free text) data entry elements. These discrete data elements may be used for research or for meeting regulatory requirements.

Data Set

A **data set** is simply a standardized group of data. There are multiple types of data sets, which may be used for billing, research, or other data uses. Data sets are used to provide a standard set of data on a patient, as well as standard definitions of data elements. Examples of data sets include the UB-04, which is standard data set required for institutional billing by federal and state governments, and the CMS-1500, which is a similar data set required for noninstitutional health-care settings. The data from both of these data sets are used by the CMS for health-care reimbursement, clinical, and population trends (Wager et al., 2017). There are several other standard data set types for specific settings or data use.

Coding

Coding is the process of taking the data in a patient's file and applying an industry-standard medical code to the data. Two basic types of coding systems are used in health care: the International Classification of Diseases (ICD; 10th revision) and Current Procedural Terminology (CPT).

The ICD-10-Clinical Modification (CM) is the system currently used for coding diagnoses in the United States. CPT is the coding system for procedures. CPT coding manuals are published by the American Medical Association every year. They are used widely in both inpatient and outpatient settings.

Both of these coding systems are used to provide information for billing, research, and other data purposes.

Data Security

Data security is a critical aspect in a health-care environment. Patient data can be lost, changed, or held hostage by viruses or malware attacks. There are several tools and methods used by health-care organizations to maintain data security. The most basic level of security includes the use of unique usernames and passwords, biometric identification, and security token identification. Unique usernames and passwords allow the system to collect an audit trail of who has accessed the system, when they did, and often which areas of the information system they accessed. Some systems are also starting to use biometric identification, such as fingerprint or retina verification, or devices that provide a randomly generated code for signature (security token identification).

Data that are transmitted can be encrypted, and firewalls can be in place to prevent unauthorized access. Data encryption is a tool used to protect information that is transferred electronically (e.g., e-mail) or physically (e.g., laptop computer). This process transforms the data into an unreadable form by using mathematical formulas (Hebda & Czar, 2009). A firewall is a mix of hardware and software that aims to prevent unauthorized access to a health-care organization's system (Hebda & Czar, 2009). This added security can also create difficulties for internal systems. A firewall must be considered when setting up an interface connection.

Nurse leaders and managers are critical to maintaining successful data security. They must take an active role in protecting a health-care organization's information assets and patient information. Nurse leaders and managers must enforce a culture that promotes and respects patient information security. They should be involved in the development and enforcement of organizational security policies that reflect rules and regulations and are designed to reduce or alleviate security risks. In addition, nurse leaders must ensure ongoing education for all staff related to information security and HIPAA.

There are also many uses for social media in health care such as Facebook, Twitter, and YouTube. These formats provide an ability to communicate and educate many patients, potential patients, and family members. Most health-care organizations utilize some type of social media; however, there need to be policies that direct how social media can be used and ways that it cannot be used. It is essential that staff are not using social media in inappropriate ways and that patients' privacy and security are not threatened.

▶ INFORMATION SYSTEMS USED IN HEALTH CARE

All nurses must understand some basics of information systems. Information systems are usually composed of several different applications that work together to provide a comprehensive record. An **application** is a computer program that performs a certain function or activity. Switching between applications can be either seamless or very apparent (e.g., selecting another application may require another login or another window to open). The following subsections describe some of the main information systems and applications used in a health-care information system.

Electronic Medication Administration Record

A common mantra in nursing school is "if it was not documented, it was not done." Documentation is the record of all assessments, treatments, and evaluations. Applications supporting documentation need to be dependable and support the clinician's workflow. The application that supports documentation of medications is the **electronic medication administration record** (eMAR). The eMAR has multiple features that enhance patient care. It provides a list of medication orders and when they are due to be administered. Once the medication is administered, it also provides a place to document medication administration. After medication administration is documented, the eMAR also provides historical information regarding medications that have been administered.

Computerized Provider Order Entry

An important application within an electronic record is the **computerized provider order entry** (CPOE). This application allows providers within a health-care organization to enter orders directly into a patient's record, thus omitting any transcription errors. It also allows integration of decision support systems (e.g., allergy alerting) and helps standardize patient care by encouraging groups of evidence-based orders (order sets). CPOE also has the potential to improve workflow among ancillary services by allowing them to receive notice of an order (e.g., from radiology) immediately, rather than depending on someone to monitor paper orders and relay the order either by fax or pneumatic tube system.

Barcode Medication Administration

Barcode medication administration is the process in which clinicians use a barcode reader to verify a patient's identity and drug information immediately before giving medication to a patient. This system requires both the patient identifier (wrist band) and drug packaging to have a barcode. Barcode medication administration is one of the best patient safety tools at the point of care (patient bedside). Barcode technology is also being used for other point of care processes to positively identify patients such as for blood administration.

Patient Portals

Many vendors of EMR systems have developed Web-based platforms for patients to access their health information online called patient portals. These portals may function across the continuum of care (inpatient and outpatient). Patient portals may allow patients to e-mail their providers, request refills, and view information such as immunizations, medications, and laboratory results (HealthIT.gov, 2015). The inpatient component of the portal provides discharge instructions, results of laboratory tests, medications, and clinician notes.

Telehealth

Telehealth and telemedicine are two related health-care technologies. It is important to differentiate these two technologies. According to HealthIT.gov (2020a), telemedicine refers specifically to remote clinical services, whereas telehealth may also include provider training, administrative meetings, and continuing medical education in addition to clinical services. **Telehealth** is the use of digital technologies to deliver medical care, health education, and public health services by connecting multiple users in separate locations. Telehealth utilizes computers and mobile devices to access health care. The person accessing the health care expertise may be another health-care provider or a patient. Health-care providers may use telehealth for specialty care or due to being in a remote location. Many patients prefer to access care in this manner (HealthIT.gov, 2020a).

The Health Resources and Services Administration (HRSA) of the U.S. Department of Health and Human Services defines *telehealth* as "the use of electronic information and telecommunications technologies to support and promote long-distance clinical health care, patient and professional health related education, public health and health administration technologies" (HealthIT.gov, 2020b). HealthIT.gov (2020a) describes the types of telehealth, including the following:

- Live video conferencing
- Store and forward (asynchronous)—transmission of a recorded health history to a health practitioner
- Remote patient monitoring—use of connected electronic tools to record personal health data in one location for review by provider in a different location, usually at a different time
- Mobile Health (mHealth)—health care as public information through mobile devices such as smartphone apps, activity trackers, automated reminders, and blood glucose monitors

Online Health Information

The number of consumers accessing health information online is growing. It is not unusual for patients to arrive for an appointment with their health-care provider equipped with information and questions based on suspect online information. This creates a need to ensure that health-care websites provide credible information. The ability to publish anything on the Internet results in information that may or may not be reliable and credible. Nurses are in the ideal position to assist patients and families in evaluating health information available online and guiding them to trusted websites (Sewell, 2016).

LEARNING ACTIVITY 10-1

Evaluating an Online Web Site

Use an online evaluation checklist and evaluate two health Web sites:

1. Score both Web sites and discuss how they compare.
2. Describe the strengths and weaknesses of each Web site.

Helpful online evaluation tools are available at https://nnlm.gov/initiatives/topics/health-websites.

▶ IMPLEMENTATION OF AN INFORMATICS PROJECT

Identifying potential issues in advance of implementation of the project is important. Superusers can help in this process. **Superusers** are generally representatives from the local nursing locations who receive enhanced training to help with implementation success and stability over the life of the system. They understand the new application and can help the staff members in the area integrate the new system or application into the future state workflow.

Once implementation begins, it is important to remember the following:

- Productivity will decrease initially while staff members are learning and becoming comfortable with the change.
- People learn at different rates and in different ways.
- Motivation to change comes from a positive assessment of the upcoming change.
- Communication is the key to successful change management.
- The environment should be one that does not expect perfection. This approach allows staff to learn and become used to the new system.

Addressing change management is essential for any informatics projects, such as the successful transition to a new EHR. Change management includes analysis of how workflow will change. A good understanding of current state and future state is important. Flow diagrams are created to illustrate the current workflow and the future workflow states (Figs. 10-1 and 10-2). Once these diagrams are created, a gap analysis is completed. Figure 10-3 illustrates a Gap Analysis Template. Finally, a Start/Stop/Continue document is created as a reference to use for staff training and implementation (Fig. 10-4). Part of this change management process is evaluation and planning for changes that will occur with the implementation.

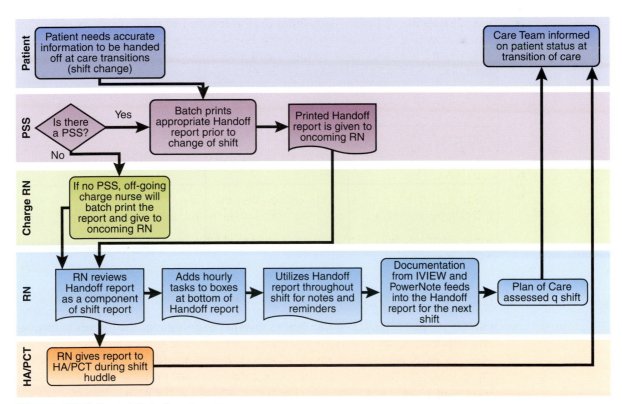

Figure 10-1 Current State flow diagram.

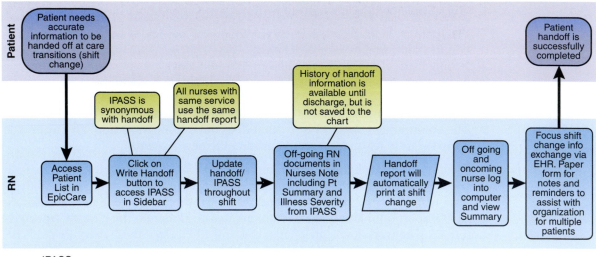

IPASS =
I – Illness Severity
P – Patient Summary
A – Action List
S – Situation Awareness & Contingency Planning
S – Synthesis by Receiver

Figure 10-2 Future State flow diagram.

Gaps	Risks	Benefits/Opportunities

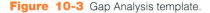

Figure 10-3 Gap Analysis template.

Nurse leaders and managers will have input into some of these documents along with the project team. It is important to review the following documents to ensure a smooth transition:

- Current State
- Future State
- Gap Analysis
- Start/Stop/Continue Documentation

Key Process	Stop	Start	Continue
Nurse			

Figure 10-4 Start/Stop/Continue template.

LEARNING ACTIVITY 10-2 | Completing a Gap Analysis and Start/Stop Continue Document

Addressing change management is essential for informatics projects, such as successful transition to a new EHR. Part of this change management process is evaluation and planning for changes that will occur with the implementation. Nursing hand-off is an important workflow from a patient safety standpoint. Evaluate Figures 10-1 and 10-2 and create a Gap Analysis using Figure 10-3. Once you have completed the Gap Analysis showing the difference between the two, create a Start/Stop/Continue document that demonstrates how handoff will be different once the new EHR is implemented using Figure 10-4.

Conversion Strategy and Conversion Planning

Conversion is that point in time when the organization switches from one system to another or turns on a new application. Conversion planning needs to take place to ensure a smooth transition. The following questions should be asked:

- Who is involved?
- Where will the system be implemented?
- When (time and date) will the conversion take place?
- Is it better to do the conversion at shift change or midshift?

- How will chart continuity be maintained?
- Will any information be backloaded into the new system?
- What activities need to be included, and who will do them?

All these items must be taken into account during the conversion. There should always be a contingency plan in case the change needs to be backed out (reversed).

Implementation Support Model

Implementation support for conversion to a new electronic system or application requires technical, vendor, education, and support resources. Most sites set up a command center that has these resources available onsite 24 hours day, 7 days a week for a designated period of time. In addition to the command center, support resources are available in the unit. Analysts and educators are placed in the units to assist with support as well as superusers. Organizations also often have vendor or consultant assistance with support, especially for "big bang" (simultaneous conversion from old to new system) implementations. This may include both "at-the-elbow" support and technical support.

Superusers play an essential role in implementation support. Different models are used at different organizations. One common model is to have three levels of superuser: expert, shift, and unit leader. The expert user is the representative who assisted with design. Shift experts on each shift help with the actual implementation. The shift expert has both clinical knowledge and supplemental computer training that is helpful as staff members transition to the new system. The role of the unit leader is to solve management issues that arise during the implementation. At the end of the implementation a plan will be put into place to convert to operational/ongoing support. Support resources will decrease at this point.

Maintenance

The system maintenance phase begins after the implementation and close of the project. Many of the project team members move on to other activities, but some team members continue to support the application and make enhancements to the system throughout the rest of the system life cycle. Each organization has a philosophy regarding the degree of software and coding enhancements that will be made during the maintenance phase. Some sites make changes only for additional regulatory requirements, whereas other sites may do a high level of customization during the maintenance phase.

Customization of the EHR may provide features that clinicians want to see; however, it may cause issues as well. Davis and Khansa (2015) suggest that personalization has allowed hospital personnel to focus on the information needed to fulfill their various roles as health-care professionals, but it has also created new barriers resulting from data inconsistency. Now that most EHR information that is used for regulatory requirements must come directly from the certified EHR, customization presents a problem. Vendors create designs that satisfy regulatory requirements, but if the EHR is customized, all the building blocks for the design may not be present.

All sites must perform upgrades to keep the code for the application up to date so that the vendor will continue to support the application. If the system is customized, configuration updates will need to be done with each upgrade to maintain customization.

System Downtime

Downtime procedures need to be developed and communicated before implementation. Staff members must know how they will obtain information when the system is down. There may be different levels of downtime that will determine what can be accessed in the system. There may be an entire network downtime, which may mean that no information is accessible. There may also be partial downtimes, which may affect certain parts of the system that will determine what information is accessible. Downtimes may also be planned or unplanned.

Planned downtimes occur when the system is taken down to make some specific changes such as an upgrade or other enhancement to the system. Planning and communication are done in advance to lessen the effects of the downtime. Backup systems are put into place to provide access to important patient data. The backup systems may be electronic or paper.

Unplanned downtimes present additional challenges. These situations do not allow the same preparation as planned downtimes. There needs to be a plan for these situations. Again, the backup plan may be another electronic system or paper. Another challenge during unplanned downtimes is communication to end users as the downtime is taking place. These communication avenues must be established before the downtime. The IT department has formal processes for determining when a downtime has occurred, when downtime processes should start, and what those processes are.

Downtime processes are becoming a focus of regulatory requirements because disruption in access to the EHR can create patient safety issues. Advanced planning by IT and operations can help to prevent these issues.

▶ SUMMARY

Nursing informatics is crucial to improving patient safety and patient outcomes. Its importance can be seen in administrative and clinical arenas. Information systems comprise a complex arrangement of hardware and software that, once successfully put in place, provide the foundation for an enhanced way of providing patient care. Electronic records provide data necessary to make clinical decisions, do research, and support regulatory requirements.

The field of informatics has expanded the potential roles for nurses. Roles for nurses in informatics span from an entry-level position (analyst or educator) to upper-level management. Nursing leaders and managers may be called on to work with a variety of these technical specialists. Nursing participation is required in all of the phases of an informatics project.

All nurses at all levels must have basic informatics skills to manage the large amount of data involved in safe and quality patient care. Nurses must be "computer fluent, information literate, and informatics knowledgeable" (Sewell, 2016,

p. 17). Nurse leaders and managers have a responsibility to ensure that adequate technological resources are available to staff to provide safe and quality nursing care.

NCLEX®-STYLE REVIEW QUESTIONS

Multiple Choice

1. How would one explain the underlying framework of nursing informatics?
    1. Nursing science and philosophical beliefs
    2. Informational technology assisting nurses to obtain information relative to patient care
    3. Combination of sciences from different disciplines such as nursing, computer, information, and information technology to provide information so as to support and effect change in nursing practice
    4. Utilization of electronic documentation in the clinical setting
    5. Helps to promote use of computer technology
2. A patient is going to a new health-care provider. Which documentation system would contain their medical record files and be brought by the patient to the scheduled office visit?
    1. Personal health record (PHR)
    2. Electronic medical record (EMR)
    3. Electronic health record (EHR)
    4. Patient does not have access to this type of information
3. Nurses on the unit are trying to find out if there is a correlation between hospital admissions for community-acquired pneumonia (CAP) and noncompliance with pneumonia vaccinations. Which action would lead to information that might help support the nurses' hypothesis?
    1. Data mining
    2. Database
    3. Data interface
    4. Demographic data related to gender
4. A nurse is admitting a patient to the hospital with congestive heart failure (CHF) using an electronic documentation system. While entering assessment data, pop-up windows are appearing asking for additional information. How would the nurse respond to this situation?
    1. Continue to chart information, then close the pop-up window and sign off note.
    2. Close the pop-up window and disable pop-up blockers from the system.
    3. Respond to the pop-up by providing the additional information that is required.
    4. Close out of the system and then sign back in to the patient's chart.

5. A nurse is taking care of a patient whose health information has been requested by a consulting physician during a phone conversation. In providing that health information to the consulting physician, which option would help prevent health information from being distributed to others in consideration of the Health Insurance Portability and Accountability Act (HIPAA)?
   1. Use encryption methods to send requested health information.
   2. Have health-care workers acknowledge a privacy disclosure statement each time they log into a medical record in the clinical setting.
   3. Send patient data via e-mail.
   4. Restrict chart access for patients on unit only to nursing staff.
6. There has been a violation of the Health Insurance Portability and Accountability Act (HIPAA) in the hospital setting. The nurse understands that violation of HIPAA would cause legal action at which level?
   1. State
   2. Federal
   3. Regional
   4. Hospital
7. With regard to the concept of meaningful use, which statement is accurate?
   1. Completion of eight core functions according to the Institute of Medicine guidelines
   2. Completion of three stages is regulated by Centers for Medicare and Medicaid Services (CMS)
   3. Certification by representatives of The Joint Commission that standards have been met
   4. Compliance with Institute of Medicine guidelines
8. Which is an example of discrete data that could be used by nurses in the research process?
   1. Narrative text describing patient's clinical response to pain medication
   2. Client's noted response as to why they were admitted to the hospital
   3. Documented patient weight
   4. Documented history and physical by health-care provider
9. A patient is reviewing an explanation of benefits (EOB) in relationship to insurance reimbursement for a medical evaluation in which he had an incision and drainage procedure performed for an infected abscess as a complication of diabetes. Which code would represent the incision and drainage procedure?
   1. Discrete data
   2. ICD (International Classification of Diseases)
   3. CPT (Current Procedural Terminology)
   4. Data sets

10. Which option would represent a method that can be used to maintain data security when using the electronic medical record system in the clinical setting by a staff nurse on a medical-surgical unit?
    1. Use a password that contains the nurse's last name.
    2. Use a random generator to come up with an access code.
    3. Use the same password while employed at the hospital.
    4. Keep logged in on the computer throughout the shift as long as a screen saver is in place.

11. Which option is *not* included in an electronic medication record (eMAR)?
    1. List of medications that the patient has been prescribed
    2. Times for medication administration
    3. Client history and physical
    4. Notation of clinical response to medication

12. A health-care provider uses the computerized provider order entry (CPOE) system to initiate a medication order for a patient. Which option is *not* included in the CPOE for the medication?
    1. Medication barcode
    2. Identification of allergies
    3. Notification of pharmacy department
    4. Transcription of name of medication

Multiple Response

13. A new nurse working on a medical-surgical unit needs some assistance with working within the electronic documentation system. Which individuals would the nurse contact to help with application of this system in the context of delivery of care? *Select all that apply.*
    1. Superuser: Expert
    2. Clinical analyst
    3. Network engineer
    4. Superuser: Shift
    5. Superuser: Unit

14. When using an electronic documentation system in the clinical environment, which situations should the nurse anticipate will occur? *Select all that apply.*
    1. Planned downtime
    2. Rolling power outages
    3. Unable to access information once a shift
    4. Periodic compromise of backup system
    5. System maintenance

15. Which criteria should a nurse use to evaluate Web sites for accuracy with regard to providing health information to the public? *Select all that apply.*
   1. Assess the sites for relative strengths and weaknesses.
   2. Make sure that there is a physician documented as providing the information.
   3. Evaluate Web sites for use of credible information supported by evidence-based practice.
   4. Web sites that require a paid subscription typically provide more accurate information.
   5. Web sites that are updated regularly provide more accurate information.

REFERENCES

American Association of Colleges of Nursing. (2021). *The essentials: Core competencies for professional nursing education.* Author. https://www.aacnnursing.org/Portals/42/AcademicNursing/pdf/Essentials-2021.pdf

American Nurses Association (ANA). (2015a). *Code of ethics for nurses with interpretive statements.* Author.

American Nurses Association (ANA). (2015b). *Nursing informatics: Scope and standards of practice* (2nd ed.). Author.

American Nurses Association (ANA). (2016). *Nursing administration: Scope and standards of practice* (2nd ed.). Author.

American Organization for Nursing Leadership. (2015a). *AONL nurse manager competencies.* Author.

American Organization for Nursing Leadership. (2015b). *AONL nurse executive competencies.* Author.

Centers for Medicare & Medicaid Services (CMS). (2016). *Eligible hospital information.* www.cms.gov/regulations-and-guidance/legislation/ehrincentiveprograms/eligible_hospital_information.html

Centers for Medicare and Medicaid Services (CMS). (2019). *Meaningful use.* https://www.cms.gov/Regulations-and-Guidance/Legislation/EHRIncentivesPrograms

Connolly, T. M., & Begg, C. E. (2005). *Database systems: A practical approach to design, implementation, and management* (4th ed.). Addison-Wesley.

Cresswell, K., Cunningham-Burley, S., & Sheikh, A. (2018). Health care robotics: Qualitative exploration of key challenges and future directions. *Journal of Medical Internet Research, 20*(7), 408.

Cronenwett, L., Sherwood, G., Barnsteiner, J., Disch, J., Johnson, J., Mitchell, P., Sullivan, D. T., & Warren, J. (2007). Quality and safety education for nurses. *Nursing Outlook, 55*(3), 122–131.

Davis, Z., & Khansa, L. (2015). Evaluating the epic electronic medical record system: A dichotomy in perspectives and solution recommendations. *Health Policy and Technology, 5,* 65–73. doi:10.1016/j.hlpt.2015.10.005

Etzioni, O., & DeCario, N. (2020, March 28). AI can help scientists find a Covid-19 vaccine. https://www.wired.com/story/opinion-ai-can-help-find-scientists-find-a-covid-19-vaccine/

Greiner, A. C., & Knebel, E. (Eds.) (2003). *Health professions education: A bridge to quality.* National Academies Press.

HealthIT.gov. (2015). *What is a patient portal?* www.healthit.gov/providers-professionals/faqs/what-patient-portal

HealthIT.gov (2020a). *Health IT playbook: Section 5 patient engagement.* https://www.healthit.gov/playbook/patient-engagement/#Telehealth

HealthIT.gov (2020b). *Telemedicine and telehealth.* https://www.healthit.gov/topic/health-it-health-care-settings/telemedicine-and-telehealth

Hebda, T., & Czar, P. (2009). *Handbook of informatics for nurses and health care professionals* (4th ed.). Pearson Prentice Hall.

Institute of Medicine (IOM). (2001). *Crossing the quality chasm: A new health system for the 21st Century.* National Academies Press.

Institute of Medicine (IOM). (2003). *Key capabilities of an electronic health record.* http://www.national academies.org/hmd/Reports/2003/Key-Capabilities-of-an-Electronic-Health-Record-System.aspx

Institute of Medicine (IOM). (2011). *The future of nursing: Leading change, advancing health.* National Academies Press.

Institute of Medicine (IOM). (2012). *Health IT and patient safety: Building safer systems for better care.* National Academies Press.

Institute of Medicine (IOM). (2019). *The future of nursing report. Where are we now?* https://www. healthleadersmedia.com/nursing/future-nursing-report-where-are-we-now

Kohn, L. T., Corrigan, J. M., & Donaldson, M. S. (Eds.). (2000). *To err is human: Building a safer health system.* National Academies Press.

Lee, S., Mohr, N. M., Street, W. N., & Nadkarni, P. (2019). Machine learning in relation to emergency medicine clinical and operational scenarios: An overview. *Western Journal of Emergency Medicine: Integrating Emergency Care With Population Health, 20*(2), 219–227. doi.org/10.5811/westjem.2019.1.41244

Luo, Y., Thompson, W. K., Herr, T. M., Zeng, Z., Berendsen, M. A., Jonnalagadda, S. R., Carson, M. B., & Starren, J. (2017). Natural language processing for EHR-based pharmacovigilance: A structured review. *Drug Safety, 40*(11), 1075–1089. doi:10.1007/s40264-017-0558-6

Newbold, S. (2013, April). *Nursing informatics boot camp.* Presentation at the meeting of Georgia Healthcare Information and Management Systems Society, Atlanta, Georgia.

Risling, T. L., & Low, C. (2019). Advocating for safe, quality and just care: What nursing leaders need to know about artificial intelligence in healthcare delivery. *Nursing Leadership, 32*(2), 31–45.

Ronquillo, C., Currie, L., & Rodney, P. (2016). The evolution of data-information-knowledge-wisdom in nursing informatics. *Advances in Nursing Science, 39*(1), E1–E18. doi:10.1097/ANS.0000000000000107

Sewell, J. (2016). *Informatics and nursing: Opportunities and challenges* (5th ed.). Wolters Kluwer.

U.S. Department of Health and Human Services. (n.d.). *Health information privacy.* www.hhs.gov/ocr/privacy

Wager, K. A., Lee F. W., & Glaser, J. P. (2017). *Health care information systems: A practical approach for health care management* (4th ed.). Jossey-Bass.

Wahoush, O., & Banfield, L. (2014). Information literacy during entry to practice: Information-seeking behaviors in student nurses and recent nurse graduates. *Nurse Education Today, 34*(2014), 208–213.

To explore learning resources for this chapter, go to FADavis.com

Part III

Leadership and Management Functions

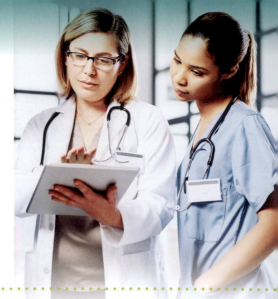

Chapter **11**

Creating and Managing a Sustainable Workforce

Elizabeth J. Murray, PhD, RN, CNE

KEY TERMS

360-degree feedback
Adjourning
Coaching
Collaboration
Constructive feedback
Corrective action
Destructive feedback
Forming
Interprofessional team
Interprofessional teamwork
Intraprofessional team
Norming
Peer review
Performance appraisal
Performing
Position description
Self-appraisal
Storming
Synergy
Teamwork

LEARNING OUTCOMES

- Outline the steps nurse leaders and managers must follow to create a sustainable workforce, including recruiting, interviewing, orienting, and retaining.
- Identify appropriate and inappropriate interview questions.
- Identify characteristics of an effective team.
- Explain the stages of team development.
- Explain the importance of collaboration among nurses of different generations.
- Describe the role of nurse leaders and managers in fostering teamwork and collaboration.
- Describe criteria used to give an effective performance appraisal.
- Explain how corrective action can be used to improve staff performance.

The Knowledge, Skills, and Attitudes Related to the Following Are Addressed in This Chapter:

Core Competencies	• Patient-Centered Care • Teamwork and Collaboration • Safety
The Essentials: Core Competencies for Professional Nursing Education (AACN, 2021)	**Domain 2: Person-Centered Care** 2.9 Provide care coordination (p. 32). **Domain 3: Population Health** 3.2 Engage in effective partnerships (p. 35). **Domain 5: Quality and Safety** 5.2 Contribute to a culture of patient safety (pp. 41–42). **Domain 6: Interprofessional Partnerships** 6.1 Communicate in a manner that facilitates a partnership approach to quality care delivery (43–44). 6.2 Perform effectively in different team roles, using principles and values of team dynamics (p. 44). 6.3 Use knowledge of nursing and other professions to address healthcare needs (p. 44). 6.4 Work with other professions to maintain a climate of mutual learning, respect, and shared values (pp. 44–45).
Code of Ethics with Interpretive Statements (ANA, 2015)	**Provision 1.1:** Respect for human dignity (pp. 1–4) **Provision 2.2:** Conflict of interest of nurses (pp. 5–7) **Provision 8.2:** Collaboration for health, human rights, and health diplomacy (pp. 31–32) **Provision 8.3:** Obligation to advance health and human rights and reduce disparities (p. 32)

Nurse Manager (NMC) Competencies (AONL, 2015a) and Nurse Executive (NEC) Competencies (AONL, 2015b)	**NMC: Human Resource Management (p. 4)**
	• Apply recruitment techniques
	• Staff selection
	• Scope of practice
	NMC: Human Resource Leadership Skills (p. 6)
	• Performance management
	• Staff retention
	NMC: Diversity (p. 6)
	• Cultural competence
	• Social justice
	• Generational diversity
	NEC: Communication and Relationship Building (p. 4)
	• Relationship management
	  • Build collaborative relationships
	• Diversity
	  • Establish an environment that values diversity (e.g., age, gender, race, religion, ethnicity, sexual orientation, culture)

Continued

The Knowledge, Skills, and Attitudes Related to the Following Are Addressed in This Chapter:—cont'd

- Establish cultural competency in the workforce
- Incorporate cultural beliefs into care delivery
- Provide an environment conducive to opinion sharing, exploration of ideas and achievement of outcomes

NEC: Business Skills (p. 10)

- Human resource management
  - Use corrective discipline to mitigate workplace behavior
  - Provide education regarding components of collective bargaining
  - Develop and evaluate recruitment, onboarding, and retention strategies
  - Develop and implement outcome-based performance management program

Nursing Administration Scope and Standards of Practice (ANA, 2016)	**Standard 2: Identification of Problems, Issues, and Trends** The nurse administrator analyzes the assessment data to identify problems, issues, and trends (p. 37). **Standard 3: Outcomes Identification** The nurse administrator identifies expected outcomes for a plan tailored to the system, organization, or population problem, issue, or trend (p. 38). **Standard 5A: Coordination** The nurse administrator coordinates implementation of the plan and associated processes (p. 41). **Standard 7: Ethics** The nurse administrator practices ethically (pp. 45–46). **Standard 8: Culturally Congruent Practice** The nurse administrator practices in a safe manner that is congruent with cultural diversity and inclusion principles (pp. 47–48). **Standard 10: Collaboration** The nurse administrator collaborates with healthcare consumers, colleagues, community leaders, and other stakeholders to advance nursing practice and healthcare transformation (p. 50). **Standard 11: Leadership** The nurse administrator leads within professional practice setting, profession, healthcare industry, and society (p. 51–52). **Standard 12: Education** The nurse administrator attains knowledge and competence that reflect current nursing practice and promotes futuristic thinking (p. 53). **Standard 14: Quality of Practice** The nurse administrator contributes to quality nursing practice (p. 55).

Source: American Association of Colleges of Nursing. (2021). *The essentials: Core competencies for professional nursing education.* Author; American Nurses Association (ANA). (2015). *Code of ethics for nurses with interpretive statements.* Author; American Nurses Association (ANA). (2016). *Nursing administration: Scope and standards of practice* (2nd ed.). Author; American Organization for Nursing Leadership (AONL). (2015a). *AONL nurse manager competencies.* Author; American Organization for Nursing Leadership (AONL). (2015b). *AONL nurse executive competencies.* Author; Cronenwett, L., Sherwood, G., Barnsteiner, J., Disch, J., Johnson, J., Mitchell, P., Sullivan, D. T., & Warren, J. (2007). Quality and safety education for nurses. *Nursing Outlook, 55*(3), 122–131; and Greiner, A. C., & Knebel, E. (Eds.) (2003). *Health professions education: A bridge to quality.* National Academies Press.

The nursing shortage is forecast to continue indefinitely as more nurses retire and as the need for health care increases, particularly because of aging Baby Boomers. It is estimated that 1.13 million registered nurses (RNs) will be needed by 2022 to fill new jobs and replace retiring nurses (American Nurses Association [ANA], 2015a). Several reasons for the ongoing nursing shortage are nurse job dissatisfaction, unhealthy work environments, lack of recognition for accomplishments, and unclear role expectations (Bryant-Hampton et al., 2010; Masters, 2014; Riley et al., 2009). The continuing nursing shortage, high turnover in nursing, complex health-care systems, increasing patient acuity, and fiscal constraints may influence nurse leaders and managers who are eager to fill nursing positions to make quick and sometimes hasty hiring decisions. However, nurse leaders and managers have a responsibility to hire safe, competent nurses with high integrity (Hader, 2005). Recruiting, developing, and retaining quality staff must be a priority for all nurse leaders and managers. In addition, addressing areas of dissatisfaction to retain experienced nurses is critical to provide the level of complex care needed today. To retain nurses, nurse leaders and managers must establish a healthy work environment that creates joy and meaning at work, creates synergy, and fosters workforce sustainability (American Association of Critical-Care Nurses, 2016; Lucian Leape Institute, 2013).

The complexity of health care globally today requires a collaborative approach to ensure patient safety and quality care. Historically, nurses have been in the habit of working alone, developing plans of care without considering the patient and their family or other health-care professionals. Nurses are called to provide patient-centered care as members of interprofessional teams, emphasizing evidence-based practice, quality improvement approaches, and informatics (Cronenwett et al., 2007; Greiner & Knebel, 2003). International evidence suggests that teams composed of various health-care professionals can maximize the strengths of health-care professionals, enhance work processes, and improve patient care outcomes (World Health Organization [WHO], 2010). Nurses must shift their mental models from working in silos to collaborating as members of the health-care team.

In this chapter, the nurse leader and manager's role in creating a sustainable workforce is covered, from the recruiting stage through retaining quality nurses. In addition, teamwork and collaboration, including the stages of team development, the characteristics of an effective team, and roles of nurse leaders and managers in fostering teamwork and collaboration, are also covered. Finally, management of staff is discussed, including the performance review process and corrective action.

► CREATING A SUSTAINABLE WORKFORCE

It is estimated that more than 1 million RNs will reach retirement age between 2025 and 2030 (Buerhaus et al., 2017; Health Resources and Service Administration [HRSA] Bureau of Health Professions, 2013). In 2018, the average age of an RN was 47.9 years, and nearly half of all RNs were over 50 years old (HRSA Bureau of Health Workforce, 2018). Buerhaus et al. (2017) propose that 1 million retiring RNs equates to an estimated loss of 2 million years of experience. This loss of knowledge and experience can result in significant negative consequences to patient safety and quality of care. Further, the acceleration of RN retirements will result in a new type of nursing shortage—a shortage of knowledge, skill, expertise, and the clinical judgment that allows a nurse to effectively care for complex patients and manage clinical and administrative challenges (Buerhaus et al., 2017).

To maintain a higher percentage of experienced nurses at the bedside, nurse leaders and managers must identify methods to increase nurse satisfaction and explore creative strategies to accommodate older nurses. Key elements of the nurse leader and manager's role related to sustaining a quality nursing workforce are displayed in Box 11-1. Nurse leaders and managers also need to bring younger nurses into the workforce to prepare for the retirement of older nurses. To achieve the goal of creating a sustainable workforce, nurse leaders and managers must be able to recruit, interview, orient, and retain quality nurses of all ages.

Recruiting

The cost of recruiting and orienting new nurses requires nurse leaders and managers to make hiring decisions carefully and to seek and select the best person for the right position. Based on the complexity of health care and high acuity of patients, some health-care organizations prefer to hire experienced nurses and/or nurses with baccalaureate degrees or advanced education. However, nurse leaders and managers should consider recruiting and hiring a balance of new nurse graduates and experienced nurses, given the increasing demand for health care, aging baby boomers, and upcoming nurse retirements (McMenamin, 2014). Nurse leaders and managers must be committed to recruiting and hiring the brightest and the best. By employing new nurse graduates and providing adequate transition-to-practice (TTP) programs, nurse leaders and managers can develop and retain increasingly experienced nurses in anticipation of the retirement of aging nurses—essentially, "growing their own" experienced nursing workforce (McMenamin, 2014). Attracting talented nurses requires providing continuing education, up-to-date technology, professional development, opportunities for advancement, and work/life balance (Gokenbach & Thomas, 2020).

Interviewing

Once a qualified applicant is identified, the nurse leader and manager should prepare for interviews by reviewing the applicant's information, resume, and letters of reference and by making notes of key questions to ask during the interview. The interview should be scheduled when the nurse leader and manager is available to

---

BOX 11-1   Key Elements to Sustaining a Quality Nursing Workforce

1. Create a vision for a healthy work environment and model it.
2. Establish a collaborative practice culture built on mutual trust and respect.
3. Promote workplace autonomy.
4. Respect nurses' rights and responsibilities.
5. Foster skilled communication to protect and advance collaboration.
6. Establish a culture of accountability.
7. Encourage shared decision making at all levels.
8. Recognize nurses for their meaningful contributions to the unit and organization.
9. Match nurses' competencies to patients' needs.
10. Advocate for patients and nurses.
11. Promote a workforce that habitually pursues excellence.
12. Promote accountability for nursing practice.

Compiled from American Association of Critical-Care Nurses, 2016; ANA, 2016; Lucian Leape Institute, 2013; Sherman & Pross, 2010.

meet for an adequate amount of time and without interruption; in addition, it is important to ensure that there is ample time for the applicant to ask questions. Some organizations may use a team approach to interviews in which applicants are also interviewed by a panel of nurses and other staff members. Involving staff can be an effective approach and reduce bias on the part of the nurse leader and manager. The focus of the interviews should be on the roles and responsibilities outlined in the position description. A **position description** reflects current practice standards and provides clear, written expectations about the roles and responsibilities of the position. It should also include the name of the person to whom the employee reports. Nurse leaders and managers must treat all applicants equally and as professionals, as well as keeping in mind that applicants may have other positions they are considering.

During the interview, the nurse leader and manager must avoid asking questions that are considered inappropriate. Although information related to the applicant's age, marital status, and medical information may be needed for payroll, benefits, and insurance purposes, the nurse leader and manager should not inquire about this information during the interview. Such information can be obtained after the employee is hired. Some of the laws discussed in Chapter 5 are relevant during the interview, including the Civil Rights Act, the Age Discrimination in Employment Act, and the Americans with Disabilities Act. Table 11-1 provides examples

Table 11-1 Interview Questions

Avoid Asking	Laws They May Violate	What to Ask Instead
• How old are you? • When did you graduate from college? • When do you plan on retiring?	Age Discrimination in Employment Act (ADEA) of 1967	• Are you old enough to do this type of work? • If hired, can you supply transcripts of your college education? • What are your long-term career goals?
• Do you have a disability? • Have you ever filed a workers' compensation claim? • Do you have a preexisting medical condition?	Americans With Disabilities Act (ADA) of 1990	• Are you able to do the duties listed in the job description without accommodations?
• Do you go to church? • What outside activities do you participate in?	Title VII of the Civil Rights Act of 1964	• What professional associations are you a member of?
• Are you married? • Do you have children? • When do you plan to start a family?	Title VII of the Civil Rights Act of 1964; Pregnancy Discrimination Act (an amendment to Title VII)	• Are you available to work evenings and weekends? • Are you available to travel on short notice?
• Are you a U.S. citizen? • What was your maiden name?	Title VII of the Civil Rights Act of 1964; Immigration Reform and Control Act	• If you are hired, are you able to provide documentation to prove you are eligible to work in the United States?
• Have you ever been arrested?	Title VII of the Civil Rights Act of 1964	• Have you ever been convicted of a crime?
• If you have been in the military, were you honorably discharged?	Uniform Services Employment and Reemployment Rights Act	• In what branch of the military did you serve?

Compiled from Society for Human Resources Management, 2015; U.S. Equal Employment Opportunity Commission, n.d.

of questions that are illegal to ask and alternative questions to ask instead. When the nurse leader and manager is interviewing several applicants for the same position, it is important to ask all applicants the same questions.

The interview is a two-way process. While the nurse leader and manager is interviewing applicants to determine whether they are qualified to fill a specific position, applicants should be assessing the interaction and gathering as much information as possible to be able to make an informed decision to accept or decline an offer. A wise applicant researches the organization before the interview. Reviewing the mission, vision, and philosophy of the organization can help nurses determine whether the organization's values and beliefs are congruent with their individual beliefs.

Orienting

Nurse leaders and managers must be dedicated to providing a proper orientation for new staff to enhance retention. When the cost of recruiting and orienting new staff is calculated, the estimated average cost of turnover is equivalent to a nurse's annual salary (Halfer, 2007). In addition, approximately 25% of new graduate nurses will leave their position within the first year (National Council of State Boards of Nursing [NCSBN], 2020). To retain new graduate nurses, orientation programs need to bridge the gap between the student nurse clinical setting and the real-world clinical setting. Programs for new nurses that focus on effective TTP and that include both competency development and role transition have been shown to improve retention rates (Halfer, 2007; Spector et al., 2015).

The NCSBN (2020) explored the issue of educating and retaining new nurse graduates since 2005 and found that the inability of new nurse graduates to transition into clinical practice has and will continue to have great consequences for the nursing profession and patient outcomes. In collaboration with more than 35 nursing organizations, the NCSBN worked to develop an evidence-based TTP model to assist new nurses as they transition from the classroom to the clinical setting (NCSBN, 2020). Structured TTP programs that are at least 6 months long and include core competencies, clinical reasoning, regular feedback on progress, self-reflection, and specialty knowledge in an area of practice improve the quality and safety practice of new graduate nurses, increase job satisfaction, decrease work stress, and decrease turnover (NCSBN, 2020; Spector et al., 2015).

When setting up orientation for new nurses as well as seasoned nurses, the nurse leader and manager must consider the characteristics of the new staff members and select an appropriate preceptor. The novice-to-expert model can assist with making successful preceptor assignments (Benner, 1984). Most new graduate nurses exhibit characteristics of the novice and advanced beginner stage, and new nurse graduates demonstrate marginally acceptable performance (NCSBN, 2011). In many cases, new nurse graduates use context-free rules to guide their actions or may begin to formulate some guidelines for their actions. New nurse graduates have not developed enough insight to discern which tasks are relevant in real-world situations (NCSBN, 2011).

The appropriate preceptor is critical to successful on-boarding of new nurses. Novices and advanced beginners do not have past experiences to base decisions on, so their approach to patient care is slow and methodical; they are very focused on being safe and efficient (Benner, 1984). In addition, the new generations of nurses need regular verbal and written feedback to build confidence and self-esteem. The best preceptor for the new nurse graduate may be a nurse who is at the competent stage (i.e., has about 3 years of experience and is able to demonstrate effective organizational, time management, and planning abilities). Competent nurses can differentiate important tasks from less important aspects of care. In addition, their time as a new nurse graduate is recent enough that they can approach the preceptorship with empathy. A less than ideal preceptor is an expert and proficient nurse because nurses at this stage make rapid decisions based on previous experiences, have difficulty putting what they know into words for the new nurse to understand, and may have less patience for the ongoing feedback the new nurse graduate requires (Benner, 1984).

EXPLORING THE EVIDENCE 11-1

Spector, N., Blegen, M. A., Silvestre, J., Barnsteiner, J., Lynn, M. R., Ulrich, B., Fogg, L., & Alexander, M. (2015). Transition to practice study in hospital settings. *Journal of Nursing Regulation, 5*(4), 24–38.

Aim
There were three aims to this study:

1. To conduct a randomized, controlled multisite study examining quality and safety, stress, competence, job satisfaction, and retention in new graduate nurses
2. To compare outcomes with a control group of hospitals that had preexisting transition to practice programs
3. To obtain diverse samples that included rural, suburban, and urban hospitals of all sizes

Methods
A randomized longitudinal multisite design was used to examine the effects of the NCSBN TTP program and other similar programs for new graduates. The researchers recruited 1,088 new RNs from 94 hospitals between July 1, 2011, and September 30, 2011, to participate.

Key Findings
This study supports that a standardized TTP program improves safety and quality outcomes. The programs in place for at least 2 years had the best outcomes over time. New nurses in hospitals with limited TTP programs had more medical errors, felt less competent, experienced more stress, reported less job satisfaction, and had twice the turnover rate than did new nurses in hospitals with TTP programs.

Implications for Nurse Leaders and Managers
This study provides significant evidence for nurse leaders and managers to support standardized TTP programs for new nurses.

Retaining

Examining strategies to retain experienced nurses is critical in finding a solution to the long-term nursing shortage. Inadequate staffing leads to nurse dissatisfaction, burnout, and turnover, all of which jeopardizes the quality of patient care. High turnover can have negative consequences on patient safety, nurse satisfaction, and the health-care organization overall as a result of low staff morale, insufficient monitoring of patients, increased errors, poor-quality care, increased patient costs, and decrease in hospital profitability (American Association of Critical-Care Nurses, 2016; Page, 2004). Moreover, high turnover threatens the overall experience level of the nursing staff, which, in turn, compromises patient safety (Page, 2004). The number one strategy to retain nurses is by creating and sustaining a healthy work environment. Accomplishing this requires strong nursing leadership at all levels of the health-care organization, but especially at the unit level, where frontline nurses and nurse leaders and managers work and where patient care is delivered (Sherman & Pross, 2010). Nurse leaders and managers must create a vision for a healthy work environment and authentically live it (American Association of Critical-Care Nurses, 2016).

A healthy work environment is one in which nurses feel safe from physiological and psychological harm and can find meaning and joy in their work. Nurse leaders and managers are responsible for creating the cultural norms and environment that result in workforce safety, meaning, and joy (Lucian Leape Institute, 2013). A work environment can be considered healthy and as one that brings meaning and joy to the worker's life when each nurse is able to answer "yes" every day to the following questions (Lucian Leape Institute, 2013, p. 15):

1. Am I treated with dignity and respect by everyone?
2. Do I have what I need so I can make a contribution that gives meaning to my life?
3. Am I recognized and thanked for what I do?

Meaningful recognition is important in retaining experienced nurses. "Nurses must be recognized and must recognize others for the value each brings to the work of the organization" (American Association of Critical-Care Nurses, 2016, p. 29). Nurses who are not recognized often feel invisible, undervalued, and disrespected, feelings that eventually can sap their motivation (American Association of Critical-Care Nurses, 2016). Nurse leaders and managers have an ethical responsibility to "establish, maintain, and promote conditions of employment that enable nurses to practice according to accepted standards" (ANA, 2015b, p. 28). Nurse leaders and managers can provide recognition, mentoring, coaching, and career or professional development opportunities to enhance the nursing workforce. Retaining experienced nurses is critical to providing safe and quality care, and a healthy work environment is paramount to retaining experienced nurses. Healthy work environments are discussed further in Chapter 12.

▶ TEAMWORK AND COLLABORATION

Nurses at all levels must gain the knowledge and develop the necessary skills and attitudes to be able to collaborate on intraprofessional and interprofessional teams. Teamwork and collaboration require "function[ing] effectively within nursing and interprofessional teams, fostering open communication, mutual respect, and shared decision-making to achieve quality patient care" (Cronenwett et al., 2007, p. 125). **Intraprofessional teams** are teams of nurses at various levels in the organization collaborating to ensure that patient care is continuous and reliable (American Association of Colleges of Nursing [AACN], 2008). When intraprofessional relationships are strong, synergy is created, and nurses at all levels function as an efficient and effective team.

Teamwork and collaboration are important to safe and quality care and a healthy work environment, whether nurse leaders and managers are building a team on the unit or across the organization. Nurses at all levels must collaborate and function on various teams important to the overall goal of delivering safe and quality care. The American Nurses Association (ANA) and the American Organization of Nurse Executives (AONE) (2012) developed the document *Principles for Collaborative Relationships Between Clinical Nurses and Nurse Managers* that outlines the necessary principles for intraprofessional teamwork and collaboration: effective communication, authentic relationships, and learning environments and culture.

Effective communication requires an understanding of the underlying context of the situation, an appreciation for the tone and emotions of a conversation, and accurate information. Principles include the following (ANA & AONE, 2012, para. 5–6):

- Engaging in active listening to understand and contemplate fully what is being relayed
- Knowing the intent of a message and the purpose and expectations of that message
- Fostering an open, safe environment
- Whether giving or receiving information, making sure that it is accurate
- Having people speak to the person they need to speak to, so the right person gets the right information

Authentic relationships bolster the profession and the quality of care patients receive. Nurses must cultivate caring relationships with each other, similar to the nurse–patient relationship, by doing the following (ANA & AONE, 2012, para. 7–8):

- Being true to yourself and being sure that actions match words and that those around you are confident that what they see is what they get
- Empowering others to have ideas, to share those ideas, and to participate in projects that leverage or enact those ideas
- Recognizing and leveraging each other's strengths
- Being honest 100% of the time with yourself and with others
- Respecting the personalities, needs, and wants of others
- Asking for what you want but staying open to negotiating the difference
- Assuming good intent from the words and actions of others and assuming that they are doing their best

A learning environment and learning culture support great nursing care and give nurses the satisfaction of knowing that their work is valuable and meaningful by doing the following (ANA & AONE, 2012, p. 9–10):

- Inspiring innovative and creative thinking
- Committing to a cycle of evaluating, improving, and celebrating, and valuing what is going well

- Creating a culture of safety, both physically and psychologically
- Sharing knowledge and learning from mistakes
- Questioning the status quo—ask "what if," not "no way"

Nurse leaders and managers must be committed to maintaining a high level of staff involvement, which will enhance job satisfaction and promote staff retention. In turn, staff satisfaction has been attributed to reduced medication errors, decreased patient falls, and a decline in patient deaths (LeBlanc, 2014; Wessel, 2015).

Interprofessional teams are teams made up of health-care professionals, the patient, and the patient's family working together to collaborate, communicate, and integrate care to ensure that patient care is continuous and reliable (AACN, 2008). Patient-centered care is closely linked to teamwork and collaboration and requires health-care professionals to actively involve or give control to the patient and the family in all health-care decisions (Disch, 2017). Nurses at all levels must promote patients' capacity for optimum involvement in their care and problem-solving (ANA, 2015c). Further, nurses must establish partnerships with other health-care professionals on interprofessional teams based on the recognition of each profession's value and contributions, mutual trust, respect, open discussion, and shared decision making (ANA, 2015c). Nurses at all levels have a responsibility to bring their unique nursing perspective to interprofessional teams to advocate for greater quality care and optimum patient outcomes and to deliver evidence-based, patient-centered care (AACN, 2008).

Teamwork is "sharing one's expertise and relinquishing some autonomy work closely with others, including patients and communities, to achieve better outcomes" (Interprofessional Education Collaborative Expert Panel [IPEC], 2011, p. 24). Teamwork involves integrating the knowledge, expertise, and experience of health-care professionals to work collaboratively in planning and delivering patient-centered care that is safe, timely, efficient, effective, and equitable (IPEC, 2011). **Interprofessional teamwork** is "the levels of cooperation, coordination and collaboration characterizing the relationships between professions in delivering patient-centered care" (IPEC, 2016, p. 8). Functioning as an effective team member requires nurses at all levels to collaborate with other team members, patients, and their families, by using available evidence to inform shared decision making and problem-solving. Inspired by a vision of interprofessional collaborative practice as key to safe, high-quality, accessible, patient-centered care, the IPEC identified four core competency domains of interprofessional collaborative practice: values and ethics for interprofessional practice; roles and responsibilities; interprofessional communication; and teams and teamwork. In 2016, IPEC updated the competencies. The updated content appears in bold (IPEC, 2016):

1. *Values and ethics for interprofessional practice* requires "work with individuals of other professions to maintain a climate of mutual respect and shared values" (p. 11).
2. The general competency statement reflecting *roles and responsibilities* is "use the knowledge of one's own role and those of other professions to appropriately assess and address the healthcare needs **of patients** and **to promote and advance the health of populations**" (p. 12).

3. *Interprofessional communication* means "to communicate with patients, families, communities, and **professionals in health and other fields** in a responsive and responsible manner that supports a team approach to **the promotion** and maintenance of health and the **prevention and** treatment of disease" (p. 13).

4. The general competency statement for *teams and teamwork* is to "apply relationship-building values and the principles of team dynamics to perform effectively in different team roles to **plan, deliver, and evaluate** patient-/population-centered care **and population health programs and policies** that **are** safe, timely, efficient, effective, and equitable" (p. 14).

Collaboration is working jointly with others in a mutually beneficial and well-defined interprofessional relationship to achieve common goals (Lukas & Andrews, 2014; Mensik, 2014). Collaboration is slowly becoming a reality in health care today. Research suggests that collaboration improves coordination, communication, quality, and safety of patient care (Robert Wood Johnson Foundation [RWJF], 2011). Health-care professionals work together on a continuum that reflects the level of intensity in the working relationship (Lukas & Andrews, 2014). Cooperation is at the lower end of intensity and involves short, informal relationships in which the parties maintain their individual goals. Next on the continuum is coordination, which is longer term and involves planning and some shared resources and goals. The highest level of intensity is collaboration, which requires commitment to shared goals by all parties. Figure 11-1 illustrates this continuum. Collaboration uses the individual and collective skills and experience of team members, and it allows them to function more effectively and deliver a higher level of services than each would be able to provide alone (RWJF, 2011, p. 1). Teamwork and collaboration require nurses at all levels to use effective communication skills to collaborate and function on interprofessional and intraprofessional teams.

Nurse leaders and managers need to foster teamwork and collaboration among staff members not only to improve patient outcomes but also to encourage growth both individually and as an organization (Hader, 2013). Improving the use of teamwork and collaboration can benefit patients, staff, and the overall organization. Teamwork benefits patients by decreasing adverse events and increasing patient satisfaction. Nurses benefit from teamwork because it decreases fatigue and burnout and improves morale and work satisfaction. The organization benefits because satisfied patients and nurses decrease litigation and turnover as well as improve the organization's reputation (The Joint Commission, 2012). Nurse leaders and

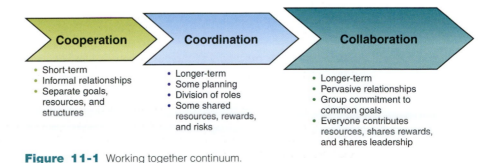

Figure 11-1 Working together continuum.

managers must engage in teamwork as both team players and team builders and provide direction to enhance the effectiveness of the team (ANA, 2016).

▶ BUILDING TEAMS

There is overwhelming evidence that the quality of teamwork and collaboration can determine whether a patient receives safe, competent, quality care in a timely manner (Wachter & Gupta, 2018). As health-care organizations are faced with increasing demands for quality, as well as pressure to control costs and increase productivity, effective team building is an optimum strategy to meet these mandates. All nurses at all levels must engage in teamwork to collaborate with patients, families, and other health-care professionals to deliver safe and quality nursing care (ANA, 2015c). Nurse leaders and managers are critical to building successful and satisfying teams (LeBlanc, 2014). Effective team building encourages staff commitment, creativity, support, and growth of individuals, the team, the unit, and the organization.

Teams are formed for different purposes. The nurse leader and manager makes hiring decisions for the purpose of building the intraprofessional nursing team for the unit. This team functions according to specific job descriptions and has clearly defined roles and responsibilities. The intraprofessional nursing team provides specific services or nursing care depending on the unit or department. Committees are formal teams within the organizational structure. The types of committees used in an organization or unit are usually determined by the mission, vision, and philosophy. Committees can be intraprofessional or interprofessional. An example of an intraprofessional committee is a nursing professional practice committee, which includes an RN from all units or departments within the organization. An example of an interprofessional committee is a hospital ethics committee, which may include RNs from several units or departments, a physician representative, social workers, a chaplain, a patient advocate, other health-care professionals, and a health-care consumer (often a former patient). Unit or department special task forces or ad hoc committees are formed to address a particular issue or project in a specific time frame. Members are designated by nurse leaders and managers and are given guidelines for the work of the team. Typically, a task force or ad hoc committee is time limited and includes several members who have expertise and/or interest in the special project. An example of a task force is a team working on a quality improvement project.

When building teams, nurse leaders and managers ask themselves several key questions (Mensik, 2014):

- What are the tasks the team needs to accomplish? Are the tasks new or have they been done before? Do the tasks require independent or interdependent work?
- Is representation from various levels of the organization needed?
- Is geographical, educational, and interprofessional diversity needed?
- What skill mix is necessary for the team to succeed? Does including team members with previous experience on successful teams help those members who do not have experience?

Finally, nurse leaders and managers should avoid asking the same reliable people to participate on teams. It may take extra effort, but encouraging new staff members to participate can bring new perspectives and avoid burnout among the more experienced staff members.

Stages of Team Development

Nurse leaders and managers must be aware of group dynamics and be prepared to facilitate the work of the team, if needed. All teams go through a series of stages as they are being formed, begin working, and accomplish their goals. Tuckman (1965) conducted a literature review to explore group process and to isolate common concepts and produce a model of group changes over time. He reviewed 55 articles and identified four stages of group development: forming, storming, norming, and performing. In 1977, Tuckman and Jensen reviewed the literature published since the original four stages were identified and added a fifth stage, adjourning (Tuckman & Jensen, 1977). Tuckman's stages have been used since the 1970s to describe the various phases of group development and team building. These stages continue to be discussed in the literature today. Some groups progress through five stages of group formation, whereas others may never progress beyond the third stage.

Forming is the initial stage when members of the team first meet each other. Members share information about themselves, learn about the purpose of the team, and begin discussion about goals. The work of the team does not start during this phase. Forming can be considered the "testing and orientation" stage (Tuckman, 1965). Members look to the leader for direction and avoid controversial topics or challenging anyone's ideas. Everyone is focused on getting along. During the forming stage, nurse leaders and managers help direct the team and assist members in understanding the purpose.

Storming occurs as the team begins to work together. Members share their opinions about how to get the work of the team accomplished, and a lack of unity commonly results as the team becomes polarized. Intragroup conflict occurs, and, sometimes, the team never progresses beyond this stage. Storming can be characterized as "conflict and polarization around interpersonal issues" (Tuckman, 1965). To move beyond this stage, the group must adopt a problem-solving mentality and let go of any personal agendas or goals. When the team is in the storming phase, nurse leaders and managers must remain positive about the work of the team, assist with resolving conflict, and coach team members through the storm.

Norming occurs once the team overcomes resistance and progresses through the storming phase. Everyone gives up individual goals and begins working as a team toward the common goal. Norming can be labeled as "development of group cohesion" (Tuckman, 1965). Group members begin to share ideas, and there is more acceptance among them. Focus becomes the work of the team. Creativity is high during this phase. Once the team is in the norming phase, nurse leaders and managers should step back and allow the team members to take responsibility and accountability for their work and progress toward the goal.

Performing is the stage in which the members understand their roles, they are flexible, and group energy is channeled into meeting the goal. Members accept each other's individual idiosyncrasies and develop group norms. The team is highly motivated to accomplish the work during this phase. This stage is characterized as "functional role-relatedness" (Tuckman, 1965). The group becomes interdependent with a strong group identity. At this point, nurse leaders and managers should not need to be involved and can focus energy on other projects.

Adjourning occurs once the work of the group is completed. Although not identified in Tuckman's original work, his subsequent work identified the notion that teams followed a life cycle model, which involved a distinct final stage (Tuckman & Jensen, 1977). The final stage can be emotional as the team disbands. When the team is beginning to adjourn, nurse leaders and managers should celebrate their successes and provide recognition to each individual.

Knowledge of group dynamics is critical for nurse leaders and managers to improve leadership competencies, facilitate team communication, and foster team cohesiveness.

Creating Synergy

As teams are formed and transition into the "norming" phase, members become interdependent and work together toward a common goal. Underlying this interdependence is the principle of synergy. Synergy catalyzes, unifies, and unleashes the greatest strengths within people. Further, it fosters creativity, imagining, and intellectual networking (Covey, 2004, p. 265). **Synergy** can be described as combining strengths of members of a team to result in remarkable outcomes that would not have been possible if members worked alone (Covey, 2004). Team synergy requires members to value their own expertise as well as others' and enables team members to be open-minded and willing to listen and learn from each other.

Nurse leaders and managers are key to successful teamwork. They must develop skills in intraprofessional and interprofessional team building and communication. Further, they must foster team synergy and model expert practice to team members and patients (ANA, 2016).

LEARNING ACTIVITY 11-1

Am I a Good Team Player?

Read the article *How To Be a Great Team Player* at https://www.mindtools.com/pages/article/newTMM_53.htm. Consider the following:

1. Are you a good/great team player?
2. Do you think being a good team player is important?
3. How could you be better?
4. Discuss with classmates strategies to improve being team players.

▶ CHARACTERISTICS OF EFFECTIVE TEAMS

Teams must do more than merely complete tasks; the members must be able to interact, coordinate, cooperate, and embrace a shared understanding of the team goals and objectives, available resources, and constraints under which the team must work (Salas et al., 2005). The following characteristics of successful teams were identified by Salas et al. (pp. 560–561):

- *Team leadership* involves the ability to direct and coordinate the activities of team members. It includes the following: assessing team performance; assigning tasks; developing team knowledge, skills, and abilities; motivating team members; planning and organizing; and establishing a positive atmosphere. All team members may lead the team once in a while. However, someone is needed to coordinate and support the work of the team.
- *Mutual performance monitoring* is the ability to develop common understandings of the team environment and apply appropriate task strategies to monitor team member performance accurately. This is critical to success of the team. Everyone needs to be aware of other team members' work; as one team member completes a task, others need to step up and help, and this approach reflects the principle of backup.
- *Backup behavior* is the ability to anticipate other team members' needs through an accurate understanding of their responsibilities. This includes the ability to shift assignments or tasks among members to achieve balance during high periods of workload or pressure.
- *Adaptability* is the ability to adjust strategies based on information gathered from the environment through the use of backup behavior and reallocation of team resources. This also involves altering the course of action in response to internal or external changing conditions.
- *Team orientation* is the ability to consider other team member's behaviors during group interactions, as well as the belief in the importance of the team goals over personal goals. Team members view their work as "our work," not "my work" (Kalisch & Schoville, 2012).
- *Shared mental models* comprise an organizing knowledge structure of the relationships among the tasks the team is engaged in and how the team members will interact. "Team members who have shared mental models have the same idea of what needs to be done, by whom, and by when" (Kalisch & Schoville, 2012, p. 53).
- *Mutual trust* is the shared belief that team members will perform their roles and protect the interests of their teammates. Team members must have trust in other team members that the work will be completed correctly and in a timely manner.
- *Closed-loop communication* is the exchange of information between a sender and a receiver irrespective of the medium. This type of communication is effective and efficient.

Salas et al. (2005) described team leadership, mutual performance monitoring, backup behavior, adaptability, and team orientation as the five core components that promote team effectiveness. They described shared mental models, mutual trust, and closed-loop communication as coordinating mechanisms that are critical to melding together the five core components. Team members who have shared mental models have an understanding of what needs to be done, by whom, and by when (Kalisch & Schoville, 2012, p. 53). Team members must communicate effectively, and there must be shared trust to feel confident that team members will complete their work in a timely manner. Nurse leaders and manager have a role in fostering all of these characteristics to ensure optimal team success.

▶ LEADING AND MANAGING TEAMS

Nurse leaders and managers serve key roles within the professional practice setting, profession, health-care industry, and society (ANA, 2016). They model "expert leadership practice to interprofessional team members and healthcare consumers" (ANA, 2016, p. 51). In fact, nurse leaders and managers are fundamental to building effective teams, but they may not always be the leader of the team. Regardless of who the team leader is, the leader must facilitate the work of the team by using effective meeting skills and frequent reminders about the team mission, goal, and accomplishments. LeBlanc (2014) suggests that the TEEAMS approach is one way in which nurse leaders and managers can create and lead successful teams. The key factors of TEEAMS are as follows:

- *Time:* Nurse leaders and managers must recognize the importance of spending adequate, quality face time with the team. LeBlanc suggests that scheduling regular time with staff members to round with them, engage in conversations, and get to know the team can be beneficial.
- *Empowerment:* Nurse leaders and managers must understand that empowerment is important to building a strong team. Empowering the team shows that nurse leaders and managers have trust in their team to make appropriate decisions with minimal intervention: "Productive teams are empowered teams!" (LeBlanc, 2014, p. 50).
- *Enthusiasm:* Nurse leaders and managers must be committed to the team's success and demonstrate enthusiasm for the individuals on the team as well as the team as a whole. Enthusiasm is contagious and results in getting team members excited about the work and the team goals.
- *Appreciation:* Appreciation is meaningful recognition of a job well done. Everyone needs recognition for their work at times. Nurse leaders and managers must show appreciation to individuals for their work toward team goals. This appreciation builds team members' self-esteem and self-image. Improved self-esteem and self-image can be translated into improved patient outcomes, increased intraprofessional and interprofessional communication, and a willingness to continue to work toward organizational goals.
- *Management:* Managing teams and holding them accountable are major roles of nurse leaders and managers. Critical to these roles is ensuring that team members are clear about their goals and understand job expectations and performance parameters. It is the nurse leader and manager's responsibility that staff members have the resources necessary to perform their duties as individuals and as members of a team.
- *Support:* All nurses at all levels need support to accomplish their work. Nurse leaders and managers must support their team including their personal, professional, and organizational needs. Strategies that nurse leaders and managers can use to support staff members include being accessible, engaging in daily

rounding, promptly returning calls, and creating an atmosphere that encourages work engagement.

Effective nurse leadership and management can have a positive impact on manager-staff relationships and team experiences, as well as enhance job satisfaction and promote staff retention. Nurse leaders and managers lead teams toward success, encourage and mentor members, provide constructive criticism, and celebrate success (Hader, 2013). Clinical nurses and nurse leaders and managers work together with the shared goal of safe and quality patient-centered care.

LEARNING ACTIVITY 11-2

Complete the Group Effectiveness Assessment

Think about a group you are involved with such as a study group or your clinical group. Visit Mindtools at https://www.mindtools.com/pages/article/newTMM_84.htm and complete the *Team Effectiveness Assessment*.

1. How did you score?
2. Were you surprised by your score?
3. Identify two to three strategies that you could implement to develop team skills.

To sustain team synergy, nurse leaders and managers must lead meetings effectively. There is nothing more deenergizing than attending a mandatory meeting where there is not a clear purpose or agenda and the meeting seems to drift aimlessly from topic to topic. Developing the competency of leading an efficient and successful meeting is critical. First and foremost, nurse leaders and managers must avoid holding unnecessary meetings. Typically, staff meetings and committee meetings are held monthly, and times may or may not vary. Best practice is to schedule monthly staff meetings on the same day (e.g., the third Monday of the month) and the same time (e.g., 7:30 a.m. for night shift staff and 7:30 p.m. for day shift). Committee meetings or task force meetings are typically scheduled monthly also.

Regardless of the type of meeting, an agenda should be prepared several days ahead of the meeting and sent to team members for review. This agenda informs members about what will be addressed and allows them to come to the meeting prepared. Meetings should begin and end on time. This shows team members that they are respected and their time is valued. Nurse leaders and managers should begin with a statement of the purpose or goals of the meeting and establish ground rules. Taking control of the meeting from the beginning sets the tone and helps keep chit chat to a minimum, thus keeping the meeting on track. In addition, team members should be reminded to show respect for those presenting by actively listening and refraining from checking telephone messages, texts, or e-mails. Throughout the meeting, the leader should encourage participation of team members. The meeting should be concluded by summarizing what was presented, describing the next steps or actions to be taken, and asking

---

EXPLORING THE EVIDENCE 11-2

Weaver, A. C., Callaghan, M., Cooper, A. L., Brandman, J., & O'Leary, K. J. (2015). Assessing interprofessional teamwork in inpatient medical oncology units. *Journal of Oncology Practice, 11*(1):19–22.

Aim

The aim of this study was to characterize teamwork among professionals in the inpatient oncology setting and to determine what barriers exist to establishing strong interprofessional collaboration.

Methods

The investigators conducted a cross-sectional study in the hematology-oncology services of an academic hospital. All nurses, residents, fellows, and attending physicians on the units were invited to participate in the study. The Safety Attitudes Questionnaire (SAQ) was distributed to 193 eligible participants.

Key Findings

Of the participants, 129 (67%) completed the study. Teamwork scores differed significantly across professional types. Physicians, residents, and hospitalists rated their collaboration with nurses as high or very high. In contrast, nurses rated collaboration with physicians, residents, and hospitalists as poor.

Barriers to collaboration were also scored differently. Nurses believed that negative communication among some professionals was the most significant obstacle to collaboration, whereas hospitalists identified difficulty reaching other providers as the major obstacle, and physicians rated teamwork and collaboration highly and did not report any major barriers.

Implications for Nurse Leaders and Managers

Although this study was conducted in the oncology setting, the researchers indicated that previous studies conducted in other hospital settings found similar results. Nurse leaders and managers need to be aware of the possible differences in the perceptions of collaboration and teamwork of interprofessional team members and encourage effective communication among all health-care professionals.

---

the team members whether they have any questions. Allow time at the end of the meeting for team members to talk about issues or concerns. A summary of the meeting should be sent out or made available to the team shortly after the meeting. An example of a typical agenda for a nursing team meeting is displayed in Table 11-2.

▶ MANAGING THE WORKFORCE

Daily and ongoing management of the workforce includes many challenges, including leveraging diversity, coaching team members, appraising performance, and using corrective action.

Table 11-2	Staff Meeting Template	

DATE/TIME:
PRESENT:

Time	Topic	Presenter
7:30 a.m.–7:35 a.m.	Welcome • Introductions • Call meeting to order • Signing of attendance sheet by everyone present • Recognition of staff achievements • Announcements for staff	Nurse leader and manager (or designee)
7:35 a.m.–7:45 a.m.	Budget report • Brief presentation of budget information staff members need to know to help them with fiscal responsibility	Nurse leader and manager (or designee)
7:45 a.m.–8:15 a.m.	New policy presentation(s)	Nurse leader and manager (or designee)
8:15 a.m. –8:45 a.m.	Team project reports • QI team • Professional Practice team	Chair, QI team Chair, Professional Practice team
8:45 a.m. –9:10 a.m.	New business • Presentation of anything new since the last meeting	Nurse leader and manager (or designee)
9:10 a.m. – 9:30 a.m.	Open discussion • The opportunity for staff to discuss issues and concerns	All
9:30 a.m.	Adjournment	Nurse leader and manager (or designee)

Leveraging Diversity

As health care becomes more globalized, nurses at all levels will be required to work more with diverse patient populations and on more diverse teams. Nurse leaders and managers are charged with working effectively with a diverse workforce, which includes leveraging differences and unique talents of team members (ANA, 2018).

Managing Generational Differences

On any nursing unit, as many as four different generations of nurses may be working side by side. Each generation has its own unique characteristics, work ethic, and expectations of the workplace (Murray, 2013). Nurse leaders and managers must identify strategies to create cohesive partnerships among the different generations to ensure safe and quality nursing care and create a healthy work environment. Stereotypes and judgmental attitudes about each generation can undermine the nursing team. For example, often there is the perception that older nurses do not like younger nurses; on the other end of the spectrum, there is sometimes the assumption by the new generation of nurses that older generations of nurses are old-fashioned and technologically challenged. When generations collide in the workplace, patient care can be compromised. In addition, nurse satisfaction can be affected, resulting in miscommunication, interpersonal tension, decreased productivity, increased absenteeism, and increased turnover. Nurse leaders and managers must foster a supportive and collegial environment that brings the various generations together to achieve their common goals. Acknowledging what each generation brings to the table and learning from the various generations can decrease tension and enhance personal and professional growth, leading to mutual respect (Murray, 2013; Weston, 2006).

Improved health and technological advances are allowing older nurses to work longer, and these expert nurses are needed for their skills and experiences to fill many essential positions (American Organization for Nursing Leadership [AONL], 2010). In fact, according to data from the HRSA Bureau of Health Workforce (2018), close to half of all RNs are more than 50 years old. Many older nurses are healthy and want to work beyond retirement years. In fact, a new view of aging is being recognized today as the average life expectancy increases and the quality of life in the final decades improves; in fact, a new middle period of life from age 50 to 70 years old is emerging, called the *third age* (Bower & Sadler, 2009). This new paradigm of successful aging is challenging the view of what is "old"— and many say, "60 is the new 40" (Bower & Sadler, 2009).

Third-age nurses are needed today to combat the current and future nursing shortage. They know the health-care system and provide a valuable resource because of their experience, knowledge, wisdom, and competence (AONL, 2010; Bower & Sadler, 2009). Nurse leaders and managers have "a vested interest in ensuring that qualified and talented nurses are not lost to traditional retirement, but instead redirected to other rewarding jobs and careers in nursing" (Bower & Sadler, 2009, p. 20). They must consider strategies to retain and develop older nurses for new and emerging roles. This approach may involve exploring environmental modifications to meet the needs of older nurses and prevent injuries because loss of strength and agility may affect older nurses' ability to turn, lift, and transfer patients, as well as tolerate the overall physical demands of the job (Page, 2004).

To leverage generational differences, nurse leaders and managers can use the following strategies to make the workplace more generationally comfortable (Murray, 2013):

- Accommodate differences by recognizing the strengths of each generation and use those strengths to build a sustainable workforce.
- Be flexible when giving options in the workplace and consider alternate scheduling options. Seek input from staff on recruitment, retention, and staffing matters that could decrease turnover and increase job satisfaction.
- Use a sophisticated management style and modify management approaches to address the differences and similarities of each generation. Keeping staff informed, providing the big picture, and using rewards, recognition, and feedback are management strategies that appeal to all generations.
- Respect competence and initiative, and value the talents and work ethics of each generation, even though they differ. For example, use the expertise and

experience of older and seasoned nurses to help develop policies and procedures and set up programs to assist new nurses. Provide younger nurses with
opportunities to solve problems and contribute to teamwork on their own
terms. Nurses of younger generations tend to be collaborators and prefer frequent feedback, so provide them with seasoned mentors who will coach them
as they launch their nursing career.

Cultural Differences

The Institute of Medicine (IOM) contends that cultural differences contribute to
ethnic and racial disparities in health care. Nurse leaders and managers must
be cognizant of these cultural issues and work toward not only increasing the
number of underrepresented minorities in the workplace but also improving
the cultural sensitivity and competency of all workers (Greiner & Knebel, 2003;
Smedley et al., 2003). According to the U.S. Census Bureau Quick Facts (July 1,
2019), the population of the United States is an estimated 328,239,523 with 18.5%
Hispanic or Latino, 13.4% Black or African American, and 5.9% Asian. To provide
safe, quality, patient-centered care, the nursing workforce should mirror the population they serve. However, there are an estimated 3,957,661 RNs in the United
States and 10.2% are Hispanic or Latino, 7.8% are Black or African American, and
5.2% are Asian. Clearly, more diversity is needed in the nursing workforce to
achieve safe, quality, patient-centered care.

Nurse leaders and managers must engage in culturally congruent practice and
develop "recruitment and retention strategies to achieve a multicultural workforce" (ANA, 2016, p. 48). Creating a diverse workforce that is reflective of the
population it serves promotes equity in health care. Further, a diverse workforce
has been linked to improved nurse–patient relationships and communication,
increased patient satisfaction, and improved health-care outcomes (Smedley et al.,
2003).

Gender Differences

Historically, nursing has been comprised primarily of women. However, trends
indicate more men are entering nursing. In 2008, approximately 7.1% of nurses were
male and in 2018, male RNs represented 9.6% of the population (HRSA Bureau of
Health Workforce, 2018). Along with the increased numbers of men in nursing
come gender differences in the workplace. These differences can be challenging.
Nurse leaders and managers need to be fair, be sensitive to the differences, understand varied perceptions, and address any issues that arise appropriately.

Coaching Staff Members

Coaching is the art of guiding another individual toward fulfilling their future;
to assist a person in achieving their goals, a coach helps them develop and prioritize viable solutions and then act on them (Narayanasamy & Penney, 2014;
Porter-O'Grady & Malloch, 2013). Coaching is a strategy used by nurse leaders and

managers to motivate and assist their staff members to improve their work performance. Part of coaching includes observing employee performance and providing ongoing feedback and constant encouragement. Effective coaching is transformative because it results in significant changes in an individual that motivate them to find achievement, fulfillment, and joy in the workplace (Narayanasamy & Penney, 2014). An effective coach assists nurses in recognizing opportunities for learning and development.

Nurse leaders and managers can use coaching when team building, in managing change, for professional development, and in career planning. The coaching relationship must be built on respect and trust. Nurses being coached must feel safe and secure, valued, and validated by the coach (Narayanasamy & Penney, 2014). To be effective coaches, nurse leaders and managers must become self-aware. Qualities of an effective coach are listed in Box 11-2. Coaching is beneficial to sustaining the workforce because it increases productivity, patient safety, quality of nursing care, and nurses' confidence and professionalism.

Appraising Performance

Nurse leaders and managers must ensure that their staff has the requisite knowledge, skills, and attitudes to perform professional responsibilities. Nurse competencies, performance standards, and educational preparation directly affect patient safety and quality outcomes. Nurse leaders and managers must set expectations for performance and address those who do not meet those expectations.

A **performance appraisal** is a formal evaluation of the work performance of an employee that is conducted by the nurse leader and manager. An effective performance appraisal can foster staff growth and development and promote retention. The employee's performance is evaluated according to the position description and established standards of practice. Nurse leaders and managers may use a performance appraisal for the following reasons:

- To assess a new employee at the conclusion of probationary status to determine whether the minimum level of performance for a position has been met
- To provide recognition for accomplishments or constructive feedback when improvement in performance is needed
- For an annual performance review of the employee's past goals, including performance related to position description, and to plan for professional development over the next year

---

BOX 11-2 Characteristics of an Effective Coach

- Be a good listener.
- Demonstrate professionalism and leadership qualities.
- Be inspiring and motivating to others.
- Be able to build confidence, self-esteem, and personal leadership in others.

- Act as a "sounding board," allowing problems and issues to be aired and redirected.
- Provide constructive feedback when necessary.
- Acknowledge work well done.
- Emphasize achievement, learning and development, and joy in work.

Compiled from Narayanasamy & Penney, 2014; Thomas et al., 2020.

As with interview questions, some of the laws discussed in Chapter 5 must be considered when conducting a performance appraisal, including the Civil Rights Act, the Age Discrimination in Employment Act, the Americans With Disabilities Act, and the Fair Labor Standards Act.

During a performance appraisal, the nurse's performance is weighed against the position description, professional standards of practice, and policies and procedures. The position description reflects legal, regulatory, and accreditation requirements; delineates the employee's roles and responsibilities; and specifies the person to whom the nurse reports. In addition, the position description outlines expected performance standards, which are often based on the ANA (2015c) *Scope and Standards of Practice* and represent the minimal level of acceptable nursing practice. Nurses working in specialty areas may have standards related to the clinical specialty included in their position description. Performance appraisals should relate only to the nurse's position description and expected performance standards and *not* to the personality of the individual.

An effective performance appraisal should promote successful work relationships and enhance employee development, as well as motivate staff to improve performance and productivity (Pearce, 2007). However, nurses may view performance appraisals as threatening, based on previous negative experiences. Providing frequent feedback on a regular basis throughout the review period can lessen fear of the process. Nurse leaders and managers should follow these steps when conducting effective performance appraisals (Pearce, 2007):

1. Prepare for the performance appraisal by keeping employee files updated with appropriate data and anecdotal notes that reflect performance observed throughout the review period. This ensures that feedback is based on facts.
2. Plan for the performance appraisal to be conducted in a formal but relaxed atmosphere. Schedule the performance appraisal at a time that is convenient for the employee and ensure there will be no interruptions.
3. Conduct the performance appraisal in such a manner as to encourage productive exchange of ideas and joint problem-solving. Review self-appraisal and peer reviews with the employee and encourage discussion.
4. Review the employee's achievements and ask whether they have achieved goals set during the previous performance appraisal.
5. Provide the employee feedback on their achievements.
6. If the performance appraisal process calls for ratings or scoring, seek input from the employee and strive for agreement.
7. Discuss plans for improvement, and assist the employee in identifying areas to work on and developing a realistic plan, but avoid actually developing the plan for the employee.
8. Address the employee's career plans, and offer realistic feedback regarding opportunities for advancements.
9. Assist the employee in developing new goals and objectives for the upcoming year by using the SMART (specific, measurable, appropriate, realistic, timed) technique.

10. Ask the employee for feedback, including how you can support the employee.
11. Provide an opportunity for the employee to add written comments on the performance appraisal.

The performance appraisal should be written and signed by the nurse leader and manager and the employee, and the employee should be provided with a copy of the signed document.

Effective nurse leaders and managers use performance appraisals as a way to provide constructive feedback regarding performance, enhance the work experience for staff, facilitate productivity, promote professionalism and career development, measure nursing performance, and, ultimately, improve the quality of nursing practice and create joy in the workplace (ANA, 2016, 2018).

LEARNING ACTIVITY 11-3   **Using SMART**

Use the SMART technique to develop five goals you would like to accomplish during the next year.

An important aspect of performance appraisal is a self-assessment or a self-appraisal. A **self-appraisal** is the process of the employee reflecting on their own personal actions and professional performance related to sense of self, values, beliefs, decisions, actions, and outcomes (Porter-O'Grady & Malloch, 2013). The self-appraisal should include a review of the employee's performance related to the previous year's goals and list specific accomplishments during the year. The employee may want to include feedback from peers as well as from patients and their families. An accountable nurse will also acknowledge areas of weakness during self-appraisal and identify strategies to make changes in practice to improve performance. Self-appraisal is part of professional autonomy, accountability, and self-regulation in nursing and "requires personal accountability for the knowledge base for professional practice, [and reflects] an individual's demonstrated personal control based on principles, guidelines, and rules deemed important" (ANA, 2010, p. 30). Nurse leaders and managers must also engage in self-appraisal of their own practice in relation to professional practice guidelines, standards, statutes, rules, and regulations on a regular basis (ANA, 2016).

Another possible element of a performance appraisal is a **peer review**, in which nurses from common practice areas assess, monitor, and make judgments about the quality of nursing care provided by a nurse peer (Haag-Heitman & George, 2011, p. 48). The peer review process also fosters accountability and supports self-regulation. Nurse leaders and managers have a critical role in establishing an effective peer review process. They may need to coach staff in the peer review process and encourage the use of constructive feedback versus destructive feedback. **Constructive feedback** is supportive, motivates the employee to succeed and grow, and involves showing respect and praising the employee for a job well done (e.g., "I really appreciate how you handled that difficult patient yesterday"), whereas **destructive feedback** includes threats and fear to control employee behavior, by criticizing the employee and making them feel humiliated (e.g., "Are you stupid? You should never walk out of the patient's room with gloves on!"). Often, nurse leaders and managers are evaluated by superiors based on peer reviews and input from staff related to employee satisfaction, successful recruitment and retention efforts, and quality outcomes.

One form of peer review is **360-degree feedback**, which is a type of constructive feedback in which nurses receive feedback from everyone around them—supervisors, peers, physicians, other health-care professionals, and even patients and their families. Typically, 360-degree feedback is anonymous. The nurse leader and manager summarizes the feedback and reviews it with the employee. The goal of 360-degree feedback is to provide specific opportunities for the employee to use in their development plan. It also provides the nurse leader and manager with particular areas in which to coach the nurse for growth and professional development.

Peer reviews and 360-degree feedback can be used not only for nurses but also for nurse leaders and managers. Informal and formal feedback on their performance from those they work with as well as from their subordinates can help nurse leaders and managers understand the effects of their leadership style and identify strengths and weaknesses in their interprofessional and intraprofessional communication skills. This feedback can be used by nurse leaders and managers in their own professional development.

Using Corrective Action

The emphasis on patient safety and quality care globally is motivating health-care organizations to focus attention on recruiting and retaining quality workers. This means keeping excellent employees (the high performers), further developing the good employees (the middle performers), and forcing the weak or poor employees (the low performers) to leave the organization (Matheny, 2005, p. 296). With regard to middle and low performers, nurse leaders and managers must address deficiencies and substandard performance immediately to avoid escalation of the behavior. Nurse leaders and managers who address poor performance in a timely manner are often perceived by staff as strong and effective; whereas nurse leaders and managers who allow poor performance are seen as unable to manage staff.

When substandard performance or deficiencies are identified, these may need to be addressed by the nurse leader and manager through **corrective action**, a progressive process used to improve poor performance.

Nurse leaders and managers must explore the deficiencies and determine whether the employee violated rules or policies and procedures or whether the deficiencies are related to lack of skill or competence. Evidence must be gathered to establish a case. Minor rule infractions such as tardiness or excessive absences should be addressed directly with the employee, and the employee should be given an opportunity to improve. Typically, this is accomplished through a written agreement between the employee and the nurse leader and manager that clearly outlines expected behavior and the consequences should the employee not meet the expectations. When a major infraction occurs, such as mistreatment of a patient, use of alcohol at work, or deferring medications from a patient, the employee should be terminated immediately (more on this later in this section). Nurse leaders and managers are bound by the ANA (2015b) *Code of Ethics for*

Nurses With Interpretive Statements to address any and all instances of incompetent, unethical, illegal, or impaired practice that compromise the safety or well-being of the patient. Further, any nurse who observes inappropriate behavior or questionable practice by another nurse that jeopardizes the rights or safety of a patient should report these concerns to the supervisor immediately (ANA, 2015b).

When establishing a corrective action plan, the nurse leader and manager must first determine the reason for the substandard performance: Is it the result of a lack of knowledge, skill, or experience, or did the employee violate policy or procedure? Next, the nurse leader and manager should address the behavior with a progressive corrective action plan according to the organization's policy and procedure; the plan may include a verbal reprimand, a written reprimand, suspension with or without pay, and termination. Corrective action should include constructive feedback to improve behavior or performance, rather than destructive feedback, which does not encourage the employee to succeed and can be detrimental to their development. Nurse leaders and managers must explore their approach to corrective action and adopt constructive techniques whenever possible. Table 11-3 outlines the nurse leader and manager's role in corrective action.

Once poor performance is addressed and the employee meets the conditions of the corrective action plan, the incident should not be held against the employee unless the behavior is repeated. It is unfair to bring up poor performance in the next performance appraisal if it has not been a problem since the employee met the conditions of the corrective action plan. However, if the employee repeats the behavior, and continued efforts to assist them in meeting the minimum standards of performance are not successful, termination may be necessary (McConnell, 2011).

Table 11-3 Corrective Action Plan

Violation	Nurse Leader and Manager's Tasks
First: An informal, verbal reprimand is given.	• Meets with employee to discuss violation or deficiency • Explores plan for improvement • Verbally discusses agreed-on plan for improvement
Second: A written reprimand is given.	• Meets with employee to discuss violation or deficiency • Establishes an agreed-on written plan for improvement • Discusses consequences if violation continues or no improvement is shown • Documents reprimand in writing
Third: Violation occurs a third time and/or there is no improvement.	• Consults with human resources • Meets with employee to discuss violation or deficiency • Suspends employee with or without pay • Encourages employee to examine the situation while away from work and determine a plan for improvement • Documents reprimand in writing
Fourth: Violation continues to occur after multiple reprimands or employee fails to improve performance to the level of standard of performance.	• Consults with human resources • Meets with employee • Terminates employee • Documents process in writing according to policy and procedures

✲ Unionization and Collective Bargaining

A union is an organization of employees who join together to have a voice and collectively negotiate for higher wages and improve working conditions (American Federation of Labor and Congress of Industrial Organizations [AFL-CIO], 2020a). The purpose behind unions is to ensure that employees have respect on the job and a voice in improving the quality of the work, products, and services. Unions also provide a counterbalance to the unchecked power of management (Teamsters, n.d.). In 1935, the National Labor Relations Act was established to support the rights of workers to form and join unions and participate in collective bargaining (AFL-CIO, 2020a). Collective bargaining is the process by which working people "negotiate contracts with their employers to determine their terms of employment, including pay, benefits, hours, leave, job health and safety policies, ways to balance work and family and more" (AFL-CIO, 2020b, para. 1). The negotiated contract or collective bargaining agreement is legally binding and enforced under federal and state law.

Unions and collective bargaining agreements represent a mechanism for nurses to gain and maintain control over professional practice and "combat management systems that threaten patient safety, quality of care, and the nurses' work environment" (Budd et al., 2004). Additional types of benefits negotiated for nurses include overtime, use of temporary nurses, provisions for continuing education and staff development, whistleblower protection, health provisions (e.g., free vaccinations), and grievance and arbitration procedures (Budd et al., 2004). The ANA supports the rights of RNs to unionize and participate in collective bargaining (ANA, 2015b).

Nurse leaders and managers have a responsibility to ensure that nurses are treated fairly and justly and that they are involved in decisions related to their practice and working conditions (ANA, 2015b, p. 24). There are several nurse unions available for nurses to join. The National Federation of Nurses (NFN; www.nfn.org) is affiliated with the American Federation of Teachers and is one of the leading national labor unions for RNs. The primary functions of the NFN are to advocate and provide a voice for RNs at the national level and to provide support, education, and assistance to member associations (Montana, Ohio, Oregon, and Washington State) (NFN, n.d.). The National Nurses United (NNU; www.nationalnursesunited.org) is the largest union for RNs and has members in every state in the United States. The NNU was formed through the merger of the California Nurses Association/National Nurses Organizing Committee, United American Nurses, and Massachusetts Nurses Association (NNU, 2010–2016). The goals of the NNU are to advance the interests of direct care nurses and patients across the United States, organize all direct-care RNs, promote effective collective bargaining representations to all NNU affiliates, expand the voice of direct care RNs, and promote accessible, quality health care for all as a human right (NNU, 2010–2016).

Terminating an employee is a painstaking process. It requires the nurse leader and manager to conduct a thorough investigation of the incident, collect pertinent data and materials related to performance (e.g., policies and procedures, position description, and standards of practice), and objectively formulate a judgment based on the facts (Cohen, 2006; Hader, 2006). The nurse leader and manager should seek advice from human resources to ensure that the necessary information and documents have been collected to support the termination before contacting the employee to set up a meeting (Cohen, 2006). Planning the meeting in three segments is a strategy the nurse leader and manager can use to present the decision in a professional manner and stay on track. First, the nurse leader and manager should state the reason for the meeting. Second, details of the incident should be presented. The nurse leader and manager must stay objective during this phase and present facts related to the event and the specific policies and procedures and standards that were violated. Third, the employee should be informed of their termination in as straightforward a manner as possible. Terminating an employee is a difficult and stressful task; following a standard procedure, including carefully reviewing all facts, remaining objective, and making an informed decision, only makes it easier (Cohen, 2006; Hader, 2006).

Nurse leaders and managers must ensure that reasonable efforts have been taken to help employees succeed. Allowing poor performance to continue without action can have a deleterious effect on the work environment. Staff morale can be negatively affected when staff members feel that the poor performance of a nurse is not dealt with in a timely manner or is ignored. In fact, nurses who are high performers may begin to slow down their performance, reduce the quality of their own work, or leave an organization if they perceive that nurse leaders and managers tolerate those who are unwilling or unable to perform at a level necessary to deliver safe and quality care (Matheny, 2005).

▶ SUMMARY

A continuing challenge nurse leaders and managers face entails recruiting and retaining new nurse graduates as well as experienced nurses. It is critical for nurse leaders and managers to balance the entry of new nurses with retirement of experienced nurses to ensure "adequate mentorship and retention of wisdom in the workplace" (ANA, 2016, p. 29). Today, it is also important for nurses to learn to work on intraprofessional and interprofessional teams to achieve the shared goal of delivering safe and quality care. Intraprofessional teamwork contributes to overall nurse satisfaction, which in turn leads to safer and higher-quality care. To work in interprofessional teams requires a shift in the health-care culture of individual experts to a cooperative and collaborative team environment. Team members integrate expertise and optimize care for patients. Nurses must be relentless in pursuing and fostering a sense of team and partnership across all health-care professions (ANA, 2010). Nurse leaders and managers can have a positive impact on the stability needed to accommodate the dynamics and complexity of the health-care system by collaborating with patients and families, intraprofessional and interprofessional colleagues, the community, and other stakeholders to achieve mutually beneficial outcomes. Nurse leaders and managers are challenged to promote a healthy work environment and implement plans to make the workplace generationally, culturally, and gender friendly in order to sustain a competent workforce.

Nurse leaders and managers must also effectively manage the workforce. To do so, nurse leaders and managers must consider the nurse's performance related to the position description and organizational performance standards. Performance appraisals can improve staff morale, productivity, and job satisfaction. Finally, nurse leaders and managers must deal with violations of policies and procedures and poor performance immediately to avoid escalation of the problem. Regardless of the reason for poor performance, the goal of corrective action should be to help the employee succeed in their position.

Nurse leaders and managers are critical to the development of successful work teams. A strong synergistic relationship between staff members and nurse leaders and managers results in safe and quality patient-centered care.

NCLEX®-STYLE REVIEW QUESTIONS

Multiple Choice

1. What action would help to promote workforce sustainability in a hospital setting?
   1. Nurse managers hiring new employees to fill positions regardless of whether they have clinical experience
   2. Allowing nursing staff to work overtime
   3. Facilitating an open communication pattern
   4. Nurse managers maintaining fiscal responsibility in budget planning
2. In order to promote clinical competencies for the new graduate nurse, which orientation strategy would be most beneficial?
   1. Didactic work in a classroom setting with other new hospital staff recruits
   2. Taking a computer training class on the hospital's electronic health record system with a designated staff superuser
   3. Working closely with other new graduate nurses to develop collegiality and professional identity
   4. Working with an experienced nurse in a mentor relationship as part of orientation training
3. Which employment option would be most beneficial for a new graduate nurse who has just passed state boards and is newly licensed as a registered nurse?
   1. Orientation training lasting 30 days for a position in an ambulatory care surgical unit
   2. Medical-surgical unit with orientation training lasting 6 months inclusive of self-review and core competencies
   3. Intensive care unit preceptorship lasting 60 days
   4. Orthopedic unit with no structured orientation process
   5. Medical oncology unit with orientation lasting 6 weeks with no assigned preceptor
4. Based on Benner's novice to expert model, which nurse would best serve as a preceptor for a new graduate nurse who is starting the orientation process on a medical-surgical unit and has no prior clinical experience other than nursing school clinical experience?
   1. Charge nurse on the unit with 20 years of experience on that unit
   2. Nurse who has just gotten off orientation but has been a nurse for about 5 years
   3. Nurse who has worked on the unit for 10 years with a varied clinical background including medical-surgical, pediatrics, and obstetrics
   4. Nurse who recently transferred from a different unit in the facility with 15 years of experience in the areas of critical care and medical-surgical settings

5. Which statement best describes what is meant by the term "third-age nurses"?
   1. Refers to individuals who already had a professional career and then went back to school to obtain a nursing license and pursue a nursing career
   2. Nurses who have three academic degrees
   3. A nurse who is within the age group of 50 to 70 years
   4. Nurses who work three 12-hour shifts to satisfy their work-week requirement

6. Nursing management has been tasked with building a new team to address methods that can be used to promote health education in the clinical setting. Members of the previous team were all from the same nursing unit in the hospital. What action should nursing management take in order to build the new team?
   1. Maintain the same member composition
   2. Limit the time allowed for the team to report
   3. Assign individual work to team members and use self-report as the basis for teamwork
   4. Invite more diverse membership

7. Which behavioral action by a charge nurse would indicate an example of *destructive feedback* if observed in a clinical setting relative to a nurse's performance?
   1. Offering the nurse a set of sterile gloves on witnessing that the gloves that the nurse is wearing to perform a procedure have a tear
   2. Telling the nurse that in all your years of nursing experience you have never seen anyone do that in front of a patient
   3. Asking the nurse to provide more detailed information related to the patient's pain assessment
   4. Telling the nurse that she is getting the next admission to the floor

8. Despite best efforts, it has been decided that a nurse is to be terminated based on several recorded action plans without noted improvement or correction of incidents. The nurse manager and the chief nursing officer of the facility are in agreement that the employee meets the criteria for termination. Which department in the facility should also be included in review of the termination procedure?
   1. Hospital Ethics Committee
   2. Medical staff
   3. Human Resources
   4. Clinical Nurse Educator

9. Which behavioral action if observed by a nurse leader would indicate effective coaching style?
   1. Providing constant feedback
   2. Keeping a low profile while looking toward inner self-reflection
   3. Acknowledging a job that is well done
   4. Focusing only on achievement of personal gain

10. You are interviewing a nurse who arrives at the interview using a walker as an assistive device for ambulation. Which question if asked would be construed as violating the American with Disabilities Act of 1990?
    1. "Can you perform the duties listed on the job description without accommodation?"
    2. "Do you need me to repeat the question?"
    3. "Do you think that you can do this job?"
    4. "Do you have a disability?"

Multiple Response

11. In a corrective plan of action, which violations would warrant documenting a written reprimand? *Select all that apply.*
    1. First
    2. Second
    3. Third
    4. Fourth
    5. All violation classes

12. Nursing students are working together in a clinical simulation activity and being monitored by nursing faculty. Which statements if observed by nursing faculty during a clinical simulation activity with nursing students would require the nursing faculty member to intervene? *Select all that apply.*
    1. "What do you think you are doing?"
    2. "I really thought you took nursing school more seriously."
    3. "What you did is so stupid that all I can do is sit here and laugh."
    4. "Do you need any help?"
    5. "Can you provide me with some more information?"

13. What components should be included in an agenda for a meeting? *Select all that apply.*
    1. Time and date of the meeting
    2. Topics to be presented
    3. Individuals who will be providing information
    4. Phone numbers of all participant members
    5. Time allotted to each topic

14. Which statements are accurate with regard to team building? *Select all that apply.*
    1. All nurses should participate in a collaborative manner.
    2. Nurse managers must participate as team leaders in order to be effective.
    3. Team building is an effective way to increase productivity.
    4. Team building is an effective way to decrease costs.
    5. Team leaders should not provide direction and allow for individual team member growth.

15. Which members would be included in an *interprofessional* team approach in the clinical setting? *Select all that apply.*
    1. Selected members from different departments throughout the hospital
    2. All of the nurses who work full time at the facility
    3. Both licensed and nonlicensed employees who work in the hospital setting
    4. A collection of individuals who work in the hospital and/or community of interest who are considered to be stakeholders
    5. Nursing staff and community health department

REFERENCES

American Association of Colleges of Nursing (AACN). (2008). *The essentials of baccalaureate education for professional nursing practice*. Author.

American Association of Colleges of Nursing. (2021). *The essentials: Core competencies for professional nursing education*. Author. https://www.aacnnursing.org/Portals/42/AcademicNursing/pdf/Essentials-2021.pdf

American Association of Critical-Care Nurses. (2016). *AACN standards for establishing and sustaining healthy work environments: A journey to excellence* (2nd ed.). Author. www.aacn.org/wd/hwe/docs/hwestandards.pdf

American Federation of Labor and Congress of Industrial Organizations (AFL-CIO). (2020a). *Unions begin with you*. www.aflcio.org/ what-unions-do

American Federation of Labor and Congress of Industrial Organizations (AFL-CIO). (2020b). *Collective bargaining*. www.aflcio.org/what-unions-do/empower-workers/collective-bargainin

American Nurses Association (ANA). (2010). *Nursing's social policy statement: The essence of the profession*. Author.

American Nurses Association (ANA). (2015a). *The nursing workforce 2014: Growth, salaries, education, demographics & trends [Fast Facts]*. https://www.nursingworld.org/~4afac8/globalassets/practiceand policy/workforce/fastfacts_nsgjobgrowth-salaries_updated8-25-15.pdf

American Nurses Association (ANA). (2015b). *Code of ethics for nurses with interpretive statements*. Author.

American Nurses Association (ANA). (2015c). *Scope and standards of practice* (3rd ed.). Author.

American Nurses Association (ANA). (2016). *Nursing administration: Scope and standards of practice* (2nd ed.). Author.

American Nurses Association (ANA). (2018). *ANA leadership: Competency model*. https://www.nursing world.org/~4a0a2e/globalassets/docs/ce/177626-ana-leadership-booklet-new-final.pdf

American Nurses Association & American Organization of Nurse Executives. (2012). *ANA/AONE principles for collaborative relationships between clinical nurses and nurse managers*. https://www.aonl.org/guiding-principles-collaborative-relationships-between-clinical-nurses-and-nurse-managers

American Organization for Nursing Leadership (AONL). (2010). *AONL guiding principles for the aging workforce*. https://www.aonl.org/system/files/media/file/2020/12/for-the-aging-workforce.pdf

American Organization for Nursing Leadership (AONL). (2015a). *AONL nurse manager competencies*. Author.

American Organization for Nursing Leadership (AONL). (2015b). *AONL nurse executive competencies*. Author.

Benner, P. (1984). *From novice to expert: Excellence and power in clinical nursing practice*. Addison-Wesley.

Bower, F. L., & Sadler, W. A. (2009). *Why retire? Career strategies for the third age nurses*. Sigma Theta Tau International.

Bryant-Hampton, L., Walton, A. M., Carroll, T., & Strickler, L. (2010). Recognition: A key retention strategy for the mature nurse. *Journal of Nursing Administration, 40*(3), 121–123.

Budd, K., Warino, L., & Patton, M. (2004). Traditional and non-traditional collective bargaining: Strategies to improve the patient care environment. *Online Journal of Issues in Nursing, 9*(1), 5.

Buerhaus, P., Auerbach, D., & Staiger, D. (2017). How should we prepare for the wave of retiring baby boomer nurses? *Health Affairs Blog,* May 3, 2017. doi:10.1377/hblog20170503.059894; https://www.healthaffairs.org/do/10.1377/hblog20170503.059894/full/

Cohen, S. (2006). How to terminate a staff nurse. *Nursing Management, 37*(10), 16.

Covey, S. R. (2004). *The 7 habits of highly effective people: Powerful lessons in personal change.* Free Press.

Cronenwett, L., Sherwood, G., Barnsteiner, J., Disch, J., Johnson, J., Mitchell, P., Sullivan, D. T., & Warren, J. (2007). Quality and safety education for nurses. *Nursing Outlook, 55*(3), 122–131.

Disch, J. (2017). Teamwork and collaboration. In G. Sherwood & J. Barnsteiner (Eds.), *Quality and safety in nursing: A competency approach to improving outcomes* (2nd ed., pp. 85–108). Wiley Blackwell.

Gokenbach, V., & Thomas, P. (2020). Maximizing human capital. In L. Roussel et al. (Eds.), *Management and leadership for nurse administrators* (8th ed., pp. 189–226). Jones & Bartlett Learning.

Greiner, A. C., & Knebel, E. (Eds.). (2003). *Health professions education: A bridge to quality.* National Academies Press.

Haag-Heitman, B., & George, V. (2011). Nursing peer review: Principles and practice. *American Nurse Today, 6*(9), 48–52.

Hader, R. (2005). How do you measure workforce integrity? *Nursing Management, 36*(9), 32–37.

Hader, R. (2006). Put employee termination etiquette to practice. *Nursing Management, 37*(12), 6.

Hader, R. (2013). Have you ever found an "I" in team? *Nursing Management, 44*(4), 6.

Halfer, D. (2007). A magnetic strategy for new graduate nurses. *Nursing Economics, 25*(1), 6–11.

Health Resources and Service Administration (HRSA) Bureau of Health Professions. (2013). *The U.S. nursing workforce: Trends in supply and education.* http://bhpr.hrsa.gov/healthworkforce/index.html

Health Resources and Service Administration (HRSA) Bureau of Health Workforce. (2018). *The national sample survey of registered nurses: Brief summary results.* https://bhw.hrsa.gov/data-research/access-data-tools/national-sample-survey-registered-nurses

Interprofessional Education Collaborative Expert Panel (IPEC). (2011). *Core competencies for interprofessional collaborative practice: Report of an expert panel.* Interprofessional Education Collaborative.

Interprofessional Education Collaborative (IPEC). (2016). *Core competencies for interprofessional collaborative practice: 2016 update.* Interprofessional Education Collaborative. https://www.ipecollalborative.org/core-competencies.html

Kalisch, B., & Schoville, R. (2012). It takes a team: Challenging the belief that each patient should be cared for by just one nurse. *American Journal of Nursing, 112*(10), 50–54.

LeBlanc, P. (2014). Leadership by design: Creating successful "TEEAMS." *Nursing Management, 45*(3), 49–51.

Lucian Leape Institute. (2013). *Through the eyes of the workforce: Creating joy, meaning, and safer health care.* National Patient Safety Foundation. http://www.ihi.org/resources/Pages/Publications/Through-the-Eyes-of-the-Workforce-Creating-Joy-Meaning-and-Safer-Health-Care.aspx

Lukas, C., & Andrews, R. (2014). *Four keys to collaboration success.* www.sagemaine.org/uploads/2/7/1/9/2719629/four_keys_to_collaboration_success.pdf

Masters, K. (2014). *Role development in professional nursing practice* (3rd ed.). Jones & Bartlett Learning.

Matheny, P. (2005). Evaluating the performance of health care employees. *Dermatology Nursing, 17*(4), 296, 300.

McConnell, C. R. (2011). Addressing problems of employee performance. *Health Care Manager, 30*(2), 185–192.

McMenamin, P. (2014). *RN retirements—tsunami warning* [Blog post]. https://community.ana.org/blogs/peter-mcmenamin/2014/03/14/rn-retirements-tsunami-warning

Mensik, J. (2014). *Lead, drive & thrive in the system.* American Nurses Association.

Murray, E. J. (2013). Generational differences: Uniting the four-way divide. *Nursing Management, 44*(12), 36–41.

Narayanasamy, A., & Penney, V. (2014). Coaching to promote professional development in nursing practice. *British Journal of Nursing, 23*(11), 568–573.

National Council of State Boards of Nursing (NCSBN). (2011). *Transition to practice: Novice to expert chart* [Preceptor Toolkit]. ncsbn.org/Preceptor-NovicetoExpertchar.pdf

National Council of State Boards of Nursing (NCSBN). (2020). *Transition to practice: Why transition to practice (TTP)?* https://www.ncsbn.org/transition-to-practice.htm

National Federation of Nurses (NFN). (n.d.) *A new day for nurses.* www.nfn.org/media/NFNbrochure-MASTER-091212-SCREEN.pdf

National Nurses United (NNU). (2010–2016). *About us.* www.nationalnursesunited.org/pages/19

Page, A. (Ed.). (2004). *Keeping patients safe: Transforming the work environment of nurses.* The National Academies Press.

Pearce, C. (2007). Ten steps to conducting appraisals. *Nursing Management, 14*(6), 21.

Porter-O'Grady, T., & Malloch, K. (2013). *Leadership in nursing practice: Changing the landscape of health care.* Jones & Bartlett Learning.

Riley, J. K., Rolband, D. H., James, D., & Norton, H. J. (2009). Clinical ladder: Nurses' perceptions and satisfiers. *Journal of Nursing Administration, 39*(4), 182–188.

Robert Wood Johnson Foundation (RJWF). (2011). *What can be done to encourage more interprofessional collaboration in health care?* [issue brief]. www.rwjf.org/content/dam/farm/reports/issue_briefs/2011/rwjf72058

Salas, E., Sims, D. E., & Burke, C. S. (2005). Is there a "big five" in teamwork? *Small Group Research, 36*(5), 555–599.

Sherman, R., & Pross, E. (2010). Growing future nurse leaders to build and sustain healthy work environments at the unit level. *Online Journal of Issues in Nursing, 15*(1), 1.

Smedley, B. D., Stith, A. Y., & Nelson, A. R. (2003). *Unequal treatment: Confronting racial and ethnic disparities in health care.* National Academies Press.

Society for Human Resources Management. (2015). *Interviewing: Guidance on appropriate questions.* www.shrm.org/templatestools/samples/powerpoints/pages/interviewingguidanceon.aspx#

Spector, N., Blegen, M. A., Silvestre, J., Barnsteiner, J., Lynn, M. R., Ulrich, B., Fogg, L., & Alexander, M. (2015). Transition to practice study in hospital settings. *Journal of Nursing Regulation, 5*(4), 24–38.

Teamsters. (n.d.). *Unions 101: A quick study of how unions help workers win a voice at work.* www.teamsters1150.org/pdfmembers_unions101.pdf

The Joint Commission. (2012). *Improving patient and worker safety: Opportunities for synergy, collaboration, and innovation.* Author. www.jointcommission.org/assets/1/18/tjc-improvingpatientandworkersafety-monograph.pdf

Thomas, P. L., McMillan, M., Barlow, P. A., & Becker, L. (2020). Executive coaching as a lever for professional development and leadership in healthcare organizations. In L. Roussel et al. (Eds.), *Management and leadership for nurse administrators* (8th ed., pp. 57–80). Jones & Bartlett Learning.

Tuckman, B. W. (1965). Developmental sequence in small groups. *Psychological Bulletin, 63*(6), 384–399.

Tuckman, B. W., & Jensen, M. C. (1977). Stages of small-group development revisited. *Group & Organization Studies, 2*(4), 419–427.

U.S. Equal Employment Opportunity Commission. (n.d.). *Prohibited employment policies/practices.* http://eeoc.gov/laws/practices/index.cfm

Wachter, R. M., Gupta, K. (2018). *Understanding patient safety* (3rd ed.). McGraw-Hill Medical.

Weaver, A. C., Callaghan, M., Cooper, A. L., Brandman, J., & O'Leary, K. J. (2015). Assessing interprofessional teamwork in inpatient medical oncology units. *Journal of Oncology Practice, 11*(1), 19–22.

Wessel, S. (2015). Start strong: What every new nurse leader should do beginning on day one. *Nurse Leader, 13*(1), 62–64.

Weston, M. J. (2006). Integrating generational perspectives in nursing. *Online Journal of Issues in Nursing, 11*(2), 2.

World Health Organization (WHO). (2010). *Framework for action on interprofessional education and collaborative practice.* www.who.int/hrh/resources/framework_action/en

 To explore learning resources for this chapter, go to FADavis.com

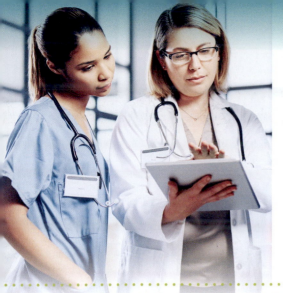

Chapter 12

Creating and Sustaining a Healthy Work Environment

Elizabeth J. Murray, PhD, RN, CNE

LEARNING OUTCOMES

- Discuss the elements of a healthy nursing work environment.
- Describe how effective techniques for safe patient handling and movement affect patient and nurse safety.
- Explore the association between nurse fatigue and patient safety.
- Describe types of workplace violence.
- Identify how nurse leaders and managers can create and sustain a healthy work environment.

KEY TERMS

Bullying
Disruptive behavior
Emergency response plan
Healthy work environment
Incivility
Lateral violence
Nurse fatigue
Security plan
Vertical violence
Workplace safety
Workplace violence

The Knowledge, Skills, and Attitudes Related to the Following Are Addressed in This Chapter:

Core Competencies	• Patient-Centered Care • Teamwork and Collaboration • Quality Improvement • Safety
The Essentials: Core Competencies for Professional Nursing Education (AACN, 2021)	**Domain 2: Person-Centered Care** 2.8 Promote self-care management (p. 32). **Domain 3: Population Health** 3.6 Advance preparedness to protect population health during disasters and public health emergencies (p. 37). **Domain 5: Quality and Safety** 5.2 Contribute to a culture of patient safety (pp. 41–42). 5.3 Contribute to a culture of provider and work environment safety (p. 42). **Domain 9: Professionalism** 9.3 Demonstrate accountability to the individual, society, and the profession (p. 53–54).
Code of Ethics with Interpretive Statements (ANA, 2015)	**Provision 1.5:** Relationships with colleagues and others (p. 4) **Provision 2.3:** Collaboration (p. 6) **Provision 3.4:** Professional responsibility in promoting a culture of safety (pp. 11–12) **Provision 4.4:** Assignment and delegation of nursing activities or tasks (p. 17) **Provision 6.2:** The environment and ethical obligation (pp. 23–24) **Provision 6.3:** Responsibility for the healthcare environment (pp. 24–25)

Nurse Manager (NMC) Competencies (AONL, 2015a) and Nurse Executive (NEC) Competencies (AONL, 2015b)	**NMC: Performance Improvement (p. 4)**
	• Monitor and promote workplace safety requirements
	NMC: Strategic Management (p. 5)
	• Contingency Plans
	  • Manage internal disaster or emergency planning and execution
	  • Manager external disaster or emergency planning and execution
	NEC: Communication and Relationship Building (p. 4)
	• Relationship management
	  • Create a trusting environment by:
	    • Following through with promises and concerns
	    • Establishing mechanisms to follow-up on commitments
	    • Communicating in a way as to maintain credibility and relationships
	• Influencing behaviors
	  • Assert views in nonthreatening, nonjudgmental ways

The Knowledge, Skills, and Attitudes Related to the Following Are Addressed in This Chapter:—cont'd

- Create a vision
- Inspire desired behaviors and manage undesired behaviors

NEC: Business Skills (p. 10)
- Human resource management
  - Evaluate the results of employee satisfaction/quality of work environment surveys
  - Support reward and recognition programs to enhance performance
  - Promote healthful work environments
  - Address sexual harassment, workplace violence, verbal and physical abuse
  - Develop and implement emergency preparedness plans

Nursing Administration Scope and Standards of Practice (ANA, 2016)	**Standard 2: Identification of Problems, Issues, and Trends** The nurse administrator analyses the assessment data to identify problems, issues, and trends (p. 37).
	Standard 5B: Promotion of Health, Education, and a Safe Environment The nurse administrator establishes strategies to promote health, education, and a safe environment (p. 42).
	Standard 14: Quality of Practice The nurse administrator contributes to quality nursing practice (p. 55).
	Standard 16: Resource Utilization The nurse administrator utilizes appropriate resources to plan, allocate, provide, and sustain evidence-based, high quality nursing services that are person, population, or community centered, culturally appropriate, safe, timely, effective, and fiscally responsible (p. 57).
	Standard 17: Environmental Health The nurse administrator practices in an environmentally safe and healthy manner (p. 59).

Source: American Association of Colleges of Nursing. (2021). *The essentials: Core competencies for professional nursing education.* Author; American Nurses Association (ANA). (2015). *Code of ethics for nurses with interpretive statements.* Author; American Nurses Association (ANA). (2016). *Nursing administration: Scope and standards of practice* (2nd ed.). Author; American Organization for Nursing Leadership (AONL). (2015a). *AONL nurse manager competencies.* Author; American Organization for Nursing Leadership (AONL). (2015b). *AONL nurse executive competencies.* Author; Cronenwett, L., Sherwood, G., Barnsteiner, J., Disch, J., Johnson, J., Mitchell, P., Sullivan, D. T., & Warren, J. (2007). Quality and safety education for nurses. *Nursing Outlook, 55*(3), 122–131; and Greiner, A. C., & Knebel, E. (Eds.) (2003). *Health professions education: A bridge to quality.* National Academies Press.

The health-care work environment can affect nurses' overall outlook as well as their own safety and the ability to provide safe and quality nursing care to patients. Unhealthy work environments create stress among nurses and can contribute to adverse events. Work environments that are unhealthy also typically lack civility, respect, and courtesy; in turn, ineffective interpersonal relationships and workplace violence are often tolerated in such climates. In contrast, a healthy work environment leads to work satisfaction, increased retention, effective organizational performance, and improved patient outcomes (Sherman & Pross, 2010). In addition, healthy work environments support meaningful work, joy in the workplace, and safer patient care delivery (Lucian Leape Institute, 2013). A healthy work environment also enhances nurse recruitment and retention and helps sustain an organization's financial viability.

Nurse leaders and managers are responsible and accountable for creating and sustaining a safe and supportive work environment for their staff and patients. However, they face extraordinary challenges in creating a healthy work environment because of the increasing demand for and decreasing supply of registered nurses, reimbursement declines, and constrained resources (Schwarz & Bolton, 2012). This chapter details the elements needed for a healthy work environment, illustrates common challenges, and identifies realistic strategies for nurse leaders and managers to use to create and sustain a healthy work environment.

▶ GUIDELINES FOR BUILDING A HEALTHY WORK ENVIRONMENT

Over the years, nursing organizations have worked to identify elements and competencies for a healthy work environment. A **healthy work environment** "is one that is safe, empowering, and satisfying [...] not merely the absence of real and perceived physical or emotional threats to health but a place of 'physical, mental, and social well-being,' supporting optimal health and safety" (American Nurses Association [ANA], n.d.). A healthy work environment supports excellent nursing care, creates a culture of physiological and psychological safety, and gives nurses the satisfaction of knowing that they are valued and their work is meaningful. The ANA has developed numerous initiatives, position statements, and brochures focusing on what is part of a healthy work environment (e.g., safe patient handling and mobility [SPHM] and healthy working hours) and what is not (e.g., bullying, workplace violence, and nurse fatigue). In 2001, the ANA developed the Nurses' Bill of Rights to help nurses improve their work environment and ensure their ability to provide safe, quality patient care (Wiseman, 2001). The ANA (n.d.) Bill of Rights outlines seven premises regarding necessary workplace expectations for sound professional nursing practice across the United States (Box 12-1). According to the document, nurses have the right to practice nursing in adherence to professional standards and ethical practice, advocate freely for themselves and their patients, and practice in a safe work environment (ANA, n.d.). Although the Bill of Rights is a statement of professional rights and not a legal document, it can assist nurse leaders and managers in the development of organizational policy and in advocating for healthy work environments for staff.

In 2002, the American Association of Colleges of Nursing (AACN) identified eight hallmarks of a work environment that foster professional nursing practice. The AACN's hallmarks represent eight characteristics of the practice setting that best support professional nursing practice and allow baccalaureate and higher degree nurses to practice to their full potential. The hallmarks are intended to apply to all professional practice settings and all types of

---

BOX 12-1 Nurses' Bill of Rights

To maximize the contributions nurses make to society, it is necessary to protect the dignity and autonomy of nurses in the workplace. To that end, the following rights must be afforded:

1. Nurses have the right to practice in a manner that fulfills their obligations to society and to those who receive nursing care.
2. Nurses have the right to practice in environments that allow them to act in accordance with professional standards and legally authorized scopes of practice.
3. Nurses have the right to a work environment that supports and facilitates ethical practice, in accordance with the *Code of Ethics for Nurses With Interpretive Statements.*
4. Nurses have the right to advocate for themselves and their patients freely and openly, without fear of retribution.
5. Nurses have the right to fair compensation for their work, consistent with their knowledge, experience, and professional responsibilities.
6. Nurses have the right to a work environment that is safe for themselves and for their patients.
7. Nurses have the right to negotiate the conditions of their employment, either as individuals or collectively, in all practice settings.

From American Nurses Association (n.d.), with permission.

---

professional nursing practice. AACN has developed a brochure outlining the eight hallmarks:

1. Manifest a philosophy of clinical care emphasizing quality, safety, interdisciplinary collaboration, continuity of care, and professional accountability.
2. Recognize the contributions of nurses' expertise on clinical care quality and patient outcomes.
3. Promote executive level nursing leadership.
4. Empower nurses' participation in clinical decision making and organization of clinical care systems.
5. Maintain clinical advancement programs based on education, certification, and advanced preparation.
6. Demonstrate professional development support for nurses.
7. Create collaborative relationships among members of the health-care team.
8. Use technological advances in clinical care and information systems.

The brochure can be accessed at https://www.aacnnursing.org/News-Information/Position-Statements-White-Papers/Hallmarks-Practice. Nurse leaders and managers in all practice settings can find these hallmarks useful. These elements are key in creating and sustaining a work environment that recognizes professional nurses for their knowledge and skills as well as ensuring retention of nurses (AACN, 2002).

In 2005, the American Association of Critical-Care Nurses developed *Standards for Establishing and Sustaining Healthy Work Environments* to promote the creation of healthy work environments that support excellence in patient care wherever nurses practice. The organization identified six essential standards for establishing and sustaining a healthy work environment (American Association of Critical-Care Nurses, 2016, p. 10):

1. *Skilled communication:* Nurses must be as proficient in communication skills as they are in clinical skills.

2. *True collaboration:* Nurses must be relentless in pursuing and fostering true collaboration.
3. *Effective decision making:* Nurses must be valued and committed partners in making policy, directing and evaluating clinical care, and leading organizational operations.
4. *Appropriate staffing:* Staffing must ensure the effective match between patient needs and nurse competencies.
5. *Meaningful recognition:* Nurses must be recognized and must recognize others for the value each brings to the work of the organization.
6. *Authentic leadership:* Nurse leaders must fully embrace the imperative of a healthy work environment, authentically live it, and engage others in its achievement.

These standards provide an "evidence-based framework for organizations to create work environments that encourage nurses and their colleagues in every health-care profession to practice to their utmost potential, ensuring optimal patient outcomes and professional fulfillment" (American Association of Critical-Care Nurses, 2016, p. 1). These standards also are interdependent (Fig. 12-1), and implementing them requires a commitment throughout the organization. In fact, all nurses have an ethical obligation to establish and sustain work environments conducive to providing safe, quality nursing care (ANA, 2015a). Nurses must promote a work environment that demands "respectful interactions among colleagues, mutual peer support, and open identification of difficult issues" (ANA, 2015a, p. 24). Further, nurses should actively participate in establishing, maintaining, and improving health-care environments and conditions of employment conducive to the provision of quality health care and consistent with the values of the profession.

The American Organization for Nursing Leadership (AONL), formerly the American Organization of Nurse Executives (AONE), met with the Emergency Nurses Association in 2014 to develop a set of guiding principles for reducing violence in the workplace. What resulted was a set of guidelines for nurse leaders and managers to use to decrease and control workplace violence in the hospital setting. The *AONL Guiding Principles: Mitigating Violence in the Workplace* (2014) offers eight principles to reduce lateral and patient and family violence systematically in the workplace (para. 3):

1. That violence can and does happen anywhere is recognized.
2. Healthy work environments promote positive patient outcomes.
3. All aspects of violence (patient, family and lateral) must be addressed.
4. A multidisciplinary team, including patients and families, is required to address workplace violence.
5. Everyone in the organization is accountable for upholding foundational behavior standards, regardless of position or discipline.
6. When members of the health-care team identify an issue that contributes to violence in the workplace, they have an obligation to address it.
7. Intention, commitment, and collaboration of nurses with other health-care professionals at all levels are needed to create a culture shift.
8. Addressing workplace violence may increase the effectiveness of nursing practice and patient care.

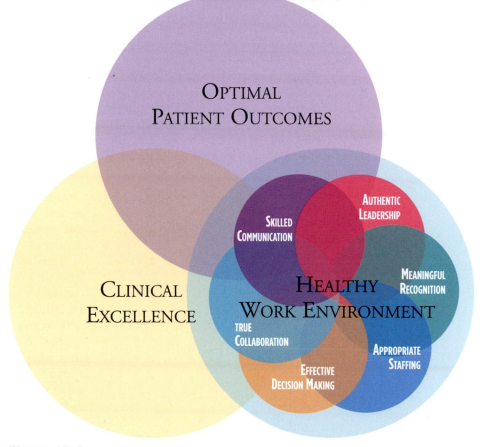

Figure 12-1 Interdependence of healthy work environment, clinical excellence, and optimal patient outcomes. *(From American Association of Critical-Care Nurses, 2016. Reprinted with permission.)*

▶ SAFETY ISSUES IN A HEALTH-CARE ENVIRONMENT

An essential element of a healthy work environment is **workplace safety**, defined by the Lucian Leape Institute (2013) as "a workplace free from risks of both physical and psychological harm" (p. 1). Yet, compared with other occupations, health-care workers have a high number of work-related injuries and illnesses (The Joint Commission [TJC], 2012). The prevalence of physiological injuries among health-care professionals is much higher than in other industries, and psychological harm such as emotional abuse, bullying, and disrespectful treatment is also common (Lucian Leape Institute, 2013). In 2011, an ANA survey completed by 4,614 registered nurses regarding health and safety issues found that major safety concerns of nurses are disabling musculoskeletal injuries and the acute and chronic effects of stress and overwork (L. C. Williams & Associates Research Group, 2011).

Although patient safety programs are prevalent throughout health-care systems, focus on nurse safety is not readily apparent: "Workforce safety in healthcare organizations tends to be considered and managed in silos often unconnected to the work of patient safety" (Lucian Leape Institute, 2013, p. 11). However, patient safety and nurse safety are linked. A systems approach that involves integration of workforce safety efforts with patient safety initiatives fosters a healthy work environment. If conditions exist in a health-care work environment that compromise the physiological and psychological health of nurses, patient safety is jeopardized. Nurse leaders and managers are responsible for ensuring a safe work environment and addressing related problems, the most common being improper patient handling and mobility, nurse fatigue, and workplace violence. In fact, accrediting agencies and the Magnet recognition program include standards that address these issues because they affect patient safety and nurse outcomes.

Safe Patient Handling and Mobility

Registered nurses risk musculoskeletal disorders (MSDs) on a daily basis through activities such as standing for extended periods of time and moving equipment. In the 2011 ANA survey, 62% of nurses reported that developing an MSD was a top concern, 56% indicated that they had experienced musculoskeletal pain that was made worse by their job, and 80% of the nurses surveyed who had pain from MSDs continued working despite experiencing frequent pain (ANA, 2015c). The most common tasks that can lead to MSDs include lifting, transferring, and repositioning patients (ANA, 2015c). In the daily handling and movement of patients, nurses jeopardize their own physical health and the physical health and well-being of their patients (Ogg, 2011). Nursing experts contend "there's no such thing as safe lifting" when nurses use their bodies as lifting mechanisms (Fitzpatrick, 2014, p. 1). Further, they contend that "old school teachings about body mechanics have been proven invalid," and nurses as well as nurse leaders and managers must change the techniques used to move, transfer, and reposition patients.

There are significant clinical consequences of improper and/or awkward patient handling and mobility techniques that can have a negative impact on the quality of care, patient safety, and patient comfort. The two principle methods for lifting and moving patients are the two-person lift and the hook-and-toss methods (TJC, 2012). Use of proper body mechanics and training in lifting techniques have been the sole methods in the United States used to prevent or minimize injuries related to moving patients, yet these methods alone continuously fail to reduce injuries during the delivery of patient care (Krill, Raven, et al., 2012), and they are still prevalent in nursing care (ANA, 2015c; TJC, 2012). Use of body mechanics is simply insufficient to protect nurses from the extremely heavy weight, uncomfortable positioning, and repetition associated with manual patient handling. Commonly, manual lifting results in microinjuries to the spine that may not be noticeable to the nurse immediately but, when cumulative, can result in a debilitating injury (ANA, 2015c).

Many barriers to eliminating the risk of harm exist. Nurses cite specifically the lack of a "no-lift" policy, the lack of adequate lifting equipment, and inadequate space on patient care units as major barriers to the development safe patient handling measures. Lack of equipment, decreased staffing levels, and the architecture of the environment are the three main modifiable attributes to improving the

E X P L O R I N G   T H E   E V I D E N C E   1 2 - 1

L. C. Williams & Associates Research Group. (2011). *American Nurses Association 2011 health and safety survey report: Hazards of the RN work environment.* http://nursingworld.org/FunctionalMenuCategories/MediaResources/MediaBackgrounders/The-Nurse-Work-Environment-2011-Health-Safety-Survey.pdf

Aim

The ANA surveyed 4,614 nurses in 2011 to determine nurses' exposure to workplace hazards and compare findings with those of a similar survey conducted in 2001.

Methods

Data were collected through a Web-based survey. A URL link to the survey was sent out to 73,500 registered nurses in the United States in July 2011.

Key Findings

The major concerns identified by nurses were as follows:

Concerns	2001	2011
1. The effects of stress and overwork	70%	74%
2. Disabling musculoskeletal injuries	59%	62%
3. Contracting an infectious disease	37%	43%
4. Threatened or experienced verbal abuse in past 12 months	57%	52%

Implications for Nurse Leaders and Managers

The findings of this study can help nurse leaders and managers as they assess the workplace for factors that affect worker safety and health. The findings of this study are important to consider when creating and sustaining a healthy work environment.

environment of care and increasing the safety of patient handling and mobility (Krill, Staffileno, et al., 2012).

Furthermore, nurses frequently do not report their injuries, most commonly because nurses believe that they would be letting their patients down, they consider injuries to be part of the profession (e.g., many nurses believe that back pain is expected), and they think that making a report would be pointless (Callison & Nussbaum, 2012).

To effect change and to ensure safer patient handling and mobility, nurse leaders and managers must implement Safe Patient Handling and Mobility (SPHM) programs and establish policies to prevent nurses and patient injuries across the care continuum. They must also gain the knowledge, skills, and attitudes to best create an environment that focuses on minimizing risk of harm to the workforce and patients alike.

A helpful resource for nurse leaders and managers is the set of interprofessional national standards for SPHM developed by the ANA (2013). The SPHM standards outline the roles of nurse leaders and managers as well as staff and encompass the following (ANA, 2013):

- A culture of safety
- A formal and sustainable SPHM program throughout the organization
- An ergonomic-specific approach
- Inclusion of SPHM technology
- An effective system of education, training, and maintaining competence
- Patient-centered assessments and plans of care adapted to meet individual patient needs
- Reasonable accommodations and postinjury return to work for staff members who have been injured
- A comprehensive evaluation system to evaluate SPHM program status

The ANA supports the adoption of "no-lift" policies and the elimination of manual handling nationwide (ANA, 2008). However, the Occupational Safety and Health Administration (OSHA) cannot enforce such policies; rather, it can only require employers to evaluate work environment safety.

As of 2016, 11 states (California, Illinois, Maryland, Minnesota, Missouri, New Jersey, New York, Ohio, Rhode Island, Texas, and Washington) have enacted safe patient handling laws. Additionally, Hawaii has a resolution in place calling for support of safe handling and mobility policies. Of these states, 10 require a comprehensive program in health-care facilities, including an established policy, guidelines for securing appropriate equipment and training, collection of data, and evaluation (Weinmeyer, 2016). In December 2015, legislation on SPHM was introduced in the House of Representatives (H.R. 4266) and the Senate (S. 2408).

The implementation of SPHM programs involving the use of patient handling equipment and devices, education, ergonomic assessment protocols, no-lift policies, and patient lift teams has facilitated the reduction in incidences of workplace injuries. These programs are believed to improve the quality of care for patients, reduce work-related health-care costs, and improve the safety of patients (Krill et al., 2012). Further, they can increase worker satisfaction and increase health-care savings as a result of reductions in worker's compensation, patient falls and pressure ulcers, and employee turnover (ANA, 2013).

LEARNING ACTIVITY 12-1   **Comparing Policies and Procedures With Safe Patient Handling and Mobility Standards**

1. Review the policies and procedures at your current clinical site.
2. Is there a specific policy on safe patient handling and mobility?
3. Compare the policy with the SPHM standards.

Nurse Fatigue

Occupations such as nursing that have extended shifts of more than 12.5 hours, rotating shifts, and higher workloads are associated with worker fatigue and sleep deprivation, both of which can lead to injuries, accidents, and performance errors (TJC, 2012). **Nurse fatigue** is the "impaired function resulting from physical labor or mental exertion" (ANA, 2014, p. 8). Fatigue can be one of three types: physiological, or reduced physical capacity; objective, or reduced productivity; and subjective, a weary or unmotivated feeling (ANA, 2014). Findings from a landmark study (Rogers et al., 2004) indicated that the number of errors and near misses registered nurses make are directly related to the number of hours worked. In addition, nurses who work more than 12.5 hours in 24 hours are three times more likely to make errors than are nurses who work less than 12.5 hours. The Institute of Medicine (Page, 2004) found that prolonged work hours resulted in negative worker performance, including slow reaction times, lapses of attention to detail, errors of omission, and compromised problem-solving. In light of this evidence, the Institute of Medicine recommended that "state regulatory bodies should prohibit nursing staff from providing patient care in any combination of scheduled shifts, mandatory overtime, or voluntary overtime in excess of 12 hours in any given 24-hour period and in excess of 60 hours per 7-day period" (Page, 2004, p. 236).

Another common situation that contributes to nurse fatigue and that can jeopardize patient safety is the lack of rest breaks during working hours. Nurses are notorious for not taking meal breaks or rest breaks during a shift. If and when a nurse takes a break, they will often not completely relinquish patient care responsibilities (TJC, 2012). Although this practice is not safe for patients or nurses, rest breaks are not mandated by federal regulations, and fewer than 25 states currently have legislation enforcing workers' legal rights to breaks (Witkoski & Dickson, 2010). Even though evidence supports recommendations that nurses take uninterrupted breaks, self-care is often sacrificed for patient care. Unfortunately, this is the current cultural attitude, and it puts both patient safety and nurse safety at risk.

There is a well-documented relationship between nurse fatigue and nurse errors that can compromise patient care and safety (ANA, 2014; Bae & Fabry, 2014; Rogers et al., 2004; Witkoski & Dickson, 2010). It is critical to safety and quality care that nurses carefully consider their level of fatigue when accepting a patient assignment that extends beyond the regularly scheduled workday or work week (ANA, 2014). In fact, nurses have an ethical obligation to practice in a manner that maintains patient and personal safety (ANA, 2014). As a patient advocate, nurses must be "alert to and take appropriate action regarding any instances of incompetent, unethical, illegal, or impaired practice by any member of the healthcare team or the healthcare system or any action on the part of others that places the rights or best interests of the patient in jeopardy" (ANA, 2015a, p. 12). Working when fatigued can place the nurse's safety, as well as the patient's, in jeopardy.

Fatigue can result in irritability, reduced motivation, inability to stay focused, diminished reaction time (TJC, 2012), increased risk for errors, decreased memory, increased risk-taking behavior, impaired mood, and ineffective communication skills. It can also have a negative impact on the health and well-being of nurses (ANA, 2014). In December 2011, TJC issued a *Sentinel Event Alert* linking healthcare worker fatigue and adverse events to high levels of worker fatigue, reduced productivity, compromised patient safety, and increased risk of personal safety and well-being (TJC, 2011, para. 1).

Nurses at all levels are obligated to seek balance between their personal and professional lives; fatigue can negatively affect both. Nurses have a responsibility to arrive at work well rested, alert, and prepared to deliver safe, quality nursing care (ANA, 2015a, 2015b). In addition, nurse leaders and managers have an ethical responsibility to foster this balance among their staff members.

Nurses and nurse leaders and managers have a joint responsibility in reducing the risk of fatigue and sleepiness in the workplace. Nurses at all levels should adopt evidence-based fatigue countermeasures and personal strategies to reduce the risk of fatigue (ANA, 2014, p. 4). Some examples include sleeping the recommended 7 to 9 hours within a 24-hour period, taking brief rest periods before work shifts, improving overall health, adopting stress management strategies, taking scheduled meal and rest breaks when working, and taking naps in accordance with organizational policies (ANA, 2014, p. 4).

Nurse leaders and managers are responsible for creating and sustaining a healthy work environment that promotes healthy work schedules. The ANA (2014) offers the following evidence-based strategies that nurse leaders and managers can use to prevent nurse fatigue (pp. 6–7):

- Limiting shifts nurses work to no more than 12 hours in 24 hours and no more than 40 hours per week
- Conducting regular audits to ensure that safe schedule policies are followed
- Ensuring that nurses are able to take scheduled meal and rest breaks
- Establishing policies to allow nurses to take naps during long shifts
- Supporting nurses' decisions to decline working extra shifts or overtime without penalizing them

Nurse leaders and managers must be change agents to develop policies that support evidence-based recommendations for dealing with nurse fatigue. They must monitor overtime to ensure that staff members are not working fatigued, develop flexible work schedules, and implement work schedules with minimal rotation of shifts (TJC, 2012). Nurse leaders and managers are "responsible for establishing a culture of safety; a healthy work environment; and for implementing evidenced-based policies, procedures, and strategies that promote health work schedules and that improve alertness" (ANA, 2014, p. 5).

Workplace Violence

The health-care industry has a long history of tolerating disrespectful behaviors that erode confidence and self-esteem. Many of these behaviors fall under the umbrella of **workplace violence** and create a culture of fear, diminish staff morale, affect patient safety and job satisfaction, and drain joy and meaning from work (Lucian Leape Institute, 2013). Further, workplace violence in health-care settings results in disrupted work relationships, miscommunication, and an unhealthy work environment, and it is linked to negative patient and nurse outcomes.

A review of the literature suggests that workplace violence is a global problem and is not unique to any one specific nursing specialty (Hockley, 2014).

Ruggiero, J. S., & Redeker, N. S. (2013). Effects of napping on sleepiness and sleep-related performance deficits in night-shift workers: A systematic review. *Biological Research for Nursing, 16*(2), 134–142.

Aim

The aim of this study was to critically review and synthesize the literature for evidence of improvements in sleepiness and sleep-related performance deficits following planned naps taken during work-shift hours by night-shift workers.

Methods

The investigators conducted searches in CINAHL, the Cochrane Library, Health and Safety Science Abstracts, MEDLINE, and PsycINFO by using the keyword *nap* along with *performance, fatigue, psychomotor vigilance, sleepiness, shift work, employment,* and *alert.* A total of 2,775 abstracts were retrieved and reviewed for eligibility to include in the systematic review. Original research reports of experimental and quasi-experimental studies included the following:

1. A specifically assigned nap (about 2 hours) taken during a night shift or simulated night shift of 7 to 13 hours in duration and beginning at 5:00 p.m. or later and ending between 6:00 a.m. and 8:00 a.m.
2. Comparison with no-nap conditions
3. The measurement of subjective sleepiness or fatigue or objective measures of sleep-related performance deficits including vigilance, cognitive functioning, logical reasoning performance, work tasks and driving, workload, and memory recall

Thirteen studies that met the criteria were analyzed by the investigators.

Key Findings

The findings of this systematic review indicated that planned naps during a night shift or simulated night shift reduced sleepiness and improved sleep-related performance deficits in some populations and in some settings. The investigators suggested that naps are safe to use in the workplace, and they recommended further research to document the effect of naps on work-specific outcomes (i.e., decision making, errors), as well as larger, randomized control trials.

Implications for Nurse Leaders and Managers

This study supports the need for scheduled rest periods for all workers. The findings provide data suggesting that actual scheduled naps can be beneficial for night-shift workers. Nurse leaders and managers can explore the findings from this study and others to identify data to support implementation of rest and nap periods in the workplace.

The United States is believed to have more workplace violence than any other industrialized nation in the world, and the incidence of violence is higher for health-care workers than for those in other occupations (Nelson, 2014). The World Health Organization, the International Council of Nurses, and Public Services International identified workplace violence as an important universal public health issue (Child & Mentes, 2010; Magnavita & Heponiemi, 2011). A meta-analysis of research studies conducted in 38 countries revealed that approximately 30% of nurses worldwide are physically assaulted and injured, and approximately 60% of nurses have experienced nonphysical violence (Spector et al., 2014).

The National Institute for Occupational Safety and Health (NIOSH) uses the following classifications for workplace violence (NIOSH, 2013):

- Type 1: The perpetrator has criminal intent and no legitimate relationship with the organization or its employees.
- Type 2: The perpetrator is the customer or client, patient, family member, or visitor and has a relationship with the organization and becomes violent while receiving services. This type of workplace violence is very common in health care.
- Type 3: The perpetrator is another coworker or commits worker-on-worker violence. This type of workplace violence includes incivility and bullying and is very common in health care.
- Type 4: The perpetrator has a relationship with a worker but no relationship with the organization. This type of workplace violence involves personal relationships (e.g., an employee is followed to work by their spouse with the intent to threaten or harm the employee).

Nonphysical workplace violence includes emotional abuse, intimidation, put-downs, harassment, humiliation, and humor at the expense of a colleague (Lucian Leape Institute, 2013). Bullying and incivility are two examples of the most prevalent nonphysical workplace violence. **Bullying** is defined as "repeated, unwanted actions intended to humiliate, offend, and cause distress in recipients" (ANA, 2015d, p. 3). Bullying harms, undermines, and degrades others and includes hostile remarks, verbal attacks, threats, taunts, intimidation, withholding of support (ANA, 2015d; McNamara, 2012; Rocker, 2012). **Incivility** is defined as "gossiping and spreading rumors and refusing to assist a coworker (ANA, 2015d, p. 2), disrespect, rudeness, and general disdain for others" (Rocker, 2012, p. 2) that often results in psychological and physiological distress for those involved (Griffin & Clark, 2014). It typically constitutes a continuum of **disruptive behavior** (Fig. 12-2), with nonverbal behavior (eye rolling) on one end of the spectrum and physical violence and tragedy on the other (Clark et al., 2015).

Types of Violence

There are several different types of workplace violence: nurse-to-nurse violence, third-party violence, nurse-to-patient violence, patient-to-nurse violence, organizational violence, external violence, sexual harassment, and mass trauma or natural disasters.

Continuum of Incivility

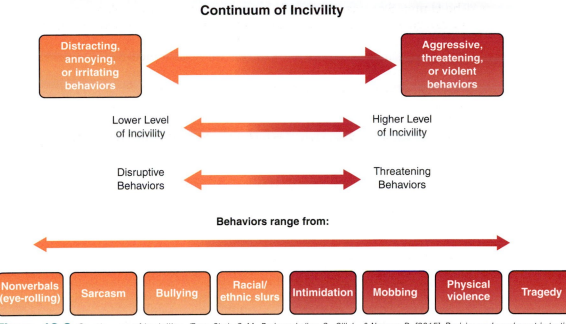

Figure 12-2 Continuum of incivility. *(From Clark, C. M., Barbosa-Leiker, C., Gill, L., & Nguyen, D. [2015]. Revision and psychometric testing of the incivility in nursing education [INE] survey: Introducing the INE-R.* Journal of Nursing Education, 54 *[6], 306–315. Reprinted with permission.)*

Nurse-to-Nurse Violence

Nurse-to-nurse violence, or physical or nonphysical violence between or among nurses who have a workplace relationship, has many other names, such as lateral violence, horizontal violence, and vertical violence. Although these terms are used interchangeably, each has a slightly different meaning, although all can be considered forms of bullying and incivility. Nurse-to-nurse violence falls under the NIOSH type 3 classification and is very common in health care. **Lateral violence** (also known as horizontal violence) consists of bullying or incivility between two or more nurses at the same level. For example, Susan, a registered nurse, is at the end of her shift and is told that Barb will be her relief. Susan says to several other nurses, "I hate to give report to Barb. She asks so many annoying questions." When Barb arrives for report, Susan rudely says, "Don't ask me any questions. I'm tired and want to go home!" The nurses who overhear all giggle. In this situation, Susan was gossiping about Barb and also spoke to her rudely. Both are examples of lateral violence.

In contrast, **vertical violence** consists of bullying or incivility between a nurse subordinate and someone at a higher level (e.g., a manager or charge nurse). For example, in a staff meeting, the nurse leader and manager is explaining to everyone about an upcoming change related to documentation. Several staff nurses ask about who made the decision to make the change. The nurse leader and manager rolls her eyes, sighs loudly, and says, "It was my decision, and I do not appreciate you questioning me!" In this situation, the nurse leader and manager was disrespectful to the nurses in the meeting. In addition, the nurse leader and manager made an important decision without discussing it with the staff members, those who are affected most by the decision. When staff members are not treated with respect, they will not feel valued or appreciated. Repeated experiences such as this can lead to avoidance, communication blocks, and distractions, which ultimately affect patient safety (Lucian Leape Institute, 2013).

Violence among nurses negatively affects the environment of care; roughly 60% of new graduate nurses leave their first nursing position within a year as a result of experiencing workplace violence (Embree & White, 2010). Nurse-to-nurse violence results in a negative community, emotional and physical aftermath, undesirable effects on patient care, and injured associations among coworkers. Nurses must keep in mind that they are called to create "an ethical environment and culture of civility and kindness, treating colleagues, coworkers, employees, students, and others with dignity and respect" (ANA, 2015a, p. 4).

Third-Party Violence

Third-party violence refers to violence that is witnessed directly or indirectly by others. This often occurs when another witnesses nurse-to-nurse violence. The person who observes the violence, the third party, can experience the same harm as the victim of the violence. When a nurse observes another nurse being rude or disrespectful to a coworker, they can experience the same physiological and/or psychological effects as the victim of the actual violence. Research shows that third-party violence jeopardizes the confidence and security of the individual witness, so the perpetrator is actually inflicting harm on secondary victims (Hockley, 2014).

Nurse-to-Patient Violence

Nurse-to-patient violence occurs when nurses are violent toward those in their professional care, with a resulting violation of the nurses' code of ethics (Hockley, 2014). The most blatant example of this type of violence is a nurse hitting a patient. Other examples can be using restraints without an order and refusing to administer pain medication in a timely manner. Often this type of violence involves nurses violating professional boundaries (e.g., asking a patient on a date). Nurses must recognize and maintain boundaries that establish appropriate limits on the nurse–patient relationship. If professional boundaries are jeopardized, nurses have an ethical responsibility to seek assistance and/or remove themselves from the situation (ANA, 2015a).

Patient-to-Nurse Violence

Patient-to-nurse violence involves a patient or family member being violent toward a nurse and falls under the NIOSH type 2 category. A patient hitting or biting a nurse is an example of this type of violence. A family member yelling at a nurse is another example. Factors such as acute disease states, alcohol or drug intoxication, self-harming behavior, or a present exacerbation of a psychiatric disease are major contributors to this type of workplace violence. Intensified states of emotion in patients or their families (e.g., nervousness, distress, despair, sorrow, irritation, or loss of control) are also considered contributing factors to the incidence of workplace violence. Typically, male patients or family members are more likely to execute both physical violence and verbal violence toward nurses who are women (Hockley, 2014). Incidences of assault against male nurses are more likely to occur in a psychiatric setting, whereas female nurses are more likely to be attacked in other specialty areas, with the highest occurrence of violence taking place within the emergency department and psychiatric care environments (Child & Mentes, 2010).

Organizational Violence

Organizational violence affects the entire health-care organization and occurs as a result of a changing work environment (Hockley, 2014). For example, excessive workloads and unsafe working conditions can be considered forms of workplace violence (International Council of Nurses, 2006). Often, this type of violence tarnishes the reputation of the organization, as well as having a negative impact on the employees.

External Violence

External violence is perpetrated by outside persons entering the workplace or when nurses are going to or from the workplace. This type of violence is type 1 according to NIOSH. It is usually random, and the perpetrators typically have criminal intent, such as rape, assault, armed robbery for drugs, or gang reprisals in emergency departments (Hockley, 2014).

Sexual Harassment

Sexual harassment has not received as much attention in recent nursing literature as workplace violence, yet it is still prevalent. Sexual harassment includes "inappropriately friendly behavior, sexually based verbal comments, vulgar, sexual language or inappropriate jokes or stories; unwelcome advances or requests for sexual favors; unwanted physical contact of a sexual nature; and sexual innuendo" (McNamara, 2012, p. 536). In a worldwide sample of 151,347 nurses, approximately one-fourth reported experiencing sexual harassment (Spector et al., 2014).

Sexual harassment in nursing occurs between nurses, between nurses and their supervisors, and between nurses and patients or family members. Many nurses take sexual harassment in stride, view it as part of the job, and decide not to report it. Nurses and nursing students have a right to a workplace free of sexual harassment, and there are legal protections. It falls on nurse leaders and managers to be knowledgeable of federal and state legislation and to ensure that policies and procedures are in place and maintained to protect staff from sexual harassment.

Mass Trauma or Natural Disasters

Workplace violence can also come in the form of mass trauma, such as biochemical attacks or terrorist attacks, and natural disasters. Nurses' work during mass trauma or natural disasters can be extremely stressful and has the potential to cause serious health and mental health issues. However, little research has been done on this type of violence (Hockley, 2014).

| LEARNING ACTIVITY 12-2 | **Reflecting on Workplace Violence During Recent Clinical Experiences** |

Reflect on recent clinical experiences you have had and respond to the following:

1. Have you observed any forms of workplace violence? What type? How did you feel?
2. Were you the victim of workplace violence? What type? How did it make you feel?
3. In the foregoing situations, did you confront the person? What was their response?
4. In the foregoing situations, did you inform your clinical instructor or supervisor? What was their response?

Contributing and Risk Factors

Workplace violence continues to occur for three reasons: because it can, because it is modeled, and because it is left unchecked (McNamara, 2012). TJC (2012) suggests that disruptive behaviors that constitute workplace violence stem from individual and systemic factors. Some individuals who may lack interpersonal coping or conflict management skills can be more prone to disruptive behavior than others. Systemic factors include increased productivity demands, cost containment, and stress from fear of litigation. Inadequate information between organization leadership and staff and a lack of staff involvement in decisions can also contribute to workplace violence (Longo, 2012).

Another contributing factor is that nurses have been expected to cope with violence and accept abuse as part of the job. The pressure, be it spoken or unspoken, put on nurses to remain silent about workplace violence (e.g., more than 80% of incidents of workplace violence go unreported [American Association of Critical-Care Nurses, 2016]) hampers development and implementation of strategies to prevent it.

In terms of which nurses are more at risk for workplace violence, risk factors involve age, gender, nursing experience, and present or previous history of involvement in an abusive relationship. Younger and less experienced nurses are more likely to be victims of workplace violence. This reality may be attributed to the fact that older, more experienced nurses are in positions of management and experience fewer patient and family interactions than younger novice nurses. Nurses in the emergency department also face an increased risk of violence, mostly related to the degree of accessibility (i.e., 24-hour access), amplified noise level, diminished security, elevated stress, and extended wait times (Child & Mentes, 2010).

Consequences

As a result of the underreporting of workplace violence incidents, there is debate on its prevalence. Research has shown that as few as 16% of nurses actually report acts of workplace violence. Some nurses ignore workplace violence because of a lack of knowledge, whereas others fear repercussion if they report it (Kaplan et al., 2010). Lack of time and inadequate administrative support have been identified as reasons that nurses fail to report events; 50% of nurses who reported acts of violence felt as if the hospital administrators neglected to act on it and in some instances that management was punitive and insinuated that the staff instigated the acts of violence (Chapman et al., 2010). Nurses who have been exposed to workplace violence perceive that organizational factors such as the environment of care as well as specific personal factors establish the frequency and character of workplace violence (Chapman et al., 2010). However, the ANA (2015d) contends that any form of workplace violence puts the nursing profession in jeopardy. Further, the ANA contends that those who witness workplace violence and do not acknowledge it, choose to ignore it, or fail to report it are actually perpetuating it (p. 2).

There are many personal consequences of workplace violence, and they can be cumulative. Nurses who are victims of workplace violence can experience physical and psychological problems as a result. Some physical effects include frequent headaches, gastrointestinal upset, weight loss or gain, sleep disturbances, hypertension, and decreased energy (Longo, 2012). The psychological effects may include stress, anxiety, nervousness, depression, frustration, mistrust, loss of self-esteem, burnout, emotional exhaustion, and fear (Longo, 2012). Health-care organizations can also be affected. Workplace violence can result in increased absenteeism, decreased worker satisfaction, and increased attrition. In addition, financial issues arise from increased use of sick pay and paying replacement workers (Longo, 2012).

Environments of care in which nurses perceive that they have a lack of control, work under authoritarian managers, have limited resources, and feel persecuted will lead to low morale and a toxic work environment, which fosters workplace violence. In contrast, a supportive environment with positive teamwork mitigates workplace violence (Embree & White, 2010; Hegney et al., 2010).

Strategies to Prevent Workplace Violence

There are strategies nurse leaders and managers can use to prevent specific kinds of workplace violence, as well as in general. First, nurse leaders and managers must examine the workplace for the presence of elements of an unhealthy environment such as tolerance of incivility and bullying, high levels of stress and frustration among staff members, and a lack of trust among staff members and between staff and management. Next, increasing awareness of workplace violence by providing information at staff meetings can help prevent workplace violence. Nurse leaders and managers can model and promote positive and professional behaviors to foster a healthy environment. In addition, nurse leaders and managers should support the development of organizational zero-tolerance workplace violence programs and policies. Methods to prevent and overcome acts of lateral violence between nurses specifically should also focus on strengthening communication among providers of care. A significant source of stress for all nurses, especially a new nurse entering practice, lateral violence among nurses prohibits the delivery of quality health care. Nurse managers and leaders must ensure that communication is open, nonbiased, and respectful at all times. Nurses must be able to trust their colleagues and believe that they work within a team. Once an incident of workplace violence occurs, nurse leaders and managers should handle the situation by acknowledging the victim, confronting the perpetrator, and informing the perpetrator that such behavior will not be tolerated.

In cases of patient-to-nurse violence, evidence suggests that implementing measures to decrease the incidence of patient and family member attacks on health-care providers has succeeded. First, violence prevention training for staff can curve the onset of an act of violence within the health-care environment and in fact decrease the overall rates of violent incidents at the hands of patients and family members (Kling et al., 2011). Second, the Alert System has been implemented and found to facilitate a reduction of the prevalence of workplace violence. The system is a violence prevention intervention that includes a risk assessment form nurses can use to assess patients and identify those at an increased risk of violence on admission into an acute care setting; if a patient is identified as such, the chart is then flagged for other providers of care so they are aware and can take precautions (e.g., wearing a personal alarm while caring for the patient, having security within the vicinity, not having objects that may potentially be used as a weapon close to the patient surroundings, and not caring for the patient without an additional staff member present) (Kling et al., 2011).

To prevent workplace violence on a wider scale, an environment of care that fosters positive collegial relationships, facilitates open communication among health-care providers, and adopts a zero-tolerance policy for abuse must be cultivated. The ANA (2020) supports a zero-tolerance policy on workplace violence. Nurse leaders and managers can enable an environment of safety that will minimize harm to patients and providers by embracing factors that create a culture of safety, such as effective communication and an organizational reporting system for incidences of workplace violence, as well as valuing the influences that have a positive impact on the quality and safety of the delivery of patient care (Cronenwett et al., 2007).

LEARNING ACTIVITY 12-3

Make a difference

#ENDNURSEABUSE: Take the pledge to reduce nurse abuse here:

• https://p2a.co/DQPJIDH

There are several resources that nurse leaders and managers can use to ensure a healthy, safe work environment. TJC (2012) set standards for addressing workplace violence or behaviors that undermine a culture of safety as well as addressing the fact that behavior that intimidates others can create an environment of hostility and disrespect that affects morale, increases staff turnover, and leads to distractions and errors, all of which compromise patient safety

EXPLORING THE EVIDENCE 12-3

Spector, P. E., Zhou, Z. E., & Che, X. X. (2014). Nurse exposure to physical and non-physical violence, bullying, and sexual harassment: A quantitative review. *International Journal of Nursing Studies, 51*(1), 72–84.

Aim

This study aimed to provide a quantitative review to estimate nurses' exposure rates to workplace violence by types of violence, setting, source, and world region.

Methods

The investigators conducted a meta-analysis of articles using the following key terms: *nurse* or *nursing* and *aggression, bullying, sexual harassment, violence,* and *workplace violence.* In all, 1,216 research reports were identified and narrowed down to 271 reports. The investigators reviewed the articles using the following criteria:

- Reports written in English
- Reports of empirical studies
- Reports related to violence against nurses

A total of 136 research studies were analyzed, including data from 151,347 nurses in 38 countries.

Key Findings

The investigators explored the rate of violence exposure by looking at the percentage of the sample that reported each type of violence and whether they were physically injured. The five types of violence were physical, non-physical, bullying, sexual harassment, and general violence (meaning nurses were asked if they were subjected to some type of violence at work). In all, 36.4% of nurses reported being physically assaulted, 67.2% reported experiencing a nonphysical assault, 37.1% were bullied, 27.9% reported sexual harassment, and 50.5% indicated that they experienced general violence in their workplace. The majority of physical violence was performed by patients and families. In contrast, health-care professionals accounted for the majority of nonphysical violence.

Implications for Nurse Leaders and Managers

This study provides an overview of the presence of workplace violence worldwide. Nurse leaders and managers can use this evidence as they implement workplace violence prevention programs. Understanding the types of violence prevalent and the initiators of the violence can help identify the type of programs necessary. Further, the authors suggested that violence prevention programs should include patients, families, physicians, nurses, and other health-care professionals.

(McNamara, 2012). Nurse leaders and managers can also use the ANA *Code of Ethics for Nurses With Interpretive Statements* (2015a), the ANA *Nursing: Scope and Standards of Practice* (2015b), and the ANA position statement *Incivility, Bullying, and Workplace Violence* (2015d) as guidelines to create and sustain a healthy work environment free of workplace violence. In addition, OSHA *Guidelines for Preventing Workplace Violence for Healthcare and Social Services Workers* (OSHA, 2015) is another valuable resource for nurse leaders and managers and provides violence prevention guidelines and effective ways to reduce risk of violence in the workplace.

Nurse leaders and managers can also look to another model that identifies and addresses quality-of-life issues, including workplace violence, for nurses (Todaro-Franceschi, 2015). The model uses the acronym ART, which stands for **A**cknowledging a problem, **R**ecognizing choices and choosing purposeful actions to take, and **T**urning toward self and others to reconnect with self and the environment in a way that fosters contentment. This model urges nurses to speak up and advocate for themselves rather than remaining silent or "going along to get along," which results in a lose-lose situation. Effective nurse leaders and managers understand that their staff members "want to be heard, understood, and respected for what they bring to the workplace" (Todaro-Franceschi, 2015).

Nurse leaders and managers are responsible to ensure they create a safe work environment, which includes establishing policies and procedures for security plans, emergency response plans, and reporting incidences and events on irregular occurrences.

▶ SECURITY AND EMERGENCY RESPONSE PLANS

All health-care facilities must have security plans in place. In addition, health care organizations should assess emergency preparedness plans, including coordination with local emergency agencies and communication with local and state public health departments. Nurses at all levels must understand their role related to security and emergency response plans.

Security Plans

A **security plan** is a formalized plan of action for addressing a security breach in a health-care facility. The plan typically addresses security issues faced by health-care facilities related to information security, infant abduction, suspicious or dangerous visitors, or admission of a dangerous individual. According to the International Association for Healthcare Security and Safety (IAHHS), security roles and responsibilities should be clearly outlined in the security plan as well as in job descriptions for all employees at all levels (IAHHS, 2018). Security plans can include specific measures such as the following:

- Electronic security systems (e.g., electronic security, intrusion alarms, video surveillance, key code access to restricted areas)

- Physical security systems (e.g., locked units with restricted access—emergency departments to prevent admission of dangerous individuals, pediatric and new-born units to prevent child abductions)
- Staff identification systems (e.g., all staff, physicians, students required to wear identification that identifies them as authorized personnel)
- Controlled access (e.g., all visitors check in and must wear an identification tag)
- Lockdown emergency system to contain a dangerous individual, shooter

Emergency Response Plans

Health-care organizations must be "adequately prepare[d] to meet the needs of patients, clients, residents, and participants during disasters and emergency situations" (TJC, 2020). An **emergency response plan** is a plan of action health-care organizations are required to have in place in the event of a disaster. Health-care organizations may face internal disasters, those occurring within the facility that can jeopardize the safety of patients, staff, and visitors. Examples of internal disasters include fire, bomb threats, active shooter, and bioterrorism. Health-care organizations may also face external disasters, those events occurring outside the organization involving mass casualties that can overload the facility. Examples of external disasters include bus accident with multiple injuries, chemical spill, explosion at a factory, and terrorism. Natural disasters such as hurricanes, tornados, floods, severe storms, wildfires, and pandemics such as Covid-19 can be considered both internal and external disasters due to the risk of danger to those within the facility as well as the community.

All health-care organizations are required to develop emergency response plans, and each state is required to implement crisis standards of care (CSC). The goal of CSC is to help health-care organizations and communities develop plans that allow them to effectively move from providing conventional care, to a contingency response, and to a crisis response when a disaster occurs (TJC, 2015). When developing an emergency response plan, the first step is conducting a risk assessment to identify potential emergencies and hazards. Nurse leaders and managers play a major role in risk assessments, as well as planning, situational response, and postemergency mitigation (ANA, 2016). Further, they must ensure that staff are aware of and prepared for their specific role during an emergency and provide them with necessary resources and training to be prepared. The AONL (2017) developed guiding principles to identify the skills and behaviors nurse leaders and managers need to effectively manage a crisis such as a mass casualty incident, technology outage, labor issues, natural disasters, biohazards, or pandemic (AONL, 2017, para. 3):

1. Nurse leaders are educated in media relations and understand the tenets of good communication.
2. Nurse leaders are skilled critical thinkers, collaborative, and able to manage ambiguity.
3. Nurse leaders project calm, confidence, and authority in all situations.

4. Nurse leaders are prepared to review and practice emergency response plans with staff.
5. The chief nursing office is a member of the organization's senior leadership team whose role is clearly defined.

Nurses at all levels have specific roles during internal and external disasters. Their roles are outlined in the organization's emergency response plan, and it is the responsibility of nurse leaders and managers to ensure everyone knows their roles before a disaster occurs. To ensure preparedness before actual emergencies, health-care organizations are required to carry out emergency drills at least twice a year (TJC, 2015).

▶ SUMMARY

An unhealthy work environment lacks safe patient mobility equipment, ignores nurse fatigue, encourages disruptive behaviors, contributes to poor patient outcomes, increases cost of care, decreases patient satisfaction, and has a negative impact on nurse retention. All nurses, regardless of role, have a responsibility to contribute to a safe and healthy environment that encourages respectful interactions with patients, families, and colleagues (ANA, 2015a). Nurses at all levels and in all settings have a moral obligation to collaborate to create an environment that fosters respect and is free from workplace violence. Nurse leaders and managers have an ethical and legal responsibility to provide a safe and healthy work environment. An environment of mutual respect promotes joy and meaning at work and enables nurses to be more satisfied and able to deliver more effective care. All factors that contribute to an unhealthy work environment must be addressed to ensure quality and promote a culture of safety for both patients and staff. Otherwise, sustaining a culture of safety becomes impossible. Nurse leaders and managers play a major role in establishing and implementing security and emergency response plans.

NCLEX®-STYLE REVIEW QUESTIONS

Multiple Choice

1. Which characteristic is included in the American Nurses Association (ANA) *Nurses' Bill of Rights*?
   1. To function as a patient/client advocate without fear of retribution
   2. Compensation for clinical practice is based solely on the fiscal budget of the employer
   3. Practice setting safety addresses patient/client only
   4. Negotiation for conditions of employment is not included as a basic right

2. Which statement is inaccurate with regard to work-related injuries and illness?
   1. Health-care workers are more likely to experience work-related injuries and illness.
   2. Stress does not play a role in work-related injuries and illness.
   3. Musculoskeletal complaints are typically seen.
   4. Working overtime appears to lead to more work-related injuries and illness.
3. A group of nurses are discussing safe patient handling and mobility on the nursing unit in relation to nurses sustaining musculoskeletal disorders (MSDs). Which statement made by one of the nurses would indicate that additional training was needed?
   1. The most common occurrence for MSDs is when nurses are transferring, lifting, or repositioning patients/clients.
   2. It is important to maintain body principles when repositioning a patient/client.
   3. If done properly, no nursing action will result in acquiring an MSD.
   4. Use of body mechanics while required does not mean that a nurse will not get an MSD.
4. A nurse has worked for over 20 years in the clinical practice setting and is experiencing considerable back pain at the present time. Questions asked by the health-care provider focus on how the nurse implemented lifting actions during the course of her career. The nurse stated that she "used safe body principles throughout her career." Based on this information, what does the health-care provider suspect might account for the nurse's physical complaints?
   1. Undiagnosed scoliosis
   2. Improper use of body mechanics
   3. Microinjuries to the spine over time
   4. Unaware of ergonomic principles as they apply to body mechanics
5. A nurse is reviewing a chart in which a medication error occurred as part of a performance improvement (PI) evaluation. Which notation if observed would indicate a potential contributory factor to the incident based on the concept of *nurse fatigue*?
   1. Clinical response to antibiotic oral medication given by the nurse was not documented.
   2. The physician's order was signed off.
   3. The pain assessment profile before medication being administered was noted as 9 out of 10.
   4. The nurse who had administered the medication was working his third shift in a row, which was considered to be an overtime shift.

6. A worker on the nursing unit has become increasingly frustrated with the work environment and is becoming more aggressive with the rest of the staff. How would this be classified according to the National Institute for Occupational Safety and Health (NIOSH)?
   1. Type 3
   2. Type 1
   3. Type 2
   4. Type 4
7. Which situation, if observed, would warrant immediate action by the nurse manager?
   1. Staff nurse asks for additional clarification from the physician related to a written order.
   2. Unit secretary asks the nurses to answer the unit phone when she is busy.
   3. Unit secretary draws caricature images of nursing staff with sarcastic comments.
   4. Two nurses who work days are switching their days for the last 2 weeks of the schedule.
8. An experienced nurse on the medical-surgical unit has a pattern of making rude statements about her coworkers. These repeated statements have become part of the unit culture. How would the nurse manager who has observed these interactions categorize this type of behavior in terms of violence?
   1. Hearsay
   2. Nurse to patient
   3. Vertical
   4. Horizontal
9. Which action would help to promote a nurse in becoming a skilled communicator?
   1. Limit reflective practices and focus on present interaction.
   2. Focus on individual thoughts and beliefs.
   3. Believe that all conversations contain credible information.
   4. Become more candid.
10. Which statement by a nursing staff member indicates that incivility has occurred on the nursing unit?
    1. "I wish that I didn't have to take that assignment."
    2. "I always end up staying late to complete my documentation and that makes me upset."
    3. "They seem to keep hiring the same type of people here, those who don't want to work and then I have to keep doing their job."
    4. "I respect my nurse manager but I don't like her as a person."

11. There was a violent incident on the medical-surgical unit that occurred between a staff worker and the worker's spouse. How would this be classified according to the National Institute for Occupational Safety and Health (NIOSH)?
    1. Type 1
    2. Type 2
    3. Type 3
    4. Type 4
12. Which observation, if noted on a performance evaluation, would require that the supervisor speak with the nurse in order to promote a healthy work environment?
    1. Works an overtime shift once every few months
    2. Follows policies and procedures
    3. Refuses to take breaks while working shifts
    4. Takes more time to document using the electronic documentation system compared with other more experienced nurses

Multiple Response

13. What factors would help to contribute to nurses being injured during delivery of client care? *Select all that apply.*
    1. Implementation of manual lifting
    2. Two-person lift
    3. One-person lift
    4. Hook-and-toss method
    5. Discontinuing "no lift" policy
14. According to the American Association of Colleges of Nursing (AACN), what hallmarks help to support a healthy work environment? *Select all that apply.*
    1. Empowerment of nurses
    2. Focusing on clinical advancement through educational programs
    3. Fostering of collaborative relationships
    4. Limiting use of technology interfaces
    5. Focusing on medical executives
15. According to the American Association of Critical-Care Nurses, what standards help to support a healthy work environment? *Select all that apply.*
    1. Closed-ended communication
    2. Adequate staffing
    3. Standards established that are independent
    4. True collaboration
    5. Authentic leadership

REFERENCES

American Association of Colleges of Nursing (AACN). (2002). *Hallmarks of the professional nursing practice environment* [white paper]. www.aacn.nche.edu/publications/white-papers/hallmarks-practice-environment

American Association of Colleges of Nursing. (2021). *The essentials: Core competencies for professional nursing education.* Author. https://www.aacnnursing.org/Portals/42/AcademicNursing/pdf/Essentials-2021.pdf

American Association of Critical-Care Nurses. (2016). *AACN standards for establishing and sustaining healthy work environments: A journey to excellence* (2nd ed.). Author. http://www.aacn.org/wd/hwe/docs/hwestandards.pdf

American Nurses Association (ANA). (n.d.). *Healthy work environment: Nurses' bill of rights.* https://www.nursingworld.org/practice-policy/work-environment/

American Nurses Association (ANA). (2008). *Elimination of manual patient handling to prevent work-related musculoskeletal disorders* [position statement]. https://www.nursingworld.org/practice-policy/nursing-excellence/official-position-statements/id/elimination-of-manual-patient-handling/

American Nurses Association (ANA). (2013). *Guide to the safe patient handling and mobility interprofessional national standards.* Author.

American Nurses Association (ANA). (2014). *Addressing nurse fatigue to promote safety and health: Joint responsibilities of registered nurses and employers to reduce risks* [revised position statement]. https://www.nursingworld.org/practice-policy/nursing-excellence/official-position-statements/id/addressing-nurse-fatigue-to-promote-safety-and-health/

American Nurses Association (ANA). (2015a). *Code of ethics for nurses with interpretive statements.* Author.

American Nurses Association (ANA). (2015b). *Nursing scope and standards of practice* (3rd ed.). Author.

American Nurses Association (ANA). (2015c). *Safe patient handling & mobility: Understanding the benefits of a comprehensive SPHM program.* https://www.nursingworld.org/~498de8/globalassets/practiceandpolicy/work-environment/health—safety/ana-sphmcover__finalapproved.pdf

American Nurses Association (ANA). (2015d). *Incivility, bullying, and workplace violence* [position statement]. http://nursingworld.org/MainMenuCategories/Policy-Advocacy/Positions-and-Resolutions/ANAPositionStatements/Position-Statements-Alphabetically/Incivility-Bullying-and-Workplace-Violence.html

American Nurses Association (ANA). (2016). *Nursing administration: Scope and standards of practice* (2nd ed.). Author.

American Nurses Association (ANA). (2020). *#Endnurseabusepanel.* https://www.nursingworld.org/get-involved/share-your-expertise/pro-issues-panel/end-nurse-abuse/

American Organization for Nursing Leadership (AONL). (2015a). *AONL nurse manager competencies.* Author.

American Organization for Nursing Leadership (AONL). (2015b). *AONL nurse executive competencies.* Author.

American Organization for Nursing Leadership (AONL). (2017). *AONL guiding principles: Role of the nurse leader in crisis management.* Author.

American Organization for Nursing Leadership (AONL). (2014). *AONL guiding principles: Mitigating violence in the workplace.* https://www.aonl.org/guiding-principles-mitigating-violence-workplace

Bae, S. H., & Fabry, D. (2014). Assessing the relationships between nurse work hours/overtime and nurse and patient outcomes: Systematic literature review. *Nursing Outlook, 62*(2), 138–156.

Callison, M. C., & Nussbaum, M. A. (2012). Identification of physically demanding patient-handling tasks in an acute care hospital: Task analysis and survey results. *International Journal of Industrial Ergonomics, 42,* 261–267.

Chapman, R., Styles, I., Perry, L., & Combs, S. (2010). Examining the characteristics of workplace violence in one non-tertiary hospital. *Journal of Clinical Nursing, 19*(3–4), 479–488.

Child, R. J., & Mentes, J. C. (2010). Violence against women: The phenomenon of workplace violence against nurses. *Issues in Mental Health Nursing, 31*(2), 89–95.

Clark, C. M., Barbosa-Leiker, C., & Gill, L., Nguyen, D. T. (2015). Revision and psychometric testing of the incivility in nursing education (INE) survey: Introducing the INE-R. *Journal of Nursing Education, 54*(6), 306–315.

Cronenwett, L., Sherwood, G., Barnsteiner, J., Disch, J., Johnson, J., Mitchell, P., Sullivan, D. T., & Warren, J. (2007). Quality and safety education for nurses. *Nursing Outlook, 55*(3), 122–131.

Embree, J. L., & White, A. H. (2010). Concept analysis: Nurse-to-nurse lateral violence. *Nursing Forum, 45*(3), 166–173.

Fitzpatrick, M. A. (2014). Safe patient handling and mobility: A call to action. *American Nurse Today, 9*(9), 1.

Greiner, A. C., & Knebel, E. (Eds.) (2003). *Health professions education: A bridge to quality.* National Academies Press.

Griffin, M., & Clark, C. M. (2014). Revisiting cognitive rehearsal as an intervention against incivility and lateral violence in nursing: 10 years later. *Journal of Continuing Education in Nursing, 45,* 535–542.

Hegney, D., Tuckett, A., Parker, D., & Eley, R. M. (2010). Workplace violence: Differences in perceptions of nursing work between those exposed and those not exposed: A cross-sector analysis. *International Journal of Nursing Practice, 16*(2), 188–202.

Hockley, C. (2014). Violence in nursing: The expectations and the reality. In C. J. Huston (Ed.), *Professional issues in nursing: Challenges and opportunities* (3rd ed., pp. 201–213). Lippincott Williams & Wilkins.

International Association for Healthcare Security and Safety (IAHHS). (2018). *Healthcare security industry guidelines.* Author.

International Council of Nurses. (2006). *Abuse and violence against nursing personnel* [ICN position statement]. Author.

Kaplan, K., Mestel, P., & Feldman, D. L. (2010). *Creating a culture of mutual respect. AORN Journal, 91*(4), 495–510.

Kling, R. N., Yassi, A., Smailes, E., Lovato, C. Y., & Koehoorn, M. (2011). Evaluation of a violence risk assessment system (the Alert System) for reducing violence in an acute hospital: A before and after study. *International Journal of Nursing Studies, 48*(5), 534–539.

Krill, C., Raven, C., & Staffileno, B. A. (2012). Moving from a clinical question to research: The implementation of a safe patient handling program. *Medsurg Nursing, 21*(2), 104–106.

Krill, C., Staffileno, B. A., & Raven, C. (2012). Empowering staff nurses to use research to change practice for safe patient handling. *Nursing Outlook, 60*(3), 157–162.

L. C. Williams & Associates Research Group. (2011). *American Nurses Association 2011 health and safety survey report: Hazards of the RN work environment.* http://nursingworld.org/FunctionalMenu Categories/MediaResources/MediaBackgrounders/The-Nurse-Work-Environment-2011-Health-Safety-Survey.pdf

Longo, J. (2012). *Bullying in the workplace: Reversing a culture.* American Nurses Association.

Lucian Leape Institute. (2013). *Through the eyes of the workforce: Creating joy, meaning, and safer health care.* http://www.ihi.org/resources/Pages/Publications/Through-the-Eyes-of-the-Workforce-Creating-Joy-Meaning-and-Safer-Health-Care.aspx

Magnavita, N., & Heponiemi, T. (2011). Workplace violence against nursing students and nurses: An Italian experience. *Journal of Nursing Scholarship, 43*(2), 203–210.

McNamara, S. A. (2012). Incivility in nursing: Unsafe nurse, unsafe patients. *AORN Journal, 95*(4), 535–540.

National Institute for Occupational Safety and Health (NIOSH). (2013). *Workplace violence prevention for nurses.* CDC Course No. WB1865-NIOSH Pub. 2013-155. www.cdc.gov/niosh/topics/violence/training_nurses.html

Nelson, R. (2014). Tackling violence against health-care workers. *Lancet, 383*(9926), 1373–1374.

Occupational Safety and Health Administration (OSHA). (2015). *Guidelines for preventing workplace violence for healthcare and social service workers.* www.osha.gov/Publications/osha3148.pdf

Ogg, M. J. (2011). Introduction to the safe patient handling and movement series. *AORN Journal, 93*(3), 331–333.

Page, A. (Ed.). (2004). *Keeping patients safe: Transforming the work environment of nurses.* National Academies Press.

Rocker, C. F. (2012). Responsibility of a frontline manager regarding staff bullying. *Online Journal of Issues in Nursing, 18*(2), 6.

Rogers, A. E., Hwang, W. T., Scott, L. D., Aiken, L. H., & Dinges, D. F. (2004). The working hours of hospital staff nurses and patient safety. *Health Affairs, 23*(4), 202–212.

Ruggiero, J. S., & Redeker, N. S. (2013). Effects of napping on sleepiness and sleep-related performance deficits in night-shift workers: A systematic review. *Biological Research for Nursing, 16*(2), 134–142.

Schwarz, D. B., & Bolton, L. B. (2012). Leadership imperative: Creating and sustaining healthy workplace environments. *Journal of Nursing Administration, 42*(11), 499–501.

Sherman, R., & Pross, E. (2010). Growing future nurse leaders to build and sustain healthy work environments at the unit level. *Online Journal of Issues in Nursing, 15*(1), 1.

Spector, P. E., Zhou, Z. E., & Che, X. X. (2014). Nurse exposure to physical and nonphysical violence, bullying, and sexual harassment: A quantitative review. *International Journal of Nursing Studies, 51*(1), 72–84.

The Joint Commission (TJC). (2011). *The Joint Commission sentinel event alert: Health care worker fatigue and patient safety* (issue 48). www.jointcommission.org/assets/1/18/SEA_48.pdf

The Joint Commission (TJC). (2012). *Improving patient and worker safety: Opportunities for synergy, collaboration and innovation.* Author. www.jointcommission.org/assets/1/18/TJC-ImprovingPatientAndWorkerSafety-Monograph.pdf

The Joint Commission (TJC). (2015). *Emergency Management: Getting started with the crisis standards of care.* https://store.jcrinc.com/emergency-management-getting-started-with-the-crisis-standards-of-care-part-1-/

The Joint Commission (TJC). (2020).*Emergency management.* https://www.jointcommission.org/resources/patient-safety-topics/emergency-management/

Todaro-Franceschi, V. (2015). The ART of maintaining the "care" in healthcare. *Nursing Management, 46*(6), 53–55.

Weinmeyer, R. (2016). Safe patient handling laws and programs for health care workers. *American Medical Association Journal of Ethics, 18*(4), 416–421. https://journalofethics.ama-assn.org/article/safe-patient-handling-laws-and-programs-health-care-workers/2016-04

Wiseman, R. (2001). The ANA develops bill of rights for registered nurses. *American Journal of Nursing, 101*(11), 55–56.

Witkoski, A., & Dickson, V. V. (2010). Hospital staff nurses' work hours, meal periods, and rest breaks: A review from an occupational health nurse perspective. *AAOHN Journal, 58*(11), 489–497.

To explore learning resources for this chapter, go to FADavis.com

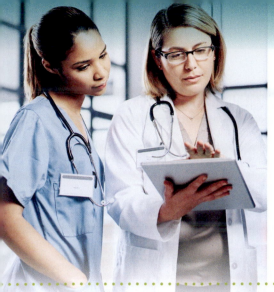

Organizing Patient Care and Staffing for Patient Safety

Elizabeth J. Murray, PhD, RN, CNE

LEARNING OUTCOMES

- Compare and contrast various care delivery models.
- Explore how innovative care delivery can affect patient, staff, and organizational outcomes.
- Apply nursing prioritization frameworks to prioritizing patient care.
- Analyze causes for the current nursing shortage and its impact on safe staffing.
- Describe the core concepts of staffing.
- Examine the relationship among nurse staffing levels, staff mix, and the quality of patient care.
- Discuss the correlation between nursing-sensitive indicators and staffing levels.
- Discuss the importance of monitoring and evaluating productivity and staffing effectiveness.

KEY TERMS

Appropriate staffing
Care delivery models
Clinical Nurse Leader Model
Differentiated Nursing Practice Model
Functional nursing
Nursing case management
Nursing-sensitive quality indicators
Partnership models
Patient acuity
Patient-centered care
Patient classification system
Patient-focused care
Primary nursing
Prioritization
Professional Nursing Practice Model
Skill mix
Staffing mix
Staffing plan
Synergy Model for Patient Care
Team nursing
Total patient care
Transforming Care at the Bedside
Unit intensity
Units of service
Workload

The Knowledge, Skills, and Attitudes Related to the Following Are Addressed in This Chapter:

Core Competencies	• Patient-Centered Care • Teamwork and Collaboration • Safety • Quality Improvement • Informatics
The Essentials: Core Competencies for Professional Nursing Education (AACN, 2021)	**Domain 2: Person-Centered Care** 2.1 Engage with the individual in establishing a caring relationship (p. 28). 2.2 Communicate effectively with individuals (pp. 28–29). 2.9 Provide care coordination (pp. 32–33). **Domain 6: Interprofessional Partnerships** 6.1 Communicate in a manner that facilitates a partnership approach to quality care delivery (p. 43). 6.2 Perform effectively in different team roles, using principles and values of team dynamics (p. 44). **Domain 7: Systems-Based Practice** 7.1 Apply knowledge of systems to work effectively across the continuum of care (p. 46). 7.3 Optimize system effectiveness through application of innovation and evidence-based practice (p. 47).
Code of Ethics with Interpretive Statements (ANA, 2015)	**Provision 2.3:** Collaboration (p. 6) **Provision 4.1:** Authority, accountability, and responsibility (p. 15) **Provision 4.2:** Accountability for nursing judgments, decisions, and actions (pp. 15–16) **Provision 4.3:** Responsibility for nursing judgments, decisions, and actions (pp. 16–17) **Provision 4.4:** Assignment and delegation of nursing activities or tasks (p. 17) **Provision 6.2:** The environment and ethical obligation (pp. 23–24)

Nurse Manager (NMC) Competencies (AONL, 2015a) and Nurse Executive (NEC) Competencies (AONL, 2015b)	**NMC: Human Resource Management (p. 4)**
	• Staffing needs
	  • Evaluate staffing patterns
	  • Match staff competency with patient acuity
	NMC: Appropriate Clinical Practice Knowledge (p. 5)
	• Each role and institution has expectations regarding the clinical knowledge and skill required of the role. These expectations should be established for the specific individual based on organizational requirements.
	NEC: Knowledge of the Health Care Environment (pp. 6–7)
	• Clinical practice knowledge
	  • Demonstrate knowledge of current nursing practice and the roles and functions of patient care teams

The Knowledge, Skills, and Attitudes Related to the Following Are Addressed in This Chapter:—cont'd

- Communication patient care standards as established by accreditation, regulatory, and quality agencies
- Delivery models/work design
  - Demonstrate current knowledge of patient care delivery systems across the continuum
  - Describe various delivery systems and age appropriate patient care models and the advantages/disadvantages of each
  - Assess the effectiveness of delivery models
  - Develop new delivery models
- Evidence-based practice/outcome measurement and research
  - Allocate nursing resources based on measurement of patient acuity/care needed

Nursing Administration Scope and Standards of Practice (ANA, 2016)	**Standard 5A: Coordination** The nurse administrator coordinates implementation of the plan and associated processes (p. 41).
	Standard 9: Communication The nurse administrator communicates effectively in all areas of practice (p. 49).
	Standard 10: Collaboration The nurse administrator collaborates with healthcare consumers, colleagues, community leaders, and other stakeholders to advance nursing practice and healthcare transformation (p. 50).
	Standard 11: Leadership The nurse administrator leads within professional practice setting, profession, healthcare industry, and society (pp. 51–52).
	Standard 14: Quality of Practice The nurse administrator contributes to quality nursing practice (p. 55).

Source: American Association of Colleges of Nursing. (2021). *The essentials: Core competencies for professional nursing education.* Author; American Nurses Association (ANA). (2015). *Code of ethics for nurses with interpretive statements.* Author; American Nurses Association (ANA). (2016). *Nursing administration: Scope and standards of practice* (2nd ed.). Author; American Organization for Nursing Leadership. (2015a). *AONL nurse manager competencies.* Author; American Organization for Nursing Leadership. (2015b). *AONL nurse executive competencies.* Author; Cronenwett, L., Sherwood, G., Barnsteiner, J., Disch, J., Johnson, J., Mitchell, P., Sullivan, D. T., & Warren, J. (2007). Quality and safety education for nurses. *Nursing Outlook, 55*(3), 122–131; and Greiner, A. C., & Knebel, E. (Eds.). (2003). *Health professions education: A bridge to quality.* National Academies Press.

Organizing patient care is a critical role for nursing leaders and managers, whether in a hospital, a skilled nursing facility, home care, or other health-care settings. The primary goal when organizing patient care is delivering safe and quality nursing care using available resources effectively. In addition, the ability to effectively prioritize nursing care is a necessary skill for nurses at all levels. Regardless of the type of model used for organizing patient care, nurse leaders and managers must make sure that appropriate staffing is implemented and sustained to ensure safe, effective, and quality nursing care is provided.

In this chapter, the major components of organizing patient care are covered, including identifying, implementing, and monitoring a care delivery model; using frameworks for prioritizing nursing care; determining staffing needs for safe, effective, and quality care; developing and implementing a staffing plan; and evaluating staffing effectiveness.

▶ CARE DELIVERY MODELS

Care delivery models are used to organize and deliver nursing care and focus on structure, process, and outcomes (Duffield et al., 2010; Neisner & Raymond, 2002; Wolf & Greenhouse, 2007). Additionally, care delivery models serve to drive assessments, decisions, planning, organization, and evaluation of structures, processes, and outcomes (Wolf & Greenhouse, 2007). These models have evolved over the past century in response to issues such as war, politics, economics, social environment, technology, and advances in health care. The care delivery model used in an organization is usually determined by nurse leaders and managers at the executive level, with the model chosen reflective of the organizational mission, philosophy, and goals. Nurse leaders and managers at the unit level should have input regarding the model chosen to ensure that it is appropriate for the unit, skill mix, number of nursing personnel available, and the acuity of the patients. Unit level leaders and managers are also responsible for implementing, monitoring, and evaluating the effectiveness, efficiency, and outcomes of the selected care delivery model. Frontline nurses should assist in monitoring and evaluating outcomes of the process.

Nursing care delivery models address five questions (Neisner & Raymond, 2002, p. 8):

1. Who is responsible for making decisions about patient care?
2. How long do that person's decisions remain in effect?
3. How is work distributed among staff members: by task or by patient?
4. How is patient care communication handled?
5. How is the whole unit managed?

Care delivery models must foster effective communication and also balance the needs of the patients with the competencies and availability of the nursing staff. Models of care provide for continuity of care across the continuum and give nurses the authority and responsibility for the provision of nursing care (Kaplow & Reed, 2008). To be effective, care delivery models should be in alignment with the organization, sustainable over time, and replicable (Wolf & Greenhouse, 2007). Regardless of the care delivery model employed, nurse leaders and managers have a responsibility to ensure that safe and quality patient care is provided by competent nursing staff. The American Organization for Nursing Leadership (AONL), formerly known as the American Organization of Nurse Executives (AONE), contends that nurse leaders and managers will need to participate in redesigning nursing care delivery in the future by focusing on patient- and family-centered care, ensuring that frontline nurses participate in the decision-making process, and optimizing nursing roles and care across the continuum (AONL, 2010). In addition, the AONL includes effective use of delivery models as a component of the knowledge of the health-care environment competency (AONL, 2015b, p. 6) in the following ways:

- Demonstrate current knowledge of patient care delivery systems across the continuum.
- Describe various delivery systems and patient care models and the advantages/ disadvantages of each.
- Assess the effectiveness of new care delivery models.
- Align care delivery models and staff performance with key safety and economic drivers.

There are many care delivery models in use today, classified as traditional, non-traditional, and contemporary models.

Traditional Models

Traditional care models are rooted in nursing's historical beginnings. The best-known traditional models of care delivery are total patient care, functional nursing, team nursing, primary nursing, and nursing case management. Many of these models are still in use today, with many newer models incorporating aspects of traditional models.

Total Patient Care

Total patient care, also known as case method, is the oldest model of care delivery. At the turn of the 20th century, nursing care took place in the patient's home. The nurse was responsible for complete nursing care of the patient as well as other duties, such as cooking and cleaning. As nursing care transitioned into the hospital in the 1930s, total patient care remained the principal care delivery model (Tiedeman & Lookinland, 2004). In the total patient care method, often used in settings such as critical care and hospice care, the nurse provides holistic care. When used in a hospital setting, total patient care is provided by one nurse during a shift; communication is hierarchical, and the charge nurse is responsible for making assignments, interfacing with physicians, and shift reports. Some variations of this method are in use today.

Functional Nursing

During World War II, a nursing shortage developed in response to increased demands for nurses abroad, resulting in a need to reorganize nursing care in hospitals stateside. **Functional nursing** was implemented as a means to accomplish patient care with the assistance of ancillary personnel. In this model, staff members work side by side and are assigned to complete specific tasks, such as passing medications, taking vital signs, and providing hygiene, for all or many patients on a unit (Tiedeman & Lookinland, 2004). Although it was intended to be used as a temporary mode of care delivery until nurses returned from the war, with the increase in population after World War II functional nursing continued in popularity because of efficient management of time, tasks, and resources. Because this model allows care to be provided by a limited number of registered nurses (RNs), it is often used today in long-term care and ambulatory care facilities. Although the functional model is viewed as efficient and cost effective, it can also result in fragmented care because nurses focus on physician's orders and necessary tasks. This model does not promote autonomy or professional development (Tiedeman & Lookinland, 2004). Communication is hierarchical, and the charge nurse is primarily responsible for assigning shifts, supervising tasks, interfacing with physicians, and writing shift reports.

Team Nursing

In response to criticism of functional nursing, **team nursing** was designed. In team nursing, licensed and unlicensed personnel collaborate to deliver total care for a group of patients under the direction of a team leader. Typically, the team leader is an RN and is responsible for the following: assigning duties to team members, based on licensure, education, ability, and competence; supervising care provided; and providing more complex care. In this model, the team leader must have effective communication skills and the necessary experience to provide strong leadership for their team (Tiedeman & Lookinland, 2004). Typically, the team leader is responsible for interfacing with physicians and providing shift reports to the oncoming team leader. In some modifications, communication can be hierarchical, and the charge nurse is responsible for related tasks directly. Some adapted versions of team nursing are still in use today on medical-surgical units.

Primary Nursing

Developed in 1968, **primary nursing** brought the RN back to the bedside. Initially, this model was developed for inpatient units on which an RN managed care for a group of patients for 24 hours a day, 7 days a week throughout their hospital stay (Manthey, 2009). When the primary nurse is not available, an associate nurse cares for the same group of patients and follows the plan of care developed by the primary nurse. In primary nursing it is feasible for a patient to be cared for by only two nurses over a 72-hour period if the nurses work 12-hour shifts; a major advantage is continuity of care.

The primary nursing model fosters a strong relationship between the nurse and the patient and their family because much of the decision making occurs at the bedside (Tiedeman & Lookinland, 2004). Primary nursing is popular in situations in which one nurse manages care for an extended number of hours or on a long-term basis, such as in ambulatory care units and home health-care settings (Manthey, 2009). In this model, communication is lateral, with the primary nurse being responsible for direct care, interfacing with physicians and other members of the health-care team, and providing shift reports.

Nursing Case Management

In an attempt to improve the cost effectiveness of patient care, **nursing case management** emerged in the late 1980s (Neisner & Raymond, 2002). Nursing case management was borrowed from social work, psychiatric settings, and community health. The goal of nursing case management is to organize patient care according to major diagnostic-related groups to achieve measurable quality outcomes while meeting predetermined time frames and costs. Case management focuses on decreasing fragmented care, improving patient self-care and quality of life, and optimizing use of resources and decreasing costs (Neisner & Raymond, 2002, p. 11). The RN functions as a case manager and is assigned to coordinate care for high-risk populations, such as patients with congestive heart failure, and manage care from admission through discharge. Historically, case management was used primarily in the hospital setting, but it now extends to community settings. The RN case manager typically has earned an advanced degree and rarely provides direct care. Case management improves communication among health-care professionals and is identified as an approach to improve patient safety while transitioning patients among levels of care.

Nontraditional Models

During the 1980s and into the 1990s, the health-care system experienced many challenges, including pressure to cut health-care expenses. In an effort to reduce costs, hospitals examined strategies to change how patient care was delivered. The result consisted of nontraditional models of nursing care that borrowed from team nursing and included the incorporation of unlicensed assistive personnel (UAPs). The most popular models of nontraditional care delivery are patient-focused care, partnership models, nonclinical models, and integrated models (Lookinland et al., 2005; Neisner & Raymond, 2002).

Regardless of the care delivery model used, nurse leaders and managers must ensure that nurses deliver culturally competent, safe, effective, and quality care. In addition, nurse leaders and managers must support nursing control of nursing practice, respect nurses' rights and responsibilities, and respect patients' rights and preferences (American Nurses Association [ANA], 2016).

Patient-Focused Care

Patient-focused care revolves around a multiskilled team approach to nursing care. In this model, the RN functions as the patient care manager and coordinates all patient-related activities. Goals of patient-focused care are to make nursing care more patient centered rather than caregiver centered, reduce the number of caregivers a patient sees during a hospital stay, and increase direct patient care time for RNs (Jones et al., 1997). In the most extreme forms of patient-focused care, all patient care services are brought to the patient. In some cases, entire units are decentralized, meaning that all staff members from housekeeping, dietary, physical therapy, and nursing are employees of that specific unit. Ultimately, patient-focused care decreases the cost of providing health care while improving the quality of services (Myers, 1998). In this model, communication is lateral, and the team interfaces with the health-care providers.

Partnership Models

Partnership models emerged in the late 1980s with the goal of decreasing the cost of nursing care while increasing productivity. Examples include Partnership in Practice (PIP), Partnership to Improve Patient Care (PIPC), and nurse extender models. In the PIP model, the RN hires the UAP, and they work as clinical partners on the same schedule; UAPs may be cross-trained to perform skills such as phlebotomy and dressing changes, thus allowing them to work with the RN to provide direct patient care (Manthey, 1989). The PIPC and nurse extender models are similar to the PIP model in that the UAPs are cross-trained to perform additional skills and typically work the same schedules as their RN partners; however, the RN is not involved in hiring (Lookinland et al., 2005). Partnership models offer more continuity of care than team nursing and are more cost effective than primary nursing. In partnership models, communication is lateral, and RNs coordinate the care, provide direct patient care, and remain accountable for all patients.

Nonclinical Models

In nonclinical models, UAPs may or may not be partnered with the RN and do not provide direct patient care. In this model, the UAP's role is supportive and includes nonclinical tasks such as assisting patients with hygiene needs, feeding patients, answering call lights, ordering supplies, and transporting patients (Lookinland et al., 2005). In the nonclinical model, RNs are responsible for coordinating care, and communication is lateral.

Integrated Models

In integrated models, UAPs provide both direct care and indirect care. In some cases, the UAP is responsible for combined duties, such as housekeeping and food service (Lookinland et al., 2005). RNs may work with only a UAP or with a licensed practical nurse (LPN)/licensed vocational nurse (LVN) and a UAP. The goal of integrated models is to relieve RNs of nonnursing tasks to improve the quality of patient care. In this model, the RN coordinates all nursing care, and communication is lateral.

Contemporary Models

Contemporary models of care, also called innovative models, are the newest approaches to organizing patient care to foster patient safety and quality outcomes. Contemporary models include the Professional Nursing Practice Model, the Differentiated Nursing Practice Model, the Clinical Nurse Leader Model, the Synergy Model for Patient Care, Transforming Care at the Bedside, and the Patient- and Family-Centered Care Model.

Professional Nursing Practice Model

The **Professional Nursing Practice Model** provides "a framework for guiding and aligning clinical practice, education, administration, and research in order to achieve positive patient and nurse staff outcomes" (Lineweaver, 2013, p. 14.) This model is identified as a core feature of Magnet hospitals (Neisner & Raymond, 2002) because Magnet hospitals typically have higher RN-to-patient ratios, and many of these hospitals are moving to all-RN staffs. In this model, RNs have greater autonomy and control over practice, and there are higher rates of patient satisfaction, lower rates of nurse burnout, and safer work environments (Neisner & Raymond, 2002). This model supports the RN's control over the delivery of nursing care as well as effective interprofessional and intraprofessional communication.

Differentiated Nursing Practice Model

The **Differentiated Nursing Practice Model** resulted from a meeting between the American Association of Colleges of Nursing (AACN) and the AONE in 1993, when members of a joint Task Force sat down together to develop a set of formal goals and recommendations regarding differentiated nursing practice (AACN-AONE Task Force, 1995). Care in this model is differentiated based on the level of education, competence, and clinical expertise of RNs: nurses with an associate degree function as technical nurses and provide the majority of bedside care; baccalaureate-prepared nurses function on a broader scale, collaborating and facilitating patient care from admission through discharge; and advanced practice nurses function within the broad health-care system and provide care across all settings throughout wellness and death. The goals of this model include the following (Neisner & Raymond, 2002, p. 11):

- Optimal nursing care matching patients' needs with the nurse's competencies
- Effective and efficient use of scarce nursing resources
- Equitable compensation
- Increased career satisfaction among nurses
- Greater loyalty to the employer
- Enhanced prestige of the nursing profession

In the differentiated nursing practice environment, nurses must be clinically competent and flexible in providing nursing care, and they must value the differing roles. Nurse leaders and managers must match the unique capabilities of nurses with patient care requirements. Differentiated nursing practice recognizes that all nurses, regardless of education, are needed to provide high-quality, comprehensive care to all patients in all settings (AACN-AONE Task Force, 1995).

Clinical Nurse Leader Model

The **Clinical Nurse Leader (CNL) Model** was developed with the goal to improve the quality of patient care across the continuum and as a way to engage highly skilled clinicians in outcome-based practice and quality improvement (AACN, 2013). The graduate of a Master's degree program, the CNL has responsibilities including designing, implementing, and evaluating patient care by coordinating, delegating, and supervising the care provided by an interprofessional team. The nurse in this role is the leader in the health-care delivery system and is not in an administrative or managerial role. "The CNL assumes accountability for patient-care outcomes through assimilation and application of evidence-based information to design, implement, and evaluate patient-care processes and models of care delivery" (AACN, 2013, para. 4). The CNL is a provider and coordinator of care and fosters interprofessional and intraprofessional communication. The CNL graduate is eligible to sit for the CNL certification offered by the Commission on Nurse Certification.

Synergy Model for Patient Care

The American Association of Critical-Care Nurses developed the **Synergy Model for Patient Care** with the core concepts that the needs of patients and families influence and drive the competencies of nurses and that synergy occurs when the needs and characteristics of the patient, clinical unit, or system are matched with the nurse's competencies (American Association of Critical-Care Nurses, n.d.a). It is a framework that can be used to organize patient care in various settings. Because each patient and family is unique, has characteristics that span the health-illness continuum, and has varying capacity for health and vulnerability to illness, the model includes eight patient characteristics (Table 13-1) and eight nursing characteristics (Table 13-2) derived from patients' needs (American Association of Critical-Care Nurses, n.d.b). Assessment data collected based on the patient characteristics can assist nurses in the development of individualized plans of nursing care. This model fosters effective communication and collaboration in achieving optimal, realistic patient and family goals. Although the model was originally developed for critical care units, it has been used in a variety of clinical settings.

Transforming Care at the Bedside

A national initiative launched by the Robert Wood Johnson Foundation and the Institute for Healthcare Improvement in 2003, **Transforming Care at the Bedside** (TCAB)

Table 13-1	Synergy Model: Characteristics of Patients and Families With Definitions
Characteristics	**Definitions**
Resiliency	The capacity to return to a restorative level of functioning using compensatory or coping mechanisms; the ability to bounce back quickly after an insult
Vulnerability	Susceptibility to actual or potential stressors that may adversely affect patient outcomes
Stability	The ability to maintain steady-state equilibrium
Complexity	The intricate entanglement of two or more systems (e.g., body, family, therapies)
Resource availability	Extent of resources (e.g., technical, fiscal, personal, psychological, and social) the patient or family brings to the situation
Participation in care	Extent to which patient or family engages in aspects of care
Participation in decision making	Extent to which patient or family engages in decision making
Predictability	A characteristic that allows one to expect a certain course of events or course of illness

From American Association of Critical-Care Nurses, n.d.b, pp. 1–3.

Table 13-2	Synergy Model: Nurse Competencies With Definitions
Competencies	**Definitions**
Clinical judgment	Clinical reasoning, which includes clinical decision making, critical thinking, and a global grasp of the situation, coupled with nursing skills acquired through a process of integrating formal and informal experiential knowledge and evidence-based guidelines
Advocacy and moral agency	Working on another's behalf and representing the concerns of the patient or family and nursing staff; serving as a moral agent in identifying and helping to resolve ethical and clinical concerns within and outside the clinical setting
Caring practices	Nursing activities that create a compassionate, supportive, and therapeutic environment for patients and staff, with the aim of promoting comfort and healing and preventing unwanted suffering
Collaboration	Working with others (e.g., patients, families, health-care providers) in a way that promotes or encourages each person's contributions toward achieving optimal or realistic patient or family goals
Systems thinking	Body of knowledge and tools that allow the nurse to manage whatever environmental and system resources exist for the patient or family and staff
Response to diversity	The sensitivity to recognize, appreciate, and incorporate differences into the provision of care
Facilitation of learning	The ability to facilitate learning for patients or families, nursing staff, other members of the health-care team, and community
Clinical inquiry (innovator/evaluator)	The ongoing process of questioning and evaluating practice and providing informed practice

From American Association of Critical-Care Nurses, n.d.b, pp. 4–8.

is a care model that empowers frontline nurses and nurse leaders and managers to accomplish the following (Lee et al., 2008; Rutherford et al., 2009):

- Improve the safety and quality of patient care on medical-surgical units
- Increase the vitality and retention of nurses
- Engage and improve patients' and their family's experiences of care
- Improve the effectiveness of the entire health-care team

The goal of TCAB is to empower nurses and other health-care team members to redesign work processes to improve the quality of patient care and decrease turnover. The initiative brings the health-care team together to collaborate on improving the quality of care. The framework includes "optimizing communication among clinicians and staff" as one of the four essential building blocks for improving staff vitality and enhancing patient safety (Lee et al., 2008, p. 4). Five themes comprise the TCAB model of care (Rutherford et al., 2009):

1. *Transformational leadership:* Leadership and management practices empower frontline staff, and this empowerment is critical to ensuring that innovations are sustained. The success of TCAB depends on the commitment of leaders and managers across the health-care system.
2. *Safe and reliable care:* Health-care teams can respond immediately to changes in a patient's condition. Processes are in place to prevent medication errors, injuries from falls, pressure ulcers, and harm from adverse events. Additionally, the care delivered is effective and equitable.

3. *Vitality and teamwork:* When the health-care team functions in a joyful and supportive environment, teamwork is effective and communication is optimized. Health-care teams strive for excellence.
4. *Patient-centered care:* Care is focused on the "whole person and family, respects individual values and choices and ensures continuity of care" (p. 13).
5. *Value-added care processes:* Patient care is free of waste, promotes continuous flow of work, and decreases redundancy. Nurses can spend more time on activities that have value for the patient and family.

Since the initiative was launched in 2007, many health-care agencies in the United States and internationally have applied improvement strategies used in TCAB for engaging frontline nurses in deciding on and implementing changes to improve patient outcomes. The TCAB model has the potential to transform care delivery and the work environment for nurses and to support interprofessional teamwork and communication at the bedside (Rutherford et al., 2009).

Patient- and Family-Centered Care Model

Health care is plagued with many problems that require systemwide solutions and partnerships with health-care professionals, administrators, planners, policy makers, and patients and their families (Conway et al., 2006). For health-care professionals to provide safe and quality care effectively, a shift is required from provider-centered care to **patient-centered care**. Additionally, as patients are becoming more knowledgeable and informed, and taking care into their own hands, nurses must be prepared to advocate strongly for patients and their families as they navigate the health-care system.

The Institute for Patient- and Family-Centered Care (IPFCC) is a nonprofit organization whose mission is to advance the understanding and practices of patient- and family-centered care and to integrate the core concepts of dignity and respect, information sharing, participation, and collaboration into all aspects of health care (IPFCC, n.d.a). The IPFCC defines patient- and family-centered care as "an approach to the planning, delivery, and evaluation of health care that is grounded in mutually beneficial partnerships among health care providers, patients, and families. […] It leads to better health outcomes, improved patient and family experience of care, better clinician and staff satisfaction, and wiser allocation of resources" (IPFCC, n.d.b, para. 1, 3).

Patient- and family-centered care places an emphasis on collaborating and planning care with patients (and their families) of all ages, at all levels of care, and in all health-care settings (Conway et al., 2006). Patient- and family-centered care should never be confused with patient-focused care mentioned earlier in this chapter. In the patient-focused care model, the RN is the coordinator and planner of care who brings as many care services to the patient as possible; in patient- and family-centered care, the patient has control over their care, and all health-care decisions are made with the RN as a collaborator in their care.

The model of patient- and family-centered care is based on four foundational concepts (Conway et al., 2006):

1. *Dignity and respect:* Health-care professionals listen to and respect the values and choices of the patient and family, and the values, beliefs, and cultural

backgrounds of the patient and family are integrated into the planning and delivery of care.

2. *Information sharing:* Health-care professionals communicate and share all information with patients and families in a timely manner. Patients and families receive comprehensive and accurate information to participate in care and decision making effectively.

3. *Participation:* Patients and families are encouraged and supported in participating in care and decision making at the level they choose.

4. *Collaboration:* Patients and families as well as health-care professionals and leaders collaborate in policy and program development, implementation, and evaluation; health-care facility design; professional education; and delivery of care (Conway et al., 2006).

Nurses are strategically positioned to be the catalysts for integrating this model into practice. The nurse-patient relationship is inherently built on mutual trust, respect, and communication. In patient- and family-centered care, nurses initiate and promote a safe healing environment, respond to individual patients' choices, recognize patients as the source of control, effectively communicate with patients and their families, and provide all necessary information for patients to make an informed health-care decision. The model of patient- and family-centered care can transform the experience of care for patients and families and of caregiving for all health-care professionals.

▶ PRIORITIZING NURSING CARE

Delivering nursing care today is a complex process that involves critical thinking, clinical reasoning, and sound clinical judgment. Nurses at all levels must have an understanding of how to prioritize nursing care, or **prioritization**. Priorities in nursing practice are determined using several frameworks such as nursing process, ABC, and Maslow's Hierarchy of Needs.

Nurses are taught the steps of the nursing process (assessment, diagnosis [analysis], outcomes identification, planning, implementation, and evaluation) during their basic nursing education. Regardless of the circumstances, nurses should begin the process by assessing the situation using these guidelines and address the following:

- Life-threatening problems or those that could result in harm to the patient if left untreated first. For example: A patient is hemorrhaging from a surgical site (life-threatening) and blood pressure 220/110 (will cause harm if left untreated).
- Actual problems and needs before potential problems or risks. For example: A patient with a temperature of 104°F (actual problem) versus a postoperative patient at risk for infection (potential problem).
- Acute problems before chronic problems. For example: A patient with status asthmaticus (an airway problem requiring immediate action) versus a patient with chronic asthma (an airway problem requiring monitoring).
- Problems identified as important to the patient.

Nurses should also assess patients using the ABCs, remembering that a patent airway is always the priority: airway, breathing, and circulation sequentially.

Nurses can use Maslow's Hierarchy to prioritize needs from the highest priority to the lowest priority or basic needs are met before moving onto the next level: physiological or biological needs, which includes the ABCs; safety and security needs; belonging and love needs; self-esteem; and self-actualization.

In addition to prioritizing and reprioritizing nursing care, nurses must also effectively prioritize and manage their time to avoid nonessential activities that could jeopardize their priorities in delivering nursing care to their patients. Nurse leaders and managers prioritize work in a similar manner. They must assess immediate needs of the unit and staff, determine the priority needs or those that are most urgent, involve staff as much as possible, and anticipate any time constraints and available resources needed to address priority needs.

▶ STAFFING FOR PATIENT SAFETY

Appropriate staffing is critical to the delivery of quality care at every practice level and every setting (ANA, 2020, p. 4). Nurse leaders and managers are responsible for making sure to have the appropriate number and mix of nursing staff at all times. Because staffing affects the ability of a nurse to deliver safe and effective care at every practice level and in all settings, staffing is a complex process (ANA, 2020). Nurse leaders and managers must understand and follow federal, state, and local regulations related to staffing and scheduling; uphold nurse practice acts; verify and track licensure of nursing staff; respect nurses' rights; ensure staff competencies; and substantiate staff compliance with regulatory and professional standards (ANA, 2016).

Safe nurse staffing enhances the delivery of safe, effective, and quality health care. Research in the United States specifically indicates that when units are staffed with more RNs, patients experience fewer complications, fewer urinary tract infections and cases of pneumonia, shorter lengths of stay, fewer adverse events, and decreased mortality rates (Aiken et al., 2002, 2017; Kane et al., 2007; Knudson, 2013; Needleman et al., 2011; Unruh, 2008). On an international scale, a Registered Nurse Forecasting (RN4CAST) study resulted in similar findings: that nurse staffing levels and the quality of the work environment were associated with patient satisfaction, quality and safety of care, and measures of nurse well-being (European Commission, 2017, para. 5). The RN4CAST study continues with hopes to improve nurse staffing worldwide; more information can be found at http://www.rn4cast.eu/about1.html.

Inadequate nurse staffing is often cited as a contributing factor when unanticipated events happen that result in patient injury, disability, or death. In addition, inadequate nurse staffing can cause nurses to experience job dissatisfaction, burnout, high "intent to quit" levels, and injury or illness (Unruh, 2008). Safe staffing fosters a positive environment for nursing practice by allowing nurses to apply the knowledge they have gained through education and practice experiences efficiently and effectively when caring for patients. Staffing must be effective to achieve positive outcomes for patients and the health-care organization.

Ensuring safe staffing is not an easy task for nurse leaders and managers, but it can be achieved by dynamic, multifaceted decision-making processes that consider a wide range of variables (ANA, 2020). The greatest challenge faced by nurse leaders and managers in maintaining safe staffing is the nursing shortage.

Shortage of Nurses

The nursing shortage is widespread globally (Knudson, 2013), and it affects all areas of nursing. This shortage is occurring at the same time the U.S. Department of Labor is suggesting that the need for nurses in outpatient settings, ambulatory care centers, outpatient surgery centers, and urgent care centers is rapidly increasing. The key to an ample supply of nurses in the future is the nation's ability to produce new nurses. The number of nurses passing the NCLEX-RN® licensure examination increased from 68,561 in 2001 to about 158,000 in 2015; however, the demand for nurses is expected to increase to 3,601,800 by 2030 (Health Resources and Services Administration [HRSA] Bureau of Health Workforce, 2017). Interestingly, the Bureau of Health Workforce report indicates that there may be an inequitable distribution of the nursing workforce across states based on local conditions such as the number of new graduates from nursing schools (HRSA Bureau of Health Workforce, 2017, p. 6).

It is anticipated that the nursing shortage will reach 1.2 million by 2022 due to the following (AACN, 2019a, pp. 2–3):

- *Nursing school enrollment is not growing fast enough to meet the projected demand for RN and advanced practice RN services.* Although there has been a 3.7% increase in enrollments in 2018, a significant segment of the nursing workforce is nearing retirement age. It has been projected that more than 1 million RNs will retire between 2019 and 2029.
- *A shortage of nursing school faculty is restricting nursing program enrollments.* Nursing schools have been forced to turn away qualified applicants because of insufficient numbers of faculty, clinical sites, classroom spaces, and clinical preceptors, as well as budget constraints, with faculty shortages noted as the major reason for not accepting qualified applicants into programs. In 2018 alone, nursing schools turned away more than 75,000 qualified baccalaureate and graduate nursing student applicants.
- *Changing demographic factors signal a need for more nurses to care for our aging population.* The demand for more nurses will increase as more baby boomers reach 60 years old. It is estimated that by 2050 the number of U.S. residents 65 and older will increase to 83.7 million.
- *Insufficient staffing is raising the stress level of nurses, affecting job satisfaction, and driving many nurses to leave the profession.* Research supports the notion that the nursing shortage increases personal stress, lowers patient care quality, and causes nurses to leave the profession.
- *High nurse turnover and vacancy rates are affecting access to health care.* Newly licensed RNs have a high rate of job change after only 1 year, and the overall RN turnover rates and vacancy rates remain close to 15%.

Shortage of Nurse Faculty

As indicated earlier, the nurse faculty shortage is identified as a major reason qualified nursing student applicants are turned away. Factors contributing to the shortage include the following (AACN, 2019b, pp. 1–2):

- *Faculty age continues to climb, narrowing the number of productive years educators teach.* In 2017, the average ages of doctorally prepared nurse faculty holding rank of assistant, associate, and full professor were 51.2 years, 57.2 years, and 62.4 years, respectively.
- *A wave of faculty retirements is expected across the United States over the next decade.* Approximately one third of the current faculty workforce is expected to retire by 2025.
- *Higher compensation in clinical and private-sector settings is luring current and potential nurse educators away from teaching.* As of 2017, the average salary of a master's-prepared assistant professor was $78,575, whereas the average salary of a nurse practitioner was $105,903.
- *Master's and doctoral programs in nursing are not producing a large enough pool of potential nurse educators to meet the demand.* Efforts to expand the number of qualified nurse educators are affected by the number of applicants to graduate and doctoral programs turned away. Again, the primary reason for not accepting applications is due to the nurse faculty shortage.

The impact of the nursing shortage is surely felt by nurse leaders and managers as they attempt to staff their patient care areas safely. To provide safe and quality care effectively, there are many factors that must be considered by nurse leaders and managers when establishing safe staffing plans.

Core Concepts of Staffing

Historically, staffing decisions were dictated by the number of patients on the unit and fixed nurse-to-patient ratios; this method did not consider the needs of the patients or the nurses' levels of education, expertise, and work satisfaction. Staffing and workload are part of a complex process that can have a negative impact on patient and nurse outcomes (Unruh, 2008). For example, when nurses believe that they cannot deliver quality care, they become dissatisfied with the work, and this can negatively affect patient satisfaction and outcomes and becomes "a vicious cycle: inadequate staffing leads to reduced job performance and diminished patient and nurse satisfaction; the resulting burnout and high turnover rates worsen staffing levels" (Unruh, 2008, p. 64).

To ensure positive patient and nurse outcomes, nurse leaders and managers must consider critical factors, such as number of patients, intensity of care, contextual issues, and level of expertise, when determining staffing needs. Although cost effectiveness is an important factor in the delivery of safe and quality care, the reimbursement structure should not influence the staffing plan. Rather, nurse leaders and managers must consider the staffing needs and staffing plan for the unit when developing the fiscal budget. It is critical that health-care organizations consider the financial impact of patient outcomes when evaluating the cost of nurse staffing.

To deal with staffing most effectively, understanding core concepts related to staffing is critical for nurse leaders and managers. Important concepts include full-time equivalent, productive time, average daily census, staffing mix, workload, units of service, nursing hours per patient day (NHPPD), unit intensity, patient acuity, and skill mix. Some of these concepts relate to the financial aspects of staffing and are addressed in Chapter 16. The concepts of staffing mix, workload and units of service, unit intensity, patient acuity, and skill mix are addressed here.

Staffing Mix

Staffing mix refers to the appropriate numbers of RNs, LPNs/LVNs, and UAPs needed on a unit, and it is based on the type of care required for specific patients and who is qualified to provide such care. Determining the staffing mix requires nurse leaders and managers to assess staff competency and make sure that all staff members have the necessary skills to carry out assigned and delegated tasks. A higher-RN staff mix provides more staffing flexibility.

Workload and Units of Service

Workload is the number of nursing staff members required to deliver care for a specific time period and is dependent on patient care needs. **Units of service** (UOS) reflect the basic measure of nursing workload based on different types of patient encounters (Table 13-3). Staffing needs vary by clinical setting. UOS assist nurse leaders and managers in determining unit-specific needs for staffing.

One example of workload is nursing hours per patient day (NHPPD), which represents the nursing care hours provided to patients by nursing personnel over a 24-hour period. NHPPD is usually based on unit census at midnight and reflects only nursing staff productive time. NHPPD is discussed further in Chapter 16.

Unit Intensity

Unit intensity considers the totality of the patients for whom care is provided and the responsibilities of nursing staff. Unit intensity is valuable in determining staffing because it takes into consideration admissions, transfers, and discharges. However, unit intensity can be difficult to measure in view of the many factors that influence it, such as severity of illness, patient dependency for activities of daily living, complexity of care, and amount of time needed to deliver care (Beglinger, 2006).

Table 13-3 Units of Service by Type of Unit or Department	
Type of Unit or Department	**Units of Service (UOS)**
Emergency department	Patient visits per month
Inpatient unit	Nursing hours per patient day
Home care	Patient visits per month
Labor and delivery	Births per month
Operating room	Minutes per case

Patient Acuity

Patient acuity represents how patients are categorized according to an assessment of their nursing care needs (Harper & McCully, 2007). It is a critical factor in determining safe staffing. Patient classification systems are tools used to determine staffing based on patient acuity. Typically, patients with more acute conditions or sicker patients receive higher classification scores to indicate that they need more direct nursing care.

Skill Mix

Skill mix refers to the varying levels of education, licensure, certifications, and experience of the staff. Skill mix can include a team made up of various numbers of RNs, LPNs, and UAPs. Determining the skill mix occurs on every shift and depends on many factors, such as the model of care delivery, patient population, patient acuity, competency requirements to care for a specific patient, levels of experience and education of staff, and licensure of staff. Nurse leaders and managers must know their staff well and understand the scope of practice for each type of staff. Appropriate staffing and skill mix can have a positive impact on patient care (Dabney & Kalisch, 2015).

RN Scope of Practice

The RN scope of practice is fairly consistent nationally and globally and includes all aspects of the nursing process. RNs are licensed personnel who have completed a specific course of study at a state-approved school of nursing and passed the NCLEX-RN® examination (National Council of State Boards of Nursing [NCSBN], 2020). The responsibilities of RNs include assessment, diagnosis, planning, intervention, and evaluation. Patient teaching, discharge planning, evaluating and monitoring changes in patient status, and complex patient care that requires special knowledge and judgment are also within the scope of practice of the RN. In addition, RNs are responsible for assigning, supervising, and delegating appropriately to other team members to ensure that safe and quality care is delivered. Teaching the theory and practice of nursing and participating in the development of health-care policies, procedures, and systems are also components of the RN's scope of practice (NCSBN, 2012).

LPN/LVN Scope of Practice

The LPN/LVN scope of practice includes physical care, taking vital signs, and administering medication, and it can vary significantly from state to state. LPNs/LVNs are licensed personnel who have completed a specific course of study of a state-approved practical or vocational nursing program and passed the NCLEX-PN® examination (NCSBN, 2020). Regardless of their scope of practice, LPNs/LVNs always work under the direction or supervision of an RN, advanced practice RN, physician, or other health-care provider designated by the state (NCSBN, 2012). Nurse leaders and managers must be cognizant of their state's nurse practice act to ensure that LPNs/LVNs are being assigned within their scope of practice.

UAP Scope of Practice

The UAP scope of practice typically includes activities of daily living, hygiene, and physical care. However, the scope of practice for UAPs also varies from state to state. UAPs are unlicensed personnel specifically trained to function in an assistive role to RNs and may or may not be regulated by a state board of nursing. UAPs perform tasks as delegated by an RN (NCSBN, 2020).

LEARNING ACTIVITY 13-1	Scopes of Practice

Scopes of Practice

Review your state nurse practice act (visit www.ncsbn.org/npa.htm). Compare the specific scopes of practice for RNs, LPNs/LVNs, and UAPs.

Staffing Approaches

Research on safe staffing has revealed that it is effective in reducing adverse events, improves quality of care received, and improves nurse satisfaction, which in turn reduces costly nurse turnover. Determining adequate staffing levels requires nurse leaders and managers to recognize unique patient care settings, patient flow (admissions, discharges, and transfers), patient acuity, and the skills, education, and experience of the available nursing staff. However, there is not a perfect method for determining staffing. The AONL (2010) calls for nurse leaders and managers to develop core staffing models that support patient-centered care and allow staff members to function at the peak of their licensure. Nurse leaders and managers can use a variety of approaches to safe staffing, such as patient classification systems, *ANA's Principles for Nurse Staffing*, the Agency for Healthcare and Research Quality nurse staffing model, and National Database of Nursing Quality Indicators staffing benchmarks.

Patient Classification Systems

A **patient classification system** (PCS) predicts patient needs and requirements for nursing care. A PCS groups patients according to acuity of illness and complexity of nursing activities necessary to care for the patients. Typically, patient acuity data are collected every shift by nursing staff and are analyzed to project nursing staff needs for the next shift. The advantage of using a PCS is that it is an objective approach to determining staffing based on patient care needs: a sicker patient requires more nursing care and therefore would have a higher acuity level. However, there are numerous issues regarding use of PCSs, including lack of standardization, lack of credibility among nurse leaders and managers, and no consideration of patient flow (Hertel, 2012).

Nurse leaders in informatics are investigating the use of information technology with PCSs to assist in effective nurse staffing (Harper, 2012). Information technology can potentially decrease costs, improve staffing efficiency, and improve quality of care and patient safety. Information technology incorporated with a

EXPLORING THE EVIDENCE 13-1

Dabney, B. W., & Kalisch, B. J. (2015). Nurse staffing levels and patient-reported missed nursing care. *Journal of Nursing Care Quality, 30*(4), 306–312.

Aim
The aim of this study was to extend previous research by exploring patient reports of missed nursing care and determine the relationship between patient reports of missed care and unit staffing levels.

Methods
A secondary analysis was used to determine the relationship between patient reports of missed care and the level of nurse staffing. The sample included 729 patients on 20 units in two hospitals. Missed nursing care was measured using the MISSCARE Survey–Patient. This tool consists of 13 questions organized according to three subscales: communication, timeliness, and basic care. Nurse staffing was measured using RNHPPD (total productive RN hours per patient day), NHPPD (total productive nursing hours per patient day, including RNs, LPNs/LVNs, and UAPs), and RN skill mix (the ratio of RNs to other nursing personnel).

Key Findings
No significant correlations were found between basic care and the nurse staffing variables or between communication and the nurse staffing variables. Significant relationships were found between missed timeliness of care and the three nurse staffing variables.

- The higher the RNHPPD, the timelier the provision of nursing care ($P = 0.0002$).
- The higher the NHPPD, the timelier the provision of nursing care ($P = 0.015$).
- The higher the RN skill mix, the timelier the provision of nursing care ($P = 0.0004$).

In addition, RN skill mix was found to be a predictor of missed timeliness. The investigators pointed out that RNs may be more focused than other nursing personnel on ensuring that patient needs are responded to quickly, and they suggested that there may also be a lack of teamwork, by citing that low levels of teamwork have been found to be predictive of missed care. Although staffing variables were not associated with communication and basic care in this study, the researchers emphasized that this finding is in contrast to finding of other studies.

Implications for Nurse Leaders and Managers
First and foremost, nurse leaders and managers must be cognizant of missed nursing care. The findings of this study provide evidence of the positive impact of appropriate staffing on patient care. Nurse leaders and managers must advocate for patients and be able to articulate to upper management that evidence shows that increased staffing, especially RN staffing, results in patient reports of more rapid responses to their needs and, in turn, can have a positive impact on patient satisfaction.

meaningful model for nurse staffing, such as the Clinical Demand Index, "can make staffing based on evidence a reality" (Harper, 2012, p. 267).

Although there are commercial PCSs for purchase, many health-care organizations design their own. Regardless of the type of PCS used, it must be reliable and valid.

American Nurses Association Principles for Safe Staffing

The ANA document *Principles for Nurse Staffing* was initially developed in 1999 and revised in 2012 and 2020 to "provide a framework to help nurses at all levels, nurse leaders, and healthcare administrators in the development, implementation, and evaluation of appropriate nurse staffing plans and activities" (ANA, 2020, p. 5). Evidence demonstrates that nursing care directly affects the quality of services and that, when RN staffing is adequate, adverse events decrease and, overall, patient outcomes improve (ANA, 2020). The evidence linking adequate nurse staffing to improved patient outcomes has continued to grow.

The updated *ANA's Principles for Nurse Staffing* identifies major elements needed to achieve appropriate nurse staffing for the delivery of safe, quality health care. The principles are focused on addressing the complexities of nurse staffing decisions and apply to all types of nurse staffing in all types of health-care settings. The principles are organized in a framework that helps detail a 21st-century context for nurse staffing that recognizes the individual contribution and added value of each individual nurse as a provider of care (ANA, 2020, p. 5). The framework includes the following five categories (ANA, 2020, pp. 7–16):

1. *The characteristics and considerations of the health-care consumer or patient:* Staffing decisions are based on the number and needs of the individual, families, and populations served.
2. *The characteristics and considerations of RNs and other interprofessional team members and staff:* The needs of the populations served determine the appropriate clinical competencies required of the RNs practicing in that clinical setting.
3. *The context of the organization and workplace culture in which the nursing services are delivered:* Health-care organizations must create work environments that value RNs and other staff as strategic assets and budgeted positions are filled in a timely manner.
4. *The overall practice environment that influences delivery of care:* Staffing is a structure and process that affects patient outcomes as well as nursing outcomes. Health-care organizations must recognize that nurse staffing is integral to a culture of safety.
5. *The evaluation of staffing plans, overall costs, effectiveness, and resources expended for nursing care:* Health-care organizations must use flexible staffing plans that demonstrate logical methods for determining staffing levels and skill mix based on evaluation data.

Agency for Healthcare Research and Quality Nurse Staffing Model

The Agency for Healthcare Research and Quality (AHRQ) nurse staffing model evolved from a meta-analysis conducted by investigators (Kane et al., 2007) under contract with the AHRQ. After reviewing 28 research studies related to the effects of nurse staffing on patient safety, the investigators found a positive correlation between adequate RN staffing levels and patient outcomes. Based on the results, these investigators developed a conceptual framework to guide nurse staffing that considers the complexity of hospital care today and accounts for the following: patient, hospital, and organizational factors; nurse characteristics; nurse staffing; medical care; and the impact of these factors on patient outcomes and length of stay (Kane et al., 2007). They also identified two key consequences of safe nurse staffing—patient outcomes and nurse outcomes—while recognizing that although patient outcomes are nurses' ultimate concern, nurse outcomes can positively or negatively affect patient outcomes and therefore must also be considered. The AHRQ model (Fig. 13-1) provides nurse leaders and managers a realistic framework for staffing because it reflects the complex relationships among patient factors, nurse staffing, nurse characteristics, hospital and organizational factors, and patient outcomes.

National Database of Nursing Quality Indicators Staffing Benchmarks

In 1994, the ANA launched the Safety and Quality Initiative to explore the empirical link between nursing care and patient outcomes (Montalvo, 2007). The ANA's findings highlighted strong links between nursing actions and patient outcomes. The focus of the initiative since the 1990s has been educating RNs about quality measurement, informing the public and policy makers about safe and quality

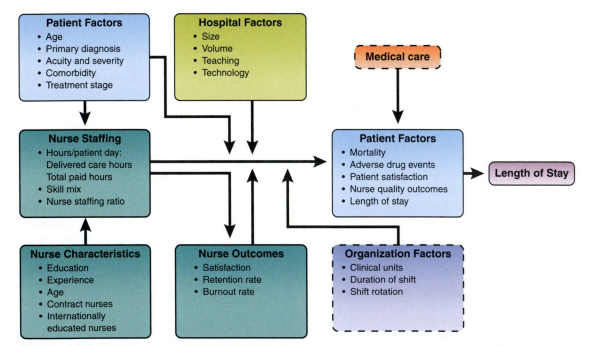

Figure 13-1 Conceptual framework of nurse staffing and patient outcomes. *(Source: Kane et al., 2007.)*

health care, and investigating research methods and data sources to evaluate safety and quality patient care empirically (Montalvo, 2007).

In 1999, the ANA joined with the University of Kansas School of Nursing and the Midwestern Research Institute to form the National Database of Nursing Quality Indicators (NDNQI), and together they work to establish definitions, data collection, and benchmarking criteria. The mission of the NDNQI is to aid RNs "in patient safety and quality improvement efforts by providing research-based national comparative data on nursing care and the relationship to patient outcomes" (Montalvo, 2007, para. 7). In addition, the NDNQI facilitates the standardization of information on nursing quality and patient outcomes across the nation. Hospitals report unit-level data quarterly, and feedback reports are provided to hospitals quarterly. The ANA developed **nursing-sensitive quality indicators** to measure patient outcomes most affected by nursing care (Montalvo, 2007). "The NDNQI provides nursing sensitive structure, process, and outcome measures to monitor relationships between quality indicators and outcomes (Press Ganey, 2019, para. 3). In-depth discussion of nursing-sensitive quality indicators and how they relate to quality care is presented in Chapter 9. The NDNQI measures characteristics of the nursing workforce related to quality of patient care, including staffing levels and turnover, as well as RN education and certification (Press Ganey, 2019).

The national database provides benchmark data for specific unit types that nurse leaders and managers can use to establish safe staffing plans. In 2014, Press Ganey Associates, Inc. acquired the NDNQI from the ANA. The NDNQI data program measures nursing quality, improves nurse satisfaction, strengthens the nursing work environment, assesses staffing levels, and improves reimbursement under current pay-for-performance policies. Currently, the NDNQI collects and evaluates unit-specific nursing-sensitive data from more than 2,000 hospitals in the United States and 95% of Magnet facilities (Press Ganey, 2019). In addition, the NDNQI RN Survey is conducted annually to "capture the voice of more than 300,000 nurses to provide hospitals with insights to drive quality improvements, reduce costly nursing turnover and improve the organization's nursing culture" (Press Ganey, 2019, para. 7).

Developing and Implementing a Staffing Plan

Nurse leaders and managers must ensure that appropriate staff members are scheduled during each shift each day to provide safe and quality nursing care. A **staffing plan** describes the number and type of nursing staff needed from shift to shift and from day to day. When considering a staffing plan, nurse leaders and managers must consider regulatory requirements (federal and state legislation, as well as state boards of nursing). Accrediting agencies such as The Joint Commission also have guidelines for effective staffing that must be considered. Additionally, nurse leaders and managers are bound by standards of practice such as those outlined in the ANA *Nursing Administration: Scope and Standards of Practice* (2016). The ANA contends that nurse leaders and managers must "explore staffing models to expand thinking beyond nurse-to-nurse ratios" (ANA, 2019, para. 1).

The ANA (2017) supports legislation to empower nurses to establish safe staffing levels that are unit specific and take into account the following (para. 4):

- RN education preparation, professional certification, and level of clinical experience
- The number and capacity of available health care personnel, geography of a unit, and available technology
- The intensity, complexity, and stability of patients

Furthermore, the ANA (2019) supports a model that establishes staffing levels that are flexible and account for changes including the following (para. 7):

- Intensity of patients' needs
- The number of admissions, transfers, and discharges during a shift
- Level of experience of the nursing staff
- Layout of the unit
- Availability of resource (e.g., ancillary staff, technology)

As of 2019, 14 states had regulation/legislation addressing nurse staffing and some type of legislation related to staffing that resembled the ANA recommendations (ANA, 2019).

Benner's Novice-to-Expert Model

Nursing leaders and managers can also look to Benner's Novice-to-Expert Model for a framework for developing and implementing staffing plans. Benner's model takes into account the tasks, competencies, and outcomes RNs can be expected to acquire based on five stages of experience (Benner, 1984):

Stage I—Novice: A novice is a nurse with no experience of situations in which they are expected to perform. Typically, the novice performs tasks from a rule-based perspective or a checklist approach. Nursing students are in the novice stage, as are nurses who change their clinical area of work to one in which they do not have previous experience (pp. 20–21).

Stage II—Advanced beginner: An advanced beginner can demonstrate marginally acceptable performance of tasks with enough experience to grasp some meaningful aspects of the situation at hand. Newly graduated nurses are considered advanced beginners and need support in the clinical setting (pp. 22–25).

Stage III—Competent: Competent nurses have 2 or 3 years of experience. The competent nurse can establish a plan of care and can determine which aspects of a situation are important and which aspects are not priorities (pp. 25–27).

Stage IV—Proficient: Proficient nurses have 3 or more years of experience. They perceive the situation as a whole rather than as aspects and use maxims, or subtle changes nurses recognize based on previous experience, as guides (pp. 27–31).

Stage V—Expert: Expert nurses operate from a deep understanding of the total situation and do not rely on analytical principles to understand the situation (pp. 31–36). They use intuitive and reflective thinking in their practice.

Nurses transition from one stage to the next as they gain more knowledge and experience, and their performance becomes fluid and flexible depending on the situation. Understanding what stage each member of the nursing staff is in can help nurse leaders and managers when developing effective staffing plans. Novice and advanced beginner nurses need more direction and coaching than competent and proficient nurses, whereas expert nurses are able to function independently and are great resources for the less experienced nurses.

Benner's model has been used over the years as a framework for teaching, as clinical ladders in health-care organizations, and for developing staffing plans. The model warns against using nurses interchangeably; rather, nurse leaders and managers should use staffing strategies that foster staffing stability and maximize expert clinical performance. Further, staffing should be such that expert nurses are available to advanced beginner nurses, competent nurses, and proficient nurses at all times for consultation to ensure safe and quality care.

LEARNING ACTIVITY 13-2

Staffing Plans

Determine how well your clinical setting staffs their unit:

- Do they use a patient classification system? What type do they use?
- Do they staff strictly by nurse-to-patient ratios? What is the typical nurse-to-patient ratio?
- What is the typical staff mix on the unit?
- Does this unit use LPNs/LVNs?

Evaluating Staffing Effectiveness

Ensuring positive patient outcomes requires nurse leaders and managers to evaluate staffing effectiveness daily, weekly, and monthly. When evaluating staffing effectiveness, nurse leaders and managers must consider many of the elements already discussed, including patient acuity trends, staffing overtime, staffing mix, patient satisfaction, and patient outcomes. Variance reports are used to evaluate staffing effectiveness by comparing planned staffing with budgeted staffing. These reports assist in identifying trends in key areas.

All nurses have a role in evaluating staffing effectiveness. Nurses are responsible for reporting to nurse leaders and managers any concerns they have related to safe staffing. In return, nurse leaders and managers have a responsibility to investigate staffing concerns identified by nursing staff and to act immediately on any issues that could have a negative impact on patient or nurse outcomes.

▶ SUMMARY

Organizing patient care to deliver safe, effective, and quality nursing care is a critical role for all nurse leaders and managers, whether organizing care for an individual patient in the hospital or at their home or whether organizing care for a group of patients in a community setting such as a skilled nursing facility. Care delivery models provide a mechanism to focus on nursing care and related outcomes. Nurses at all levels use guidelines such as the nursing process, ABCs, and Maslow's Hierarchy of Needs for making clinical judgments and prioritizing patient care.

Nurse leaders and managers must anticipate patient volume, complexity of patient care needed, admissions, discharges, and transfers when establishing staffing plans to provide safe and quality nursing.

NCLEX®-STYLE REVIEW QUESTIONS

Multiple Choice

1. In terms of traditional care models, what is the *primary* difference between total patient care and functional nursing?
   1. Inclusion of ancillary personnel to complete patient care tasks
   2. Type of clinical setting
   3. Educational background
   4. Length of shift
2. Which type of traditional care model is most similar to the total patient care model?
   1. Functional
   2. Team
   3. Bedside
   4. Primary
3. Which nursing care model's *primary* focus is on reducing the cost of nursing care while at the same time looking to improve productivity?
   1. Primary
   2. Partnership
   3. Patient-focused
   4. Team
4. A registered nurse (RN) is working on a medical-surgical care unit with a five-patient assignment. Helping the RN with completion of direct and nondirect tasks is an unlicensed assistive personnel (UAP). Based on this information, what type of patient care model is being implemented?
   1. Primary
   2. Integrated
   3. Nonclinical
   4. Team
5. Which theme is not included in the initiative, *Transforming Care at the Bedside (TCAB)* model?
   1. Safe care
   2. Vitality and teamwork
   3. Limited value
   4. Transformational leadership

6. Based on current clinical research, which statement represents support for promoting adequate staffing?
   1. Adequate staffing places little demand on the budgeting of nursing units.
   2. Staffing practices are unrelated to nursing fatigue.
   3. Adequate staffing helps to promote both patient and nurse satisfaction.
   4. Staffing patterns do not affect hospital infection rate.
7. Which clinical environment is reporting an increased need for nursing staff?
   1. Ambulatory care
   2. Obstetrical units
   3. Intensive care units
   4. Medical-surgical units
8. Which factors play an important role in being able to academically prepare students to become future nurses?
   1. Increase in available clinical sites combined with an increase in nursing school enrollment
   2. Increased enrollment in graduate nursing programs and preceptors
   3. Decreased student's interest to pursue a nursing degree along with decreased classroom space
   4. Decreased number of nursing faculty
9. According to clinical research findings, with what is a lower registered nurse (RN) skill mix associated?
   1. Increased productivity
   2. Fewer patient complications
   3. Increased efficiency
   4. Poorer time management
10. Which statement is correct with regard to scope of practice for both registered nurses (RNs) and licensed vocational/practical nurses (LVNs and LPNs)?
   1. Work under the direction of the RN in the clinical setting
   2. Passed a national licensing examination
   3. Administer all medications to patients in the clinical setting
   4. Graduated from an accredited nursing program
11. In terms of regulation, which statement is accurate with regard to unlicensed assistive personnel (UAPs)?
   1. Consistent state regulation of responsibilities
   2. May or may not be regulated by a state board of nursing
   3. Can perform tasks in the absence of delegation
   4. Has a nursing license

12. The charge nurse on the unit is getting ready to prepare staffing and assignments for the upcoming shift. The charge nurse reviews the following information: number of patients on the unit, corresponding patient acuity, and present level of staffing pattern. What type of process is the charge nurse implementing to make this decision?
    1. Nursing assessment
    2. Evidence-based practice
    3. Patient classification system
    4. Budgeting

Multiple Response

13. According to Benner's *novice-to-expert theory*, which statements are true? *Select all that apply.*
    1. A nursing student is considered to be an advanced beginner.
    2. Proficient nurses look at the entire picture rather than individual elements.
    3. Competent nurses use intuition and reflective practice.
    4. A new graduate would not be categorized as a novice nurse.
    5. Competent nurses use checklists to differentiate tasks.

14. According to Benner's *novice-to-expert theory*, which statements are false? *Select all that apply.*
    1. Proficient nurses have the largest amount of clinical experience.
    2. Competent nurses have at least 10 years of clinical experience.
    3. Competent nurses are able to identify priorities based on their established plan of care.
    4. Advanced beginners need to be mentored in the clinical setting.
    5. An experienced nurse does not become a novice when transferring to another clinical unit in which they have no experience.

REFERENCES

Aiken, L. H., Clarke, S. P., Sloane, D. M., Sochalski, J., & Silber, J. H. (2002). Hospital nurse staffing and patient mortality, nurse burnout, and job dissatisfaction. *Journal of the American Medical Association, 288*(16), 1987–1993.

Aiken, L. H., Sloane, D., Griffiths, P., Rafferty, A. M., Bruyneel, L., McHugh, M., Maier, C. B., Moreno-Casbas, T., Ball, J. E., Ausserhofer, D., & Sermeus, W. (2017). Nursing skill mix in European hospitals: Cross-sectional study of the association with mortality, patient ratings, and quality of care. *British Journal of Quality and Safety, 26*(7), 559–568.

American Association of Colleges of Nursing. (2021). *The essentials: Core competencies for professional nursing education.* Author. https://www.aacnnursing.org/Portals/42/AcademicNursing/pdf/Essentials-2021.pdf

American Association of Colleges of Nursing (AACN). (2013). *Competencies and curricular expectations for clinical nurse leader education and practice.* Author. https://www.aacnnursing.org/News-Information/Position-Statements-White-Papers/CNL

American Association of Colleges of Nursing (AACN). (2019a). *Nursing shortage fact sheet.* https://www.aacnnursing.org/News-Information/Fact-Sheets/Nursing-Shortage

American Association of Colleges of Nursing (AACN). (2019b). *Nursing faculty shortage fact sheet.* https://www.aacnnursing.org/News-Information/Fact-Sheets/Nursing-Faculty-Shortage

American Association of Colleges of Nursing (AACN)–American Organization of Nurse Executives (AONE) Task Force. (1995). *A model for differentiated nursing practice.* American Association of Colleges of Nursing.

American Association of Critical-Care Nurses. (n.d.a). *The AACN synergy model for patient care.* https://www.aacn.org/nursing-excellence/aacn-standards/synergy-model

American Association of Critical-Care Nurses. (n.d.b). *The AACN synergy model for patient care.* https://www.aacn.org/~/media/aacn-website/nursing-excellence/standards/aacnsynergymodel forpatientcare.pdf?la=en

American Nurses Association (ANA). (2015). *Code of ethics for nurses with interpretive statements.* Author.

American Nurses Association (ANA). (2016). *Nursing administration: Scope and standards of practice* (2nd ed.). Author.

American Nurses Association (ANA). (2017). *Safe staffing.* https://ana.aristotle.com/SitePages/safestaffing.aspx

American Nurses Association (ANA). (2019). *Nurse staffing advocacy.* https://www.nursingworld.org/practice-policy/nurse-staffing/nurse-staffing-advocacy/

American Nurses Association (ANA). (2020). *ANA's principles for nurse staffing* (3rd ed.). Author.

American Organization for Nursing Leadership (AONL). (2010). *AONL guiding principles for future patient care delivery.* https://www.aonl.org/system/files/media/file/2020/12/future-patient-care-delivery.pdf

American Organization for Nursing Leadership (AONL). (2015a). *AONL nurse manager competencies.* Author.

American Organization for Nursing Leadership (AONL). (2015b). *AONL nurse executive competencies.* Author.

Beglinger, J. E. (2006). Quantifying patient care intensity: An evidence-based approach to determining staffing requirements. *Nursing Administration Quarterly, 30*(3), 193–202.

Benner, P. (1984). *From novice to expert: Excellence and power in clinical nursing practice.* Addison-Wesley.

Conway, J., Johnson, B., Edgman-Levitan, S., Schlucter, J. Ford, D., Sodomka, P., & Simmons, L. (2006). *Partnering with patients and families to design a patient- and family-centered health care system: A roadmap for the future.* Institute for Patient- and Family-Centered Care. www.ipfcc.org/pdf/Roadmap.pdf

Cronenwett, L., Sherwood, G., Barnsteiner, J., Disch, J., Johnson, J., Mitchell, P., Sullivan, D. T., & Warren, J. (2007). Quality and safety education for nurses. *Nursing Outlook, 55*(3), 122–131.

Dabney, B. W., & Kalisch, B. J. (2015). Nurse staffing levels and patient-reported missed nursing care. *Journal of Nursing Care Quality, 30*(4), 306–312.

Duffield, C., Roche, M., Diers, D., Catling-Paull, C., & Blay, N. (2010). Staffing, skill mix, and the model of care. *Journal of Clinical Nursing, 19*(15–16), 2242–2251.

European Commission. (2017). *RN4CAST report summary: More support for nursing resources.* https://cordis.europa.eu/article/id/86323-more-support-for-nursing-resources

Greiner, A. C., & Knebel, E. (Eds.). (2003). *Health professions education: A bridge to quality.* National Academies Press.

Harper, E. M. (2012). Staffing based on evidence: Can health information technology make it possible? *Nursing Economics, 30*(5), 262–267, 281.

Harper, K., & McCully, C. (2007). Acuity systems dialogue and patient classification system essentials. *Nursing Administration Quarterly, 31*(4), 284–299.

Health Resources and Services Administration (HRSA) Bureau of Health Workforce. (2017). *Supply and demand projections of the nursing workforce: 2014-2030* https://bhw.hrsa.gov/sites/default/files/bureau-health-workforce/data-research/nchwa-hrsa-nursing-report.pdf

Hertel, R. (2012). Regulating patient staffing: A complex issue. *MedSurg Matters, 21*(1), 3–7.

Institute for Patient- and Family-Centered Care (IPFCC). (n.d.a). *About us.* https://www.ipfcc.org/about/index.html

Institute for Patient- and Family-Centered Care (IPFCC). (n.d.b). *Patient- and family-centered care.* https://www.ipfcc.org/about/pfcc.html

Jones, K. R., DeBaca, V., & Yarbrough, M. (1997). Organizational culture assessment before and after implementing patient-focused care. *Nursing Economics, 15*(2), 73–80.

Kane, R. L., Shamliyan, T., Mueller, C., Duval, S., & Wilt, T. J. (2007). *Nurse staffing and quality of patient care: Evidence report/technology assessment No. 151* (prepared by the Minnesota Evidence-based Practice Center Under Contract No. 290-02-0009). AHRQ Publication No. 07-E005. Agency for Healthcare Research and Quality. https://www.researchgate.net/profile/Sue_Duval/publication/6076607_Nurse_Staffing_and_Quality_of_Patient_Care/links/02bfe513686476e80a000000.pdf

Kaplow, R., & Reed, K. D. (2008). The ACCN synergy model for patient care: A nursing model as a force of magnetism. *Nursing Economics, 26*(1), 17–25.

Knudson, L. (2013). Management connections: Nurse staffing levels linked to patient outcomes, nurse retention. *AORN Journal, 97*(1), C1, C8–C9.

Lee, B., Shannon, D., Rutherford, P., & Peck, C. (2008). *Transforming care at the bedside how to guide: Optimizing communication and teamwork.* Institute for Healthcare Improvement.

Lineweaver, L. (2013). *Nurse staffing 101: A decision-making guide for the RN.* American Nurses Association.

Lookinland, S., Tiedeman, M. E., & Crosson, A. E. (2005). Nontraditional models of care delivery: Have they solved the problems? *Journal of Nursing Administration, 35*(2), 74–80.

Manthey, M. (1989). Practice partnerships: The newest concept in care delivery. *Journal of Nursing Administration, 19*(2), 33–35.

Manthey, M. (2009). The 40th anniversary of primary nursing: Setting the record straight. *Creative Nursing, 15*(1), 36–38.

Montalvo, I. (2007). The National Database of Nursing Quality Indicators® (NDNQI®). *Online Journal of Issues in Nursing, 12*(3), 2.

Myers, S. M. (1998). Patient-focused care: What managers should know. *Nursing Economics, 16*(4), 180–188.

National Council of State Boards of Nursing (NCSBN). (2012). *NCSBN Model Act.* https://www.ncsbn.org/14_Model_Act_0914.pdf

National Council of State Boards of Nursing (NCSBN). (2020). *Definition of nursing terms.* https://www.ncsbn.org/nursing-terms.htm

Needleman, J., Buerhaus, P., Pankratz, V. S., Leibson, C. L., Stevens, S. R., & Harris, M. (2011). Nurse staffing and inpatient hospital mortality. *New England Journal of Medicine, 364*(11), 1037–1045.

Neisner, J., & Raymond, B. (2002). *Nurse staffing and care delivery models: A review of the evidence.* Kaiser Permanente. www.kpihp.org/wp-content/uploads/2012/12/nurse_staffing.pdf

Press Ganey. (2019). *Solution summary: Turn nursing quality insights into improved patient experiences.* https://www.pressganey.com/resources/program-summary/ndnqi-solution-summary

Rutherford, P., Moen, R., & Taylor, J. (2009). TCAB: The "how" and the "what": Developing an initiative to involve nurses in transformative change. *American Journal of Nursing, 100*(11), 5–17.

Tiedeman, M. E., & Lookinland, S. (2004). Traditional models of care delivery. *Journal of Nursing Administration, 34*(6), 291–297.

Unruh, L. (2008). Nurse staffing and patient, nurse, and financial outcomes. *American Journal of Nursing, 108*(1), 62–71.

Wolf, G. A., & Greenhouse, P. K. (2007). Blueprint for design: Creating models that direct change. *Journal of Nursing Administration, 37*(9), 381–387.

To explore learning resources for this chapter, go to FADavis.com

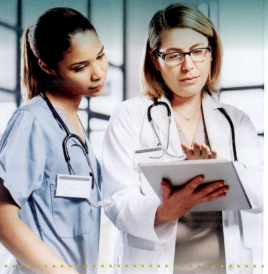

Chapter **14**

Delegating Effectively

Lynne Portnoy, MSN, RN, CNE
Elizabeth J. Murray, PhD, RN, CNE

LEARNING OUTCOMES

- Describe how the concepts of accountability, assignment, authority, prioritization, responsibility, and supervision pertain to delegation.
- Outline what can and cannot be delegated and who can and cannot delegate.
- Describe the five rights of delegation.
- Explain the four steps of the delegation decision-making process.
- Identify potential barriers to effective delegation and strategies to overcome them.
- Describe the nurse leader and manager's role in effective delegation.
- Explain how nursing judgment affects delegation.

KEY TERMS

Accountability
Assignment
Authority
Delegate
Delegation
Delegator
Mindful communication
Nursing judgment
Overdelegation
Prioritization
Responsibility
Supervision
Underdelegation

The Knowledge, Skills, and Attitudes Related to the Following Are Addressed in This Chapter:

Core Competencies	• Patient-Centered Care • Teamwork and Collaboration • Safety
The Essentials: Core Competencies for Professional Nursing Education (AACN, 2021)	**Domain 2: Person-Centered Care** 2.6 Demonstrate accountability for care delivery (p. 31). **Domain 6: Interprofessional Partnerships** 6.1 Communicate in a manner that facilitates a partnership approach to quality care delivery (p. 43). 6.2 Perform effectively in different team roles, using principles and values of team dynamics (p. 44). **Domain 9: Professionalism** 9.3 Demonstrate accountability to the individual, society, and the profession (p. 53).
Code of Ethics with Interpretive Statements (ANA, 2015)	**Provision 1.5:** Relationships with colleagues and others (p. 4) **Provision 2.3:** Collaboration (p. 6) **Provision 3.4:** Professional responsibility in promoting a culture of safety (pp. 11–12) **Provision 4:** The nurse has authority, accountability, and responsibility for nursing practice: makes decisions; and takes action consistent with the obligation to promote health and to provide optimal care (pp. 15–17)

Nurse Manager (NMC) Competencies (AONL, 2015a) and Nurse Executive (NEC) Competencies (AONL, 2015b)	**NMC: Human Resource Management (p. 4)**
	• Scope of practice
	  • Develop role definitions for staff consistent with scope of practice
	NMC: Relationship Management and Influencing Behaviors (p. 6)
	• Promote team dynamics
	• Mentor and coach staff and colleagues
	• Apply communication principles
	NEC: Communication and Relationship Building (p. 4)
	• Relationship management
	  • Build collaborative relationships
	  • Create a trusting environment
	• Influencing behaviors
	  • Facilitate consensus building
	  • Promote decisions that are patient-centered

Nursing Administration Scope and Standards of Practice (ANA, 2016)	**Standard 5A: Coordination** The nurse administrator coordinates implementation of the plan and associated processes (p. 41). **Standard 7: Ethics** The nurse administrator practices ethically (pp. 45–46). **Standard 9: Communication** The nurse administrator communicates effectively in all areas of practice (p. 49).

The Knowledge, Skills, and Attitudes Related to the Following Are Addressed in This Chapter:—cont'd

Standard 10: Collaboration The nurse administrator collaborates with healthcare consumers, colleagues, community leaders, and other stakeholders to advance nursing practice and healthcare transformation (p. 50).

Standard 11: Leadership The nurse administrator leads within professional practice setting, profession, healthcare industry, and society (pp. 51–52).

Standard 14: Quality of Practice The nurse administrator contributes to quality nursing practice (p. 55).

Source: American Association of Colleges of Nursing. (2021). *The essentials: Core competencies for professional nursing education.* Author; American Nurses Association (ANA). (2015). *Code of ethics for nurses with interpretive statements.* Author; American Nurses Association (ANA). (2016). *Nursing administration: Scope and standards of practice* (2nd ed.). Author; American Organization for Nursing Leadership (AONL). (2015a). *AONL nurse manager competencies.* Author; American Organization for Nursing Leadership (AONL). (2015b). *AONL nurse executive competencies.* Author; Cronenwett, L., Sherwood, G., Barnsteiner, J., Disch, J., Johnson, J., Mitchell, P., Sullivan, D. T., & Warren, J. (2007). Quality and safety education for nurses. *Nursing Outlook, 55*(3), 122–131; and Greiner, A. C., & Knebel, E. (Eds.). (2003). *Health professions education: A bridge to quality.* National Academies Press.

Nurses at all levels and in all settings are required to assign and delegate tasks to and supervise other health-care workers. Nurses must develop skills in delegation, prioritization, and oversight of nursing care (American Association of Colleges of Nursing [AACN], 2008). Florence Nightingale first talked about delegation in 1860:

> *But again, to look to all these things yourself does not mean to do them yourself [...] But can you not insure that it is done when not done by yourself? Can you insure that it is not undone when your back is turned? [...] The former only implies that just what you can do with your own hands is done. The latter that what ought to be done is always done (Nightingale, 1860, p. 29).*

Effective delegation is considered a core skill for professional nursing practice globally (American Nurses Association [ANA] & National Council of State Boards of Nursing [NCSBN], 2019; International Council of Nurses [ICN], 2012). The ICN (2008) maintains that nurses are responsible for the delegation of nursing care and supervision of assistive personnel. The ANA recognizes delegation as an important skill for nurses to deliver safe and effective care: The nurse "delegates according to the health, safety, and welfare of the healthcare consumer and considering the circumstance, person, task, direction or communication, supervision, evaluation, as well as the state nurse practice act regulations, institution, and regulatory entities while maintaining accountability for care" (ANA, 2015a, p. 61). Moreover, the ANA's *Code of Ethics for Nurses With Interpretive Statements* states that "nurses are accountable and responsible for the assignment or delegation of nursing activities. Such assignment or delegation must be consistent with state practice acts, organizational policy, and nursing standards of practice" (ANA, 2015b, p. 17).

Delegation is essential to effective leadership and management as well as managerial productivity. As a management principle, delegation is necessary to obtaining desired outcomes through the work of nursing staff (NCSBN, 1997). Nurse leaders and managers must delegate many routine tasks to allow themselves time to handle more complex activities that require a higher level of expertise.

In this chapter, the key principles of delegation are outlined, including what can be delegated and by whom. Next, the five rights of delegation are covered, followed by a breakdown of the delegation process.

▶ KEY PRINCIPLES OF DELEGATION

Delegation requires problem-solving skills, critical thinking skills, and clinical judgment. Development of delegation skills begins early in a nurse's academic career, but proficiency is achieved with education and experience. Indeed, delegation can be difficult for novice nurses because they are still acquiring foundational knowledge and skills, have limited experience, and are in the early stages of developing critical thinking skills (Duffy & McCoy, 2014). **Delegation** is defined as the act of transferring to a competent individual the authority to perform a selected nursing task in a selected situation, the process for doing the work while retaining accountability for the outcomes (ANA, 2015a). Additionally, the individual delegating the task retains accountability for the outcome (ANA, 2015a, p. 86). Nurses delegate tasks based on patient needs, potential for harm, stability of a patient's condition, complexity of the task, and predictability of the outcome. Also taken into consideration are the qualifications and skill level of the person to whom the task is delegated (ANA, 2012). Nurses must be familiar with their state nurse practice acts to ensure that they delegate within legal parameters. Most state nurse practice acts prohibit nurses from delegating certain aspects of the nursing process to enrolled nurses (ENs), licensed practical nurses (LPNs), licensed vocational nurses (LVNs), and unlicensed assistive personnel (UAPs). In addition, an individual cannot delegate a task that is not in their own scope of practice (ANA & NCSBN, 2019). Delegation is a management principle used to obtain the desired outcomes through the work of others (NCSBN, 1997). When delegation is used effectively, nurse leaders and managers can expand access to nursing care, promote safe and quality nursing care, and facilitate effective use of health-care resources.

In the delegation process, the **delegator** is the one who is delegating the nursing responsibility and is a licensed nurse; the delegator may be an advanced practice registered nurse (APRN), a registered nurse (RN), or an LPN/LVN (ANA & NCSBN, 2019). The delegator must have the appropriate qualifications, education, and authority to delegate as determined by the state nurse practice act, other regulatory agencies, and organization policy and procedures. The **delegate** (also referred to as the *delegatee*) is the person to whom the nursing responsibility is being delegated, and they must also have the appropriate education, skills, and competence to carry out the activity. RNs may delegate nursing activities to other RNs, LPNs or LVNs, and UAPs.

Accountability means "to be answerable to oneself and others for one's own choices, decisions, and actions as measured against a standard such as that established by the ANA Code of Ethics" (ANA, 2015b, p. 41). In the process of delegation, an RN must comply with the state nurse practice act or regulating bodies and is accountable for the quality of nursing care provided. Nurses have a professional accountability and obligation not to abuse trust and to be able to justify professional actions (Royal College of Nursing, 2015). Nurses are accountable for the decision to delegate and for the tasks delegated to others. In addition, "nurses are accountable for their professional practice and image as well as the outcomes of their own and delegated nursing care" (AACN, 2008, p. 9). The health-care organization and leadership are also accountable for delegation. Organizational accountability involves providing sufficient resources for nurses to provide nursing care effectively and safely, including the following (ANA & NCSBN, 2019, p. 3):

- Determining nursing responsibilities that can be delegated, to whom, and under what circumstances
- Developing delegation policies and procedures
- Periodically evaluating delegation processes
- Promoting a positive culture/work environment

Nurse leaders and managers are accountable for providing "a safe environment that supports and facilitates appropriate assignment and delegation" (ANA, 2015a, p. 17). They set the expectations for appropriate delegation and ensure that RNs, LPNs/LVNs, and UAPs are aware of individual roles (Duffy & McCoy, 2014; Hughes et al., 2018). Additionally, nurse leaders and managers are accountable for establishing systems to assess, monitor, verify, and communicate ongoing competence requirements in areas related to delegation (ANA, 2012, p. 7).

A licensed nurse has legitimate authority by virtue of their professional licensure to delegate specific tasks to other licensed nurses or UAP. In the delegation process, nurses have authority to make assessments, diagnose, plan nurse care, implement and evaluate nursing care, and exercise nursing judgment. **Authority** is a "legal source of power; the right to act or command the actions of others and to have them followed" (Porter-O'Grady & Malloch, 2013, p. 432). A nurse must have the authority or the right to act or command the actions of others to carry out patient care activities safely. Authority is based on the state nurse practice act and should also be reflected in a nurse's job description. The organization must give the nurse the authority to direct the work of others. Nurse leaders and managers have the authority to determine how staff resources will be distributed on the unit based on patient needs.

Responsibility is the obligation one has to accomplish work. Additionally, responsibility involves the individual's obligation to perform competently at the person's level of education. In the delegation process, the nurse is responsible to assess the situation, determine the competence of the delegate and appropriateness of delegation, supervise the delegate, evaluate the performance of the delegate, and manage the results (Porter-O'Grady & Malloch, 2013). Delegates accept responsibility when they agree to perform tasks delegated to them (ANA, 2012; Weydt, 2010). The delegate is responsible for their own actions and for accepting only tasks for which they are qualified and providing feedback to the delegator as directed (Porter-O'Grady & Malloch, 2013).

Supervision is the active process of guiding, directing, and influencing the outcome of an individual's performance of a task (ANA, 2012, p. 6). The nurse supervises the activities delegated by monitoring the delegate's performance of the task or function and ensuring compliance with standards of practice and policies and procedures. Organizational policies and procedures must be in place to support the nurse delegating a task. In the event the activity is being done inappropriately, there must be policy in place to allow the nurse to assess the situation and take back control of the task if necessary (ANA & NCSBN, 2019). Nurses engaged in "supervision of patient care should not be construed as managerial supervisors on behalf of the employer under federal labor laws" (ANA, 2012, p. 4).

Assignment describes the "routine care, activities, and procedures that are within the authorized scope of practice" of each staff member during a given time period (ANA & NCSBN, 2019). When making an assignment, a nurse designates an individual to be responsible for specific patients or selected responsibilities the individual is already authorized to take on through the nurse practice act (Porter-O'Grady & Malloch, 2013). During the assignment process, a transfer of responsibility and accountability for the activity occur. The nurse assigning tasks must ensure that the activity is within the individual's scope of practice. For example, the charge nurse of a unit typically makes the assignment of patient care for nurses on the shift. The charge nurse is accountable for their decisions related to the assignments but transfers the accountability for care to the assigned nurses.

Prioritization is another important principle of delegation. Although nurses are accustomed to prioritizing nursing care, delegation also requires effective prioritization. **Prioritization** is deciding which patient needs or problems require immediate action and which are not urgent and can be addressed at a later time.

What Can and Cannot Be Delegated

Many state nurse practice acts, regulatory agency guidelines, and institutional policies specify nursing activities that may be delegated. Delegated tasks may involve monitoring patients, collecting specimens, reporting, providing care, and documenting data. The decision to delegate "must be based on the needs of the patient, the stability and predictability of the patient's condition, the documented competence of the delegate, and the ability of the licensed nurse to supervise the delegated responsibility and its outcome" (ANA & NCSBN, 2019, p. 7). The UAP may take vital signs, measure intake and output, and report the information to the nurse. The nurse interprets the reported information as part of the assessment and then makes clinical judgments and uses the data to establish a plan of care.

Tasks that should not be delegated include aspects of the nursing process (e.g., performing an assessment, formulating a nursing diagnosis, developing and updating a plan of care for a patient, and evaluating the patient's progress toward achieving goals), as well as communicating with health-care providers, implementing orders from health-care providers, providing teaching to patient and/or family, evaluating patient status, and triage (ANA, 2015a; Anderson et al., 2006; Duffy & McCoy, 2014). Table 14-1 displays role-specific nursing activities for professional nurses, LPNs or LVNs, and UAPs. In general, any nursing activity that requires patient education, specialized nursing knowledge, or

Table 14-1	Specific Nursing Activities of Registered Nurses, Licensed Practical Nurses or Licensed Vocational Nurses, and Unlicensed Assistive Personnel	
RNs	**LPNs or LVNs**	**UAPs**
Can do all activities that can be done by LPNs or LVNs and UAPs plus the following: • Activities requiring specialized nursing knowledge or nursing judgment • Care for unstable patients with unpredictable outcomes • All aspects of the nursing process: assessment, diagnosis, planning, implementation, and evaluation • Administration of all medications • Initiation and maintenance of intravenous fluids • Administration of intravenous medications • Blood transfusions • Complex dressing changes • Sterile procedures	Under the direction of RNs, can do all activities that can be done by UAPs plus the following: • Care for stable patients with predictable outcomes • Collection of patient data and reporting to RNs • Updating of initial RN assessment • Implementation of patient care • Reinforcement of patient education • Basic dressing changes • Medication administration (excluding intravenous medications in some states) • Administration of enteral feedings • Insertion of urinary catheters • Tracheostomy care • Monitoring of intravenous infusions, blood transfusions, and intravenous sites	Under the direction of the RN, can do the following: • Assisting a patient with activities of daily living • Assisting a patient with hygiene • Bed making • Assisting with ambulation, positioning, and transferring • Dressing • Feeding of patients without swallowing precautions • Collecting specimens • Collecting patient data (e.g., vital signs, weights, and intake and output) and reporting to the RN

LPNs, licensed practical nurses; LVNs, licensed vocational nurses; RNs, registered nurses; UAPs, unlicensed assistive personnel.

nursing judgment *cannot* be delegated. **Nursing judgment** is defined as the educated, informed, and experienced process that a nurse uses to form an opinion and reach a clinical decision based on the analysis of available information (NCSBN, 2005). Further, nursing judgment includes conscious decision making and intuition.

Who Can and Cannot Delegate

As mentioned earlier, RNs may delegate to other RNs, LPNs or LVNs, and UAPs. In addition, LPNs or LVNs may delegate to a UAP if directed to do so by an RN. An LPN or LVN cannot assign or delegate to an RN.

LPNs or LVNs can perform tasks that UAPs are not qualified to do. State nurse practice acts dictate the scope of practice for LPNs or LVNs, although the scope of practice varies from state to state. Often the role of the LPN or LVN can be confusing for new nurses or those who have not worked with them before, so all nurses must be knowledgeable about the nurse practice act in their state. Monitoring patients' health status and providing basic nursing care under the direction of an RN comprise the duties of LPNs or LVNs. Common tasks LPNs or LVNs can perform include those of the UAP in addition to updating initial assessments performed by the RN, reinforcing teaching, and monitoring patient status.

UAPs are health-care workers who provide low-risk care that does not require nursing knowledge or nursing judgment. UAPs typically assist patients with activities of daily living, such as bed making, bathing, and assisting with dressing, and they provide basic care under the supervision of an RN. Usually, UAPs do not hold a license; however, they may be certified.

According to the NCSBN and the ANA (2019, pp. 2–3), regardless of the delegator, key points related to delegation include the following:

- The delegate is allowed to perform a specific nursing task that is beyond the delegate's traditional role and the delegate does not routinely perform the task.
- The delegate has obtained additional education, training, and validated competency to perform the task.
- The licensed nurse cannot delegate nursing judgment or critical decision making.
- The delegated task is within the scope of practice of the delegator.
- Nursing responsibilities are delegated by someone who has the authority to delegate.
- The delegated task must be within the scope of practice of the delegate as outlined by the state nurse practice act.

LEARNING ACTIVITY 14-1   **Review your state nurse practice act, and determine the following:**

- Does it address delegation?
- Does it describe specific tasks that can or cannot be delegated?
- Does it describe who can and cannot delegate?

▶ THE FIVE RIGHTS OF DELEGATION

Nurse leaders and managers must work collaboratively with staff nurses to maintain the integrity of patient care (NCSBN, 1997). The five rights of delegation can be used as a guide for nurses to clarify critical elements of the delegation decision-making process: The *right task* is assigned to the *right person* under the *right circumstances* with the RN providing the *right direction or communication* and the *right supervision*. The five rights of delegation delineate accountability for nurses at all levels.

Right Task

In the nurse's best judgment, the right task is one that can be safely delegated to a specific delegate for a specific patient. Appropriate activities for consideration for delegation include those that (NCSBN, 1997):

- Frequently occur in the daily care of patients
- Are within the scope of practice of the LPN or LVN
- Do not require the UAP to exercise nursing judgment
- Do not require application of the nursing process
- Do not have risks that are predictable or beyond minimal
- Use a standard and unchanging procedure

Nurse leaders and managers are responsible for ensuring that appropriate activities for consideration in the delegation process are identified in the LPN or LVN and UAP job description. In addition, nurse leaders and managers must describe the expectations and limitations of activities in organizational policies and procedures and in standards of practice (NCSBN, 1997).

Right Circumstances

When delegating, the nurse must consider the patient setting, available resources, and other relevant factors. Effective delegation requires the nurse to assess the status of patients, analyze the data, and identify patient-specific goals and nursing care needs. In addition, the nurse must match the complexity of the task with the competency level of the delegate and the amount of supervision needed. Nurse leaders and managers are responsible for assessing the needs of the patient population on the unit or in the department and identifying collective nursing care needs, priorities, and resources. Further, ensuring appropriate staffing and skill mix, as well as providing sufficient equipment and supplies, is critical for effective delegation. The issue of safe staffing levels is a concerning and continuing problem effecting safe delegation. Encouraging collaboration and participation in decision making enhances relationships and builds stronger staffing plans (Halm, 2019).

Right Person

It is important for nurses to know the competency levels of those on the patient care team to delegate on an individual and patient-specific basis. Nurse leaders and managers must establish organizational standards consistent with state laws to ensure educational requirements and competencies of RNs, LPNs or LVNs, and UAPs. Nurse leaders and managers should ensure that competence standards related to delegation are integrated into organizational policies and should assess RN, LPN or LVN, and UAP performance routinely. Performance evaluations should be based on standards, and nurse leaders must initiate steps to remedy any failure to meet standards (NCSBN, 1997). Further, it is inappropriate for nurse leaders and managers to require nurses to delegate when, in the nurse's professional judgment, delegation is unsafe. The decision whether or not to delegate is based on the nurse's judgment concerning the patient condition, competence of the team members, degree of supervision that may be required, and that the delegated activity is ethical and can be safely carried out (ANA & NCSBN, 2019).

Presenting an opportunity for the UAP, LPN, LVN, or RN to express their opinion and share decisions related to their work has been identified as enhancing workplace empowerment and can lead to safer patient outcomes (Conger & Kanungo, 1988; Hui, 1994; Laschinger et al., 1999; The Joint Commission, 2019).

Right Direction or Communication

Communication is critical to effective delegation. The nurse must provide a clear, concise description of the task, including its objective, limits, and expectations (ANA & NCSBN, 2019). Communication between the delegator and the delegate is essential to safe patient care. Situation-specific communication includes the following (NCSBN, 1997, p. 24):

- Specific data to be collected and method and timelines for reporting
- Specific activities to be performed and any patient-specific instruction and limitations
- The expected result or potential complications and timelines for communicating such information

Nurse leaders and managers are responsible for communicating acceptable activities, competencies, and qualifications of all staff members through standards of practice, role descriptions, and policies and procedures (NCSBN, 1997). Further, nurse leaders and managers must facilitate open communication with all staff members and encourage them to express concerns or refuse an assignment, without fear of reprisal, if they believe that they do not possess the required skills needed to perform the task safely (ANA, 2015a).

Right Supervision or Evaluation

The nurse provides feedback to the delegate as well as appropriate monitoring, evaluation, and intervention as needed. The nurse may supervise the activity or assign supervision to another licensed nurse. The nurse must provide specific directions and clear expectations of how the task is to be performed; in addition, the nurse should monitor the performance, obtain and provide feedback, intervene if needed, and ensure proper documentation (NCSBN, 1997). Finally, the nurse must evaluate the entire delegation process and provide feedback to all involved, including the patient. Nurse leaders and managers are responsible for ensuring that adequate human resources are available to provide for sufficient supervision. Nurse leaders and managers also must evaluate the outcomes of the patient population and use information to develop quality improvement programs and risk management plans (NCSBN, 1997).

LEARNING ACTIVITY 14-2

What to Consider When Delegating

Taylor is a new charge nurse on a busy medical-surgical unit. She is having some difficulties with her organizational and time management skills. Today, there are five new admissions and four patients scheduled for surgery. She is assigning patients to the teams. One team consists of an RN, LPN, and UAP. Nursing students will be on the unit and one is assigned to each team.

1. What does the charge nurse need to consider when making assignments to LPNs, UAPs, and the nursing students?
2. Using the five rights of delegation, list two activities that Taylor could delegate to:
   a. RN
   b. LPN
   c. UAP
   d. Nursing student

▶ THE DELEGATION PROCESS

When a task is delegated, decisions must be made with the goal of delivering safe and quality patient care. The nurse must assess the knowledge, skill, and experience of the delegate, as well as the following (Snyder et al., 2004, p. 10):

- *Potential for harm:* The nurse must determine how much risk the activity can cause the individual patient.
- *Complexity of the task:* The more complex the task, the less desirable it is to delegate. Only an RN should perform complex tasks.
- *Amount of problem-solving and innovation needed:* Activities that require special attention, adaptation, or an innovated approach should not be delegated.
- *Unpredictability of outcome:* It is not advisable to delegate an activity if the patient's response is unknown or unpredictable.
- *Level of patient interaction:* The nurse should avoid delegating activities that may interfere with the nurse's developing a trusting relationship with the patient.

Delegation is a complex but necessary process requiring skill in clinical judgment to accomplish safe and effective nursing care in a timely manner. The delegation process includes assessment and planning, communication, surveillance and supervision, and evaluation and feedback.

Delegation is based on patient needs and available resources. During the assessment and planning steps of the delegation process, the nurse plans for care and specifies the knowledge and skills required to accomplish the task (ANA & NCSBN, 2019). The nurse determines whether there are any cultural modifications needed, whether the patient's condition is stable and predictable, and whether the environment in which care will be provided is stable (Duffy & McCoy, 2014). Next, the nurse develops a plan of care with the patient and their family. If the nurse determines that patient needs will be met without jeopardizing safety, the nurse will then proceed to the next step.

Clear directions must be given to the delegate, including unique patient information and expectations *regarding what to do, what to report, and when to ask for assistance* (ANA & NCSBN, 2019; NCSBN, 2005). Communication must be a two-way process, with the nurse assessing the delegate's understanding of expectations and providing clarification if needed. Communication should be mindful (Anthony & Vidal, 2010). **Mindful communication** is an active process in which those involved are focused on attending to, responding to, and perceiving information. In mindful communication, information is continually analyzed and categorized, thus allowing for dynamic information processing. The communication process is discussed in depth in Chapter 8.

Surveillance and supervision of delegation are related to the nurse's responsibility for patient care and include determining the level of supervision required for the specific situation. Surveillance is the process of observing and staying attuned to the patient's status and staff performance and, if necessary, following up on a changing situation. The nurse must supervise the delegate by monitoring the task and ensuring compliance with standards of practice and policies and procedures (NCSBN, 2005).

Finally, evaluation and feedback are used to assess the effectiveness of the delegation and the outcome and to determine whether there is a need to modify the plan of care. The nurse evaluates the patient's response to the delegated task, including feedback from the patient and/or family during this step. Evaluation is an important step in the process that is sometimes left out. The nurse should be prepared to provide feedback to the delegate regarding whether the care provided was performed correctly, whether the desired patient outcome was achieved, and any areas for improvement (NCSBN, 2005). Evaluation should be continuous during the delegation process. When evaluating and providing feedback, the nurse must consider accepting variations in the style in which tasks are performed as long as standards of care are met and patient outcomes are appropriate. A nurse leader who effectively delegates improves the skills and knowledge of the LPN, LVN, UAP, and RN and ensures that appropriate resources are available to them (The Joint Commission, 2019). The nurse monitors the delegation process, provides feedback to the delegate, obtains feedback from the delegate, considers the initial assessment, evaluates the patient outcome, and modifies the plan of care if necessary. It is important to avoid confusing delegation with assignment. Nurse leaders and managers assign tasks, routine care activities, and procedures that are within the scope of practice for licensed nurses and UAPs. These activities are often outlined in the state nurse practice act. The delegation process for RNs delegating tasks to UAPs is illustrated in Figure 14-1.

LEARNING ACTIVITY 14-3

Delegation Decision Making

Use Figure 14-1 and Table 14-1 and determine whether you as the RN would delegate the following tasks to a UAP:

- Feeding a patient with difficulty swallowing
- Measuring intake and output
- Ambulating a patient for the first time after abdominal surgery
- Evaluating a patient's pain level after receiving pain medication
- Emptying a urinary drainage bag
- Checking nasogastric tube placement
- Monitoring intravenous fluids
- Administering enteral feedings
- Performing colostomy care
- Giving discharge instructions

▶ BARRIERS TO EFFECTIVE DELEGATION

Delegation can be very challenging for both the delegator and the delegate, and there are numerous reasons that delegation can be unsuccessful. Unfortunately, ineffective delegation can jeopardize the provision of safe and quality patient care in a timely manner and can result in missed care or omitted care (e.g., ambulating and turning patients, providing hygiene, documenting input and output, patient teaching, discharge planning) (Kalisch, 2006). Nurse leaders and managers must

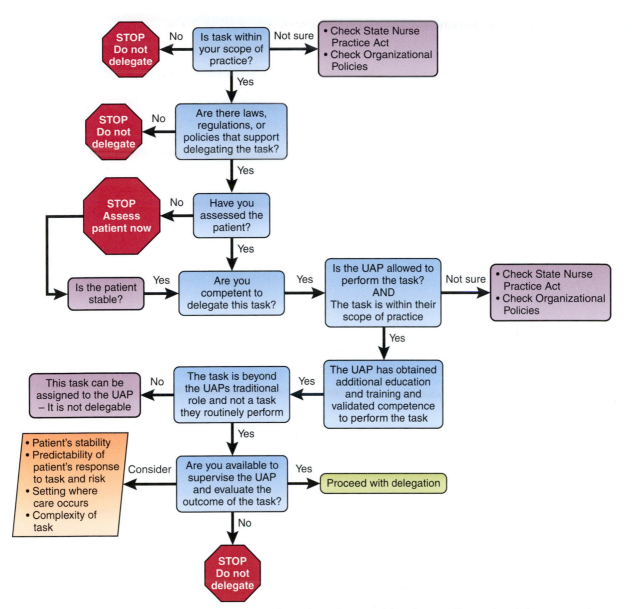

Figure 14-1 Delegation decision-making algorithm for registered nurses delegating to unlicensed assistive personnel (UAPs). (Adapted from American Nurses Association. [2012]. *ANA's principles for delegation.* Author; National Council of State Boards of Nursing. [2016]. National guidelines for nursing delegation. *Journal of Nursing Regulation, 7*(1), 5–14; and National Council of State Boards of Nursing & American Nurses Association. [2019]. *National guidelines for nursing delegation: Joint statement on delegation.* https://www.ncsbn.org/13546.htm)

implement strategies to diminish factors contributing to poor delegation (Gravlin & Bittner, 2010). Recognizing potential barriers is the first step in overcoming them (Snyder et al., 2004). Major barriers to effective delegation can be related to the delegator, the delegate, and to leadership and management. There are times when delegation can result in conflict between the delegator and the delegate. In a study to understand the differences in the perceptions of delegation between nurses and UAPs, investigators found that when conflict occurred during the delegation process, nurses and UAPs had different perceptions of the cause of the conflict (Potter et al., 2010). The importance of clear and concise communication cannot be overstated. Concerns regarding appropriate delegation can arise in professional malpractice cases as well. As more health care is delivered in a community setting, issues regarding delegation will become entangled in standards-of-care concerns following unexpected outcomes (Miller, 2018). Effective delegation can enhance patient outcomes (Wagner, 2018).

E X P L O R I N G   T H E   E V I D E N C E   1 4 - 1

Wagner, E. (2018). Improving patient care outcomes through better delegation-communication between nurses and assistive personnel. *Journal of Nursing Care Quality, 33*(3), 187–193.

Aim

The purpose of a quality improvement (QI) project was to determine whether improving the delegation-communication practices among nurses and UAPs influenced effective delegation techniques, reduced falls and pressure injury rates, and improved patient satisfaction with care on an adult acute care pulmonary/medical/surgical unit.

Methods

A single group pretest-posttest design used to determine the effect of a delegation-communication learning intervention for both RNs and UAPs preparedness to delegate, knowledge level, use of delegation, mindfulness, supervision issues, and delegation decision making.

Outcomes focused on their ability to use delegation-communication to reduce patient falls and the incidence of pressure injuries and improve patient satisfaction with care.

Baseline observations were made of RNs and UAP on two occasions over 8 hours each to assess the delegation-communication practices common on the unit. Communication appeared to occur only when there was a change in patient status or there was movement on or off the unit.

After the observation period there was a pretest survey to assess knowledge deficits related to delegation, competency, role knowledge, supervision issues, mindful communication techniques, and delegation decision making followed by an online lecture and techniques for mindful communication.

Key Findings
- Preparedness for delegation
  - RNs:
    - Before the learning intervention RNs tended to delay the decision to delegate and were more likely to delegate tasks usually expected in the UAP job description (e.g., bathing, bed making).

- After the learning intervention RNs' results showed significant differences (improvement) after the learning intervention in four items: explaining performance appraisals, facilitating clearer communication, explaining tasks, and seeking feedback.
- UAPs:
  - After the learning intervention items improved with the learning intervention, but only one area was significant: losing respect because of delegation (preintervention mean 2.86; postintervention mean 1.86, $P = 0.39$).
- Patient outcomes:
  - Before the learning intervention the fall rate was 2.17 per 1,000 patient days during the month before the project. The fall rate decreased to 0 during the 4-month project and remained there for 2 months after the project. Hospital-acquired pressure injury rate, stage II, before the intervention was 3.7%. During the project this rate fluctuated from 4.17% to 0%. This rate remained at 0% for the 2-month postproject period. The Press-Ganey patient satisfaction remained static with little change. One month after the project there was an improved promptness to call buttons (pre 86.7%, post 88.7%), slightly poorer pain control rate (pre 86.3%, post 85.5%), and an unchanged rate of staff working together to care for them (pre 90.2%, post 90.2%).

Implications for Nurses and Nurse Managers

Nurses and UAPs need continued support and education related to delegation techniques and communication for safe and effective management of care in acute care settings. A team approach is necessary to reach desired patient outcomes and can be improved with effective communication and delegation practices. Nurse leaders and managers should consider including education regarding communication and roles and responsibilities related to delegation during new-hire orientation and annually. In addition, using a care delivery model that builds relationships between RNs and UAPs can improve communication techniques, delegation practice, and patient outcomes.

Delegator-Related Barriers

Nurses may not delegate because they are not team players, prefer to work alone, or believe they can perform certain tasks better than others. Insecurity, lack of experience, and poor organizational skills are other reasons nurses do not delegate. The nurse may experience fear when considering delegation (e.g., that it will result in a negative outcome or that the safety of the patient could be jeopardized) (Snyder et al., 2004). Other nurses fear criticism from other nurses or delegates.

Nurses may also delegate too many tasks to a delegate or delegate to only a few select delegates. **Overdelegation** occurs when the workload is more than the delegate can accomplish in the allotted time frame. In addition, overdelegation can overwork some delegates while leaving others with little to do. Nurses may overdelegate when they feel uncomfortable performing certain tasks, are unorganized, or are inexperienced with delegation. Nurse leaders and managers often overdelegate when they are unfamiliar with certain responsibilities, especially if staff members are comfortable with the task.

In contrast, **underdelegation** is the failure to transfer authority for a task or the failure to provide clear direction to the delegate. Underdelegation occurs for a variety of reasons. Some nurses fear losing control or authority and recognition. In some cases, nurses underdelegate because of a lack of willingness to accept variations in the style in which tasks are performed. Nurse leaders and managers may underdelegate because they feel insecure or are concerned that more experienced staff members may resent them. In addition, they may believe that they can accomplish the task quicker or do not want to take the time to explain, observe, and evaluate the delegate (Duffy & McCoy, 2014; Porter-O'Grady & Malloch, 2013). Other reasons for underdelegation are fear of the task being done incorrectly or poorly and of depending on others (Porter-O'Grady & Malloch, 2013). New nurses often underdelegate because they are inexperienced with using authority to delegate, fear being disliked, or fear making a mistake in the delegation decision-making process (Duffy & McCoy, 2014).

Delegate-Related Barriers

The delegate must be reliable and willing to accept delegated tasks; in fact, some delegates may refuse to accept a delegated task. Lack of confidence or fear of failure on the part of the delegate can affect the delegation process. The delegate may lack experience or confidence. Nurses should consider the following potential reasons for refusal and attempt to work with the delegate if possible (Porter-O'Grady & Malloch, 2013, p. 441):

- Lack of willingness to do the task
- Lack of skill or comfort with the skill required for the task
- Feeling overworked or perception of an unfair assignment
- Physical inability to do the work

Leadership- and Management-Related Barriers

Leadership and management at the organizational and unit level that do not promote effective delegation can have a negative impact on patient outcomes. A lack of guidelines that address who can delegate and what tasks can be delegated does not provide support for effective delegation. There must be policies and procedures in place that allow input from nurses and support delegation as a nurse's right and responsibility. Policies should protect the nurses from inappropriate assignments and delegation of inappropriate nursing activities or responsibilities (ANA, 2015b).

Job descriptions for RNs, LPNs or LVNs, and UAPs should address the delegation process to allow nurses to have the authority to delegate. The nurse's job description must reflect the nurse's authority, responsibility, and accountability for delegation. The delegate's job description should indicate the type of nursing tasks and skills that they can take on. Nurses must also be knowledgeable about the delegate's job description. Nurse leaders and managers are responsible for validating delegate credentials and qualifications and keeping staff nurses informed.

Lack of a supportive environment, poor staffing levels, lack of tolerance for mistakes, and the absence of processes for validation of competencies for delegation can pose major barriers to effective delegation. The quality of delegation practices on a unit can influence patient safety.

Breaking Down Barriers

Fostering trusting and respectful relationships among RNs, LPNs or LVNs, and UAPs is critical to effective delegation (Bittner & Gravlin, 2009). Establishing guidelines, policies, and procedures to support the delegation process promotes delegation and offers guidance for nurses engaging in delegation. Including delegation in the job descriptions of all nursing personnel establishes the authority, accountability, and responsibility for delegation. In addition, this allows nurse leaders and managers to hold all staff members accountable to principles related to delegation that are addressed in the job description. Nurse leaders and managers can provide periodic feedback related to the delegation process to RNS, LPNs or LVNs, and UAPs to promote the development of effective delegation skills.

Nurse leaders and managers must focus efforts on creating a supportive environment that promotes effective communication and teamwork. Creating a supportive environment for delegation can facilitate patient care and reduce risks for adverse events and near misses (Potter et al., 2010). Nurse leaders and managers should create "a culture of quality and safety that ensures attention to detail and honest reporting of omissions of nursing care" (Kalisch, 2006, p. 312). Nurse leaders and managers are accountable for compromised standards of care resulting from poor delegation practices. Therefore, nurse leaders and managers must promote reporting missed care followed by root cause analysis to determine underlying causes of the problem and identify strategies to improve the delegation process.

EXPLORING THE EVIDENCE 14-2

Hughes, M., Kirk, R., & Dixon, A. (2018). New Zealand nurses' storied experiences of direction and delegation. *Nursing Praxis in New Zealand, 34*(3), 32–45.

Aim
To examine nurses' observations about the practice of delegation and experiences of enrolled nurses' (new nurses') and RNs' delegation-communication interactions.

Methods
Narrative inquiry was chosen to facilitate the ability to place nurses, conditions, and exchanges into a whole story. Purposive sampling was used to select

Continued

EXPLORING THE EVIDENCE 14 - 2—cont'd

the 36 nurses. Inclusion criteria included all nurses holding a current practicing certificate who were registered with the Nursing Council of New Zealand. Enrolled nurses (ENs) were nurses enrolled.

Key Findings
- A lack of guidance, evidence, and in-service education regarding the delegation process was voiced by RNs.
- RNs expressed dissatisfaction with the lack of leadership from their nursing seniors in providing information about their professional responsibility in delegating to ENs.
- Communicating thoroughly and proficiently is critical to the success of a delegation collaboration.
- There is confusion about the definition of delegation in relation to differing roles of nursing personnel, and this lack of clarity affects the timing of care.
- A one size fits all approach does not meet nurses' knowledge needs regarding delegation.
- Delegation and direction training is as important as other compulsory in-service training sessions such as fire-training, fall prevention, and SBAR.
- A mentor or "dedicated buddy" is recommended to ensure that the core competency of delegation is communicated.
- Results found that working in a team differs from working as a team.
- RNs found that at times the primary nursing model was easier when busy, and that team nursing with its attendant delegation could be counterproductive to the team model of nursing required for safe and effective care.
- ENs felt that communication was not always inclusive and the way a task was communicated was as important as the task being delegated.
- ENs believed that developing a relationship between RNs and ENs was an essential part of good delegation experiences.

Implications for Nurse Leaders and Managers
Effective communication is key in all delegation interactions. Nurse leaders and managers must ensure that policies and procedures related to delegation are clear and made available to all team members. Further, they should assess the delegation skills of team members regularly to make sure nurses are comfortable with the delegation process and new nurses understand their roles and responsibilities related to delegation.

▶ SUMMARY

Delegation is a complex process in nursing practice that requires nursing knowledge, nursing judgment, and final accountability for patient care. Effective delegation requires all nurses as well as nurse leaders and managers to be knowledgeable about the principles of delegation, the associated risks and benefits of delegation, and state regulations governing nursing practice. Effective delegation is critical to safe and quality patient care because it frees the nurse to be able to do more specialized tasks that involve making nursing judgments and coordinating patient care. Organizations must support nurse leaders and managers in the coordination, supervision, and delegation of care as needed. Effective leadership and management at the organizational and unit or department level foster successful delegation.

NCLEX®-STYLE REVIEW QUESTIONS

Multiple Choice

1. A registered nurse (RN) is working on a medical-surgical unit functioning as a team leader for five patients with a licensed practical nurse (LPN) and a certified nurse's aide (CNA). Which action should *not* be delegated to the CNA?
    1. Positioning the patient for comfort by raising the head of the bed
    2. Performing a pain assessment
    3. Assisting the patient with transfer from bed to chair
    4. Offering the patient fluids
2. Which statement best reflects the concept of accountability with regard to delegation of tasks?
    1. Nursing state practice acts do not require nurses to be held accountable for their actions.
    2. Accountability exists at both nursing and organizational levels.
    3. An organization's obligation to accountability is based on its ability to offer quality care regardless of nurse staffing.
    4. The competency of the nurse is not considered as being relevant to accountability.
3. Which situation provides an example of the *right circumstances* as defined by the five rights of delegation?
    1. Completion of the task does not require nursing judgment
    2. Assessing needs of the population in the context of available resources
    3. Identifying competency level
    4. Providing correct information to a patient
4. A nurse manager is educating a staff nurse with regard to the five rights of delegation. Which statement by the staff nurse indicates that additional training is needed with regard to *right supervision or evaluation*?
    1. Once a task has been delegated, the nurse is absolved of responsibility.
    2. Nurses should provide feedback relative to task completion.
    3. It is important to provide clear directions relative to task delegation.
    4. Performance of the delegated task should be monitored.

5. Which observation, if made by a registered nurse (RN) who is working with a licensed practical nurse (LPN) and an unlicensed assistive personnel (UAP), would require *immediate* intervention based on the delegation process?
   1. UAP was transferring a patient out of bed who was 2 days postoperative laparoscopic surgery
   2. LPN was administering oral pain medication following performing a pain assessment
   3. LPN was monitoring a blood transfusion
   4. UAP was providing information to a patient who was just placed on isolation relative to neutropenic precautions

6. A physician has ordered a rectal suppository to be administered to a 25-year-old male patient. The registered nurse (RN) delegates this task to the licensed practical nurse (LPN). The LPN would prefer not to complete this task. The RN tells the nurse manager about this issue. How would the nurse manager interpret this refusal by the LPN to perform a delegated task?
   1. Underdelegation
   2. Possibility of a delegate-related barrier
   3. Overdelegation
   4. Possibility of a delegator-related barrier

7. A group of nurse managers are reviewing a new job description for a staff nurse on a medical-surgical unit. Which observation if found would indicate that the job description needs revision with regard to delegation?
   1. Delineation of roles and responsibilities
   2. A listing of tasks that the nurse can complete
   3. No mention of the nursing position authority
   4. Listing of minimum qualifications for the nursing position

8. Nonlicensed staff members (unlicensed assistive personnel [UAP]) have asked for a meeting with the nurse manager as they are unhappy with how one of the nursing staff (registered nurse [RN]) has been delegating tasks with regard to patient care. Which statement, if made by a nonlicensed staff member, would indicate that additional instruction is needed for the nursing staff with regard to effective delegation principles?
   1. "The RN told me that I couldn't obtain a urine specimen from a patient."
   2. "I was told by the RN that I had to wait until the order was written in the patient's chart before I could act on it."
   3. "The RN told me that I should wait until after lunch before I gave the patient AM care as the patient had just been medicated for pain."
   4. "The RN told me that I had to change all of the bed linen for the patients before I went home at the end of the shift."

9. Which task should *not* be delegated to a licensed vocational nurse (LVN) by a registered nurse (RN) who is working with an LVN and unlicensed assistive personal (UAP) as part of the team?
   1. Performing oral hygiene for a patient who has oral ulcerations
   2. Feeding a patient with dysphagia
   3. Transferring a patient from the bed to a chair
   4. Monitoring a blood transfusion

10. Which patient activity could be performed by either a registered nurse (RN) or a licensed practical nurse (LPN) or delegated as a task even if there is an unlicensed assistive personnel (UAP) present on the unit?
    1. Initiation of blood transfusion
    2. Tracheostomy care
    3. Assisting a patient with feeding
    4. Obtaining daily weight

11. A registered nurse (RN) refuses to delegate any patient care tasks to other members of the nursing unit staff, preferring to complete all tasks herself. What type of delegation practice would this demonstrate?
    1. Underdelegation
    2. Effective delegation
    3. Overdelegation
    4. Recognition of right person

12. A registered nurse (RN) delegated specimen collection to an unlicensed assistive personnel (UAP) for a patient who had a urine analysis ordered by the physician. The UAP did not obtain the specimen. When checking the patient's chart later in the shift, the RN noticed that there was no documentation that a urine specimen was collected. The RN asked the UAP to provide an explanation for why the specimen was not obtained. The UAP told the RN that she was going to obtain the specimen from the patient after lunch. Which stated action would correlate with the delegation right of right communication?
    1. The RN followed up later in the shift, checking the patient's chart for documentation of the specimen collection.
    2. The RN delegated the task to the UAP.
    3. The UAP told the RN that she was going to obtain the specimen from the patient after lunch.
    4. The RN monitored the task completion process.

Multiple Response

13. Which examples represent improper use of delegation in the clinical setting by a registered nurse (RN), licensed practical nurse (LPN), or unlicensed assistive personnel (UAP)? *Select all that apply.*
    1. UAP delegating a task to an LPN
    2. RN delegating a task to a UAP or an LPN
    3. LPN delegating a task to an RN
    4. RN delegating a task to an RN
    5. UAP delegating a task to an RN

14. Which aspects are included in how nurses develop nursing judgment? *Select all that apply.*
    1. Academic experience
    2. Use of experience to help form an opinion
    3. Analysis of information to help arrive at a decision
    4. Leadership style
    5. Level of administrative experience as opposed to being a staff nurse
15. Which actions should *not* be delegated to a licensed vocational nurse (LVN) on a medical unit in a hospital setting by a registered nurse (RN)? *Select all that apply.*
    1. Initiating a blood transfusion
    2. Inserting a urinary catheter
    3. Administering chemotherapy infusion
    4. Completing initial admission assessment
    5. Performing postoperative dressing changes

REFERENCES

American Association of Colleges of Nursing (AACN). (2008). *The essentials of baccalaureate education for professional nursing practice*. Author.

American Association of Colleges of Nursing. (2021). *The essentials: Core competencies for professional nursing education*. Author. https://www.aacnnursing.org/Portals/42/AcademicNursing/pdf/Essentials-2021.pdf

American Nurses Association (ANA). (2012). *ANA's principles for delegation by nurses to unlicensed assistive personnel (UAP)*. Author.

American Nurses Association (ANA). (2015a). *Nursing: Scope and standards of practice* (3rd ed.). Author.

American Nurses Association (ANA). (2015b). *Code of ethics for nurses with interpretive statements*. Author.

American Nurses Association (ANA). (2016). *Nursing administration: Scope and standards of practice* (2nd ed.). Author.

American Nurses Association (ANA) & National Council of State Boards of Nursing (NCSBN). (2019). *National guidelines for nursing delegation*. https://www.nursingworld.org/~4962ca/globalassets/practiceandpolicy/nursing-excellence/ana-position-statements/nursing-practice/ana-ncsbn-joint-statement-on-delegation.pdf

American Organization for Nursing Leadership (AONL). (2015a). *AONL nurse manager competencies*. Author.

American Organization for Nursing Leadership (AONL). (2015b). *AONL nurse executive competencies*. Author.

Anderson, P. S., Twibell, R. S., & Siela, D. (2006, November). Delegating without doubts. *American Nurse Today*, 54–57.

Anthony, M. K., & Vidal, K. (2010). Mindful communication: A novel approach to improving delegation and increasing patient safety. *Online Journal of Issues in Nursing, 15*(2), 2.

Bittner, N. P., & Gravlin, G. (2009). Critical thinking, delegation, and missed care in nursing practice. *Journal of Nursing Administration, 39*(3), 142–146.

Conger, J. A., & Kanungo, R. N. (1988).The empowerment process: Integrating theory and practice. *Academy of Management Review, 13*(3), 471–482.

Cronenwett, L., Sherwood, G., Barnsteiner, J., Disch, J., Johnson, J., Mitchell, P., Sullivan, D. T., & Warren, J. (2007). Quality and safety education for nurses. *Nursing Outlook, 55*(3), 122–131.

Duffy, M., & McCoy, S. F. (2014). *Delegation and you: When to delegate and to whom*. American Nurses Association.

Gravlin, G., & Bittner, N. P. (2010). Nurses' and nursing assistants' reports of missed care and delegation. *Journal of Nursing Administration, 40*(7/8), 329–335.

Greiner, A. C., & Knebel, E. (Eds.). (2003). *Health professions education: A bridge to quality.* National Academies Press.

Halm, M. (2019). The influence of appropriate staffing and healthy work environments on patient and nurse outcomes. *American Journal of Critical Care, 28,* 152–156.

Hughes, M., Kirk, R., & Dixon, A. (2018). New Zealand nurses' storied experiences of direction and delegation. *Nursing Praxis in New Zealand, 34*(3), 32–45.

Hui, C. (1994) Effects of leader empowerment behaviors and followers' personal control, voice, and self efficacy on in-role and extra-role performance: An extension of Conger and Kanungo's empowerment process model. (Unpublished doctoral dissertation). Proquest Information and Learning (UMI No. 9418834). Indiana University, Indianapolis.

International Council of Nurses (ICN). (2008). *Assistive nursing personnel* [position statement]. www.icn.ch/images/stories/documents/publications/position_statements/B01_Assistive_Support_Nsg_Personnel.pdf

International Council of Nurses (ICN). (2012). *The ICN code of ethics for nurses.* www.icn.ch/images/stories/documents/about/icncode_english.pdf

Kalisch, B. J. (2006). Missed nursing care: A qualitative study. *Journal of Nursing Care Quality, 21*(4), 306–311.

Laschinger, H. K., Wong, C., McMahon, L., & Kaufmann, C. (1999). Leader behavior impact on staff nurse empowerment, job tension and work effectiveness. *Journal of Nursing Administration, 29*(5), 28–39.

Miller, L. A. (2018). Delegation: Legal issues for clinicians. *Journal of Perinatal & Neonatal Nursing, 32*(2), 104–106. doi:10.1097/JPN.0000000000000327

National Council of State Boards of Nursing (NCSBN). (1997). *Report of the unlicensed assistive personnel (UAP) task force.* www.ncsbn.org/1997_part6.pdf

National Council of State Boards of Nursing (NCSBN). (2005). *Working with others: A position paper.* www.ncsbn.org/Working_with_Others.pdf

National Council of State Boards of Nursing (NCSBN). (2016). National guidelines for nursing delegation. *Journal of Nursing Regulation, 7*(1), 5–14. https://www.journalofnursingregulation.com

National Council of State Boards of Nursing (NCSBN) & American Nurses Association (ANA). (2019). *National guidelines for nursing delegation: Joint statement on delegation.* https://www.ncsbn.org/13546.htm

Nightingale, F. (1860 [reprinted 1969]). *Notes on nursing: What it is and what it is not.* Dover Publications.

Porter-O'Grady, T., & Malloch, K. (2013). *Leadership in nursing practice: Changing the landscape of health care.* Jones & Bartlett Learning.

Potter, P., Deshields, T., & Kuhrik, M. (2010). Delegation practices between registered nurses and nursing assistive personnel. *Journal of Nursing Management, 18,* 157–165.

Royal College of Nursing. (2015). *Accountability and delegation.* www.rcn.org.uk/__data/assets/pdf_file/0003/381720/003942.pdf

Snyder, D. A., Medina, J., Bell, L., & Wavra, T. A. (Eds.). (2004). *AACN delegation handbook* (2nd ed.). www.aacn.org/wd/practice/docs/aacndelegationhandbook.pdf

The Joint Commission. (2019, July). Developing resilience to combat nurse burnout. *Quick Safety (50).* https://www.jointcommission.org/-/media/tjc/newsletters/quick_safety_nurse_resilience_final_7_19_19pdf.pdf

Wagner, E. A. (2018). Improving patient care outcomes through better delegation-communication between nurses and assistive personnel. *Journal of Nursing Care Quality, 33*(2), 187–193. doi:10.1097/NCQ.0000000000000282

Weydt, A. (2010). Developing delegation skills. *Online Journal of Issues in Nursing, 15*(2), 1.

 To explore learning resources for this chapter, go to FADavis.com

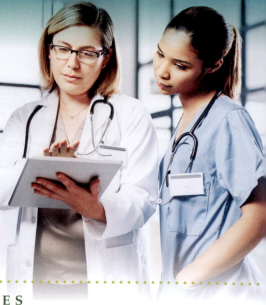

Chapter *15*

Leading Change and Managing Conflict

Elizabeth J. Murray, PhD, RN, CNE

KEY TERMS

Change
Change agent
Chaos theory
Conflict
Empirical-rational strategy
Innovation
Learning organization
Negotiation
Normative-reeducative strategy
Planned change
Power-coercive strategy
Unplanned change

LEARNING OUTCOMES

- Compare and contrast traditional change theories and models.
- Discuss emerging change theories.
- Describe the nurse leader and manager's role in the change process.
- Identify common human responses to change.
- Explain five approaches to managing conflict.
- Examine key elements of effective negotiation.

The Knowledge, Skills, and Attitudes Related to the Following Are Addressed in This Chapter:

Core Competencies	• Teamwork and Collaboration • Quality Improvement • Evidence-Based Practice
The Essentials: Core Competencies for Professional Nursing Education (AACN, 2021)	**Domain 3: Population Health** 3.5 Demonstrate advocacy strategies (p. 37). **Domain 4: Scholarship for Nursing Practice** 4.2 Integrate best evidence into nursing practice (pp. 39–40). **Domain 7: Systems-Based Practice** 7.3 Optimize system effectiveness through application of innovation and evidence-based practice (p. 48).
Code of Ethics with Interpretive Statements (ANA, 2015)	**Provision 1.5:** Relationships with colleagues and others (p. 4) **Provision 2.1:** Primacy of the patient's interests (p. 5) **Provision 2.3:** Collaboration (p. 6)

Nurse Manager (NMC) Competencies (AONL, 2015a) and Nurse Executive (NEC) Competencies (AONL, 2015b)	**NMC: Strategic Management (p. 5)**
	• Facilitate change
	• Project management
	• Demonstrate negotiation skills
	NMC: Relationship Management and Influencing Behaviors (p. 6)
	• Manage conflict
	• Situation management
	• Influence others
	  • Act as change agent
	NEC: Communication and Relationship Building (p. 4)
	• Relationship management
	  • Build collaborative relationships
	  • Exhibit effective conflict resolution skills
	  • Create a trusting environment
	• Influencing behaviors
	  • Facilitate consensus building
	NEC: Leadership (p. 8)
	• Change management
	  • Adapt leadership style to situation needs
	  • Use change theory to implement changes
	  • Serve as a change agent

Continued

The Knowledge, Skills, and Attitudes Related to the Following Are Addressed in This Chapter:—cont'd

Nursing Administration Scope and Standards of Practice (ANA, 2016)	**Standard 7: Ethics** The nurse administrator practices ethically (pp. 45–46).
	Standard 8: Culturally Congruent Practice The nurse administrator practices in a safe manner that is congruent with cultural diversity and inclusion principles (pp. 47–48).
	Standard 9: Communication The nurse administrator communicates effectively in all areas of practice (p. 49).
	Standard 10: Collaboration The nurse administrator collaborates with healthcare consumers, colleagues, community leaders, and other stakeholders to advance nursing practice and healthcare transformation (p. 50).
	Standard 17: Environmental Health The nurse administrator practices in an environmentally safe and healthy manner (p. 59).

Source: American Association of Colleges of Nursing. (2021). *The essentials: Core competencies for professional nursing education.* Author; American Nurses Association (ANA). (2015). *Code of ethics for nurses with interpretive statements.* Author; American Nurses Association (ANA). (2016). *Nursing administration: Scope and standards of practice* (2nd ed.). Author; American Organization for Nursing Leadership (AONL). (2015a). *AONL nurse manager competencies.* Author; American Organization for Nursing Leadership (AONL). (2015b). *AONL nurse executive competencies.* Author; Cronenwett, L., Sherwood, G., Barnsteiner, J., Disch, J., Johnson, J., Mitchell, P., Sullivan, D. T., & Warren, J. (2007). Quality and safety education for nurses. *Nursing Outlook, 55*(3), 122–131; and Greiner, A. C., & Knebel, E. (Eds.). (2003). *Health professions education: A bridge to quality.* National Academies Press.

Change and conflict are ever present in health care today, thanks to constant-ly evolving technology, new regulations, changing public expectations, increasing environmental concerns, and heavy demand on scarce resources. In turn, nurses must be knowledgeable about the change process and understand that conflict can result when the process is ineffective. In the dynamic environment of health care, change is inevitable and unpredictable, and it affects staff, patients, and the organization overall. Historian and critical feminist Joan Wallach Scott states, "Those who expect moments of change to be comfortable and free of conflict have not learned their history" (Quote Garden, 2016). Change in the work environment can create uncertainty and elicit emotional responses from employees (Bowers, 2011). Most people do not like change, and when experiencing change, not all people respond in the same way.

Nurses at all levels must develop a basic understanding of change theories and models to fulfill the social mandate for nursing practice outlined in the American Nurses Association (ANA, 2010) *Nursing's Social Policy Statement,* which states that nurses must be open to changes and willing to apply new evidence in practice as it emerges. In addition, nurses must embrace change to ensure that safe and quality nursing care is provided.

Change can be difficult and is often met with resistance, which can result in conflict. Nurse leaders and managers are instrumental in facilitating successful change at both the unit and organizational levels. Successfully leading and managing the change process are vital leadership skills (Stefancyk et al., 2013). Nurse leaders and managers are called to "take a leadership role and become early adopters in leading change, removing barriers, challenging the status quo, and creating innovative solutions to address nursing workforce issues that contribute to the health of America" (ANA, 2016, p. 16).

Although change is a very common cause of conflict, wise nurse leaders and managers recognize that conflict is always present in the workplace (Porter-O'Grady & Malloch, 2013). Further, conflict is dynamic and does not disappear; rather, it can only be managed. When conflict is managed effectively, the results can be innovative solutions and better relationships (Smith-Trudeau, 2019). Nurse leaders and managers have a responsibility to acquire the knowledge, skills, and attitudes to manage and lead change, as well as engage staff in consensus building and conflict management (ANA, 2016).

▶ CHANGE THEORIES

Change is a dynamic process that results in altering or making something different. Change can be planned or unplanned. **Planned change** is purposeful, calculated, and collaborative, and it includes the deliberate application of change theories (Mitchell, 2013; Roussel et al., 2020). Change that is purposeful and planned is usually well received by staff. In contrast, **unplanned change** occurs when the need for change is sudden and necessary to manage a crisis. Unplanned change can cause anxiety and stress among staff members. Successful nurse leaders and managers manage unplanned change "through effective communication, adaptability, coordination, and the ability to remain grounded" (Erickson, 2014, p. 125). Highly effective nurse leaders and managers develop high-functioning, empowered teams whose members know what is expected, remain calm during crisis, and do what is right for the patients (Erickson, 2014). Closely related to and frequently an integral part of change is **innovation**, the process of creating something new after thoughtful analysis of a phenomenon or situation.

Implementing change can be very challenging and yet is necessary for progress. Often, the change process fails because those executing the change neglect to take a structured approach. Planned change is best carried out using a theoretical framework or model (Mitchell, 2013; Shirey, 2013). The situation at hand and the type of change being implemented help determine the appropriate theory or framework to apply, lead, and manage the process, and this approach can result in a sustainable change (Shirey, 2013). Because not all theories fit all nursing situations, nurse leaders and managers must be familiar with various change theories to be able to select a framework wisely. The most common change theories and models used fall into two categories: (1) traditional theories and models and (2) emerging theories.

Traditional Change Theories and Models

Traditional change theories and models are linear and suggest that change occurs in a sequential manner. For the change to be successful, the organization or unit must progress through each stage. These theories require ongoing work to ensure that goals are met and change is sustained. Table 15-1 provides a comparison of traditional change theories.

Lewin's Force-Field Model (1951)

Lewin's Force-Field theory is one of the most widely used theories. Lewin believed that change results from two field or environmental forces: (1) driving forces (helping forces) that attempt to facilitate the change and move it forward and (2) restraining forces (hindering forces) that attempt to impede change and maintain the status quo. Successful change requires the driving forces to be greater than the restraining forces. This three-step change model involves unfreezing the status quo, moving toward the new way, and refreezing or stabilizing the change for sustainability (Lewin, 1951; Mensik, 2014; Shirey, 2013):

1. The *unfreezing stage* is the point at which it is determined that change is needed, and driving and restraining forces are identified. The change agent must create

Table 15-1 Comparison of Traditional Change Theories and Models				
	Lewin (1951)	**Lippitt et al. (1958)**	**Rogers (1995, 2003)**	**Kotter (1996)**
Theory and/or Model	Force-Field Model	Phases of Change Model	Innovation-Decision Process	Eight-Stage Process of Creating Major Change
Components in Model	• Unfreezing	• Diagnosing the problem • Assessing motivation and capacity for change • Assessing the change agent's motivation and resources	• Knowledge • Persuasion	• Establishing a sense of urgency • Creating the guiding coalition • Developing a vision and strategy • Communicating the change vision
	• Moving	• Selecting progressive change objectives • Choosing an appropriate role for the change agent	• Decision • Implementation	• Empowering broad-based action • Generating short-term wins
	• Refreezing	• Maintaining the change after it has started • Terminating the helping relationship	• Confirmation	• Consolidating gains and producing more change • Anchoring new approaches in the culture
When to Use	General model useful for problem-solving and most situations and planned change	General model useful for most planned change and changing processes	Model useful in individual and organizational change and very useful when implementing technological change	Effective model for rapidly changing organizations and for learning organizations

Compiled from Kotter, 1996; Lewin, 1951; Lippitt et al., 1958; Rogers, 1995, 2003.

a sense of urgency to change, strengthen the driving forces, and weaken the re-straining forces for successful change. During this stage, nurse leaders and man-agers can help prepare staff members for the change by helping them recognize the need for change, building trust, and actively engaging staff in the change process. Motivation to change occurs in this stage.

2. The *moving stage* begins the initiation of the desired change. Information is gath-ered, the change is planned, and movement toward changing begins in this stage. During the moving stage, the new innovation is examined, accepted, and tried. This stage requires unfreezing and moving toward a new way of thinking and behaving. Nurse leaders and managers can facilitate movement by coach-ing those affected by the change to overcome fears and engage them in prob-lem-solving and working toward the desired outcome.

3. The *refreezing stage* involves stabilizing the change and achieving equilibrium. The innovation is incorporated into the routine. The change becomes the new norm. In this stage, nurse leaders and managers should reinforce the change through formal and informal processes including policies, procedures, stan-dards of care, and other common tools used throughout the organization. This stage is crucial to sustaining change over time.

Throughout the process, the nurse leader and manager must employ strategies to increase driving forces and/or decrease restraining forces for the change to be successful. Many other theories are based on Lewin's theory.

Lippitt's Phases of Change Model (1958)

Lippitt et al. (1958) expanded Lewin's original theory by identifying additional stages of the change process. The Phases of Change Model uses language similar to the nursing process and focuses more on the people involved in the change process than on the change process itself. This model stresses the importance of communication and rapport with those involved in the process. The model follows these seven steps (Lippitt et al., 1958; Mensik, 2014; Mitchell, 2013):

1. *Diagnosing the problem* involves identifying the need for the change and recruit-ing others to assist with data collection. Effective communication is critical in the first phase to avoid miscommunication through the grapevine. Nurse lead-ers and managers can spearhead drafting a plan for change at this time.

2. *Assessing the motivation and capacity for change* is actually assessing the unit or organization for readiness to change. Nurse leaders and managers must com-municate with those affected by the change, respond to concerns, provide ratio-nale for the change, and identify possible resistance to the change.

3. *Assessing the change agent's motivation and resources* must be done for successful change to occur. The change agent must be willing to commit to the change and see the process through to the end. This phase requires nurse leaders and man-agers to identify their role in the change process. They must be realistic about the time commitment necessary and recruit assistance.

4. *Selecting progressive change objectives* involves clearly defining the change, es-tablishing realistic goals, and developing a plan for change. Nurse leaders and

managers actively assess their team and delegate appropriate responsibilities during this phase of the process.

5. *Choosing an appropriate role for the change agent* and implementing the plan for change comprise one of the final steps. It is important that nurse leaders and managers remain flexible during this stage.

6. *Maintaining the change after it has started* and as it is being incorporated into the unit or organization culture is critical. Nurse leaders and managers monitor the stability of the change as it becomes part of the system. Communication and feedback are critical during this phase to avoid regressing to the previous state.

7. *Terminating the helping relationship* once the process has stabilized occurs when the change agent withdraws from the process and the change is evaluated. Nurse leaders and managers continue monitoring and evaluating the change for sustainability.

The role of the change agent is extremely important in Lippitt's model. Nurse leaders and managers most often function in the change agent role and are responsible to drive "the innovation into everyday practice" (Mensik, 2014, p. 64).

Rogers' Innovation-Decision Process (1995)

Rogers (1995) broadened Lewin's theory and developed a five-stage innovation-decision process, which consists of a series of actions and choices over time that an individual or decision-making unit must follow. Further, recognizing the common behavioral responses to change that individuals may experience can facilitate change. The five stages are as follows (Rogers, 1995; Shirey, 2006):

1. *Knowledge* occurs when an individual or decision-making unit is exposed to an innovation and gains understanding of how it functions. Nurse leaders and managers create the need for the innovation and increase motivation among staff members to learn more about the innovation.

2. *Persuasion* occurs when an individual or decision-making unit forms a favorable or unfavorable attitude toward the innovation. The perceived attributes of the innovation are key in this stage. Nurse leaders and managers can engage staff members to share positive experiences with the innovation with their peers to promote favorable attitudes.

3. *Decision* occurs when an individual or decision-making unit engages in activities to adopt or reject the innovation. To facilitate adoption, nurse leaders and managers may want to pilot the innovation on a specific unit. Staff members can then experience the desirable qualities of the innovation.

4. *Implementation* occurs when an individual or decision-making unit begins using an innovation. Nurse leaders and managers must ensure that adequate technical support and proper infrastructure are available during implementation to avoid stalling the innovation.

5. *Confirmation* occurs when an individual or decision-making unit seeks reinforcement of a decision made or reverses a previous decision to adopt or reject innovation (Rogers, 1995, p. 162). Overall, staff members desire to avoid conflict and work to keep the innovation going. Nurse leaders and managers may provide

encouragement and validate that the decision was the correct one (Shirey, 2006). Long-term support may be needed to stabilize the change and help those involved develop self-reliance during this phase.

Rogers suggests that, for change to be successful, everyone involved with the change and/or affected by the change must be committed to the change. In addition, nurse leaders and managers must deal with behavioral responses to change and attempt to figure out how to channel negative responses into support for the change or innovation (Rogers, 1995). Nurse leaders and managers are involved in creating a shared vision for the innovation and provide the leadership needed to sustain the change (Mensik, 2014).

Kotter's Eight-Stage Process of Creating Major Change (1996)

Kotter (1996) suggested that successful change involves a multistep process that overcomes all sources of resistance and must be directed by high-quality leadership. He describes eight stages of the change process that can help nurse leaders and managers manage change cognitively as well as emotionally (Kotter, 1996):

1. *Establishing a sense of urgency* involves examining the competition or need for change to improve quality and/or safety. During this stage, nurse leaders and managers must discuss major opportunities and potential crises identified and present convincing evidence for the need to change.
2. *Creating the guiding coalition* means putting together a group with the necessary power to lead the change and getting everyone to work together. Identifying key staff members and empowering them to participate in the change process is important for nurse leaders and managers during this stage.
3. *Developing a vision and strategy* means creating a vision to direct the change effort. Nurse leaders and managers spend time during this stage making the vision clear and understandable for everyone.
4. *Communicating the change vision* to everyone involved in or affected by the change is important, as is having the leader or manager model the behavior expected of employees. The goal for nurse leaders and managers is to persuade as many staff members as possible to embrace the vision.
5. *Empowering broad-based action* involves changing systems or structures that undermine the vision, getting rid of obstacles, and encouraging risk taking and nontraditional ideas. Nurse leaders and managers must actively confront opponents. In addition, they can provide information and assist staff members to embrace the vision.
6. *Generating short-term wins* consists of planning for and creating improvements in performance, or "wins," and visibly recognizing and rewarding those responsible for the "wins." The focus is on lessening the impact of the cynics, pessimists, and skeptics by rewarding and motivating staff members embracing the change (Salmela et al., 2013).
7. *Consolidating gains and producing more change* include using increased credibility to change systems and processes that do not fit the vision. This stage also involves hiring, promoting, and developing those who can implement the vision, as well as reinvigorating the process with new projects and themes.

8. *Anchoring new approaches in the culture* is creating better performance through productivity orientation and through better and more effective leadership and management. In this stage, the connection between behavior and organizational success is emphasized, as well as ensuring leadership development and succession (Kotter, 1996, p. 21). Nurse leaders and managers focus on sustaining the change or innovation.

Nurse leaders and managers are seen in Kotter's model as important during the various phases of the process because of their keen communication skills, ability to anchor the vision of the change, and skill in persuading staff members to embrace the change (Salmela et al., 2013).

Emerging Change Theories

Traditional theories are useful in providing structure and direction for change. However, the linear models do not recognize the dynamic context in which change occurs and the unanticipated human actions and responses. Newer theories are emerging that are more complex than the traditional theories. Systems theory provides the foundation for emerging theories of change. Using a systems approach to change and innovation results in a comprehensive view and realization that systems are complex. Human beings, families, organizations, cities, and nations are all systems with interrelationships among members, and a close look at those interrelationships reveals infinite complexity.

Emerging theories are cyclical rather than linear and require organizations to react with speed and flexibility. The newer theories provide another perspective from which to view change and innovation based on complexity science. Complexity science recognizes that the world is in continual motion and that a change in one area can result in numerous changes in other areas. Change and innovation from the perspective of complexity science are highly interrelated, dynamic, and unpredictable (Porter-O'Grady & Malloch, 2013). Understanding complex systems when leading and managing change results in a collective commitment to the change created. Two theories based on complexity science and systems theory, chaos theory and learning organization theory (discussed in detail in Chapter 7), are actually used to understand organizational behavior. Chaos theory and learning organizations theory are also used to understand change and innovation. Nurse leaders and managers who understand these theories in relation to change and innovation can assist staff through the change process successfully.

Chaos Theory

Many relate chaos to complete randomness. In fact, the word *chaos* is derived from the Greek language and means "formless matter." However, even when a system may appear chaotic and disorderly, there is actually an underlying complex order. **Chaos theory** is nonlinear and unpredictable, and it explains why a small change in one area can have a large affect across an organization. This is also known as the

EXPLORING THE EVIDENCE 15-1

Salmela, S., Eriksson, K., & Fagerström, L. (2013). Nurse leaders' perceptions of an approaching organizational change. *Qualitative Health Research, 23*(5), 689–699.

Aim

The aim of this study was to understand nurse leaders' perceptions of an approaching organizational change (a merger between a health-care center and a hospital).

Methods

This study was a qualitative study using a hermeneutical design and Kotter's Eight-Stage Process of Creating Major Change as a theoretical framework. Seventeen nurse leaders participated in semistructured interviews. The interviews sought to obtain information related to nurse leaders' views of the following:

- Change and the approaching merger and change process
- Their roles as leaders during the change process
- Their previous change experiences

Data from the interviews were analyzed using a hermeneutical interpretive process.

Key Findings

The study resulted in three main themes:

1. *Positive and active engagement in continuous change:* Nurse leaders in the study indicated an understanding of change as part of the daily routine, and they were very willing to participate and influence staff members as nurse leaders.
2. *Confidence in change and adaptation without deeper engagement:* Nurse leaders in the study had positive attitudes, which enabled them to see the possibilities, and understood that change is necessary.
3. *Feelings of insecurity and anxiety:* Nurse leaders in the study were experiencing uncertainty about their roles as leaders and anxiety related to the demands placed on them currently and anticipated in the future. They also felt as if they were spectators in the change process.

Implications for Nurse Leaders and Managers

Nurse leaders and managers are great resources for organizational change. However, according to the authors of the study, nurse leaders and managers are not always included by upper administration when organizational change is being implemented. The findings of this study suggest that nurse leaders and managers are in critical positions to influence organizational change for a positive outcome. Further, including nurse leaders and managers at all levels can facilitate the change process across the organization.

"butterfly effect," or the notion that the flapping of a butterfly's wings in one part of the world can have a major impact, such as a hurricane or tsunami, on the other side of the world (Crowell, 2016; Mensik, 2014; Porter-O'Grady & Malloch, 2010). Nurse leaders and managers must be aware of the complexity of health care, the unit, and the organization. Further, they must understand that, because of multiple factors, decisions made can result in changes that were unintended.

Learning Organization Theory

Learning organization theory was first described by Senge (1990), who suggested that to excel, future organizations will need to "discover how to tap people's commitment and capacity to learn at all levels in an organization" (p. 4). He called on leaders to move away from traditional authoritarian "controlling organizations" to learning organizations. In a learning organization, all staff members are involved in problem-solving and implementing change and innovation, and this involvement enables the organization to respond quickly to chaos. Senge (1990) defined a **learning organization** as an "organization where people continually expand their capacity to create the results they truly desire, where new and expansive patterns of thinking are nurtured, where collective aspiration is set free, and where people are continually learning how to learn together" (p. 3). Senge identified systems thinking, personal mastery, mental models, building shared vision, and team learning as five disciplines that organizations need to adopt and practice to become learning organizations.

Members of a learning organization are continually practicing the five disciplines and are continually learning. The more learning that occurs, the more aware the members become of what they can still learn. In health care, adopting the five disciplines has the potential to result in high-quality and safe patient care. Nurse leaders and managers who help staff members see the larger system build an understanding of complex problems. This understanding enables staff members to develop long-term changes and work together to improve the whole system, rather than pursuing symptomatic fixes to parts of the whole (Senge et al., 2015). In turn, change and innovation can be sustained over time.

▶ MANAGING CHANGE AND INNOVATION

Managing change and innovation requires nurse leaders and managers to know the who, why, what, when, and how of change (Porter-O'Grady & Malloch, 2013):

- *Who:* The who of change are the key stakeholders (e.g., patients and families, employees, communities) related to the work to be changed. To be able to change or motivate stakeholders, nurse leaders and managers must understand their own comfort and competence related to change. Nurse leaders and managers must be self-aware regarding their knowledge or lack of knowledge of the change process, personal comfort with change and risk taking, relationships, conflict, and negotiation skills.

- *Why:* The why of change is a reasonable rationale for the change. A lack of understanding for the reason for change can result in resistance and unsuccessful implementation of the change and innovation. Given the complexity of health care and the limited resources today, change and innovation should be evidence based and linked to patient safety, quality health care, and improving the work environment.

- *What:* The what of change is the actual change or innovation being implemented. Identifying what to change is determined after the rationale for the change is clear. Change and innovation may involve revising or creating policies, processes, procedures, and/or standards. Keep in mind that implementing the specific change may require additional resources and technology as well as education and competency development for staff.
- *When:* The when of change is determining at what point to start the change process and how long it will take to achieve the change. The timing for change can be directed by the impetus behind the change. However, when to change is best determined by those who will be most involved with or affected by the outcome of the change.
- *How:* The how of change involves the techniques or processes needed for successful and sustainable change.

Facilitating change and innovation is more than establishing and implementing a plan. It requires four specific competencies (Porter-O'Grady & Malloch, 2013, p. 51):

1. Personal knowledge of and accountability for one's own strengths and limitations specific to change and innovation, including technical capability and computer literacy
2. Understanding the essence of change and innovation concepts as well as the tools of innovation
3. The ability to collaborate and fully engage team members
4. Competence in embracing vulnerability and risk taking

Nurse leaders and managers are responsible for designing innovations to effect change in practice and outcomes (ANA, 2016).

Effective nurse leaders and managers should be concerned with both people and productivity during the change process. Nurse leaders and managers must value staff and create an environment that supports the change. Managing change means being a change agent, responding effectively to change, adopting change, and being prepared to deal with barriers to change.

Becoming a Change Agent

Nurses at all levels can facilitate change. A **change agent** is one who leads and manages the change process, including management of group dynamics, resistance to change, continuous communication, and the momentum toward the desired outcome. The responsibilities of a change agent can include the following:

- Gathering data necessary to identify a problem that needs to be changed
- Informing members of the group that change is needed and facilitating them to recognize and acknowledge the need for change
- Setting goals and objectives for the change and developing a plan

- Identifying those who will be affected by the change and including them in the process
- Identifying resisting and driving forces
- Implementing the change
- Communicating continuously during the process
- Providing support during the process
- Evaluating the change and make modifications to the plan as necessary
- Staying involved/available after the change process for a significant amount of time to ensure sustainability

Change agents need to be effective communicators and must excel at interpersonal skills. Change agents need to develop the knowledge, skills, and attitudes to align people, processes, and purposes to achieve the change and innovation. Nurse leaders and managers often find themselves functioning as change agents. As change agents, nurse leaders and managers are responsible to manage change and assist staff in the change process.

When nurse leaders and managers model a positive and enthusiastic approach to change and innovation, they can inspire staff.

Responding to Change

Resistance to change is common. Many people are not comfortable with change. Various factors can affect a person's ability to handle change and innovation, such as adaptability, comfort with the status quo, perceptions of the benefits of the change, and how threatened a person feels by the change. Effective change agents anticipate human responses to change and include strategies to manage the responses in the plan. Staff members need time to adjust to the thought of change and time to adjust to the actual change. Nurse leaders and managers can help staff cope with change by making sure the rationale for the change is clear and allowing staff members to verbalize concerns and express their emotions. During the change process, nurse leaders and managers can also help staff members cope by ensuring open communication, providing feedback on a regular basis, and empowering them throughout the change process.

As change agents, nurse leaders and managers can use several strategies when dealing with resistance. Different strategies work in different situations, so change agents must consider which strategy is most appropriate for the change or innovation to be successful. Chinn and Benne (1969) described three common change strategies that can be useful for nurse leaders and managers during the change process. The **normative-reeducative strategy** focuses on the relationship needs of staff members, uses peer pressure, and relies on staff members' desires to have satisfactory work relationships (Chinn & Benne, 1969). The normative-reeducative strategy is used when some resistance is expected but nurse leaders and managers believe that staff will succumb to peer pressure rather than resist the change. The **empirical-rational strategy** assumes that staff members are essentially self-interested and providing information and education will assist staff in changing behavior and adopting the change or innovation (Chinn & Benne, 1969). Typically, when a change is being implemented the first step is to explain the need for the change.

Once staff members understand the need for change and perceive personal benefit, they will embrace it. The empirical-rational strategy is useful when minimal resistance is expected. The **power-coercive strategy** is based on power and authority and assumes that staff will respond to authority and threats of job loss (Chinn & Benne, 1969). This strategy is used when resistance is expected but nurse leaders and managers plan to implement the change regardless of how the majority feels. The power-coercive strategy results in rapid change and is often perceived by staff members as they must accept the change or find a new place to work.

Adopting Change

In general, people adopt change at different times during the process. Rogers (1995) suggested that people adopt change in various stages and can be categorized into five groups, as he illustrated the categories on a bell curve. Figure 15-1 illustrates the categories of change adopters. The first 2.5% of people to adopt change are the "innovators," also known as venturesome. Innovators are willing to take risks. The next 13.5% to embrace the innovation are called "early adopters"; they are more discerning when choosing to adopt an innovation. The "early majority" makes up the next 34% to adopt the change. Known to be deliberate, the early majority usually interacts with the early adopters before making decisions. The "late majority" comprises the next 34%, who are skeptical and reluctant to adopt an innovation until most others have done so. Finally, the last to accept change are the "laggards" at 16%, who are stuck in the past traditions. Each category has specific characteristics. Nurse leaders must understand each group and how to focus time and energy appropriately to maximize the change effort. Table 15-2 lists the categories of change adopters and related characteristics.

Dealing With Barriers to Change

Change will happen. Continually facilitating staff to focus on the change or innovation must be a priority for nurse leaders and managers. However, 75% of all change initiatives fail (Manion, 2011, p. 230). Change initiatives typically

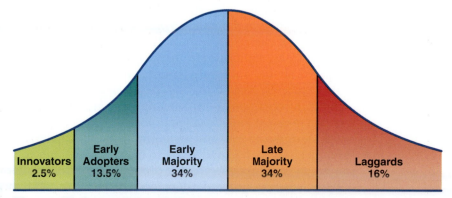

Figure 15-1 Five adopter categories.

Table 15-2	Rate of Adoption, Category of Adopters, and Related Characteristics	
Percentage	**Category**	**Characteristics**
2.5%	Innovators (venturesome)	• Inherently eager to try new things • Embracing change • Willing to take risks • Able to cope with uncertainty • Often not respected by others; seen as outliers
13.5%	Early adopters (respectable)	• Open and receptive to change • Often sought out by change agents • Role models • Considered by peers as "the person to check with" before adopting change • More integrated with the social system
34%	Early majority (deliberate)	• Preferring the status quo • Rarely taking the lead • Comfortable as followers • Adopting change before the majority
34%	Late majority (skeptical)	• Skeptical and cautious • Needing to feel safe • Tending to adopt change after the majority • Adopting because of peer pressure
16%	Laggards (traditional)	• Suspicious of change and change agents • Using the past as a point of reference • Holding traditional values • Last to adopt

Compiled from Rogers, 1995, 2003.

fail because of poor coordination, ineffective communication, and lack of staff cooperation. Thoughtful planning and ongoing communication can help overcome barriers to change. Nurse leaders and managers must position themselves to be in the forefront of change and innovation (Shirey, 2006). Further, they must be the coaches, encouragers, and positive role models for change (Anderson, 2014).

Nurse leaders and managers must be committed to and exhibit an attitude that supports the change or innovation. When change or innovation is imposed on the staff in an authoritarian manner, resistance is inevitable. Nurse leaders and managers should anticipate barriers to change and implement strategies to ward of resistance. By identifying the change resisters early on, much resistance can be avoided. Effective nurse leaders and managers will engage and empower nurses who are resistant in the change process so the planned change is not impeded.

Savvy nurse leaders and managers recognize that there are different strategies for managing change and strive to match approaches to their particular circumstances to optimize the change process. Ineffective leaders try to make change happen, whereas system leaders focus on creating conditions that can create sustainable change (Senge et al., 2015).

How Do You Respond to Change?

Think about a recent experience that involved some type of change on your part.

1. What category of adopters do you fall under? (See Table 15-2.)
2. Do you believe you need improvement in how you respond to change?
3. List two or three strategies you can use to improve your response to change.

▶ ## MANAGING CONFLICT

The health-care system is complex and constantly changing, and various demands in the workplace can generate conflict among staff members and others. **Conflict** is a state of disharmony among people and occurs when people have differing views. A little conflict is good and can result in organizational growth. In contrast, too much conflict can paralyze an organization or unit. Conflict, if not managed, can result in stress for all involved, interfere with the ability to work together, and have a negative impact on patient care. Further, unmanaged conflict can result in decreased staff morale, increased turnover, poor-quality patient care, increased health-care costs, and patient dissatisfaction (Losa Iglesias & De Bengoa Vallejo, 2012). Common factors that result in conflict can be related to personnel issues, personal issues, work environment, power struggles, differing value systems, and leadership and management styles (Padrutt, 2010). Therefore, all nurses at all levels must understand conflict and how it can be managed.

Nurse leaders and managers must strive to promote "ongoing evaluation and continuous improvement of conflict resolution skills" (ANA, 2016, p. 49). Nurse leaders and managers spend close to one-fourth of their time in conflict management activities (Padrutt, 2010; Rundio et al., 2016; Valentine, 2001). It is imperative for nurse leaders and managers to learn how to deal with conflict and role model effective conflict management for staff. When managed effectively, conflict can provide a mechanism through which work can be accomplished. Findings from one study suggest that interpersonal conflicts in the workplace should be confronted directly, constructively, and together with those involved (Mahon & Nicotera, 2011). However, nurses in general are highly unlikely to confront conflict and respond by avoidance or withdrawal (Mahon & Nicotera, 2011). Poorly managed conflict can pose additional problems in the workplace such as job dissatisfaction, depression, increased turnover, compromised patient safety, and aggression.

Types of Conflict

Conflict management requires nurse leaders and managers to assess the situation, identify the type of conflict, and explore perceptions about the conflict with those involved. The type of conflict directs the conflict management strategy that is used.

Intrapersonal Conflict

Intrapersonal conflict is an internal conflict, or a conflict coming from within a person. An individual may be confronted with an issue or situation that creates a sense of discomfort within. An example of intrapersonal conflict is a nurse trying to make a decision to go back to school for an advanced degree who may experience conflict between personal and professional goals (e.g., balancing family life and pursuing professional advancement). An individual nurse's intrapersonal conflict can affect others on the unit, thus resulting in interpersonal conflict (Padrutt, 2010).

Interpersonal Conflict

Interpersonal conflict occurs when there is a disagreement between or among two or more people. The disagreement can be related to differing values, ethics, goals, beliefs, or priorities. Interpersonal conflict is very common in the workplace. An example of interpersonal conflict is a difference of opinion between a nurse and a family member regarding a patient's living will.

Intergroup Conflict

Also common in the workplace is conflict that occurs between groups of people, also called intergroup conflict. For example, the emergency department staff may complain that patients are not moved to the intensive care unit in a timely manner, and in turn, staff members in the intensive care unit complain that the emergency department staff is always demanding to transport patients before patients are discharged, thereby making beds available.

Organizational Conflict

Organizational conflict can result when there is disagreement between staff and organizational policies and procedures, standards, or changes being made. For example, administration implements a new procedure for nurses to use when documenting nursing care without input from the nurses. This can cause organizational conflict because administration implements a change without consulting those it affects most, nurses at the bedside.

Conflict Management Strategies

There are five common strategies for conflict management (Thomas & Kilman, 1977), and each is used successfully to manage conflict in different situations. Typically, most people use a combination of strategies when dealing with conflict. The five strategies are as follows (Thomas & Kilman, 1977):

1. The *avoiding* strategy involves withdrawing or hiding from the conflict. The strategy is not always effective in resolving conflict and just postpones the conflict. Because the conflict is not resolved, it may reappear again later.

2. *Accommodating* involves sacrificing one's own needs or goals and trying to satisfy another's desires, needs, or goals. This strategy does not resolve conflict and may result in future conflict.

3. Individuals who use the *competing* strategy pursue their own needs, desires, or goals at the expense of others. The competitor wants to win and is not cooperative. This strategy is power driven and can result in aggression.

4. *Compromising* is an effective conflict management strategy. When compromising, everyone gives something up, and everyone gets something they want in return. However, to be effective, those involved must be on an even playing field.

5. *Collaborating* is the best strategy to use in conflict management because it involves a shared approach to resolving conflict. Shared goals are identified, and a commitment to working together is implemented by those involved. Collaborating is time consuming, but it results in the best chance of a resolution (Padrutt, 2010).

Effective conflict management requires those involved to use a variety of strategies based on the situation (Sportsman & Hamilton, 2007). A nurse's perceptions, values, beliefs, and attitudes play a role in the conflict process and how conflict is managed (Whitworth, 2008). Effective nurse leaders and managers recognize the differences in personalities of staff members and their methods of handling conflict and understand the impact the differences can have in the workplace. Ineffective conflict management can result in excessive stress for those involved and negatively affect interpersonal relationships. In contrast, effective conflict management results in positive outcomes, including improved work relationships and increased productivity.

Role of Nurse Leaders and Managers in Addressing Conflict

Nurse leaders and managers are challenged to learn to deal with conflict in a way that will manage the issues at hand while maintaining positive relationships among staff members. Establishing open communication and employing active listening skills can help nurse leaders and managers manage conflict on the unit. Often, challenging individuals can cause conflict among staff. Nurse leaders and managers need to work to engage all staff members as a team to create safe, quality patient outcomes. In addition, nurse leaders and managers must encourage positive interactions among staff members and health-care providers as part of a healthy work environment (Sportsman & Hamilton, 2007). A healthy work environment is discussed in Chapter 12.

Nurse leaders and managers need to mediate when interpersonal or intergroup conflict occurs to avoid negative effects on nursing care and patient outcomes. Elements that should be explored include the following (Porter-O'Grady & Malloch, 2013):

- *Mutual respect:* Those involved in the conflict may need a reminder to be respectful and focus on the issue and not the other person.
- *Needs versus wants:* The nurse leader and manager must help those involved differentiate between what they need and what they want.

- *Compassion and empathy:* Those involved in the conflict may need assistance understanding each other and hearing the other person's position.
- *Staying in the "I":* The nurse leader and manager reminds those involved to focus on "I" statements and avoid using "you" statements and avoid blaming.

When dealing with conflict among staff members, nurse leaders and managers should avoid criticizing or passing judgment on others' opinions. Instead, they must focus goals on how team members' behaviors have affected team outcomes, and building consensus. A successful nurse leader and manager identifies conflict, works with those involved to manage and/or resolve the issues, and moves on (Porter-O'Grady & Malloch, 2013). An important skills for nurse leaders and managers to master is negotiation.

Negotiation

According to Filho et al. (2019), **negotiation** "is the art of making choices and offering others benefits that they want in order to get what we need in return in a voluntary and consensual manner" (p. 49). Negotiation focuses on managing differing points of view related to an issue that needs to be resolved (Cleary et al., 2018). It can be an emotional process and requires effective communication skills to keep differences from escalating, resulting in avoiding the situation, or ending in a complete communication breakdown (Cleary et al., 2018). Nurse leaders and managers can employ four key principles for successful negotiations (Rundio et al., 2016, p. 74):

1. Separating the people from the problem
2. Focusing on interests, not positions
3. Inventing options for mutual gains
4. Insisting on objective criteria

Nurse leaders and managers should learn the art of negotiation to enhance their roles in relation to managing and sustaining a health work environment, collaboration and teamwork, building relationships, performance reviews, and career advancement (Cleary et al., 2018; Smith-Trudeau, 2019).

LEARNING ACTIVITY 15-2   **Leading Change and Managing Conflict**

Review this scenario and respond to the questions that follow:

The nursing division has just approved a change in the intravenous (IV) pumps throughout your hospital. The new IV pumps are very high-tech smart pumps. You have scheduled a meeting with your staff to discuss this change and the change process. You have some concerns about your older staff members who are not keen on high-tech equipment. During the meeting, the nurses complained that they do not see the need to change the IV pumps. They complained that the new pumps were difficult to use and difficult to read the screens. Several younger nurses shared their excitement about the change and indicated they thought the new pumps would save time and be more efficient when noting intake and clearing pumps.

1. According to Lewin's Model of Change, in which phase are the older nurses? In which phase are the younger nurses?
2. What strategies could you use to engage the nurses who are resistant?
3. How could you capitalize on the enthusiasm of the younger nurses?

▶ **SUMMARY**

The rapidly changing health-care environment today requires nurse leaders and managers to develop knowledge and skills in leading and managing change and innovation. Nurse leaders and managers must be skilled in understanding change theory, serving as change agents, and supporting staff during the change process. Regardless of how important a change or innovation is, nurse leaders and managers must consider human response and include strategies to help staff members cope with change in the overall plan. Further, nurse leaders and managers must understand that conflict can result from change and be willing to apply strategies to manage change as needed. Nurses at all levels must also understand that conflict is part of change, it can be healthy, and it allows for new ideas to emerge.

NCLEX®-STYLE REVIEW QUESTIONS

Multiple Choice

1. Which characteristic is always included when considering making changes in any type of nursing setting?
    1. It is often met with resistance.
    2. It does not lead to conflict.
    3. As long as stakeholders are vested in the process, there will be no problems with implementation.
    4. All changes lead to improved outcomes.
2. In the clinical setting, the hospital organization has changed to a different electronic health record (EHR) system after reviewing several different types of available systems. Of what type of change is this an example?
    1. Planned change
    2. Unplanned change
    3. Innovation
    4. Crisis resolution
3. Which aspect of change takes place in the refreezing stage of Lewin's Force-Field Model?
    1. Determination that change is needed
    2. Achievement of equilibrium
    3. Exhibiting motivation to change
    4. Gathering of information occurs

4. Which information is represented by the framed question, "why" of change?
   1. Participant stakeholders
   2. Rationale
   3. Timing
   4. Technique

5. Which statement is accurate with regard to the Phases of Change Model?
   1. Change always occurs in a comprehensive manner.
   2. Communication and feedback are critical elements.
   3. Time does not affect potential for change.
   4. Realistic goals are often not achieved.

6. Staff nurses in response to a suggested change on the unit have displayed no resistance and are embracing the change. Which example of change strategy is represented by this scenario?
   1. Normative-reeducative
   2. Empirical-rational
   3. Power-coercive
   4. Anticipated due to peer pressure

7. In a hospital setting, there appears to be conflict between the hospital's administrative personnel regarding hospital performance objectives. What type of conflict could be applied to this situation?
   1. Intrapersonal
   2. Organizational
   3. Interpersonal
   4. Intergroup

8. A nurse manager attempts to resolve conflict on the unit between staff members by bringing all sides to the table to have a discussion. What type of conflict management strategy is being displayed?
   1. Accommodating
   2. Competing
   3. Avoidance
   4. Collaborating

9. Which action, if used by a nurse manager, would lead to increased conflict in the clinical setting?
   1. Assessment of needs versus wants
   2. Reminding staff that every member should be treated with respect
   3. Emphasizing the importance of listening
   4. Using statements that focus on the individual performing the behavior indicating "we" or "you"

10. Nurses in the emergency department (ED) are complaining about how the medical-surgical unit nurses are responding to them when patients are being transported to the floor. The ED nurses state that the medical-surgical nurses do not want to do their job at times. The medical-surgical unit nurses state that the ED nurses always bring the patients near change of shift. What type of conflict is represented by this situation?
    1. Interpersonal
    2. Intergroup
    3. Organizational
    4. Intrapersonal
11. Which percentage represents the amount of time nurse leaders and managers spend in helping to resolve conflicts within the clinical setting according to clinical research?
    1. Approximately 25%
    2. Varies between 50% and 100%
    3. 99%
    4. Less than 10%
12. Which characteristic is *not* attributed to Emerging Change Theories?
    1. Linear in nature
    2. Inherent complexity
    3. Exhibit flexibility
    4. Focus on innovation

Multiple Response

13. Which information is consistent with the chaos theory of change? *Select all that apply.*
    1. It is nonlinear.
    2. It contains formed matter.
    3. It may also be referred to as the "butterfly effect."
    4. It reflects randomness.
    5. It can be predicted.
14. When comparing traditional change theories and models, which statements are accurate with regard to when to apply specific models? *Select all that apply.*
    1. Force-field model when problem-solving
    2. Eight-stage process when rapid change is required for learning organizations
    3. Force-field model when planned change is anticipated
    4. Innovation-decision process when implementing technological changes
    5. Phases of change when organizational change is warranted
15. Which behaviors, if utilized by nurse managers, would help to establish change in the clinical environment? *Select all that apply.*
    1. Rewarding consistent actions at the expense of anticipated change
    2. Helping to build trust
    3. Instilling confidence
    4. Anticipating that change is inevitable
    5. Not allowing staff to transfer off unit

REFERENCES

American Association of Colleges of Nursing. (2021). *The essentials: Core competencies for professional nursing education.* Author. https://www.aacnnursing.org/Portals/42/AcademicNursing/pdf/Essentials-2021.pdf

American Nurses Association (ANA). (2010). *Nursing's social policy statement: The essence of the profession.* Author.

American Nurses Association (ANA). (2015). *Code of ethics for nurses with interpretive statements.* Author.

American Nurses Association (ANA). (2016). *Nursing administration: Scope and standards of practice* (2nd ed.). Author.

American Organization for Nursing Leadership (AONL). (2015a). *AONL nurse manager competencies.* Author.

American Organization for Nursing Leadership (AONL). (2015b). *AONL nurse executive competencies.* Author.

Anderson, R. (2014, August). Thrive or survive: Healthcare reform from the perspective of a nurse CE. *Nurse Leader, 25–27.*

Bowers, B. (2011). Managing change by empowering staff. *Nursing Times, 107*(32/33). www.nursingtimes.net/nursing-practice/clinical-zones/management/managing-change-by-empowering-staff/5033731.article

Chinn, R., & Benne, K. D. (1969). *General strategies for effecting changes in human systems.* In W. Bennis, K. Benne, & R. Chinn (Eds.). *The planning of change* (pp. 32–59). Harcourt, Rinehart, & Winston.

Cleary, M., Lees, D., & Sayers, J. (2018). The art of negotiation. *Issues in Mental Health Nursing, 39*(10), 910–912.

Cronenwett, L., Sherwood, G., Barnsteiner, J., Disch, J., Johnson, J., Mitchell, P., Sullivan, D. T., & Warren, J. (2007). Quality and safety education for nurses. *Nursing Outlook, 55*(3), 122–131.

Crowell, D. M. (2016). *Complexity leadership: Nursing's role in health care delivery* (2nd ed.). F. A. Davis.

Erickson, J. I. (2014). Leading unplanned change. *Journal of Nursing Administration, 44*(3), 125–126.

Filho, W. C., Padua, I. C., & Fernandes, N. S. (2019). Negotiation: Techniques, strategies, and approaches to medical professionals. *International Journal of Healthcare Management, 12*(1), 48–53.

Greiner, A. C., & Knebel, E. (Eds.). (2003). *Health professions education: A bridge to quality.* National Academies Press.

Kotter, J. P. (1996). *Leading change.* Harvard Business School Press.

Lewin, K. (1951). *Field theory in social science.* Harper Brothers.

Lippitt, R., Watson, J., & Wesley, B. (1958). *The dynamics of planned change.* Harcourt Brace.

Losa Iglesias, M. E., & De Bengoa Vallejo, R. B. (2012). Conflict resolution styles in the nursing profession. *Contemporary Nurse, 43*(1), 73–80.

Mahon, M. M., & Nicotera, A. M. (2011). Nursing and conflict communication: Avoidance as preferred strategy. *Nursing Administration Quarterly, 35*(2), 152–163.

Manion, J. (2011). *From management to leadership* (3rd ed.). Jossey-Bass.

Mensik, J. (2014). *Lead, drive & thrive in the system.* American Nurses Association.

Mitchell, G. (2013). Selecting the best theory to implement planned change. *Nursing Management, 20*(1), 32–37.

Padrutt, J. (2010). Resolving conflict: Now more important than ever. *Nursing Management, 40*(1), 52–54.

Porter-O'Grady, T., & Malloch, K. (2010). *Innovation leadership: Creating the landscape of health care.* Jones & Bartlett Publishers.

Porter-O'Grady, T., & Malloch, K. (2013). *Leadership in nursing practice: Changing the landscape of health care.* Jones & Bartlett Learning.

Quote Garden. (2016). *Questions about change.* www.quotegarden.com/change.html

Rogers, E. M. (1995). *Diffusion of innovations* (4th ed.). Free Press.

Rogers, E. M. (2003). *Diffusion of innovations* (5th ed.). Free Press.

Roussel, L., Thomas, P. L., & Harris, J. L. (2020). *Management and leadership for nurse administrators* (8th ed.). Jones & Bartlett Learning.

Rundio, A., Wilson, V., & Meloy, F. A.(2016). *Nurse executive review and resource manual* (3rd ed.). Nursing Knowledge Center, American Nurses Association.

Salmela, S., Eriksson, K., & Fagerström, L. (2013). Nurse leaders' perceptions of an approaching organizational change. *Qualitative Health Research, 23*(5), 689–699.

Senge, P. M. (1990). *The fifth discipline: The art and practice of the learning organization.* Doubleday.

Senge, P., Hamilton, H., & Kania, J. (2015, Winter). The dawn of system leadership. *Stanford Social Innovation Review,* 27–33.

Shirey, M. R. (2006). Evidence-based practice: How nurse leaders can facilitate innovation. *Nursing Administration Quarterly, 30*(3), 252–265.

Shirey, M. R. (2013). Lewin's theory of planned change as a strategic resource. *Journal of Nursing Administration, 43*(2), 69–72.

Smith-Trudeau, P. (2019, January, February, March). Solving problems creatively and negotiating collaboratively. *Vermont Nurse Connection,* 4–5.

Sportsman, S., & Hamilton, P. (2007). Conflict management styles in the health professions. *Journal of Professional Nursing, 23*(3), 157–166.

Stefancyk, A., Hancock, B., & Meadows, M. T. (2013). The nurse manager: Change agent, change coach? *Nursing Administration Quarterly, 37*(1), 13–17.

Thomas, K. W., & Kilman, R. H. (1977). Developing a forced-choice measure of conflict-handling behavior: The "mode" instrument. *Educational and Psychological Measurement, 37*(2), 309–325.

Valentine, P. E. (2001). A gender perspective on conflict management strategies of nurses. *Journal of Nursing Scholarship, 33*(1), 69–74.

Whitworth, B. S. (2008). Is there a relationship between personality type and preferred conflict-handling styles? An exploratory study of registered nurses in southern Mississippi. *Journal of Nursing Management, 16,* 921–932.

To explore learning resources for this chapter, go to FADavis.com

Chapter 16

Managing Finances

Elizabeth J. Murray, PhD, RN, CNE

KEY TERMS

Break-even analysis
Capital budget
Direct expenses
Fixed expenses
Full-time equivalent
Incremental budgeting
Indirect expenses
Necessary care activities
Nonproductive time
Non–value-added care activities
Nursing hours per patient day
Operating budget
Performance budgeting
Personnel budget
Productive time
Productivity
Units of service
Value-added care activities
Variable expenses
Variances
Workload
Zero-based budgeting

LEARNING OUTCOMES

- Understand why budgeting is a critical skill for nurse leaders and managers.
- Examine issues nurse leaders and managers face when attempting to balance cost containment, cost effectiveness, and quality care.
- Define basic budget terminology.
- Explain the steps in the budget process.
- Describe different types of budgets.
- Compare and contrast different budgeting methods.

The Knowledge, Skills, and Attitudes Related to the Following Are Addressed in This Chapter:

Core Competencies	• Patient-Centered Care • Teamwork and Collaboration • Evidence-Based Practice • Informatics
The Essentials: Core Competencies for Professional Nursing Education (AACN, 2021)	**Domain 7: Systems-Based Practice** 7.2 Incorporate consideration of cost-effectiveness of care (pp. 46–47).
Code of Ethics with Interpretive Statements (ANA, 2015)	**Provision 2.2:** Conflict of interest for nurses (pp. 5–6) **Provision 2.3:** Collaboration (p. 6)

Nurse Manager (NMC) Competencies (AONL, 2015a) and Nurse Executive (NEC) Competencies (AONL, 2015b)	**NMC: Financial Management (p. 4)**
	• Recognize the impact of reimbursement on revenue
	• Anticipate the effects of changes on reimbursement programs for patient care
	• Maximize care efficiency and throughput
	• Understand the relationship between value-based purchasing and quality outcomes with revenue and reimbursement
	• Create a budget
	• Monitor a budget
	• Analyze a budget and explain variance
	• Conduct ongoing evaluation of productivity
	• Forecast future revenue and expenses Capital budgeting
	  • Justification
	  • Cost benefit analysis
	NMC: Technology (p. 5)
	• Information technology (IT): Understand the effect of IT on patient care and delivery systems to reduce workload
	  • Use information systems to support business decisions
	NEC: Knowledge of the Health Care Environment (pp. 6–7)
	• Health care economics and policy
	  • Understand regulation and payment issues that affect an organization's finances
	  • Describe individual organization's payer mix, CMI and benchmark database

Continued

The Knowledge, Skills, and Attitudes Related to the Following Are Addressed in This Chapter:—cont'd

- Align care delivery models and staff performance with key safety and economic drivers (e.g., value-based purchasing, bundled payment)
- Take action when opportunities exist to adjust operations to respond effectively to environmental changes in economic elements
- Use knowledge of federal and state laws and regulations that affect the provision of patient care (e.g., tort reform, malpractice/negligence, reimbursement)
- Participate in legislative process on health care issues through such mechanisms as membership in professional organization and personal contact with officials
- Educate patient care team members on the legislative process, the regulatory process and methods for influencing both
- Interpret impact of legislation at the state and federal level on nursing and health care organizations
- Evidence-based practice/outcome measurement and research
  - Allocate nursing resources based on measurement of patient acuity/care needed

NEC: Business Skills (p. 10)
- Financial management
  - Develop and manage an annual operating budget and long-term capital expenditure plan
  - Use business models for health care organizations and apply fundamental concepts of economics
  - Interpret financial statements
  - Manage financial resources
  - Ensure the use of accurate charging mechanisms
  - Educate patient care team members on financial implications of patient care decisions
  - Participate in the negotiation and monitoring of contract compliance (e.g., physicians, service providers)
- Human resource management
  - Analyze market data in relation to supply and demand
  - Contribute to the development of compensation programs

Nursing Administration Scope and Standards of Practice (ANA, 2016)

Standard 1: Assessment The nurse administrator collects pertinent data and information relative to the situation, issue, problem, or trend (pp. 35–36).
Standard 3: Outcomes Identification The nurse administrator identifies expected outcomes for a plan tailored to the system, organization, or population problem, issue, or trend (p. 38).

The Knowledge, Skills, and Attitudes Related to the Following Are Addressed in This Chapter:—cont'd

Standard 4: Planning The nurse administrator develops a plan that defines, articulates, and establishes strategies and alternatives to attain expected, measurable outcomes (p. 39).

Standard 5: Implementation The nurse administrator implements the identified plan (p. 40).

Standard 7: Ethics The nurse administrator practices ethically (pp. 45–46).

Standard 11: Leadership The nurse administrator leads within professional practice setting, profession, healthcare industry, and society (pp. 51–52).

Standard 16: Resource Utilization The nurse administrator utilizes appropriate resources to plan, allocate, provide, and sustain evidence-based, high quality nursing services that are person-, population-, or community-centered, culturally appropriate, safe, timely, effective, and fiscally responsible (pp. 57–58).

Source: American Association of Colleges of Nursing. (2021). *The essentials: Core competencies for professional nursing education.* Author; American Nurses Association (ANA). (2015). *Code of ethics for nurses with interpretive statements.* Author; American Nurses Association (ANA). (2016). *Nursing administration: Scope and standards of practice* (2nd ed.). Author; American Organization for Nursing Leadership (AONL). (2015a). *AONL nurse manager competencies.* Author; American Organization for Nursing Leadership (AONL). (2015b). *AONL nurse executive competencies.* Author; Cronenwett, L., Sherwood, G., Barnsteiner, J., Disch, J., Johnson, J., Mitchell, P., Sullivan, D. T., & Warren, J. (2007). Quality and safety education for nurses. *Nursing Outlook, 55*(3), 122–131; and Greiner, A. C., & Knebel, E. (Eds.). (2003). *Health professions education: A bridge to quality.* National Academies Press.

In today's health-care delivery system, all nurses have a duty to provide value-added and cost-effective nursing care (Seifert, 2012), and there is added pressure to do so in keeping with the current trend to move to a value-driven budget process that focuses on patient-centered outcomes. In their ongoing commitment to the profession, nurses should use "their skills, knowledge, and abilities to act as visionaries, promoting safe practice environments, and supporting resourceful, accessible, and cost-effective delivery of health care to serve the ever changing needs of the population" (American Nurses Association [ANA], 2010, p. 26). In addition, nurses must participate in and lead efforts to minimize costs and unnecessary duplication of services as well as conserve resources. However, it falls to nurse leaders and managers to actually balance and align budgets. Nurse leaders and managers must become astute financial planners with a keen understanding of fiscal planning, budget forecasting, and cost containment. In turn, they have a tremendous amount of influence on costs related to managing personnel, supplies, and lengths of stay. In this chapter, nurse leaders and managers discover why budgeting skill is a necessary core competency, develop an understanding of how budgeting directly affects patient safety, and learn the basics of the budgeting process.

▶ ORGANIZATIONAL AND UNIT-BASED FINANCES

Financial management for health-care organizations has become extremely complex and the market has become very competitive. Enactment of the Affordable Care Act and continuing health-care reform have put pressure on organizations to reduce costs, improve quality of care across the continuum, decrease gaps, and reduce redundancies (Thomas & Roussel, 2020).

Organizational financial management involves three major functions: planning, control, and decision making (Jones et al., 2019):

- Planning is critical for efficient management of the organization. Effective planning allows the organization to set goals; determine, allocate, or obtain resources to meet the goals; and move forward.
- Control is important once the plan is established. The plan must be implemented, and control is necessary to carry out the plan, assess the progress, evaluate related income and expenses, and establish strategies for when progress is unsatisfactory.
- Decision making is an ongoing process for all levels of financial management in an organization. Decision making is needed during planning and during control.

Nurses at all levels have a role in organizational and unit-based financial management. Nurse leaders and managers have a "central role in determining the human and fiscal resources required to accomplish work" (Thomas & Roussel, 2020, p. 156).

Chief Nurse Executive

The Chief Nurse Executive (CNE) is the senior level nurse in an organization and is considered a member of the senior administrative team and must have a good understanding of financial management. The CNE has responsibility for the financial management at the organizational level as well as for the nursing division. The CNE has the authority and responsibility for revenue earned and expenses incurred by the nursing division. The CNE negotiates and establishes the amount of resources available for nursing and is held accountable for spending above or below the planned budget (Jones et al., 2019).

Midlevel Managers/Clinical Directors

Midlevel managers report to the CNE and are often responsible for an area of the division of nursing that includes two or more units. For example, the Clinical Director of Critical Care may be responsible for several intensive care units (ICUs) (e.g., surgical ICU, medical ICU, cardiac ICU, and trauma ICU). Typically, the midlevel manager is responsible for guiding the first-line managers of the units they oversee in the budget process. Therefore, they are held accountable by the CNE for expenditures above and below the budgeted amounts.

First-line Managers

First-line managers are responsible for the unit-based financial management and must answer to the midlevel managers for any variances in the established budget. Nurse leaders and managers at this level must be knowledgeable about creating a budget, monitoring a budget, analyzing a budget, and conducting ongoing evaluation of productivity (Jones et al., 2019). Nurse leaders and managers must understand sources of health-care financing and reimbursement, including government, insurance, self-pay, and private and philanthropic gifts (ANA, 2016, p. 15).

Staff Nurses

Staff nurses should have some basic knowledge of the unit budget. They need to understand how their daily actions in providing patient care influence health-care costs (Jones et al., 2019).

▶ BUDGETING AS A CORE COMPETENCY

In any industry, including health care, the overall goal of the budgeting process is to gain high-quality value for every dollar spent (Porter-O'Grady & Malloch, 2013). Budgeting is an ongoing activity that requires nurse leaders and managers to develop fiscal literacy to monitor the financial status of a specific unit or units and ultimately provide quality cost-effective nursing care. Nurse leaders and managers are responsible and accountable for operating and capital budgets as well as daily, weekly, and annual productivity. Nurse leaders and managers may be responsible for an individual cost center or several cost centers depending on their role within the organization. For example, the manager of a surgical intensive care unit is responsible for the cost center for just that unit; the director of critical care services is responsible for overseeing the cost centers of the surgical intensive care unit, medical intensive care unit, cardiac care unit, and cardiac telemetry unit; and the chief nursing officer is responsible for managing all nursing cost centers. No matter how many cost centers they oversee, nurse leaders and managers must have adequate knowledge of the process to be effective.

The main purpose of a nursing budget is to determine how to allocate the fiscal resources necessary to accomplish the objectives, programs, and activities of nursing services; the budgeting process provides nurse leaders and managers with the necessary tools to ensure that resources benefit patients and the organization, rather than being wasted (Finkler & McHugh, 2008; Swansburg, 1997). The budgeting process has a direct effect on the quantity and quality of the nursing care provided. Nurses at all levels should be involved in the budget process to ensure that adequate and appropriate resources are available to deliver safe, quality care. To budget effectively, nurse leaders and managers must develop specific knowledge in fiscal management and financial outcomes and skills in budgeting and monetary management (ANA, 2016). In addition, nurse leaders and managers must ensure that resources are allocated "to optimize the provision of quality, safe, and cost-effective care" (ANA, 2016, p. 57).

The American Organization for Nursing Leadership (AONL) identifies financial management as a core competency for nurses in management or executive positions. Financial management falls under the domain of business skills and includes the following components (AONL, 2015b, p. 10):

- Articulate business models for health-care organizations and fundamental concepts of economics.
- Describe general accounting principles and define basic accounting terms.
- Analyze financial statements.
- Manage financial resources by developing business plans.
- Establish procedures to ensure accurate charging mechanisms.
- Educate patient care team members on financial implications of patient care decisions.

▶ COST CONTAINMENT AND EFFECTIVENESS

Nurse leaders and managers are charged with developing, implementing, evaluating, and monitoring a cost-effective budget. It is crucial for nurse leaders and managers to make sound fiscal decisions and spend their budgets wisely when it comes to activities that affect safe and quality patient care, patient satisfaction, and nurse satisfaction (Swearingen, 2009). New policies and reimbursement structures in the current health-care system directly affect the nursing budget. As the cost of health care continues to rise, the health-care system is focusing more on improving patient outcomes, controlling costs, and providing financial rewards to health-care organizations that can do both (Anderson & Danna, 2013). Nurse leaders and managers must be knowledgeable about the changing reimbursement based on quality. In fact, the link between quality performance measures and reimbursement requires nurse leaders and managers to be vigilant in monitoring and increasing nurses' time delivering direct care when necessary (Swearingen, 2009). Nurse leaders and managers have a direct impact on patient care outcomes, the costs associated with patient care, and the financial stability of the nursing unit or department.

Effective nurse leaders and managers recognize that they have control over unit activities that contribute to the budget, such as supply costs and the amount of waste that occurs. Further, expenditures and waste result from the actions of all individuals working on the unit. Engaging staff members in the budget process and emphasizing the financial impact on the unit when supplies are wasted or not charged can enable managers to maintain better control over the budget (Waxman, 2005). In fact, nurse leaders and managers have minimal success in controlling the budget without the cooperation of all unit staff members (Finkler & McHugh, 2008). Although there are aspects of the budget that managers cannot control, such as the amount of revenue generated, patient acuity, and benefit packages for staff (Waxman, 2005), nurse leaders and managers must focus time and energy on the areas they can control, rather than activities that are out of their reach. Technology and automation have helped nurse leaders and managers manage the budget process and make informed cost-effective decisions. Tools such as variance reports, staffing spreadsheets, forecasting software, and dashboards can help nurse leaders and managers oversee the unit budget, monitor trends, and make informed budget changes as needed.

Although the implications of effective budgeting are important, budgeting is a complicated process that may not come naturally to all nurses. In turn, nurse leaders and managers must make it a priority to become experts in the basics of the budgeting process to be able to advocate for and allocate resources for safe, timely, effective, efficient, equitable patient-centered care.

▶ THE BUDGET PROCESS

A nursing budget is a systematic plan that provides the best estimate of nursing expenses and revenues, and it is most effectively stated in terms of attainable objectives. A prerequisite for the nurse leader and manager to setting a budget is understanding budget terminology and basic formulas. Basic budget terminology and related formulas are listed in Table 16-1.

Nurse leaders and managers should have a road map to help with the planning process. The budget process can be compared with the nursing process. Similar to the nursing care plan, the budget plan is expressed in financial terms and carried out within a specific time frame. To deliver quality care, nurses must know how to develop and implement a nursing care plan. In turn, nurse leaders and managers must know how to develop, implement, and manage a budget plan (Anderson & Danna, 2013). To forecast a budget, it is necessary first to assess the current needs in terms of operating expenses, labor, supplies, and equipment. The second step is to diagnose or determine a cost-effective budget that maximizes the use of resources as well as ensures safe, quality care. Third is to plan and develop a realistic budget. Implementing the budget is the fourth step and includes ongoing monitoring and analysis of the monthly budget to identify any variances. The last step is control and feedback, which is similar to evaluation (Jones et al., 2019).

Table 16-1	Basic Budget Terminology and Formulas	
Terminology	**Description**	**Formula**
Average daily census (ADC)	The average number of patients on the unit on any given day over a period of time	Total patients on the unit in 1 year/ 365 days
Break-even quantity	The number of patients needed to break even	Fixed costs/variable costs per patient
Cost per unit of service (CPUOS)	Total cost divided by units of service	Total staff numbers worked in 24 hours × average hourly rate × hours per shift/ADC
Full-time equivalent (FTE)	The equivalent of one full-time employee working for 1 year; can be a combination of employees working part-time to equal one full-time employee	1 employee working 8 hours per day × 5 days × 52 weeks = 2,080 hours/year
Nursing hours per patient day (NHPPD)	The amount of productive nursing care hours per patient day in a 24-hour period	Productive nursing hours worked in 24 hours/patient census for 24 hours
Productivity	Measure of the input required for the output	Output × 100 input
Variance	Deviation from the projected budget	Monthly budgeted expense − monthly actual expense = variance in $ Variance in $/monthly budgeted expense = % of variance

Assessment

During the assessment phase, nurse leaders and managers must gather data and assess the needs for the upcoming fiscal year. This process includes determining workload and patient care hours, forecasting nonproductive work hours, estimating costs of supplies and services, and projecting unit capital expenses. Additionally, nurse leaders and managers should examine the present nursing activities as well as those planned for the future. Typically, expenses and revenues are analyzed from the previous fiscal year, and any deviations from the projected budget the previous year are examined closely to avoid similar deviations in the future.

Diagnosis

The diagnosis phase involves determining the nursing productivity goal for the upcoming fiscal year. Productivity is related to the delivery of nursing care as well as the effectiveness of that care relative to patient outcomes. Nurse leaders and managers must evaluate unit goals from the previous year to ensure that these goals are in alignment with the organization's current mission and philosophy, and they must revise or develop new goals for the future year if necessary. The projected budget is based on programs and activities needed to accomplish the nursing productivity goal as well as the organization's broader goals and fiscal projections.

Planning

A successful budget provides an annual plan that guides effective use of human and material resources, nursing services, and management of the environment to improve productivity. In addition, a good budget considers the needs of the unit as well as the organization and places available resources in the appropriate places where the accomplishment of goals will be greatest (Finkler et al., 2014). Budget worksheets are used during the planning step to assist nursing leaders and managers in preparing their budgets. The planning stage is key to ensuring that patients receive cost-effective and safe nursing care from satisfied nursing staff members. Ideally, the budget is somewhat flexible to allow for fluctuations in patient numbers and acuity.

During the planning process, nurse leaders and managers may need to determine whether a program or service will lose money, make money, or break even. The process used to determine the profitability of a service is called **break-even analysis** (Finkler & McHugh, 2008). Break-even analysis is useful in forecasting revenues for a specific unit or service. If total revenues are greater than total expenses, there is a profit, and if total revenues are less than total expenses, there is a loss. When revenues are equal to expenses and there is not a profit or a loss, the program or service will just break even (Finkler & McHugh, 2008). In nursing, the break-even quantity is the number of patients needed to break even (see Table 16-3 for the formula to calculate break-even quantity). The price is the cost for each patient or the average amount collected per patient. When the variable costs per patient are lower than the break-even quantity, there is a loss, and when they are higher, there is a profit. The break-even analysis is also useful to determine direct care hours for the nursing unit.

Implementation

On each unit, the nurse leader and manager directs, evaluates, and executes all budget-related activities. During implementation phase, the nurse leader and manager must attempt to keep the unit functioning within the budget plan. Prioritization is critical, and it is important for nurse leaders and managers to engage all staff members in the process and motivate them to work within the constraints of the budget. To promote fiscal awareness among all nursing staff members, nurse leaders and managers should meet with staff early in the implementation stage to explain the budget or the upcoming year, discuss variances that occurred in the previous budget year, and encourage input regarding any deviations. The more informed the staff members are about the budget goals and the plans to meet those goals, the more likely it is that the budget goals will be met.

Evaluation (Control and Feedback)

The evaluation phase of the budget process begins once the budget is implemented and continues through the next year when a new budget is set. Control involves taking action to ensure that the budget plan is followed. Feedback relates to using results to improve the accuracy of the budget. Because the nursing budget establishes the financial standards for the unit, nurse leaders and managers are accountable to address any deviations in the budget and take appropriate action to avoid excess or inadequate money at the end of the budget year. Expense and revenue reports as well as comparisons between projected budget and actual budget are often provided to nurse leaders and managers by the financial department on a regular basis, usually monthly and quarterly. During the evaluation phase, nurse leaders and managers must review reports on a regular basis for any deviations, or **variances**, from the projected budget. The actual results are compared with budgeted expectations and the difference between the two results in the variance and are analyzed to determine cause, with corrective action taken when necessary. The goal of variance analysis is to strengthen the accuracy of budget forecasting and minimize crisis management when a deviation does occur (Porter-O'Grady & Malloch, 2013). Ideally, a flexible budget was set during the planning stage to allow for some variances on a monthly basis. Should variances become significant, adjustments may be necessary.

Variations occur most often in the areas of finances, staffing, and supplies (Porter-O'Grady & Malloch, 2013). Variances can be positive, meaning better than expected, or negative, meaning not as good as expected. Regardless of the type of variance, nurse leaders and managers must provide a written explanation to upper management, explaining or justifying why the numbers are greater or less than the budgeted amount; this amount can be a percentage or a dollar amount. Table 16-2 illustrates a typical unit budget report for 1 month.

Table 16-2   Monthly Variance Report*

Date Budgeted Items	Monthly Budgeted Expense ($)	Monthly Actual Expense ($)	Variance in $	Variance in %	Year-to-Date Budget	Year-to-Date Actual	Year-to-Date Variance
IV solutions	2,250	3,628	(1,378)	(61.2)	9,000	8,242	758
IV primary sets	1,110	1,990	(880)	(79)	4,440	4,340	100
Oxygen cannulas	550	500	50	9	2,200	2,310	(110)
Suction catheters	750	600	150	20	3,000	3,100	(100)
Sterile water	1,200	1,124	76	6.3	3,920	3,750	170
Sterile saline	1,200	1,010	100	8.3	3,920	3,770	150

*The monthly expenses for IV solutions and IV primary sets were higher than the budgeted expenses, with variances of ($1,378) or (61.2%) and ($880) or (79%), respectively. However, the year-to-date actual and variance are within the budgeted expense. The nurse leader and manager must explain this variance and identify causes of the overage to ensure that the overall budget for the year is met.
IV, intravenous.

Although all variances are important to analyze, staffing variances are typically the greatest concern for nurse leaders and managers. Nurse leaders and managers vigilantly monitor the required number of nursing staff needed to care for patients safely and compare those numbers with the actual nursing staff available. Staffing variances occur when there is a difference between required nursing care hours and actual nursing care hours. A staffing variance can fall at either end of the spectrum: not enough staff to care for patients safely or too many staff members scheduled for the number and acuity of patients on the unit. Nurse leaders and managers must analyze the causes of the individual staff variances as well as variances in total nursing care hours (Porter-O'Grady & Malloch, 2013). When variances become significant, strategies to avoid them in the future should be implemented and documented. In addition, nurse leaders and managers should monitor trends in variances to assist in addressing workload issues.

Productivity

As part of the ongoing evaluation of the budget, nurse leaders and managers must monitor productivity. **Productivity** is the ratio of output (e.g., products or services) to input (e.g., resources used). Output factors depend on the particular health-care agency and the type and frequency of services it provides (e.g., procedures, deliveries, clinic visits, admissions, home visits); output factors also include patient satisfaction and patient outcomes. Input factors include the skill level and experience of staff and can be affected by patient acuity, unit layout, and nursing management. To maintain or increase productivity, the nurse leader and manager must examine factors that affect both output and input, by keeping in mind that decreasing outputs or increasing inputs typically increases productivity.

Productivity related to staffing reflects the efficiency of a nursing staff in delivering nursing care and the effectiveness of the care delivered relative to its quality and appropriateness. To measure productivity related to staffing would use the ratio of required hours (output) to the provided staffing hours (input). The formula would be:

$$Productivity = required\ staff\ hours \div provided\ staff\ hours \times 100\%$$

Productivity should ideally be the perfect blend of efficiency and safe care. Even small variations up or down can affect these factors. Consider the following example: If the standard of care is 6 nursing hours per patient day (NHPPD) and the census of the unit is 32 patients, then 192 hours of care per day are needed to care for the patients. To reach 100% productivity, the nurse manager needs 192 hours of care provided by their staff:

$$192\ hours\ needed/192\ hours\ provided \times 100 = 100\%\ productivity$$

If the number of hours provided decreases for some reason, according to the equation, productivity actually rises:

$$192\ hours\ needed/175\ hours\ provided \times 100 = 110\%\ productivity$$

However, fewer hours of care provided will likely mean that the quality of care may not be adequate. If the hours provided are increased according to

$$192\ hours\ needed/200\ hours\ provided \times 100 = 96\%\ productivity,$$

then, although the quality of care may be greater with more hours of care provided, productivity is decreased and therefore is less efficient. The key is finding a balance between safe, quality patient care and cost containment. Nurse leaders and managers have a major challenge today balancing safe and quality care with meeting organizational productivity requirements. They must monitor staff productivity and evaluate staffing effectiveness on a regular basis. Productivity can be improved by decreasing provided staff hours and maintaining or increasing required staff hours.

Efficiency, or taking care not to waste resources such as supplies, equipment, and human capital, is obviously critical when considering productivity. Another important element is effectiveness, or providing care based on evidence and avoiding underuse and overuse of resources. Evaluating system inefficiencies and eliminating outdated processes can help increase effectiveness and efficiency (Porter-O'Grady & Malloch, 2013). When considering efficiency and effectiveness, nurse leaders and managers must take into account necessary care activities, value-added care activities, and non–value-added care activities (Upenieks et al., 2008).

Necessary Care Activities

Necessary care activities are those activities that are "essential in delivering patient care and do not directly benefit the patient" (Upenieks et al., p. 295). Calling primary care providers, transcribing orders, and documenting medication administration are examples of necessary care activities. When nurses are engaged in necessary care activities, they are not providing patient care, yet the activity is important to patient safety and quality care.

Value-Added Care Activities

Nursing activities that are performed by registered nurses (RNs), are patient centered, and directly benefit the patient are considered **value-added care activities** (Upenieks et al., 2008). Some examples of value-added activities, which are typically performed by RNs, include direct care activities such as the following: assessment; taking of vital signs; wound care; medication administration; communication with the patient, family, and care team; and care rounds. Indirect care activities that are also value added include chart review, handoffs, and care conferences (Upenieks et al., 2008).

Non–Value-Added Care Activities

Nursing activities that are performed by RNs and do not benefit the patient and are not necessary to delivering patient care are **non–value-added care activities** (Upenieks et al., 2008). Non–value-added activities include looking for equipment or people, waiting for telephone calls, and waiting for patient transport. Such activities constitute wasted time that could possibly be avoided if systems and processes worked more efficiently (Storfjell et al., 2009). Nurse leaders and managers often overlook decreasing or eliminating non–value-added work when making adjustments for variances. Non–value-added care activities can lead to increased costs and nurse dissatisfaction, both of which affect patient safety and quality of care (Storfjell et al., 2009).

EXPLORING THE EVIDENCE 16-1

Twigg, D. E., Geelhoed, E. A., Bremner, A. P., & Duffield, C. M. (2013). The economic benefits of increased levels of nursing care in the hospital setting. *Journal of Advanced Nursing, 69*(10), 2253–2261.

Aim

The aim of this study was to assess the economic impact of increased nursing hours of care on health outcomes in adult teaching hospitals.

Methods

This study had a longitudinal design with a retrospective analysis of a cohort of multiday-stay patients admitted to adult teaching hospitals in Perth, Australia. The investigators conducted a secondary analysis of data obtained in 2010 on hospital morbidity and staffing from September 2000 through June 2004 to analyze nursing-sensitive outcomes after implementing staffing using the nursing hours per patient day (NHPPD) staffing method.

Key Findings

NHPPD increased from 3,466,811.84 registered nurse (RN) hours to 3,876,798.96 RN hours after implementation. In all, 1,357 nursing-sensitive outcomes were prevented after implementation, including the following:

- 145 surgical wound infections
- 173 pulmonary failures
- 541 ulcers, cases of gastritis, episode of upper gastrointestinal bleeding
- 343 episodes of shock or cardiac arrest
- 155 cases of failure to rescue

Based on the nursing-sensitive outcomes prevented, the investigators estimated that the net cost savings as a result of implementing the NHPPD staffing method was $12,108,948 Australian dollars, and the cost per life gained was $4,324 Australian dollars.

Implications for Nurse Leaders and Managers

Implementing the NHPPD staffing method resulted in increasing RN staffing and decreasing adverse nursing-sensitive outcomes. The findings of this study discount the common belief that increasing staffing is not cost effective. Nurse leaders and managers can use this type of research to support increasing staffing as a cost-effective patient safety intervention. The investigators emphasized that these results fall within the cost-effectiveness thresholds of the United States, the United Kingdom, and Sweden.

▶ TYPES OF BUDGETS

The budget process is basically the same, no matter the budget, and in fact, different budgets are needed for different purposes, although they are generally prepared at the same time because decisions about one type of budget may affect another. Three major types of budgets make up a nursing budget: operating budget, personnel budget, and capital budget.

Operating Budget

The **operating budget** is the overall plan for a nursing department and accounts for expenses and revenues related to the day-to-day operation of the nursing unit for a fiscal year, which is a 12-month period that either typically coincides with the calendar year or runs from July 1 to June 30. The operating budget includes all unit expenses (e.g., costs related to providing care to patients) and revenues (e.g., income from providing such services).

Expenses

Expenses include the total cost of running the nursing unit. The two main categories of expenses are as follows: personnel salaries, which include normal wages, overtime, paid holidays, benefits, shift differentials, and other paid time; and nonsalary expenses, which include medical and surgical supplies, office supplies, equipment rental, and repair and maintenance of equipment.

Expenses are typically broken down into line items, which represent specific categories of costs such as office supplies, surgical supplies, and medications. Common expenses or costs included in the operating budget are either fixed or variable and can be direct or indirect:

- **Fixed expenses** do not change over the budget period, regardless of the volume of patients or activity level of the organization. Examples of fixed expenses include administrative salaries, rental or mortgage payments, insurance premiums, utilities, and taxes.
- **Variable expenses** fluctuate depending on patient volume and acuity or on activity level of the organization. Examples of variable expenses include patient care supplies, medications, linen, and food. If the number or acuity level of patients increases, more supplies, medications, linens, and food will be needed, resulting in higher variable expenses. The personnel budget is also an example of a variable expense because staffing can vary depending on the patient census and level of acuity.
- **Direct expenses** directly affect patient care and include the costs of providing patient care. Examples of direct expenses include personnel salaries, medical and surgical supplies, and medications.
- **Indirect expenses** are necessary for daily operations of the organization but do not affect patient care. Examples of indirect expenses include utilities, building maintenance, and salaries of ancillary staff members such as security guards or parking attendants.

Revenues

Revenue is income from services provided and varies depending on the type of unit and organization. Although nursing is not considered a revenue-producing industry, revenue is generated and is projected for a nursing unit from the average daily census (ADC) or number of procedures done. Nursing revenue in a hospital is included with the room charges. However, nursing revenue can be generated in other ways, such as by patient visits or procedures (Anderson & Danna, 2013). Other sources of revenue can include grants, donations, gifts, third-party payers, Medicaid, Medicare, and income from gift shops, parking fees, and vending machines.

Personnel Budget

The **personnel budget** allocates expenses related to nursing personnel. This budget is part of the operating budget and is typically the largest budget in the organization.

This budget is also very time-consuming to establish and manage. The personnel budget is directly related to the ability of nurse leaders and managers to supervise their staff and requires vigilant monitoring of fluctuating patient census and acuity to avoid overstaffing or understaffing. Nurse leaders and managers must consider the staffing needs and staffing plan for the unit when developing the fiscal budget. The personnel budget includes expenses for regular salaries, hourly differentials, overtime, and nonproductive time.

Nurse leaders and managers must consider some of the core staffing concepts such as full-time equivalent, productive time, and nonproductive time. A **full-time equivalent** (FTE) is a unit that measures the work of one full-time employee for 1 year (or 52 weeks) based on a 40-hour work week, equating a total of 2,080 paid hours per year. An FTE may comprise one person working full-time or several people sharing the full-time hours. For example, two nurses working 20 hours/week equate to one FTE. **Productive time** refers to the actual hours worked on the unit caring for patients. In contrast, **nonproductive time** refers to benefit time, such as vacation hours, holiday time, sick hours, education time, and jury duty. When determining staffing needs, the manager accounts for nurses who are using benefit time and who in turn need to be replaced by additional staff. To determine available productive time for each FTE, the manager must subtract nonproductive time from the total hours a full-time employee works.

To develop the personnel budget, nurse leaders and managers must first determine the FTEs needed to staff their unit to maintain safe, quality patient care for 24 hours per day, 7 days per week, 52 weeks per year (Finkler & McHugh, 2008). An FTE position equals 40 work hours per week for 52 weeks a year, or 2,080 hours per year.

Next, the nurse leader and manager must forecast staffing needs based on the ADC. The ADC provides a measure of the unit activity and is calculated by averaging the census at midnight each day over a period of time. In forecasting FTEs, the nurse leader and manager must also consider staffing for days off and calculate nonproductive time (i.e., paid time when staff members are not providing patient care) to determine an estimate of the number of FTEs needed to replace staff. Table 16-3 illustrates how to calculate FTE requirements for nonproductive time. The steps for calculating FTEs for a telemetry unit are illustrated in Box 16-1.

Table 16-3 Full-Time Equivalent Requirements for Nonproductive Time

Paid Nonproductive Time per Employee	Number of Days	Number of Hours
Annual leave	10	80
Holiday leave	6	48
Jury duty	1	8
Sick leave	10	80
Personal leave	1	8
Total	28	224

To calculate the number of additional full-time equivalents (FTEs) needed when staff members are on paid time off:

Number of nonproductive hours ÷ FTE hours

224 ÷ 2,080 = 0.1076

PART III

LEADERSHIP AND MANAGEMENT FUNCTIONS

BOX 16-1   Determining Full-Time Equivalents Needed on a Unit

Example: A 32-bed telemetry unit with an average daily census of 32 patients uses a nurse-to-patient ratio of 1:4. The unit is staffed with registered nurses working 8-hour shifts.

To calculate the number of full-time equivalents (FTEs) needed to staff this unit:

STEP 1: CALCULATE NURSING HOURS PER PATIENT DAY (NHPPD)

Per 1:4 ratio, 8 nurses are needed for each shift:

8 nurses × 3 shifts = 24 nurses needed for 24 hours

24 nurses × 8 hours = Nurses will work a total of 192 hours in 24 hours

192 hours/32 patients = 6 NHPPD

STEP 2: CALCULATE THE NUMBER OF FTES NEEDED TO COVER DAYS OFF

8 nurses per shift × 7 days per week/Number of shifts each FTE works

8 nurses per shift × 7 days/5 = 11.2 FTEs per shift are needed to cover days off

11.2 × 3 shifts per day = 33.6 FTEs per day to cover days off

24 + 33.6 = 57.6 FTEs needed to provide coverage 24 hours/day and 7 days/week

STEP 3: CALCULATE THE NUMBER OF FTES NEEDED FOR NONPRODUCTIVE TIME

Number of nurses times the factor to determine number of FTEs needed (from Table 16-3):

24 × 0.11 = 2.64 additional FTEs are needed to work when nurses are on paid time off

RESULT

57.6 + 2.64 = 60.24 FTEs are needed to budget for the telemetry unit

---

Once FTEs are determined, they must be converted to dollar values to make realistic cost-effective decisions in the budget process (Rohloff, 2006). When converting FTEs to costs, the hourly rate, shift differentials, projected overtime, and orientation time must be considered. Again, the nurse leader and manager refers to the previous year to forecast these additional labor costs.

Finally, workload must be used as the basis for quantifying the productive hours needed to deliver nursing care. **Workload** is the number of nursing staff members required to deliver care for a specific time period and is dependent on patient care needs. Workload is measured differently depending on the clinical setting (e.g., in the operating room, it is based on minutes per surgical case; and in home care, it is measured by the number of nursing visits per month). **Units of service** (UOS) reflect the basic measure of nursing workload based on different types of patient. Staffing needs vary by clinical setting. UOS assist nurse leaders and managers in determining unit-specific needs for staffing. Although tools to measure workload in outpatient and ambulatory care centers are limited, numerous tools are available to measure workload in the acute care setting (Dickson et al., 2010). How workload in acute care settings is measured varies depending on how the organization calculates workload measures and the type of unit and agency. For example, in a hospital medical-surgical unit, workload may be based on acuity by using a patient classification system (see Chapter 13).

Another example of workload is **nursing hours per patient day** (NHPPD), which represents the nursing care hours provided to patients by nursing personnel over a 24-hour period. NHPPD is usually based on unit census at midnight and reflects only nursing staff productive time. The formula to calculate NHPPD is illustrated in Box 16-2 through the calculation of NHPPD for an inpatient medical-surgical unit.

BOX 16-2 Calculation of Nursing Hours per Patient Day (NHPPD)	
(Nursing staff hours available)/(24-hour census) = NHPPD	In this unit, RNs work 8-hour shifts, and there are four RNs per three daily shifts.
Example:	12 RNs each working 8 hours = 96 hours worked in 24 hours
In a 30-bed medical unit, census at midnight is 28.	96 working hours/28 patients = 3.43 NHPPD

Using NHPPD based on the previous budget year to forecast staffing needs for the upcoming year is an appropriate and cost-effective approach (Porter-O'Grady & Malloch, 2013; Twigg et al., 2013).

LEARNING ACTIVITY 16-1 Calculating Full-Time Equivalents for Your Unit Using Nursing Hours per Patient Day

You are the manager of a 50-bed medical-surgical unit. Over the past year, the unit has had an average daily census of 48. You staff your unit using nursing hours per patient day (NHPPD). Complete the following tasks:

1. Calculate the NHPPD.
2. Based on the NHPPD, calculate the full-time equivalents needed to staff the unit:
   - Daily
   - Weekly
   - Monthly

Capital Budget

The **capital budget** includes equipment, furniture, technology (hardware and software), and building renovations, and it is separate from the operating and personnel budget processes. The minimum value of a capital item can vary depending on the organization, and any item costing less than the minimum is considered a routine expense. Typically, items that are included in the capital budget have a minimum value of $1,000 and have an expected performance life of more than 1 year. To compile a capital budget, nurse leaders and managers should seek input from staff to identify items that meet the cost limit and have a multiyear life. In addition, nurse leaders and managers must develop an understanding of the financial implications of leasing versus purchasing equipment, the expected life of equipment, and estimated costs of maintenance (Contino, 2004). Other considerations include projected patient needs, how the budget will affect revenues and expenses, and funds available. Once the decision is made regarding the needed capital items or assets, the request goes through a separate review and approval process at the organizational level (Finkler & McHugh, 2008).

LEARNING ACTIVITY 16-2

Comparing Budgets

Describe the differences among an operating budget, a personnel budget, and a capital budget. What comprises each type of budget?

▶ BUDGETING METHODS

Different health-care organizations may use different budgeting methods. The type of method is determined by the administration and aligns with the organization's mission and goals. The three common types of budgeting methods are incremental budgeting, performance budgeting, and zero-based budgeting.

Incremental Budgeting

Also called the flat-percentage method, **incremental budgeting** involves multiplying the current year's budget by a predetermined figure based on the cost of living, consumer price index, or inflation rate and then using that number to project for the next fiscal year. The major advantages of incremental budgeting are that it is very simple and it requires little expertise (Jones et al., 2019). However, this method is inefficient and does not encourage prioritization of needs for the future, nor does it facilitate motivation to contain costs. Incremental budgeting is commonly used in determining household or personal budgets because those budgets are usually based on annual income and are adjusted according to increases in annual income.

Performance Budgeting

Performance budgeting emphasizes outcomes and results rather than activities and outputs. Typical budgeting processes do not reflect goals related to cost-effectiveness, patient safety, and quality of nursing care. Performance budgeting, also called outcome budgeting, can help determine the amount of money needed to provide value-added nursing care, non–value-added nursing care, and quality nursing care, as well as to ensure patient and staff satisfaction and to control costs. Performance budgeting measures multiple outcomes of the nursing unit. Rather than focusing on the resources used, it provides a picture of where resources are used and their relationship with the goals of the nursing unit as well as the organization (Finkler & McHugh, 2008).

Although performance budgeting can be time consuming, by using this method of budgeting, nurse leaders and managers can easily demonstrate quality of nursing care and its relation to budget cuts. Performance budgeting evolves from the operating budget and links outcomes to the consumption of financial resources.

Zero-Based Budgeting

In **zero-based budgeting**, nurse leaders and managers start the budget from zero each year as if each item or program was brand new. Zero-based budgeting requires nurse leaders and managers to prioritize and justify or rejustify requested funds meticulously on an annual basis. Supporting rationale must be provided for each planned revenue and expense. The goal is to have zero funds left at the end of the fiscal year. Therefore, rather than basing the budget on the past year, nurse leaders and managers are required to provide a rationale for all expenditures (Finkler et al., 2014). The advantage of zero-based budgeting is that it forces managers to set priorities—all functions must stand on their own merits (Jones et al., 2019). Zero-based budgeting also encourages communication and coordination between managers and their staff. A major disadvantage of zero-based budgeting is that it is labor intensive. In addition, zero-based budgeting requires nurse leaders and managers to have special training in the budget process.

LEARNING ACTIVITY 16-3	**Analyzing Budget Variances**

You are the manager of a medical-surgical unit. The following is your monthly medical-surgical supply budget report.

Month	Budgeted Expenses ($)	Actual Expenses ($)	Variance in $	Variance in %
January	82,500	91,421	(8,921)	(10.81)
February	82,500	90,382	(7,882)	(9.55)
March	78,950	77,014	1,936	2.45
April	78,950	76,002	2,948	3.73

Answer the following:

1. Which month(s) is the variance over budget?
2. Which month(s) is the variance under budget?
3. What could some of the causes be for being over or under budget?

▶ SUMMARY

The budget process is ongoing and cyclical, much like the nursing process. When planning a budget, nurse leaders and managers are required to think ahead, anticipate changes, establish goals, and coordinate realistic plans. An important element to the budgeting process is forecasting. Nurse leaders and managers must have a clear understanding of the following to manage their unit budgets effectively: the budgeted ADC for the unit, the process the organization uses to measure unit productivity, the organization's policies, and the state regulations (Waxman, 2005).

Involving staff nurses in the budget process helps them understand the relationship between health-care costs and delivery of safe, quality patient care. Additionally, nurse leaders and managers who maintain transparency in the budget process and encourage staff participation in managing cost-effective work practices foster positive nurse outcomes. Nurse leaders and managers as well as staff must engage in the process by identifying patient outcomes and eliminate interventions that do not add value to those outcomes. The budget process is ongoing and requires all nurses to strive for cost containment without jeopardizing safe, quality patient care.

NCLEX®-STYLE REVIEW QUESTIONS

Multiple Choice

1. What would be considered to be a key component of the budgeting process for a nursing unit?
   1. To provide cost-effective care
   2. Efficiency independent of quality
   3. Keeping costs contained independent of quality
   4. Maintaining cost and quality at minimum levels
2. Which aspects of the budget are *not* within a nurse manager's control?
   1. Staffing assignment
   2. Staffing pattern
   3. Patient acuity
   4. Cost of supplies
3. When calculating *break-even quantity*, which information is needed?
   1. Total cost divided by units of service
   2. Fixed costs divided by variable costs per patient
   3. Measure of the input provided by the output
   4. Deviation from the projected budget
4. Which situation would take *priority* when reviewing the nursing unit budget for the past year?
   1. No increase in productivity rate
   2. Increasing patient/patient satisfaction
   3. Increase in reported staffing variance
   4. Change in several of the manufacturers related to products and supplies
5. The nurse manager is observing an experienced nurse who is new to the unit perform a dressing change. The experienced nurse is using sterile gauze, but the orders for the dressing change indicate that it is a clean dressing change. The time to complete the procedure was under 5 minutes. The patient tolerated the procedure without complaints. How would the nurse manager interpret this situation?
   1. The experienced nurse is demonstrating decreased productivity.
   2. The patient was satisfied with the demonstrated task.
   3. The experienced nurse is not demonstrating efficiency.
   4. The experienced nurse can teach other nurses how to do the dressing.

6. A nurse is looking on the unit for an infusion pump to use for the patient. How would the nurse manager classify this nurse activity?
   1. Value care
   2. Necessary care
   3. Non–value-added care
   4. Indirect care

7. Which is an example of a fixed expense in a budget for a nursing unit?
   1. Medications
   2. Supplies
   3. Administrative salaries
   4. Salaries for nursing staff

8. The nursing unit is asking for a new Hoyer lift to be used to assist staff in the transfer of patients in the clinical setting. Which type of budget request would be needed to obtain this piece of equipment?
   1. Personnel budget
   2. Capital budget
   3. Personal budget
   4. Would be considered as a variable request

9. Which budgeting method uses projections based on the current year's budget multiplied by a predetermined amount to arrive at a new budget proposal?
   1. Zero-based
   2. Performance
   3. Operational
   4. Flat percentage

10. What type of nursing activity is noted when a registered nurse (RN) administers medication to a patient who is experiencing nausea?
    1. Value-added nondirect care
    2. Necessary care
    3. Value-added direct care
    4. Non–value-added care

11. Even though nursing is not considered to be revenue generating in terms of health care, how is revenue projected on a nursing unit?
    1. Viewed as being separate from the room charge
    2. Determined by patient satisfaction
    3. Based on average daily census or number of procedures done
    4. Related to the number of nurses in the facility

Multiple Response

12. A nurse manager has to submit requests for the capital budget for the medical-surgical unit. Which considerations should the nurse manager include when planning the capital budget? *Select all that apply.*
    1. Recommendations from unit staff
    2. Items that cost less than $500
    3. Items that you anticipate with a performance life of 1 year
    4. Financial implications relative to buying versus leasing
    5. Projected maintenance costs for the item

13. Which activities would be included in the assessment phase of budget planning? *Select all that apply.*
    1. Estimating cost of supplies
    2. Determining workload
    3. Gathering relevant data
    4. Comparing actual versus projected results
    5. Starting once the budget has been implemented
14. Which statements reflect accurate information related to the concept of productivity? *Select all that apply.*
    1. It is not affected by output or input.
    2. It should be a blend of efficiency and safety.
    3. It is determined only by input.
    4. It has to be monitored to be determined.
    5. Input refers to resources used.

REFERENCES

American Association of Colleges of Nursing. (2021). *The essentials: Core competencies for professional nursing education.* Author. https://www.aacnnursing.org/Portals/42/AcademicNursing/pdf/Essentials-2021.pdf

American Nurses Association (ANA). (2010). *Nursing's social policy statement: The essence of the profession.* Author.

American Nurses Association (ANA). (2015). *Code of ethics for nurses with interpretive statements.* Author.

American Nurses Association (ANA). (2016). *Nursing administration: Scope and standards of practice* (2nd ed.). Author.

American Organization for Nursing Leadership (AONL). (2015a). *AONL nurse manager competencies.* Author.

American Organization for Nursing Leadership (AONL). (2015b). *AONL nurse executive competencies.* Author.

Anderson, B., & Danna, D. (2013). Budgeting principles for nurse managers. In L. Roussel, *Management and leadership for nurse administrators* (6th ed., pp. 435–478). Jones & Bartlett Learning.

Contino, D. S. (2004). Leadership competencies: Knowledge, skills, and aptitudes nurses need to lead organizations effectively. *Critical Care Nurse, 24*(3), 52–64.

Cronenwett, L., Sherwood, G., Barnsteiner, J., Disch, J., Johnson, J., Mitchell, P., Sullivan, D. T., & Warren, J. (2007). Quality and safety education for nurses. *Nursing Outlook, 55*(3), 122–131.

Dickson, K. L., Cramer, A. M., & Peckham, C. M. (2010). Nursing workload measurement in ambulatory care. *Nursing Economics, 28*(1), 37–43.

Finkler, S. A., Jones, C. B., & Kovner, C. T. (2014). *Financial management for nurse managers and executives* (4th ed.). Elsevier.

Finkler, S. A., & McHugh, M. L. (2008). *Budgeting concepts for nurse managers* (4th ed.). Saunders.

Greiner, A. C., & Knebel, E. (Eds.). (2003). *Health professions education: A bridge to quality.* National Academies Press.

Jones, C. B., Finkler, S. A., Kovner, C. T., & Mose, J. N. (2019). *Financial management for nurse managers and executives* (5th ed.). Elsevier.

Porter-O'Grady, T., & Malloch, K. (2013). *Leadership in nursing practice: Changing the landscape of health care.* Jones & Bartlett Learning.

Rohloff, R. M. (2006). Full-time equivalents: What needs to be assessed to meet patient care and create realistic budgets. *Nurse Leader, 4*(1), 49–54.

Seifert, P. C. (2012). The business of nurses *is* business. *AORN Journal, 95*(2), 181–183.

Storfjell, J. L., Ohlson, S., & Omoike, O., Fitzpatrick, T., & Wetasin, K. (2009). Non–value-added time: The million dollar nursing opportunity. *Journal of Nursing Administration, 39*(1), 38–45.

Swansburg, R. C. (1997). *Budgeting and financial management for nurse managers.* Jones & Bartlett Publishers.

Swearingen, S. (2009). A journey to leadership: Designing a nursing leadership development program. *Journal of Continuing Education in Nursing, 40*(3), 107–112.

Thomas, P. L., & Roussel, L. (2020). Procuring and sustaining resources: The budgeting process. In Roussel, L., Thomas, P. L., & Harris, J. L., *Management and leadership for nurse administrators* (8th ed., pp. 155–188). Jones & Bartlett Learning.

Twigg, D. E., Geelhoed, E. A., Bremner, A. P., & Duffield, C. M. (2013). The economic benefits of increased levels of nursing care in the hospital setting. *Journal of Advanced Nursing, 69*(10), 2253–2261.

Upenieks, V. V., Akhavan, J., & Kotlerman, J. (2008). Value-added care: A paradigm shift in patient care delivery. *Nursing Economics, 26*(5), 294–301.

Waxman, K. T. (2005, February). Creating a culture of financially savvy nurse leaders. *Nurse Leader,* 31–35.

To explore learning resources for this chapter, go to FADavis.com

Part IV

Managing Your Future
in Nursing

Chapter 17
Transitioning From Student to Professional Nurse and Beyond

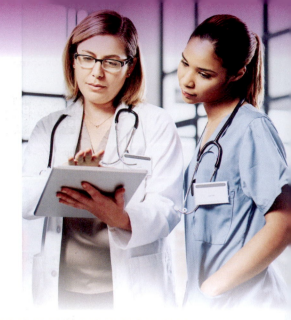

Chapter 17

Transitioning From Student to Professional Nurse and Beyond

Elizabeth J. Murray, PhD, RN, CNE

KEY TERMS

Competence
Healthy nurse
Lifelong learner
Mentor
Plausible future
Possible future
Preceptor
Preferable future
Probable future
Professional socialization
Reflective learning
Résumé
Self-care
Specialty certification

LEARNING OUTCOMES

- Describe the process of professional socialization.
- Develop a career plan for the future.
- Identify strategies for professional growth.
- Discuss what it means to be a lifelong learner.
- Identify several self-care techniques to use when beginning a career in nursing.

The Knowledge, Skills, and Attitudes Related to the Following Are Addressed in This Chapter:

Core Competencies	• Patient-Centered Care • Teamwork and Collaboration • Evidence-Based Practice
The Essentials: Core Competencies for Professional Nursing Education (AACN, 2021)	**Domain 10: Personal, Professional, and Leadership Development** 10.1 Demonstrate a commitment to personal health and well-being (p. 56). 10.2 Demonstrate a spirit of inquiry that fosters flexibility and professional maturity (pp. 56–57). 10.3 Develop capacity for leadership (pp. 57–58).
Code of Ethics with Interpretive Statements (ANA, 2015a)	**Provision 4.3:** Responsibility for nursing judgments, decisions, and actions (pp. 16–17) **Provision 5.1:** Duties to self and others (p. 19) **Provision 5.2:** Promotion of personal health, safety, and well-being (p. 19) **Provision 5.5:** Maintenance of competence and continuation of professional growth (p. 22) **Provision 5.6:** Continuation of personal growth (p. 22)

Nurse Manager (NMC) Competencies (AONL, 2015a) and Nurse Executive (NEC) Competencies (AONL, 2015b)	**NMC: Human Resource Leadership Skills (p. 6)**
	• Staff development
	  • Facilitate staff education and needs assessment
	  • Ensure competency validation
	  • Promote professional development
	NMC: Relationship Management and Influencing Behaviors (p. 6)
	• Promote professional development
	  • Apply principles of self-awareness
	  • Encourage evidence-based practice
	NEC: Professionalism (p. 9)
	• Personal and professional accountability
	  • Promote leader and staff participation in lifelong learning and educational achievement
	  • Promote professional certification for staff
	• Career planning
	  • Coach others in developing their own career plans

Continued

The Knowledge, Skills, and Attitudes Related to the Following Are Addressed in This Chapter:—cont'd

NEC: Business Skills (p. 10)
- Human resource management
  - Ensure development of educational programs to foster workforce competencies and development goals

Nursing Administration Scope and Standards of Practice (ANA, 2016)	**Standard 2: Identification of Problems, Issues, and Trends** The nurse administrator analyses the assessment data to identify problems, issues, and trends (p. 37). **Standard 7: Ethics** The nurse administrator practices ethically (pp. 45–46). **Standard 11: Leadership** The nurse administrator leads within professional practice setting, profession, healthcare industry, and society (pp. 51–52). **Standard 12: Education** The nurse administrator attains knowledge and competence that reflect current nursing practice and promotes futuristic thinking (p. 53). **Standard 15: Professional Practice Evaluation** The nurse administrator evaluates one's own and others' nursing practice (p. 56).

Source: American Association of Colleges of Nursing. (2021). *The essentials: Core competencies for professional nursing education.* Author; American Nurses Association (ANA). (2015a). *Code of ethics for nurses with interpretive statements.* Author; American Nurses Association (ANA). (2016). *Nursing administration: Scope and standards of practice* (2nd ed.). Author; American Organization for Nursing Leadership (AONL). (2015a). *AONL nurse manager competencies.* Author; American Organization for Nursing Leadership (AONL). (2015b). *AONL nurse executive competencies.* Author; Cronenwett, L., Sherwood, G., Barnsteiner, J., Disch, J., Johnson, J., Mitchell, P., Sullivan, D. T., & Warren, J. (2007). Quality and safety education for nurses. *Nursing Outlook, 55*(3), 122–131; and Greiner, A. C., & Knebel, E. (Eds.). (2003). *Health professions education: A bridge to quality.* National Academies Press.

Today—and in the years to come—nurses have unique opportunities to influence health care in the United States and globally. The Institute of Medicine (2011) report *The Future of Nursing: Leading Change, Advancing Health* suggested that the envisioned future of health care is one that makes quality care accessible to the diverse populations of the United States, intentionally promotes wellness and disease prevention, reliably improves health outcomes, and provides compassionate care across the life span (p. 2). To meet this envisioned future will require raising educational levels and competencies of nurses and fostering intraprofessional and interprofessional collaboration to improve patient safety and quality of care. The Quality and Safety Education for Nurses (QSEN) initiative continues to gain momentum and has been integrated into nursing textbooks, accreditation and certification standards, and licensure examinations. Entry-level nurses are educated using a core set of nursing competencies to promote patient safety and quality care. However, retention of new nurse graduates is a major issue for the profession that has grave consequences for nurse safety, patient safety, and quality of nursing care.

This chapter outlines how nurses can develop a career plan for the future. Strategies for professional growth are also covered, as is what it means to be a lifelong learner. Finally, self-care techniques to use when beginning a career in nursing are discussed.

▶ PROFESSIONAL SOCIALIZATION

Nursing is a learned profession based on science and art (American Nurses Association [ANA], 2010). The science of nursing is based on a core body of knowledge "that requires judgment and skill based on principles of the biological, physical, behavioral, and social sciences" (ANA, 2015b, p. 6) and "the art of nursing is based on caring and respect for human dignity" (ANA, 2015b, p. 11) and embraces the values, culture, and standards of the profession. Nursing students learn to think and act like a nurse in nursing school through classroom and clinical experiences with the goal of developing professionalism (Mariet, 2016). **Professional socialization** in nursing encompasses the process by which students learn the science and art of nursing; internalize the values, attitudes, culture, and goals of the profession; and develop a sense of professional identity (Dinmohammadi et al., 2013; Mariet, 2016; Masters & Gilmore, 2020).

Professional socialization is a personal, interactive, and ongoing process that begins when a student enters nursing school and continues through their career. There are many models of professional socialization and all have similar elements. Regardless of the model, professional socialization involves the process of acquiring the knowledge and skills of the profession and internalizing the attitudes, values, culture, and standards of the profession into one's own behavior.

In nursing school, students focus on learning specific knowledge and skills that are reinforced through traditional teaching strategies used by faculty. Teaching students content knowledge, "what they need to know," step-by-step tasks, time management skills, and classroom and clinical rules results in what is known as external socialization or formal socialization to the profession (Day & Sherwood, 2017; Mariet, 2016). External socialization may allow students to be successful academically, but it does not necessarily make a graduate from nursing school a good nurse. In contrast, informal socialization includes learning that occurs incidentally as students are exposed to situations and experiences that help them value professional behavior. These experiences help students internalize attitudes, beliefs, values, and standards of the profession (Mariet, 2016; Masters & Gilmore, 2020). Informal socialization experiences may be more powerful and memorable because it is through interactions with professional nurses that professional identity and internalization of professional values and culture occurs (Dinmohammadi et al., 2013; Mariet, 2016).

Benner et al. (2010) refer to the informal socialization process as formation. During formation, there is a shift from learning the knowledge and skills to actually applying them in service to patients, families, and communities rather than to achieve a grade on an examination or in a course (Benner et al., 2010; Day & Sherwood, 2017). In other words, the student is transformed from just *"acting* like a nurse to *being* a nurse" (Benner et al., 2010, p. 177).

Professional socialization is important in nursing because it includes acquiring the knowledge, skills, and attitudes of the profession, developing the sense of professional identity, developing the ability to cope with professional roles, and a commitment to the profession and lifelong learning. These are the necessary values and characteristics to promote safe, effective, and quality patient-centered care. Professional socialization continues beyond nursing school. As new nurses begin planning for their future career, they must keep in mind their obligation to "continue to learn about new concepts, concerns, controversies, and healthcare ethics relevant to the current and evolving scope and standards of nursing practice" (ANA, 2015a, p. 22).

▶ CAREER PLANNING AND DEVELOPMENT

The current job market is promising for new nurse graduates. According to the ANA (2014a), the percentage of job offers at the time of graduation for nurses with a baccalaureate degree in nursing (BSN) is 59% compared with other college graduates (29.3%). A total of 1.13 million new registered nurses (RNs) will be needed by 2022 to fill new jobs and to replace retiring nurses (ANA, 2014a).

Finding the right position at an organization where education is valued and advanced education is supported and promoted is essential to long-term success and job satisfaction as a nurse. The American Association of Colleges of Nursing (AACN, n.d.a) identified hallmarks or characteristics of the practice setting that best support professional nursing practice (Box 17-1). When present, these hallmarks allow baccalaureate and higher-degree nurses to practice to their full potential. These eight hallmarks are included in the AACN (n.d.b) brochure *What Every Nursing Student Should Know When Seeking Employment* to assist nursing students and new nurse graduates in making the best decision on where to seek employment following graduation.

Preparing a Strategic Career Plan

Besides considering where they want to work for their first nursing position, new nurse graduates should be preparing a strategic career plan before graduating from nursing school. A strategic career plan is the roadmap to a nurse's success. The initial step in strategic career planning in nursing is developing specific, measurable, achievable, realistic, and timely, or SMART, goals. Using the SMART technique to outline a plan for the future can be valuable to new nurse graduates as they begin career planning and development. Once goals are established, nurses should identify specific action steps necessary to meet each goal and set a timeline for completing each step. Before implementing the action steps, nurses

BOX 17-1 Hallmarks of the Professional Nursing Practice Environment

These hallmarks are present in health-care systems, hospitals, organizations, or practice environments that:

1. Manifest a philosophy of clinical care emphasizing quality, safety, interdisciplinary collaboration, continuity of care, and professional accountability. For example:
   - The organization has a philosophy and mission statement that reflect these criteria.
   - Nursing staff members have meaningful input into policy development and operational management of issues related to clinical quality, safety, and clinical outcomes evaluation.
   - Nurse staffing patterns have an adequate number of qualified nurses to meet patients' needs, including consideration of the complexity of patient care.
   - Nursing is represented on the organization's staff committees that govern policy and operations.
   - The organization has a formal program of performance improvement that includes a focus on nursing practice, safety, continuity of care, and outcomes.
   - Nursing staff members assume responsibility and accountability for their own nursing practice.
2. Recognize contributions of nurses' knowledge and expertise to clinical care quality and patient outcomes. For example:
   - The organization differentiates the practice roles of nurses based on educational preparation, certification, and advanced preparation.
   - The organization has a compensation and reward system that recognizes role distinctions among staff nurses and other expert nurses (e.g., based on clinical expertise, reflective of nursing practice, education, or advanced credentialing).
   - The organization's performance improvement program has criteria to evaluate whether nursing care practices are based on the most current research evidence.
   - Professional and educational credentials of members of all disciplines, including nurses, are recognized by title on name tags and reports.
   - Nurses and members of other disciplines participate in media events, public relations announcements, marketing of clinical services, and strategic planning.
   - Nurses are encouraged to be mentors to less experienced colleagues and to share their enthusiasm about professional nursing within the organization and the community.
   - Advanced nursing roles, including clinical nurse specialists, nurse practitioners, scientists, educators, and other advanced practice roles, are used in the organization to support and enhance nursing care.
3. Promote executive level nursing leadership. For example:
   - The nurse executive participates in the governing body.
   - The nurse executive reports to the highest-level operations or corporate officer.
   - The nurse executive has the authority and accountability for all nursing or patient care delivery, financial resources, and personnel.
   - The nurse executive is supported by adequate managerial and support staff.
4. Empower nurses' participation in clinical decision making and organization of clinical care systems. For example:
   - A decentralized, unit-based program or team organizational structure exists for decision making.
   - Organization or system-wide committee and communication structures include nurses.
   - Nurses have a demonstrated leadership role in performance improvement of clinical care and the organization of clinical care systems.
   - A utilization review system is in place for nursing analysis and correction of clinical care errors and patient safety concerns.
   - Staff nurses have the authority to develop and execute nursing care orders and actions and to control their practice.
5. Maintain clinical advancement programs based on education, certification, and advanced preparation. For example:
   - Financial rewards are available for clinical advancement and education.
   - Opportunities are available for promotion and longevity related to education, clinical expertise, and professional contributions.
   - Peer review and patient, collegial, and managerial input are available for performance evaluation on an annual or routine basis.

Continued

BOX 17-1 Hallmarks of the Professional Nursing Practice Environment—cont'd

- Individuals in nursing leadership and management positions have appropriate education and credentials aligned with their role and responsibilities.
6. Demonstrate professional development support for nurses. For example:
  - Professional continuing education opportunities are available and supported.
  - Resource support exists for advanced education in nursing, including registered nurse (RN)–to–bachelor of science in nursing (BSN) completion programs and graduate degree programs.
  - Preceptorships, organized orientation programs, retooling or refresher programs, residency programs, internships, or other educational programs are available and encouraged.
  - Incentive programs exist for RN education for interested licensed practical nurses and nonnurse health-care personnel.
  - Long-term career support program targeted to specific populations of nurses, such as older individuals, home care or operating room nurses, or nurses from diverse ethnic backgrounds.
  - Specialty certification and advanced credentials are encouraged, promoted, and recognized.
  - Advanced practice nurses (APNs), nurse researchers, and nurse educators are employed and used in leadership roles to support clinical nursing practice.

- Linkages are developed between health-care institutions and baccalaureate or graduate schools of nursing to provide support for continuing education, collaborative research, and clinical educational affiliations.
7. Create collaborative relationships among members of the health-care provider team. For example:
  - Professional nurses, physicians, and other health-care professionals practice collaboratively and participate in standing organizational committees, bioethics committees, the governing structure, and the institutional review processes.
  - Professional nurses have appropriate oversight and supervisory authority of unlicensed members of the nursing care team.
  - An interdisciplinary team peer review process is used, especially in the review of patient care errors.
8. Use technological advances in clinical care and information systems. For example:
  - Documentation is supported through appropriate application of technology to the patient care process.
  - Appropriate equipment, supplies, and technology are available to optimize the efficient delivery of quality nursing care.
  - Resource requirements are quantified and monitored to ensure appropriate resource allocation.

Modified from American Association of Colleges of Nursing (n.d.a).

---

need to take inventory of available resources and consider who and what will help implement each step. The last step is identifying the indicators of success. This step requires nurses to determine the indicators that will help evaluate whether or not the goals were met (Donner & Wheeler, 2001). Career plans are dynamic and should be reviewed and revised as personal and professional circumstances change. Career planning is important for nurses at all levels because it can be useful to evaluate a nurse's present work situation and shape their future in the nursing profession.

Developing a Résumé

A **résumé** is a record of a nurse's education, employment history, accomplishments, and achievements. A well-designed and well-thought-out résumé can help a new nurse graduate gain an advantage over others. As a new graduate, a nurse should develop a résumé that includes any work experience in health care, volunteer experiences, and special accomplishments during education such as awards and honors received, scholarly assignments, memberships in student organizations, and any leadership positions held. Keep in mind that every activity does not belong on the résumé. In fact, most nurse leaders and managers spend approximately 30 seconds reviewing the typical résumé (Hood, 2014). Therefore, a résumé must present a concise picture of the nurse's strengths, accomplishments, and experiences. Headings guide the nurse leader and manager in finding specific information. The résumé should be written and revised to showcase specific experiences and accomplishments that match the position for which a nurse is applying. For an example of a résumé for a new nurse graduate, see Figure 17-1.

In addition to an effective résumé, the new nurse graduate needs to develop a cover letter. A cover letter should always accompany the résumé. The cover letter is how the nurse introduces themselves to the prospective employer. An effective cover letter is addressed to a specific person and includes the following:

- The reason the nurse is applying for a specific position
- A brief statement of the nurse's qualifications for the position, including strengths and experiences related to the position
- A statement expressing appreciation to the prospective employer for consideration

For an example of a cover letter for a new nurse graduate see Figure 17-2.

LEARNING ACTIVITY 17-1   **Visit the American Nurses Association Career Center**

Available at https://www.nursingworld.org/resources/individual/welcome-to-the-profession/

- Register for the Welcome to the Profession Kit.
- Access the toolkit.
- Review the Web site.

Interviewing

The interview process can be stressful for all nurses. To lessen anxiety, nurses should prepare for the interview by learning about the organization ahead of time. Seeking out the following information can be very helpful in preparing for the interview and lessening anxiety:

- The organization's mission, vision, and philosophy (see Chapter 9 for more information)
- Accreditation status and Magnet status
- Length of orientation or residency program
- Nurse-to-patient ratio and professional practice model
- Whether the nursing service uses a shared governance model

NAME
Street address
City, State Zip code
Telephone number
Email address

GOAL
To obtain a position as a professional registered nurse in the emergency department.

EDUCATION
20XX-present: Name of College/University, City, State
Anticipated date of graduation
Degree: Bachelor of Science in Nursing
List other colleges and universities attended in chronological order and include years attended and major.

WORK EXPERIENCE
Patient Care Technician
20XX-present: Medical-surgical unit, St. John's Hospital, City, State
• List duties

Candy Striper
20XX-present: St. John's Hospital, City, State
• List duties

PROFESSIONAL ORGANIZATIONS
20XX-present: Student Nurse's Association, Name of College/University, City, State
20XX-present: National Student Nurse's Association Certifications

CERTIFICATIONS
20XX-present: Basic Life Support Provider through the American Heart Association

AWARDS
List any awards, scholarships, recognition received, Dean's list.

REFERENCES AVAILABLE ON REQUEST

Figure 17-1 Example résumé for new nurse graduate.

Address
City, State Zip code
Phone
Email address

Date

Ms. Angela Smith, BSN, RN
Director, Emergency Department
St. John's Hospital
Address
City, State Zip code

Dear Ms. Smith:

I am requesting an opportunity to discuss my career goals with you. I will be graduating on May 1, 20XX, with my baccalaureate degree in nursing from the (name of school). I am scheduled to take the NCLEX-RN examination on June 26, 20XX.

I look forward to hearing from you soon to set up an interview appointment. If you have any questions, please feel free to contact me.

Sincerely,

Signature

Name

Figure 17-2 Example cover letter for new nurse graduate.

If unable to determine this information beforehand, the nurse should plan to ask about it during the interview. Preparing a few questions to ask during the interview process is appropriate and shows forethought. In fact, asking thoughtful questions specific to the organization, unit, and position shows the prospective employer that the nurse has put forth effort to learn about the organization and is sincerely interested in the position. Additionally, the nurse should plan to arrive to the interview a few minutes early. It is a good idea to ask for clear directions to the facility, specific building, and office where the interview will take place. If the interview is in an area the nurse is not familiar with, visiting the site a few days before, identifying the building, and checking out the parking can be helpful. Professional dress is a must, as is comfort. This is not the time to be tugging on a jacket that does not fit properly or limping because of blisters from new shoes.

Remember, the interview is a two-way process. The employer is determining whether the applicant is qualified to meet the needs of the unit, and the applicant is deciding whether the position meets their personal and professional needs. To prepare for possible questions that may be asked by the prospective employer during the interview, see Chapter 11.

▶ TRANSITION TO PRACTICE

Transitioning from a student to a newly licensed RN is very exciting as well as challenging, and it can cause feelings of uncertainty and stress. The basic education of new nurse graduates cannot ensure that they will be confident and competent as they transition into a professional role. Factors such as the increasing complexity of health care, the nursing shortage, high-acuity patients, and the looming retirement of many experienced nurses support the critical need for the successful transition of new nurse graduates from the academic setting to the clinical practice setting. One of the recommendations of the IOM (2011) is to implement "nurse residency programs to provide nurses with an appropriate transition to practice and develop a more competent nursing workforce" (p. 148).

According to the National Council of State Boards of Nursing (NCSBN, 2021), new nurses care for patients in a complex health-care environment and experience high levels of stress that cause 25% of these nurses to leave a position within the first year of nursing practice. These factors negatively influence safe and quality care and result in poor health-care outcomes. In an integrative review, Rush et al. (2013) found that transition to practice (TTP) programs that integrate formal and informal education, preceptorships, mentorships, and unit-specific orientations are significantly effective in retraining new nurse graduates. The NCSBN developed an evidence-based TTP model to ensure successful transition from the academic setting to the practice setting. The model integrates education, practice, and regulations for successful transition from the classroom to the clinical practice setting and beyond (NCSBN, 2021).

Recent research suggests that residency programs can reduce turnover rates in the first year of practice and promote growth in clinical decision making and leadership skills (Al-Dossery et al., 2013). Spector et al. (2015) conducted a study to examine the impact of the NCSBN TTP program on quality and safety and new nurse graduate stress, competence, job satisfaction, and retention. These investigators found a substantial improvement in quality and safety outcomes as well as in self-reported stress, competence, and job satisfaction. Based on comprehensive research, the NCSBN developed the TPP® Program that consists of one course for preceptors and five courses for new nurses. The program is designed to help nurses become competent professionals. More information about the TPP® Program is available at https://www.ncsbn.org/transition-to-practice.htm.

Nurse leaders and managers are vital to the success of TTP programs. They provide support for knowledge acquisition and build new nurse graduates' confidence in skills (D'Addona et al., 2015). In addition, nurse leaders and managers are critical in the socialization of new nurse graduates by providing a safe environment where new nurses can share concerns and receive support.

▶ PRECEPTORS AND MENTORS

An effective orientation program can be critical to retaining new nurses. The most common form of orientation program for new nurse graduates involves the use of preceptors. Typically, a **preceptor** is a staff nurse who is recognized for their clinical competence, leadership abilities, organizational skills, and desire to orient new nurse graduates. The role of the preceptor is to ensure that the new nurse graduate expands their basic nursing education and further develops the knowledge, skills, and attitudes necessary to function competently in the nursing position. The preceptor serves as a role model as well as provides the new nurse graduate an orientation to the unit, socialization within the unit culture, assistance with skill mastery, and a resource regarding policies and procedures.

The new nurse graduate typically demonstrates marginally acceptable performance as an advanced beginner, according to Benner's (1984) Novice-to-Expert model. The competent nurse, the third stage of Benner's model, is an appropriate preceptor for the novice or advanced beginner (NCSBN, 2021) because they experience a sense of mastery in the clinical setting and can discern relevant from irrelevant assessment data (Benner, 1984).

Different from a preceptor, a **mentor** is an experienced individual, who may or may not be a nurse, who is willing to maintain a long-term relationship, empowering, nurturing, advising, and guiding the new nurse graduate throughout their professional career. The mentoring relationship can benefit nurses at all levels, not just new nurse graduates. When selecting a mentor, nurses should consider someone who is easy to communicate with and willing to commit time to the mentoring relationship. "All nurses have a responsibility to mentor those who come after them, whether by helping a new nurse become oriented or by taking on more formal responsibilities as a teacher of nursing students or a preceptor" (IOM, 2011, p. 244). An effective mentor inspires and challenges the new nurse to a high level of professionalism. The mentoring relationship can be mutually beneficial and result in growth for both the new nurse and the mentor (Grossman & Valiga, 2013).

▶ STRATEGIES FOR PROFESSIONAL GROWTH

Nurses today cannot stop learning just because they have earned their degree, attained licensure, and become working nurses (Johnson, 2015). Health care is rapidly changing and requires nurses to keep up with those changes to provide safe, evidence-based, and quality care. Patients deserve to have highly competent nurses who are adept at caring for them across all settings (IOM, 2011). For nurses to thrive in this complex environment, they must be committed to lifelong learning. It is imperative that nurses maintain current knowledge by reading professional journals, attending continuing education offerings, and seeking certification in their specialties to enhance and validate their knowledge and skills in clinical practice (Johnson, 2015). **Competence** is situational and dynamic and requires performing at an expected level that integrates knowledge, skills, attitudes, and nursing judgment (ANA, 2015b, p. 44). Nurses must attain and maintain competencies after graduating from nursing school. Competence is both an ongoing process and an outcome (ANA, 2014b, 2015b). Therefore, attaining and maintaining competence are important. Being a competent nurse has both legal and ethical implications. "The ability to perform at the expected level requires a process of lifelong learning. Registered nurses must continually reassess their competencies and identify needs for additional knowledge, skills, personal growth, and integrative learning experiences" (ANA, 2015b, p. 45). Competence affects not only the safety and quality of care but also self-respect, self-esteem, and meaningfulness of work (ANA, 2015a).

Ensuring that nurses maintain competence is the shared responsibility of the profession, individual nurses, professional organizations, regulatory agencies, credentialing agencies, and nurse leaders and managers (ANA, 2010, 2014b). Nurse leaders and managers must be committed to providing an environment that is conducive to competent nursing practice. "Employers who provide opportunities for professional development and continuing education promote a positive practice environment in which nurses can maintain and enhance skills and competencies" (ANA, 2015b, p. 47). In essence, nurses at all levels must embrace a culture of nursing competence, a culture in which shared beliefs, attitudes, and values promote lifelong learning result in an environment of safe and quality care (Porter-O'Grady & Malloch, 2013).

Becoming a Lifelong Learner

Inherent in the ability to provide competent, safe, quality nursing care is a commitment to lifelong learning. A **lifelong learner** is one who seeks continuing education opportunities to increase their knowledge and skills and improve their attitudes throughout their professional and personal life. According to Provision 5.1 of the ANA *Code of Ethics for Nurses With Interpretive Statements*, nurses have a responsibility to maintain competence and continuation of professional growth, which requires a commitment to lifelong learning (ANA,

2015a). In an address to her nursing students in May, 1872, Florence Nightingale said:

> *For us who Nurse, our Nursing is a thing, which, unless in it we are making progress every year, every month, every week, take my word for it we are going back. [. . .] The more experience we gain, the more progress we can make. The progress you make in your year's training with us is as nothing to what you must make every year after your year's training is over. [...] A woman who thinks in herself: "Now I am a 'full' Nurse, a 'skilled' Nurse, I have learnt all that there is to be learnt": take my word for it, she does not know what a Nurse is, and she never will know; she is gone back already. [...] Conceit and Nursing cannot exist in the same person, any more than new patches on an old garment. [...] Every year of her service a good Nurse will say: "I learn something every day." (Florence Nightingale to her nurses, 1914, p. 1.)*

Lifelong learning includes learning about new concepts, issues, and controversies relevant to evolving nursing practice. Learning can occur through many activities such as continuing education, networking with colleagues, reading professional literature, achieving specialty certification, and pursuing advanced degrees in nursing (ANA, 2015a).

To attain and maintain the knowledge, skills, and attitudes necessary for evidence-based professional practice, nurses must engage in continuous formal, informal, and reflective learning activities (ANA, 2014b). Formal learning occurs through engaging in structured, academic, and professional development activities, whereas informal learning is related to the experiential learning that occurs in the workplace, community, and home settings (ANA, 2014b). According to the ANA, **reflective learning** "represents recurrent thoughtful personal self-assessment, analysis, and synthesis of strengths and opportunities for improvement" (2014b, p. 4). Weaknesses and opportunities identified through reflective learning should be what drive a nurse's plan for career development and lifelong learning. One way nurses at all levels can maintain currency in practice is through continuing education activities.

Continuing Education

Once licensed, RNs must maintain current licensure to continue nursing practice. Depending on the state, the requirements for license renewal may include renewal fees, current work address, current home address, notification of criminal activities, and proof of a specific number of continuing education hours. Nurses attain and maintain competencies during their professional career through continuing education activities. Continuing education is often provided by hospitals, community agencies, professional organizations, and professional meetings and can be provided in various formats (i.e., face to face, online, self-study, conferences, workshops, and seminars). The American Nurses Credentialing Center is responsible for accrediting standards of continuing education programs and courses. Continuing education credits reflect the length of programs. One credit of continuing education is equivalent to 50 minutes. In some states, university and college coursework may meet continuing education requirements. Different states may have different numbers of continuing education hours required for license renewal.

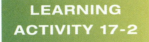

LEARNING ACTIVITY 17-2   Visit the NCSBN website available at www.ncsbn.org/contact-bon.htm to find a list of State Boards of Nursing. Then identify the continuing education requirements of the state where you plan to practice after graduation.

Specialty Certification

Specialty certification validates specific knowledge, skills, and attitudes demonstrated by a nurse in a specialized area of practice (Box 17-2). Certified nurses are role models of professional accountability (Altman, 2011). By becoming certified, nurses demonstrate they are responsible for their own practice by seeking further education and being motivated to provide high-quality nursing care. In addition, nurses who continually renew their certification demonstrate their commitment to increasing their knowledge in their nursing specialty (Foster, 2012).

Nurse leaders and managers prefer to hire certified nurses if possible because they have a proven knowledge base, documented experience in their clinical specialty, and a demonstrated commitment to lifelong learning and career advancement (Altman, 2011; Stromborg et al., 2005). In addition, research suggests that specialty certification improves patient safety outcomes (Boltz et al., 2013; Kendall-Gallagher & Blegen, 2009). Nurse leaders and managers can promote certification by seeking certification themselves and advocating for organizational support for certification such as financial incentives, public recognition, and including credentials on name tags. Specialty certification has a positive impact on staff, patients, and the organization (Altman, 2011).

BOX 17-2   Specialty Certifications

NURSE PRACTITIONER (NP) CERTIFICATIONS

Adult-Gerontology Acute Care NP

Adult-Gerontology Primary Care NP

Family NP

Psychiatric-Mental Health NP (across the life span)

CLINICAL NURSE SPECIALIST (CNS) CERTIFICATIONS

Adult-Gerontology CNS

SPECIALTY CERTIFICATIONS

Ambulatory Care Nursing

Cardiac Vascular Nursing

Care Coordination and Transition Management

Gerontological Nursing

Informatics Nursing

Medical-Surgical Nursing

Nurse Executive

Nurse Executive–Advanced

Nursing Case Management

Nursing Professional Development

Pain Management Nursing

Pediatric Nursing

Psychiatric-Mental Health Nursing

INTERPROFESSIONAL CERTIFICATIONS

National Healthcare Disaster

Compiled from American Nurses Credentialing Center, 2020.

EXPLORING THE EVIDENCE 17-1

Boltz, M., Capezuti, E., Wagner, L., Rosenberg, M., & Secic, M. (2013). Patient safety in medical-surgical units: Can nurse certification make a difference? *Medsurg Nursing, 22*(1), 26–37.

Aim

The purpose of this study was to examine the relationship between nurse certification and unit-level nursing-sensitive quality indicators that primarily serve older adults.

Methods

A descriptive retrospective design and multivariate regression technique were used to study units involved in the Nurses Improving Care for Health system Elders (NICHE). The sample included 35 medical units and 9 medical-surgical units in 35 hospitals. The investigators collected data on the following:

- Nurse certification: the percentage of RNs certified in any specialty and the percentage certified by the American Nurses Credentialing Center in Gerontological Nursing
- Nursing-sensitive unit-level quality indicators from the previous quarter including patient fall rates, patient falls with injuries, presence of pressure ulcers, and use of restraints
- Unit-level data such as RN staffing, nursing care hours per patient day, skill mix, percentage of RNs with bachelor's degrees, and percentage of RN hours supplied by contract or agency nurses

Key Findings

The researchers found a significant inverse relationship between nurse certification and fall rates ($p = 0.05$) but no significant relationship between nurse certification and falls with injury, pressure ulcers, and use of restraints. The investigators discussed the small sample size as a limitation and the reason for the lack of significant findings.

Implications for Nurse Leaders and Managers

The researchers concluded that nursing-sensitive outcomes in hospitalized older adults may be affected by nurse certification. Nurse leaders and managers should consider nurse certification as a strategy to improve patient outcomes in hospitalized older adults. Further, certification can promote nurse satisfaction.

Advanced Degrees

Safe and quality care depends on nurse leaders and managers hiring a well-educated workforce. Research indicates that care provided by nurses at the baccalaureate level and higher results in lower mortality rates, fewer medication errors, and better patient outcomes (AACN, 2019). In its report *The Future of Nursing,* the IOM recognized that associate degree nurses are essential for the current health-care system. However, the IOM recommended that 80% of all nurses obtain a baccalaureate degree or higher by 2020 and that the number of nurses with doctorates double by 2020 (IOM, 2011). Increasing the percentage of baccalaureate-prepared nurses to 80% by 2020 is "necessary to move the nursing workforce to an expanded set of competencies, especially in the domains of community and public health, leadership, systems improvement and change, research, and health policy" (IOM, 2011, p. 173). According to the AACN Fact Sheet: *The Impact of Education on Nursing Practice* (2019), progress has been made toward this goal. The percentage of RNs with a baccalaureate degree or higher was 56% in 2019, up from 49% in 2010.

Nurse leaders and managers play a pivotal role in the educational future of nursing. First and foremost, nurse leaders and managers must seek advanced degrees themselves. Next, nurse leaders and managers must support other nurses who want to pursue further education. The AACN encourages nurse leaders and managers to "foster practice environments that embrace lifelong learning and offers incentives to nurses seeking to advance their education to the baccalaureate and higher degree levels" (AACN, 2019, para. 2). Further, the AACN encourages BSN graduates to seek out employers who value their level of education and competence.

Nurse leaders and managers can become involved at the organizational level by spearheading initiatives to establish or increase tuition reimbursement programs for nurses with a desire to return to school and other staff members who are pursuing additional education in nursing or another health-care field.

Contributing to the Nursing Profession

Membership in professional nursing organizations can provide many opportunities to contribute to the profession. Part of being a professional is belonging to a professional organization. Nursing professional organizations are vital to the profession today and in the future. Members of professional organizations work collectively to "define and promote standards of behavior and practice" (Beyers, 2013, p. 388).

The primary roles of professional organizations include professional development, advancing the profession, developing and promoting health-care policy, and advocacy for members and consumers of health care. All nurses at all levels must contribute to "the advancement of the profession through knowledge development, evaluation, dissemination, and application to practice" (ANA, 2015b, p. 27). In fact, nurses are expected to use current research and evidence in their practice. Nurses should also contribute to the profession by leading and serving on institutional or health policy committees. Nurse leaders and managers should participate in the promotion and implementation of health policies. Nurse leaders and managers are responsible to ensure that the organization supports nursing research and evidence-based practice. They must become involved at the administrative level to promote and create processes and structures that are conducive to scholarly inquiry (ANA, 2015a). In addition, nurse leaders and managers should promote communication of information and advancement of the profession through writing, publishing, and presentations for professional or lay audiences (ANA, 2016). Nurse leaders and managers are also responsible for promoting the advancement of the profession by participating and encouraging staff participation in professional organizations.

▶ BALANCING PERSONAL AND PROFESSIONAL LIFE

Nurses at all levels are responsible for delivering high-quality, safe, patient care in a complex health-care environment. To be able to meet this responsibility consistently, nurses must engage in a lifestyle that promotes their own health and well-being (ANA, 2015a). Yet, nurses are less healthy than the average American (ANA, 2020a, para. 2). Nurses are very focused on caring for others, often to their own detriment. Caring for others before oneself can result in an environment that saps energy and jeopardizes personal health. What many nurses do not understand is that caring for oneself is foundational to being able to care for others (Cranick et al., 2015). **Self-care** is "choosing behaviors that balance the effects of emotional and physical stressors. These behaviors can include exercising, eating nutritious foods, getting enough sleep, practicing self-centering activities, abstaining from substance abuse, and pursuing creative outlets" (Richards et al., 2014, p. 3). Nurses have a duty to take care of their own health and safety just as they care for their patients (ANA, 2015b). Provision 5 of the ANA *Code of Ethics for Nurses With Interpretive Statements* states that "the nurse owes the same duties to self as to others, including the responsibility to promote health and safety, preserve wholeness of character and integrity, maintain competence, and continue personal and professional growth" (ANA, 2015a, p. 19). Sadly, many nurses easily become trapped in an unhealthy cycle of putting others before themselves and depleting their energy and time for self-care. The resulting fatigue from the lack of self-care is linked to an increased risk of errors, memory deficits, impaired mood, miscommunication, and overall poor performance that can jeopardize patient safety and quality of nursing care (ANA, 2014a).

Personal wellness is important. Nursing students should begin self-care during their educational program. Habits developed early in one's career can have lasting effects. "As the largest subset of health care workers, nurses are critical to America's health care system"; further, "the well-being of nurses is fundamental to the health of our nation" (ANA, 2020a, para. 1). The Healthy Nurse Healthy Nation Grand Challenge (HNHN GC) was launched by the ANA to "transform the health of the nation by improving the health of the nation's 4 million registered nurses" (ANA, 2020b, para. 2). There are three goals of the HNHN Challenge (ANA, 2020b):

1. Engage nurses on three levels: individual, organization, and interpersonal.
2. Improve their health in key areas: physical activity, rest, nutrition, quality of life, and safety.
3. Create a **healthy nurse** population, which, in turn, will create a healthy nation.

Nurses at all levels have a responsibility to engage in evidence-based self-care strategies to reduce the risk of fatigue. Richards et al. (2014) suggest that self-care should focus on six areas:

1. *Physical self-care:* "Physical self-care includes proper nutrition, emphasizing disease prevention and management, regular cardiovascular and strength building

exercise, adequate sleep and rest, and an understanding of personal self-care routines" (p. 9).

2. *Mental self-care:* "Mental self-care focuses on flexibility, stress-reducing practices, open-mindedness, and constant learning: these are the pillars of a healthy mental environment" (p. 17).

3. *Emotional self-care:* Emotional self-care involves identifying where unresolved emotional pain is eroding self-care and focuses on understanding inaccuracies, challenging negative beliefs, and changing how one thinks (p. 25).

4. *Spiritual self-care:* Spiritual self-care is a reflection of the belief in a higher power that provides a connection to the universe. Beliefs may or may not be based in organized religion, but the spirit reflected is unique to the individual (p. 27).

5. *Relationship self-care:* An individual's life is affected, either positively or negatively, by the quality of the relationships in which they are involved. Self-care can be challenged by toxic relationships. Therefore, to be a healthy nurse may require eliminating toxic people from one's life (p. 29).

6. *Choice self-care:* When nurses make choices from self-compassion, the choices are in line with core values. Choosing to create a life of improved self-care may take some work, but nurses will have a renewed sense of freedom (p. 30).

Nurses at all levels should model health maintenance and health promotion measures for their patients, seek health care when needed, and avoid unnecessary health or safety risks in personal and professional activities (ANA, 2015b).

Nurse leaders and managers have an ethical responsibility to foster balance within their units by promoting healthy lifestyles and encouraging nurses to make time for self-care (ANA, 2015b; Cranick et al., 2015). The ANA identifies five healthy constructs that are important to foster a work environment conducive to supporting healthy nurses (ANA, 2015a, p. 24):

1. *Calling to care:* Caring is the interpersonal, compassionate offering of self by which the healthy nurse builds relationships with patients and their families.

2. *Priority to self-care:* Self-care and supportive environments enable the healthy nurse to increase the ability to manage the physical and emotional stressors of the work and home environments effectively.

3. *Opportunity to role model:* The healthy nurse confidently recognizes and identifies personal health challenges in themselves and in the patients, thereby enabling the nurse and the patients to overcome these challenges in a collaborative, nonaccusatory manner.

4. *Responsibility to educate:* Using nonjudgmental approaches, considering adult learning patterns and readiness to change, the healthy nurse empowers themselves and others by sharing health, safety, and wellness knowledge and skills, resources, and attitudes.

5. *Authority to advocate:* The healthy nurse is empowered to advocate on numerous levels including personally, interpersonally, within the work environment and the community, and at the local, state, and national levels in policy development and advocacy.

EXPLORING THE EVIDENCE 17-2

Cranick, L., Miller, A., Allen, K., Ewell, A., & Whittington, K. (2015). Does RN perception of self-care impact job satisfaction? *Nursing Management, 46*(5), 16–18.

Aim

The purpose of this study was to determine whether engaging in self-care has a positive impact on a nurse's level of job satisfaction.

Methods

A descriptive study was conducted using an online survey that was e-mailed to RNs working in a rural multihospital system to determine the relationship of how nurses feel about their participation in self-care with their personal feelings of job satisfaction. The questionnaire included four categories of questions: interpersonal relationships with other nurses, nurses' assessments of their own ability to perform the job effectively, personal feelings about how the organization promotes self-care, and personal habits regarding self-care and well-being in their private lives.

Key Findings

The investigators reported that 182 RNs responded to the survey. A positive correlation was found between a nurse's job satisfaction and the amount of self-care participated in each week. In addition, there was a significant correlation with various factors related to job satisfaction such as experiencing anxiety ($p \leq 0.01$), looking forward to coming to work ($p \leq 0.01$, and being in a good mood while at work ($p \leq .0.01$). However, only 4.42% of the participants indicated that they were satisfied with their organization's efforts to promote self-care.

Implications for Nurse Leaders and Managers

Nurse leaders and managers must understand that job satisfaction is one determinant of nursing turnover and that higher job satisfaction can have a positive impact on patient outcomes. Two strategies supported by this study are reinforcing healthy lifestyles for nurses and encouraging self-care attitudes and methods in the workplace. Nurse leaders and managers should assist staff in recognizing the importance of self-care and encourage staff members to support each other to ensure uninterrupted break times.

Nurse leaders and managers should implement evidence-based policies, procedures, and strategies that promote healthy work schedules, improve alertness, and discourage nurses from working extra hours that may contribute to fatigue (ANA, 2014a, p. 5).

LEARNING ACTIVITY 17-3	Join the Healthy Nurse Healthy Nation Grand Challenge

Available at https://www.healthynursehealthynation.org/en/

- Take the health assessment survey and identify your risks.
- Pick your focus areas, make a commitment, and participate with others.
- Get a classmate to join also to share your successes.

▶ FUTURE DIRECTIONS

Conceptualizing the future can be difficult and demanding. In a classic article by Henchey (1978), four types of futures are presented, each with different characteristics and purposes. Interestingly, they are still relevant to consider today. The **plausible future**, or what could be, focuses on what may occur based on current and projected trends. The **probable future** is what will likely occur and actually reflects the present state with minimal changes. Looking at the probable future is the catalyst that motivates people to want and explore possible futures (Henchey, 1978). The **possible future**, or what may be, considers all possible situations that could occur. The possibilities inspire people to explore the perfect future or what Henchey calls the preferable future. The **preferable future** is what should be and begins with a vision and a roadmap to get there. Nurses and nurse leaders and managers can shape the preferable future.

The preferred future is one in which nurses provide safe, quality care in a healthy work and optimal healing environment. The Lucian Leape Institute (2013) described the future healthy and safe workplace:

> *Innovation, critical thinking, and technological and scientific advancement would be intrinsic to the work, without loss of compassion and relationship. Each day, all members of the workforce would learn something new and experience a sense of meaning and joy. All members of the workforce would be able to identify their contributions to the minute. Management would hold workforce safety and experience as a nonnegotiable requirement. [...] Patients and families would participate as partners in their care. They would enter the health care organization with a sense of relief and confidence that they would be respected, cared for, and safe in the hands of inspired care teams who clearly find their work meaningful (pp. 22–23).*

Nurse leaders and managers can contribute significantly to this preferred future by honoring and respecting staff and protecting the physical, psychological, and emotional safety of these staff members. This culture of respect creates joy and meaning in the workplace, which results in safe and quality health care.

Nurse leaders and managers must be aware of possible trends in the future so that the profession can be influenced positively. Ideally, nurse leaders and managers will be a leading force in creating the future of health care, not just reacting and adapting to future changes (Grossman & Valiga, 2016).

For nurses to thrive in the anticipated increasingly complex health-care environment of the future will require the following (Johnson, 2015, pp. 90–91):

- Lifelong learning through formal and informal education
- Ability to implement practice changes rapidly and well
- Focus on outcomes and process improvements to influence the direction of health care
- Recognizing that the patient and their family must be at the center of care
- Partnership with other health-care professionals to improve patient care through teamwork and collaboration

▶ **SUMMARY**

Nursing students begin the process of professional socialization when they enter nursing school and continue the process throughout their nursing career. Nurses at all levels should be involved in ongoing career planning and development that includes personal and professional self-assessment, envisioning the future, and establishing realistic goals to get there. Whatever goal a nurse pursues, the key is planning to obtain the necessary experience, the proper education, and specialty certification, if appropriate, to develop the knowledge, skills, and attitudes that will prepare the nurse for a long-term career in a dynamic, complex health-care environment. Continued competence is critical to the nursing profession as well as ensuring safe, quality nursing care. Nurses have a professional responsibility to engage in lifelong learning and self-reflection (AACN, 2021). All nurses should strive for balance between personal life and professional life. Further, all nurses should support each other's needs for balance between personal and work life. No one can predict the future. However, visualizing or envisioning several possibilities and developing goals for a preferable future will allow nurses to shape their future.

NCLEX®-STYLE REVIEW QUESTIONS

Multiple Choice

1. What component is *not* included in the SMART technique acronym?
   1. Specific
   2. Realistic
   3. Talented
   4. Measurable
2. A nursing student who is going to graduate from a bachelor of science in nursing (BSN) program is preparing a résumé. What fact should the nurse pay attention to when preparing the document?
   1. Most employers who read résumés spend little time reviewing the document.
   2. All activities should be included in the document regardless of whether they relate to the job position.
   3. The document should be presented in a comprehensive narrative format.
   4. Language style used is not important.

3. Which information should *not* be included in a cover letter?
   1. Should serve as an introduction
   2. Quotes from references
   3. Reason why you are applying for the position
   4. Brief summary of qualifications
4. An experienced nurse is applying for a new job position, and an interview has been scheduled. What *priority* information should the experienced nurse use to help prepare for the upcoming interview?
   1. Review of the hospital's Web site
   2. Whether the hospital has achieved Magnet status
   3. Review of organization's mission, values, and goals
   4. Type of staffing pattern utilized by the facility
5. Which statement indicates the primary purpose for *nurse residency* programs?
   1. To decrease the stress level for new graduates
   2. To provide a transition program that leads to competent practice
   3. To allow for new nurses to learn basic information
   4. To provide continuing education credits for initial licensure
6. Which statement reflects the difference between a preceptor and a mentor?
   1. Preceptors provide a lifelong learning relationship, whereas mentors provide shorter-term learning relationships.
   2. Mentors do not have to be nurses but preceptors do.
   3. A mentoring relationship exists only at the beginning graduate nurse level, whereas preceptors occur across experience levels.
   4. It is the type of communication pattern that is maintained.
7. Which statement is accurate with regard to the concept of *competence* as applied to nursing practice?
   1. Competence is not considered to be an outcome.
   2. Competence is a static variable.
   3. Nurses must continue to maintain competence following graduation from nursing school.
   4. Once competence has been assessed, it is achieved and does not need to be reevaluated.
8. How many minutes is equivalent to one credit of continuing education credit?
   1. 25
   2. 60
   3. It varies from state to state.
   4. 50
9. Which self-care area is included in helping nurses to limit fatigue in the clinical setting?
   1. Educational
   2. Spiritual
   3. Flexible
   4. Individual

10. A group of nurses are discussing unit policies and procedures. Based on a consensus of opinion, the nurses suggest minimal changes in the near future. What type of future is demonstrated by this statement?
    1. Preferable
    2. Plausible
    3. Possible
    4. Probable
11. What elements are included in the hallmarks of a professional nursing practice environment?
    1. Minimal staffing patterns
    2. Nursing staff members who have limited input
    3. A formal program for performance improvement
    4. Limited accountability but with increased responsibility
12. Which certification degree represents an acute care nurse practitioner?
    1. Adult health clinical nurse specialist
    2. Informatics nursing
    3. Adult psychiatry, mental health
    4. Nurse executive—advanced

Multiple Response

13. Which components are included in a résumé? *Select all that apply.*
    1. Contact information for the applicant
    2. A listing of personal friends
    3. A listing of educational degrees
    4. Related work history
    5. Personal preferences related to job description
14. Which statements describe differences between licensure and certification? *Select all that apply.*
    1. Certification is based on meeting additional criteria as opposed to licensure, which is based on meeting minimal competency.
    2. In order to become licensed, one must meet certification standards.
    3. The licensure period typically lasts longer than certification periods.
    4. Licensure represents general knowledge, whereas certification represents specialized knowledge.
    5. Licensure is renewable as long as criteria are met, whereas certification is not renewable.
15. Which statements are true with regard to continuing education (CE) credit requirements for registered nurses? *Select all that apply.*
    1. CEs are not required once the nurse has achieved licensure.
    2. CE requirements may vary from state to state.
    3. It is the individual nurse's responsibility to continue to take CEs.
    4. CEs are limited in how they are presented.
    5. CEs courses are accredited.

REFERENCES

Al-Dossery, R., Kitsana, P., & Maddox, P. J. (2013). The impact of residency programs on new nurse graduates' clinical decision-making and leadership skills: A systematic review. *Nurse Education Today, 34*(6), 1024–1028.

Altman, M. (2011). Let's get certified: Best practices for nurse leaders and managers to create a culture of certification. *AACN Advanced Critical Care, 12*(1), 68–75.

American Association of Colleges of Nursing (n.d.a). *Hallmarks of the professional nursing practice environment.* https://www.aacnnursing.org/News-Information/Position-Statements-White-Papers/Hallmarks-Practice

American Association of Colleges of Nursing (AACN). (n.d.b). *What every nursing student should know whenseekingemployment.*https://www.aacnnursing.org/Portals/42/Publications/Brochures/SeekingEmployment.pdf

American Association of Colleges of Nursing (AACN). (2019). *The impact of education on nursing practice* [fact sheet]. www.aacn.nche.edu/media-relations/fact-sheets/impact-of-education

American Association of Colleges of Nursing. (2021). *The essentials: Core competencies for professional nursing education.* Author. https://www.aacnnursing.org/Portals/42/AcademicNursing/pdf/Essentials-2021.pdf

American Nurses Association (ANA). (2010). *Nursing's social policy statement: The essence of the profession.* American Nurses Association.

American Nurses Association (ANA). (2014a). *The nursing workforce 2014: Growth, salaries, education, demographics, & trends* [fast facts]. www.nursingworld.org/MainMenuCategories/ThePracticeofProfessionalNursing/workforce/Fast-Facts-2014-Nursing-Workforce.pdf

American Nurses Association (ANA). (2014b). *Professional role competence* [position statement]. www.nursingworld.org/position/practice/role.aspx

American Nurses Association (ANA). (2015a). *Code of ethics for nurses with interpretive statements.* Author.

American Nurses Association (ANA). (2015b). *Nursing: Scope and standards of practice* (3rd ed.). Author.

American Nurses Association (ANA). (2016). *Nursing administration: Scope and standards of practice* (2nd ed.). Author.

American Nurses Association (ANA). (2020a). *Healthy Nurse Healthy Nation: About the HNHN GC.* https://www.healthynursehealthynation.org/en/about/about-the-hnhn-gc/

American Nurses Association (ANA). (2020b). *Healthy Nurse Healthy Nation Grand Challenge.* https://www.healthynursehealthynation.org/en/

American Nurses Credentialing Center. (2020). *ANCC Certification Center.* https://www.nursingworld.org/ancc/

American Organization for Nursing Leadership (AONL). (2015a). *AONL nurse manager competencies.* Author.

American Organization for Nursing Leadership (AONL). (2015b). *AONL nurse executive competencies.* Author.

Benner, P. (1984). *From novice to expert: Excellence and power in clinical nursing practice.* Addison-Wesley.

Benner, P., Stutphen, M., Leonard, V., & Day, L. (2010). *Educating nurses: A call for radical transformation.* Jossey-Bass.

Beyers, M. (2013). Nursing's professional associations. In C. J. Huston (Ed.), *Professional issues in nursing: Challenges & opportunities* (3rd ed.). Wolters Kluwer, Lippincott Williams & Wilkins.

Boltz, M., Capezuti, E., Wagner, L., Rosenberg, M., & Secic, M. (2013). Patient safety in medical-surgical units: Can nurse certification make a difference? *Medsurg Nursing, 22*(1), 26–37.

Cranick, L., Miller, A., Allen, K., Ewell, A., & Whittington, K. (2015). Does RN perception of self-care impact job satisfaction? *Nursing Management, 46*(5), 16–18.

Cronenwett, L., Sherwood, G., Barnsteiner, J., Disch, J., Johnson, J., Mitchell, P., Sullivan, D. T., & Warren, J. (2007). Quality and safety education for nurses. *Nursing Outlook, 55*(3), 122–131.

D'Addona, M., Pinto, J., Oliver, C., Turcotte, S., & Lavoie-Tremblay, M. (2015). Nursing leaders' perceptions of a transition support program for new nurse graduates. *Health Care Manager, 34*(1), 14–22.

Day, L., & Sherwood, G. (2017). Quality and safety education in clinical learning environments. In G. Sherwood & J. Barnsteiner (Eds.), *Quality and safety in nursing: A competency approach to improving outcomes* (2nd ed., pp. 253–264). Wiley Blackwell.

Dinmohammadi, M., Peyrovi, H., & Mehrdad, N. (2013). Concept analysis of professional socialization in nursing. *Nursing Forum, 48*(1), 26–34.

Donner, G. J., & Wheeler, M. M. (2001). *It's your career: Take charge career planning and development.* International Council of Nurses.

Florence Nightingale to her nurses: A selection from Miss Nightingale's address to probationers and nurses of the Nightingale School at St. Thomas's Hospital. (1914). Macmillan. www.archive.org/stream/ florencenighting00nighiala/florencenighting00nighiala_djvu.txt

Foster, C. W. (2012). Institute of medicine the future of nursing report, lifelong learning, and certification. *Medsurg Nursing, 21*(2), 115–116.

Greiner, A. C., & Knebel, E. (Eds.). (2003). *Health professions education: A bridge to quality.* National Academies Press.

Grossman, S. C., & Valiga, T. M. (2016). *The new leadership challenge: Creating the future of nursing* (5th ed.). F. A. Davis.

Henchey, N. (1978). Making sense of future studies. *Alternatives, 7,* 24–28.

Hood, L. J (2014). *Leddy and Pepper's conceptual basses of professional nursing* (8th ed.). Wolters Kluwer Health.

Institute of Medicine (IOM). (2011). *The future of nursing: Leading change, advancing health.* National Academies Press.

Johnson, S. (2015). *What would Florence do?* American Nurses Association.

Kendall-Gallagher, D., & Blegen, M. A. (2009). Competence and certification of registered nurses and safety of patients in intensive care units. *American Journal of Critical Care, 18*(2), 106–113.

Lucian Leape Institute. (2013). *Through the eyes of the workforce: Creating joy, meaning, and safer health care.* http://www.ihi.org/resources/Pages/Publications/Through-the-Eyes-of-the-Workforce-Creating-Joy-Meaning-and-Safer-Health-Care.aspx

Mariet, J. (2016). Professional socialization models in nursing. *International Journal of Nursing Education, 8*(3), 143–148. doi:10.5958/0974-9357.2016.00107.0

Masters, K., & Gilmore, M. (2020). Education and socialization to the professional nursing role. In K. Masters (Ed.), *Role development in professional nursing practice* (5th ed.). Jones & Bartlett Learning.

National Council of State Boards of Nursing (NCSBN). (2021). *Transition to practice program (TTP).* www.ncsbn.org/transition-to-practice.htm

Porter-O'Grady, T., & Malloch, K. (2013). *Leadership in nursing practice: Changing the landscape of health care.* Jones & Bartlett Learning.

Richards, K., Sheen, E., & Mazzer, M. C. (2014). *Self-care and you: Caring for the caregiver.* American Nurses Association.

Rush, K. L., Adamack, M., Gordon, J., Lilly, M., & Janke, R. (2013). Best practices of formal new graduate nurse transition programs: An integrative review. *International Journal of Nursing Studies, 50*(3), 345–356.

Spector, N., Blegen, M. A., Silvestre, J., Barnsteiner, J., Lynn, M. R., Ulrich, B., Fogg, L., & Alexander, M. (2015). Transition to practice study in hospital settings. *Journal of Nursing Regulation, 5*(4), 24–38.

Stromborg, M. F., Niebuhr, B., & Prevost, S. (2005). Specialty certification: More than a title. *Nursing Management, 36*(5), 36–46.

To explore learning resources for this chapter, go to FADavis.com

NCLEX®-Style Review Questions Answer Key

 Answers with rationales for each question are available in the learning resources on **FADavis.com**

Chapter 1
1. 3
2. 4
3. 3
4. 1
5. 4
6. 3
7. 4
8. 2
9. 1
10. 2
11. 1, 3, 5
12. 2, 4, 5
13. 2, 3, 4
14. 1, 4, 5

Chapter 2
1. 4
2. 3
3. 2
4. 3
5. 4
6. 2
7. 3
8. 1, 3
9. 2, 3, 5
10. 1, 3

Chapter 3
1. 4
2. 2
3. 2
4. 2
5. 4
6. 3
7. 2
8. 3
9. 2

10. 2
11. 3
12. 1, 2, 5
13. 2, 3, 4

Chapter 4
1. 2
2. 3
3. 2
4. 3
5. 3
6. 3
7. 2
8. 1, 3, 4
9. 1, 2, 3, 4, 5
10. 2, 3, 5

Chapter 5
1. 3
2. 1
3. 2
4. 4
5. 2
6. 3
7. 2
8. 4
9. 1, 2, 4, 5
10. 2, 3, 4, 5

Chapter 6
1. 1
2. 4
3. 1
4. 2
5. 3
6. 3
7. 3
8. 1
9. 2
10. 3
11. 1, 2, 4, 5
12. 2, 3

Chapter 7
1. 3
2. 2
3. 1
4. 2
5. 1
6. 4
7. 3
8. 3
9. 2
10. 1
11. 3
12. 1, 4, 5

Chapter 8
1. 1
2. 2
3. 1
4. 1
5. 2
6. 1
7. 3
8. 1
9. 2
10. 1, 2, 4
11. 1, 2, 3
12. 2, 4, 5

Chapter 9
1. 3
2. 1
3. 3
4. 2
5. 3
6. 4
7. 2
8. 1

9. 4
10. 1, 3, 4
11. 2, 3, 4

Chapter 10
1. 3
2. 1
3. 1
4. 3
5. 1
6. 2
7. 2
8. 3
9. 3
10. 2
11. 3
12. 1
13. 1, 4, 5
14. 1, 5
15. 1, 3

Chapter 11
1. 3
2. 4
3. 2
4. 2
5. 3
6. 4
7. 2
8. 3
9. 3
10. 4
11. 2, 3, 4
12. 1, 2, 3
13. 1, 2, 3, 5
14. 1, 3, 4
15. 1, 3, 4

Chapter 12
1. 1
2. 2
3. 3
4. 3
5. 4
6. 1
7. 3

8. 4
9. 4
10. 3
11. 4
12. 3
13. 1, 3, 5
14. 1, 2, 3
15. 2, 4, 5

Chapter 13
1. 1
2. 4
3. 2
4. 2
5. 3
6. 3
7. 1
8. 4
9. 4
10. 2
11. 2
12. 3
13. 2, 4
14. 1, 2, 5

Chapter 14
1. 2
2. 2
3. 2
4. 1
5. 4
6. 2
7. 3
8. 1
9. 3
10. 2
11. 1
12. 3
13. 1, 3, 5
14. 1, 2, 3
15. 1, 3, 4

Chapter 15
1. 1
2. 1
3. 2

4. 2
5. 2
6. 2
7. 2
8. 4
9. 4
10. 2
11. 1
12. 1
13. 1, 3, 4
14. 1, 2, 3, 4
15. 2, 3, 4

Chapter 16
1. 1
2. 3
3. 2
4. 3
5. 3
6. 3
7. 3
8. 2
9. 4
10. 3
11. 3
12. 1, 4, 5
13. 1, 2, 3
14. 2, 4, 5

Chapter 17
1. 3
2. 1
3. 2
4. 3
5. 2
6. 2
7. 3
8. 4
9. 2
10. 4
11. 3
12. 3
13. 1, 3, 4
14. 1, 4
15. 2, 3, 5

Index

Note: Page numbers followed by f indicate figures, those followed by t indicate tables.